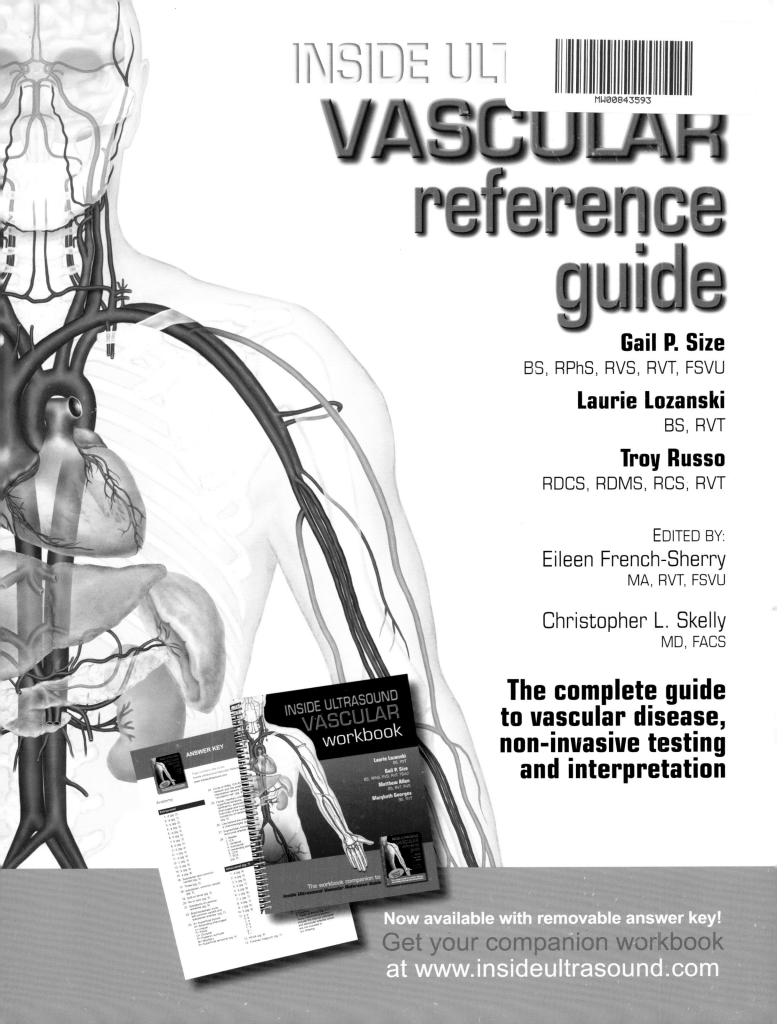

INSIDE ULT
VASCULAR
reference guide

Gail P. Size
BS, RPhS, RVS, RVT, FSVU

Laurie Lozanski
BS, RVT

Troy Russo
RDCS, RDMS, RCS, RVT

EDITED BY:
Eileen French-Sherry
MA, RVT, FSVU

Christopher L. Skelly
MD, FACS

The complete guide to vascular disease, non-invasive testing and interpretation

MW00843593

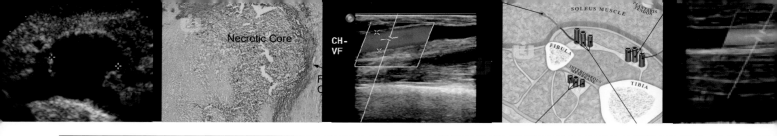

This book is dedicated to the
memory of two very special people:

To our dear friend,
Andrea Michelle Griffin, RDMS, RVT

We loved your mix of innocence, energy and frank honesty. You were a gifted sonographer and passionate teacher. Although your time with us was short, your lessons will live on for years to come. We loved you dearly, Missy.

To Gail's beloved sister,
Sharon Schoen

Thank you for years of inspiration and always telling me how proud you were of me; those words helped me become the person I am today, you are missed everyday.

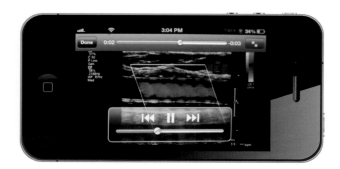

QR codes can be found throughout this book, which will allow you to view video clips of various pathology or duplex findings using your smartphone or tablet. To access these files, use the camera on your device and a QR code reader. Your device must have internet to use this feature.

There are many free QR code readers available for download, please check your app store for more information.

Gail P. Size, BS, RPhS, RVS, RVT, FSVU
Inside Ultrasound's Vascular Reference Guide

©2013-2021 by Inside Ultrasound, Inc., First Edition
June 2021

Inside Ultrasound, Inc
13303 S. Desert Dawn Drive
Pearce, AZ, 85625
Phone 520-642-1303
Fax 520-642-1304
www.insideultrasound.com

ISBN: 978-0-9747694-3-1

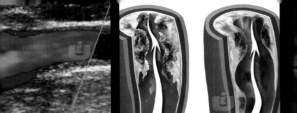
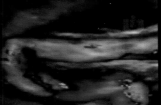
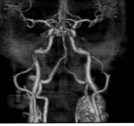

TABLE OF CONTENTS

CME Information

Go to www.insideultrasound.com, from the bookstore, pick product IU400CME and make your purchase. Upon receiving your receipt, in the upper right corner click on download, this will give you further instructions. Your exam will be available within two business days. Watch your email; you will be receiving a message from admin@exambuilder.com with instructions and a link to access the exam. You should add this address to your contacts so that it does not go into your spam. The exam contains 100 multiple choice questions. The passing grade is 70%. Each candidate will be allowed three attempts to successfully complete the exam. Upon successful completion you will be able to download your certificate.

Successful candidates will earn 20 hours of CME awarded from the Society of Vascular Ultrasound (SVU). This program meets the criteria for SVU-CMEs which are accepted by:

- American Registry of Diagnostic Medical Sonographers® (ARDMS®)
- Cardiovascular Credentialing International (CCI)
- American Registry of Radiologic Technologists (ARRT) for Category A credit
- Intersocietal Accreditation Commission (IAC - Vascular) for laboratory accreditation.
- American College of Radiology (ACR) for laboratory accreditation.

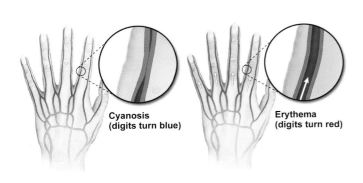

Cyanosis
(digits turn blue)

Erythema
(digits turn red)

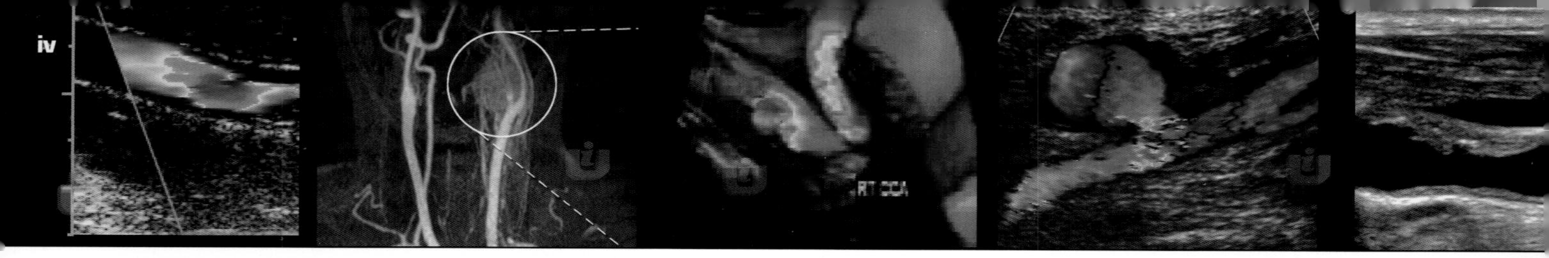

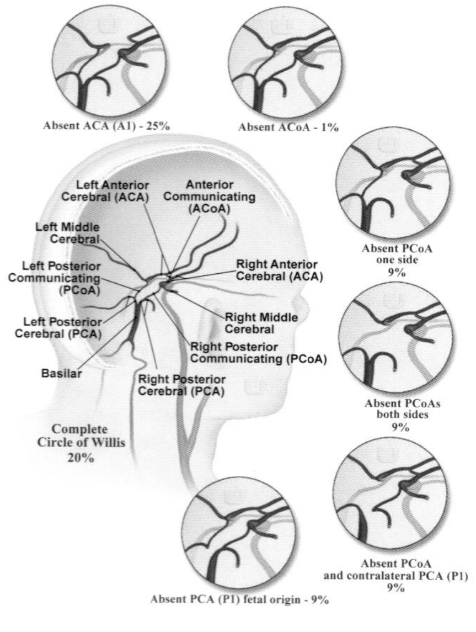

Absent ACA (A1) - 25%

Absent ACoA - 1%

Left Anterior Cerebral (ACA)

Anterior Communicating (ACoA)

Left Middle Cerebral

Left Posterior Communicating (PCoA)

Right Anterior Cerebral (ACA)

Left Posterior Cerebral (PCA)

Right Middle Cerebral

Right Posterior Communicating (PCoA)

Basilar

Right Posterior Cerebral (PCA)

Complete Circle of Willis 20%

Absent PCoA one side 9%

Absent PCoAs both sides 9%

Absent PCoA and contralateral PCA (P1) 9%

Absent PCA (P1) fetal origin - 9%

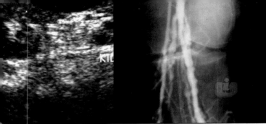
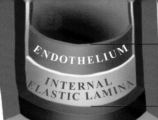
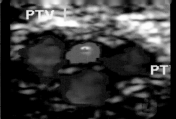

TYPICAL   TORTUOUS   KINKED   COILED

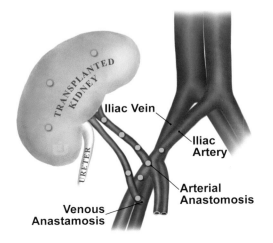

TRANSPLANTED KIDNEY

Iliac Vein

Iliac Artery

URETER

Arterial Anastomosis

Venous Anastamosis

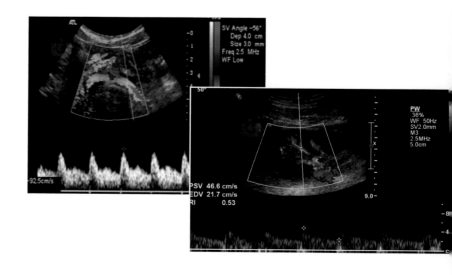

vi

RACH
V GRFT
BYPS

.6 cm/s
.550 cm

Brachial

Right   Left

138   140

PT   155   154
DP   152   141

131   TBI   116
0.94   0.83

1.11   ABI   1.10

LIST OF TABLES

Volume Pulse Recording

Lower Extremity Digital Evaluations: Toe Pressures (TBI) and Photoplethysmography (PPG)

Exercise and Stress Testing of the Extremities

Lower Extremity Arterial Duplex

Arterial Bypass and Stent Surveillance

Arterial Testing (Upper Extremity)

Upper Extremity Segmental Pressures and Doppler Waveforms

Upper Extremity Digital Evaluations: Pressure and Photoplethysmography (DBI) and (PPG)

Upper Extremity Arterial Duplex

Thoracic Outlet Testing

Cold Immersion Testing for Raynaud's Phenomenon

Additional Arterial Testing

Pseudoaneurysm Duplex

Duplex of Arteriovenous Fistulas and Grafts for Hemodialysis Access

Penile Testing

Venous Testing

Lower Extremity Venous Duplex Ultrasound Examination

Lower Extremity Venous Insufficiency Duplex Examination

Duplex Imaging for Venous Ablation

Upper Extremity Venous Duplex Ultrasound Examination

IVC and Iliac Venous Scanning

Upper and Lower Extremity Venous Duplex Mapping

Francis Loth, PhD
Associate Professor
F. Theodore Harrington Endowed
Chair, Department of Mechanical
Engineering
The University of Akron
Akron, OH

Susan McCormick, PhD
Assistant Professor, Vascular Research
Section of Vascular and Endovascular
Therapy
University of Chicago Medical Center
& Biological Sciences
Chicago, IL

Terry Reynolds, BS, RDCS
President, R² Publishing, Inc.
Consultant
Phoenix, AZ

Heather Roberts, RPh
Pharmacy Manager, Walgreen's
Prescott Valley, AZ

Rita Shugart, RN, RVT, FSVU
President, Shugart Consulting
Greensboro, NC

Faye Temple, Grad. Dip. U/S (RMIT)
Sonographer in charge
Sonographer tutor at Royal Melbourne
Institute of Technology and Monash
University
St Vincents Public Hospital
Fitzroy, Melbourne
Australia

Section Editors:

Hisham Bassiouny, MD FACS
Professor and Chief,
Vascular Surgery and Endotherapy
Dar Al Fouad Hospital, 6th of October
City, Egypt

Sharon Blattner, M.Ed., PA-C
Assistant Professor/Director of Clinical
Education
Northwestern University – Feinberg
School of Medicine
Physician Assistant Program
Chicago, IL

Robert De Jong, RDMS, RDCS, RVT
Radiology Technical Manager,
Ultrasound,
The Johns Hopkins Medical
Institutions
Baltimore, MD

Richard K. Duncan, BA, RDCS
President, Echo-Web, LLC
Jacksonville, FL

Marge Hutchisson, LPN, RVT,
RDCS
Director of Accreditation – IAC
Vascular Testing
Ellicott City, MD

Nicos Labropoulos, PhD, DIC, RVT
Professor of Surgery and Radiology
Director, Vascular Laboratory
Department of Surgery
Stony Brook University Medical
Center
Stony Brook, NY

Jose Montalvo Jr., RN, RVT
Vascular Consultant
University of Illinois at Chicago
Vascular Laboratory
Chicago, IL

Terry Needham, RVT
President, Needham Vascular
Consulting
Chattanooga, TN

Marsha Neumeyer, BS, RVT,
FSDMS, FSVU, FAIUM
International Director
Vascular Diagnostic Educational
Services
Harrisburg, PA

Richard Palma, BS, RDCS, RCS,
APS, FASE
Director and Clinical Coordinator,
Hoffman Heart Institute School of
Cardiac Ultrasound
St. Francis Hospital and Medical
Center
Hartford, CT

Donald Ridgway, BA, RVT
Professor Emeritus
Grossmont College Cardiovascular
Technology Program
El Cajon, CA

Janice Hickey Scharf, CRGS,
RDMS, BSc. MRT
Chairperson, Canadian Association
of Registered Diagnostic Ultrasound
Professionals (CARDUP)
Clinical Applications Specialist,
Ultrasound
Philips Healthcare, Canada

Robert Scissions, RVT, FSVU
Technical Director Jobst Vascular
Laboratory
Toledo, OH

Patrick Washko, BSRT, RDMS, RVT
Technical Director
Rex Hospital (UNC Healthcare)
Vascular Diagnostic Center
Raleigh, NC

Allen Tabor, RVT
Product Applications Specialist
Philips Healthcare
Seattle, WA

Cindy Weiland, RVT, RRT
Chief Compliance Officer
Intersocietal Accreditation
Commission (IAC)
Ellicott City, MD

Ajay Zachariah, BS, RVT, RDCS,
RDMS, FSVU
Consultant
Vascular Diagnostic Services
Mercer Island, WA

Book Introduction

This first edition of *Inside Ultrasound Vascular Reference Guide* provides the cardiovascular professional with a comprehensive easy to follow vascular reference. The book contains a detailed table of contents, list of tables and a comprehensive index for easy reference. Each chapter is organized with:

- A definition
- Etiology of disease
- Risk factors
- Indications and contraindications for exam
- Mechanism of disease
- Location of disease
- Patient history and physical exam
- Full protocols and summary protocols
- Normal and abnormal criteria
- Differential diagnosis
- Correlation
- Medical, surgical and endovascular treatments
- Comprehensive points to remember in each section

The book is filled with extra hints and tips, over 160 reference tables and 950 illustrations and images.

One of the most exciting elements in this book is the use of Quick Response Codes (QR Code), allowing us to share images and videos with you. When you find a QR code imbedded in an image, simply use a QR scanner from your mobile device and you will immediately be connected to an image or video! It's that easy!

The full ePub version of this guide will be available in the near future. The ePub edition will include embedded video, search topics, assess definitions and embedded note taking capabilities.

Acknowledgements

I wish to thank some of my mentors, those who saw something in me and took the time and energy to help me grow. First, thanks to Dr. Fileno Nicoletti, who in the early 80's asked me to open the hospital's first "Blood Flow Lab," and consequently I was honored to be trained in my home town of Chicago by Donna Blackburn and Drs. John Bergan and James Yao at Northwestern University's Blood Flow Lab. Secondly, my thanks to Dr. Morris Bernstein, one of my great teachers, who insisted I stay at his side through every vascular surgery and every follow up visit, it was at that time that I received my intense education and training on the vascular patient. The third person I would like to thank is Dr. Joseph Caprini, who had the confidence in me to allow me to open his vascular laboratory and be a part of his research team along with Dr. Juan Arcelus. Finally, my thanks to my dear friend Dr. Nicos Labropoulos who made it all fun and connected the loose ends for me.

I am grateful to all my colleagues through the years, especially the wonderful medical and technical staff members at the University of Chicago vascular laboratory, without their help and guidance this project could not have become a reality. This reference guide "took a village" to complete, and I am so blessed to have so many wonderful people in my village. Thank you, to my co authors, Laurie Lozanksi and Troy Russo, Chellie Buzzeo our graphic designer who's endless dedication and energy made this project happen, Denise Eggman, our medical illustrator who created the beautiful medical anatomy and graphic drawings, Dolores Nowak and Veda Miller for their years and years of proof reading, Iva McKay, my fantastic administrative assistant and to Kathleen Benyak and Ray Klumb for the generous use of their office space when my world was so busy I needed to escape.

A special thank you to my family, my dear husband John, who unconditionally loved and encouraged me through the years but especially through this project. Thank you Angie, for understanding why I missed so many of your games at school this winter and spring!

– Gail

Frontal View of the Extracranial and Intracranial Arterial System

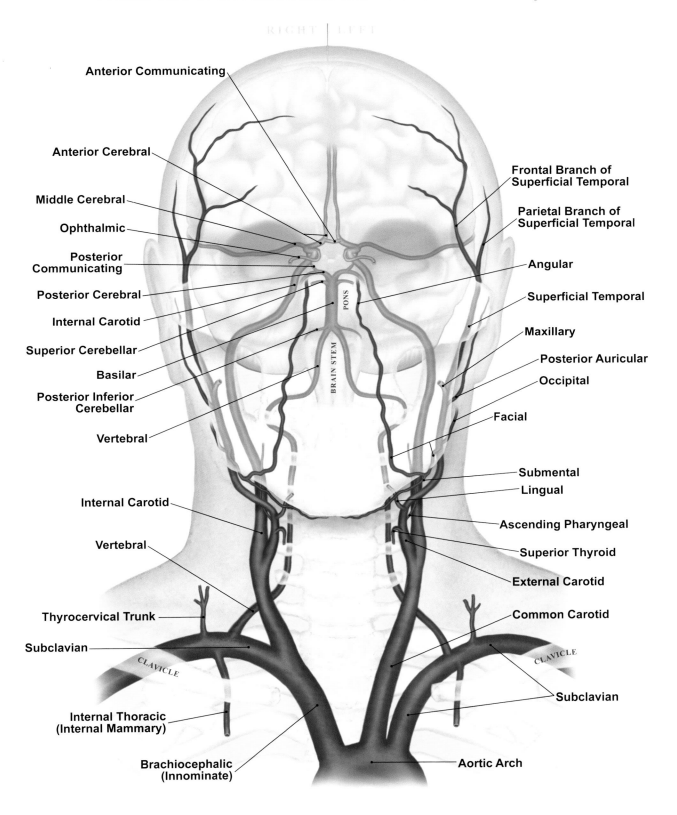

RIGHT | LEFT

Anterior Communicating

Anterior Cerebral

Middle Cerebral

Ophthalmic

Posterior Communicating

Posterior Cerebral

Internal Carotid

Superior Cerebellar

Basilar

Posterior Inferior Cerebellar

Vertebral

Internal Carotid

Vertebral

Thyrocervical Trunk

Subclavian

Internal Thoracic (Internal Mammary)

Brachiocephalic (Innominate)

Frontal Branch of Superficial Temporal

Parietal Branch of Superficial Temporal

Angular

Superficial Temporal

Maxillary

Posterior Auricular

Occipital

Facial

Submental

Lingual

Ascending Pharyngeal

Superior Thyroid

External Carotid

Common Carotid

Subclavian

Aortic Arch

PONS

BRAIN STEM

CLAVICLE

CLAVICLE

Extracranial Anatomy

Within the cerebrovascular arterial system, arteries are considered extracranial or intracranial. The extracranial vessels lay outside the skull or cranium. The intracranial vessels lay within the skull or cranium.

- The common carotid artery is classified as an extracranial vessel.
- The external carotid artery is classified as an extracranial vessel.
- The internal carotid artery is classified as an extracranial and intracranial vessel.
- The vertebral artery is classified as an extracranial and intracranial vessel.

Aortic Arch and Great Vessels

- The arteries supplying the extracranial and intracranial arteries originate off the aortic arch.
- The first vessel and largest branch originating off the aortic arch is the brachiocephalic trunk (innominate artery), which is sometimes referred to as the brachiocephalic artery.
  - The brachiocephalic trunk is approximately 4-5 cm in length, branching off the aortic arch at the level of the upper border of the second right costal cartilage.
  - The brachiocephalic artery travels upward, bifurcating into the right subclavian and right common carotid arteries.
  - The right brachiocephalic trunk and the proximal segments of the right common carotid and subclavian arteries are often rather tortuous.[1]
- The second vessel originating off the aortic arch is the left common carotid artery and the third vessel is the left subclavian artery.
- The brachiocephalic trunk, left common carotid and subclavian arteries are commonly referred to as the "great vessels". This is one of the very few places where there is an anatomical variation between the right and left sides of the body.
- Redundancy and buckling of the great vessels usually occurs in females and is associated with hypertension.[2]

Subclavian Arteries

The subclavian artery is not considered a part of the intra or extracranial system. Since many testing centers include the subclavian artery in the carotid duplex exam, this section is included as a review

- The brachiocephalic trunk travels upward, bifurcating into the right subclavian and right common carotid arteries.
- The left subclavian artery originates from the aortic arch.

Internal and External Carotid Anatomy

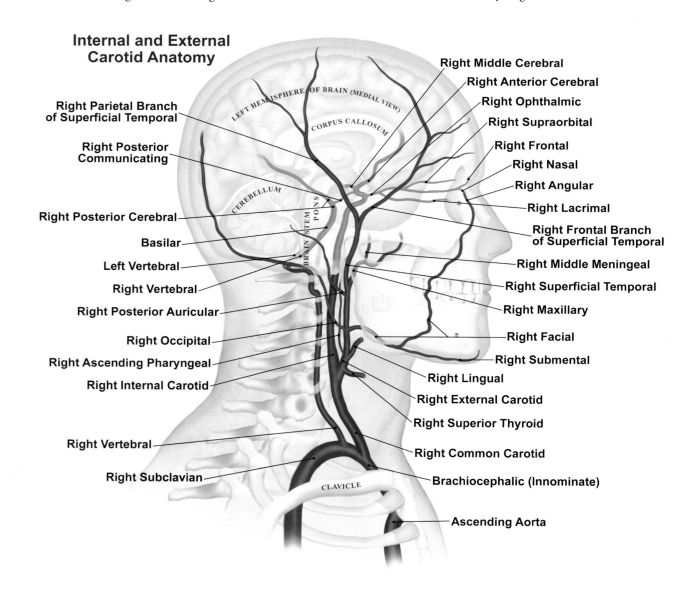

Right Middle Cerebral
Right Anterior Cerebral
Right Ophthalmic
Right Supraorbital
Right Frontal
Right Nasal
Right Angular
Right Lacrimal
Right Frontal Branch of Superficial Temporal
Right Middle Meningeal
Right Superficial Temporal
Right Maxillary
Right Facial
Right Submental
Right Lingual
Right External Carotid
Right Superior Thyroid
Right Common Carotid
Brachiocephalic (Innominate)
Ascending Aorta

Right Parietal Branch of Superficial Temporal
Right Posterior Communicating
Right Posterior Cerebral
Basilar
Left Vertebral
Right Vertebral
Right Posterior Auricular
Right Occipital
Right Ascending Pharyngeal
Right Internal Carotid
Right Vertebral
Right Subclavian

LEFT HEMISPHERE OF BRAIN (MEDIAL VIEW)
CORPUS CALLOSUM
CEREBELLUM
BRAIN STEM
PONS
CLAVICLE

Anatomy

Extracranial and Intracranial

- Both subclavian arteries pass just above the dome of the pleura.
- Branches of the subclavian arteries include the thryocervical, dorsal scapular, mammary (internal thoracic) and costocervical. All of these branches are capable of providing collateral circulation to the arm in the event of an arterial occlusion.
- The right subclavian can be tortuous and can mimic aneurysmal dilation. This condition is often seen in elderly hypertensive females.
- The subclavian arteries have three segments:
  - The first segment runs from its origin to the medial border of the anterior scalene (scalenus) muscle.
  - The second segment travels behind the anterior scalene muscle.
  - The third segment runs from the lateral margin of the scalene muscle to the first rib's outer border.
- Due to the close proximity of the subclavian artery to the clavicle, first rib and scalene muscle, a compression syndrome, "thoracic outlet syndrome" can occur.

Common Carotid Artery

- The right common carotid artery (CCA) typically originates from the brachiocephalic trunk and the left CCA arises directly from the aortic arch.
- The CCA moves upward on the anterolateral aspect of the neck to the level of the thyroid cartilage (vertebrae C2-C3), where it bifurcates into the internal carotid artery (ICA) and external carotid artery (ECA).
- The normal diameter of the CCA is 0.75 to 1.25 cm.

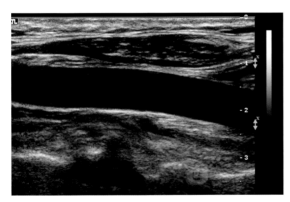

Common carotid artery

Carotid Bifurcation

- At the level of the carotid bifurcation the vessel becomes enlarged. This area, referred to as the carotid bulb or sinus, contains sensory nerve endings acting as baroreceptors. The *carotid body* (a baroreceptor) lies behind the artery and has a chemoreceptor function, making it sensitive to changes in pH, O_2 and CO_2 levels, so it can actually decrease the heart rate.

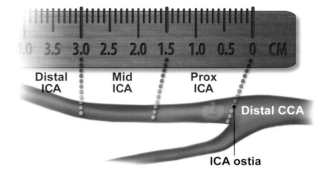

Carotid bifurcation anatomy
Note: Many labs have different definitions of location and configuration of the carotid bulb.

- There is variation in the level of the bifurcation from side to side:[1]
  - 28% of carotid arteries bifurcate at the same level.
  - 50% of left neck bifurcations are higher that the right.
  - 22% of right neck bifurcations are higher than the left.
- Anatomical variations can occur at the level of the carotid bifurcation and can include the CCA, ICA, ECA or any combination of these arteries.
  - The usual anatomical configuration is that the ECA lies more medial and anterior to the ICA artery.
  - The most common variation is the ECA artery lying posterior and lateral to the ICA.
  - The second most common variation is the ECA lying posterior and medial to the ICA.
  - The third most common is the ECA and ICA lie side by side.
- The bifurcation is the most common location for atherosclerotic lesions to occur due to the complicated flow patterns associated with the configuration.

Common Carotid Artery and Adjacent Anatomy

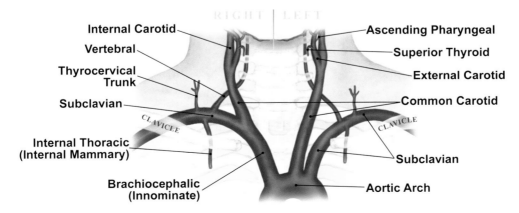

External Carotid Artery

- The external carotid artery (ECA) begins at the carotid bifurcation and travels upward terminating as the superficial temporal artery (STA).
- The ECA is smaller than the ICA and usually takes an anterior and medial course after the carotid bifurcation.
- The ECA has several branches which supply the face, neck and skull:
  - **Anterior branches:**
    - **Superior thyroid:** branches off the anterior portion and near the origin of the ECA then courses downward to the thyroid
    - **Lingual:** branches off the anterior ECA
    - **Facial:** branches off the anterior ECA, above the lingual artery
  - **Posterior branches:**
    - **Occipital:** branches off the posterior portion of the ECA opposite the facial artery
    - **Posterior Auricular:** branches off the posterior portion of the ECA just distal to the maxillary artery
  - **Ascending pharyngeal branch**:
    - Ascending pharyngeal branches off the posterior ECA and supplies the pharynx
  - **Terminal branches**:
    - **Superficial temporal artery (STA)** is the terminal ECA and divides into the frontal branch of the STA (anterior branch) and the parietal branch of the STA (posterior branch).
    - **Internal maxillary** is the terminal anterior branch of the STA
- ECA branches are important sources of collateral blood supply in carotid and vertebral disease. Common collateral pathways include:
  - Facial, maxillary and orbital branches
  - Superficial temporal artery and branches of the ophthalmic artery
  - Ascending pharyngeal branches and muscular branches of the vertebral artery
- The ECA diameter ranges from 0.25 to 0.70 cm.

> *The first major branch of the ECA is the superior thyroid artery. This branch helps distinguish the ECA from the ICA.*

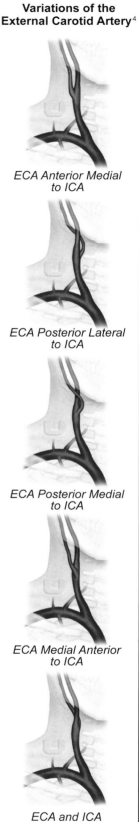

Variations of the External Carotid Artery[4]

ECA Anterior Medial to ICA

ECA Posterior Lateral to ICA

ECA Posterior Medial to ICA

ECA Medial Anterior to ICA

ECA and ICA Side-by-Side ECA Lateral to ICA

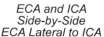

Variations taken from Gerlock, A. et al. 1988 Applications of Non-invasive Vascular Techniques. Philadelphia Saunders p126.

External Carotid Artery Anatomy

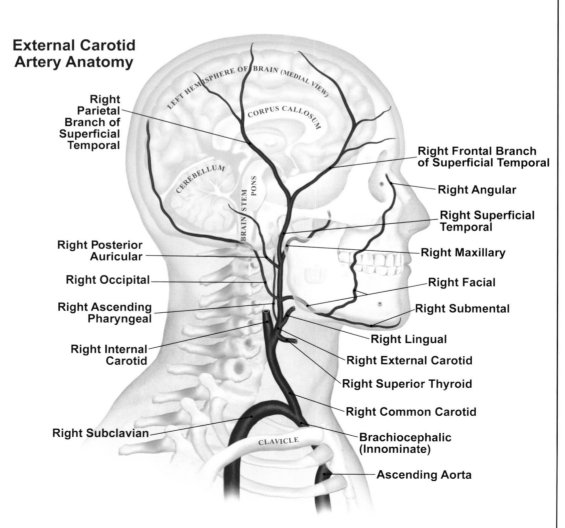

LEFT HEMISPHERE OF BRAIN (MEDIAL VIEW)

CORPUS CALLOSUM

CEREBELLUM

PONS

BRAIN STEM

CLAVICLE

- Right Parietal Branch of Superficial Temporal
- Right Posterior Auricular
- Right Occipital
- Right Ascending Pharyngeal
- Right Internal Carotid
- Right Subclavian
- Right Frontal Branch of Superficial Temporal
- Right Angular
- Right Superficial Temporal
- Right Maxillary
- Right Facial
- Right Submental
- Right Lingual
- Right External Carotid
- Right Superior Thyroid
- Right Common Carotid
- Brachiocephalic (Innominate)
- Ascending Aorta

Internal Carotid Artery

- The ICA begins at the carotid bifurcation and moves upward as a single vessel until it enters the cranium and terminates, bifurcating into the middle cerebral artery (MCA) and anterior cerebral artery (ACA).

- The ICA is classified as both an extracranial and intracranial vessel.

- The ICA usually takes a posterior and lateral course after the carotid bifurcation.

- The ICA has no branches within the neck area.

- Approximately 75% (200-400 ml/min) of the blood supply to the brain flows through the internal carotid arteries.

- The ICA supplies most of the anterior circulation of the cerebrum.

- The ICA diameter ranges from 0.5 to 1.0 cm

- Shape distortions can be described as tortuous, kinked, coiled, s-shaped, c-shaped, z-shaped, and u-shaped.

- Variations result from embryologic, pathologic, and aging effects.[2] The three most common distortions are:
  - **Tortuosity:** multiple turns or twists of the vessel, S-shaped elongation or curvature. Typically congenital and asymptomatic.
  - **Kinking:** reveals a sharp angle of 90 degrees or less usually located 2-4 cm above the carotid bifurcation.
  - **Coiling:** occurs when the arterial segment forms a complete circle from its longitudinal axis.

- The most important difference between a tortuous, coiled and kinked vessel is that the kinked vessel is most often associated with symptoms of cerebral ischemia.

- The ophthalmic artery is considered the first branch of the ICA supplying the eye. This branch occurs at the level of the carotid siphon.

Internal Carotid Artery Anatomy

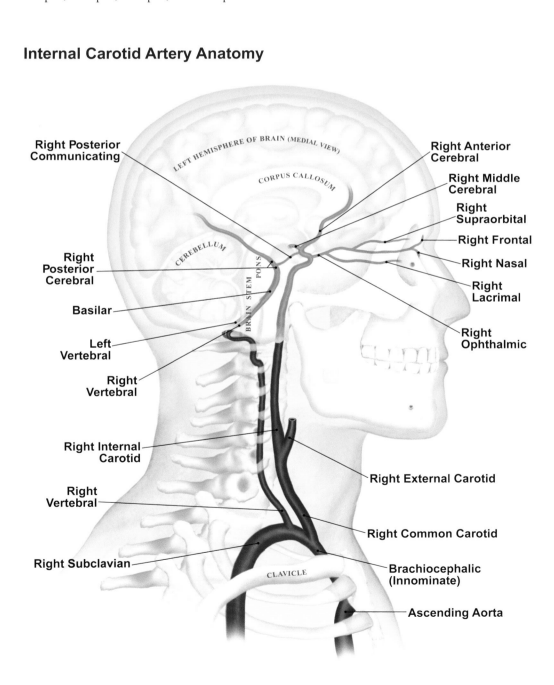

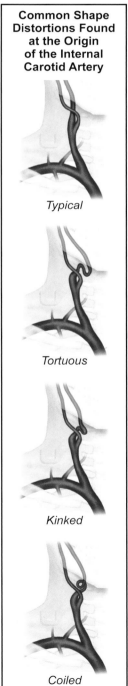

Common Shape Distortions Found at the Origin of the Internal Carotid Artery

Typical

Tortuous

Kinked

Coiled

- The ICA is divided into four major segments:
  - **Cervical:** begins at the carotid bifurcation and terminates when the internal carotid artery enters the skull. This is the longest segment of the ICA.
  - **Petrous:** begins once the ICA enters the carotid canal and courses vertically and then anteromedially through the canal.
  - **Cavernous:** located between the two dural layers that form the floor and roof of the cavernous sinus. The ICA bends forward along the sphenoid sinus and then turns backward; this is the S-shaped curve known as the carotid siphon. The ophthalmic artery is located in this segment. The proximal portion of the ICA siphon is the parasellar segment, followed by the genu and the supraclinoid segments.
  - **Cerebral:** short segment which divides into the anterior and middle cerebral arteries.

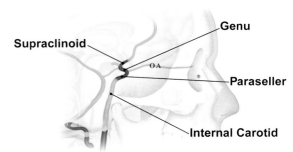

Anatomy of the carotid siphon

Intracranial Anatomy

The Circle of Willis includes: the internal carotid, middle cerebral, anterior cerebral and anterior communicating arteries. The vertebral arteries, basilar arteries, posterior cerebral arteries, and the posterior communicating arteries are also part of the Circle of Willis.

Anatomy of the Intracranial Circulation

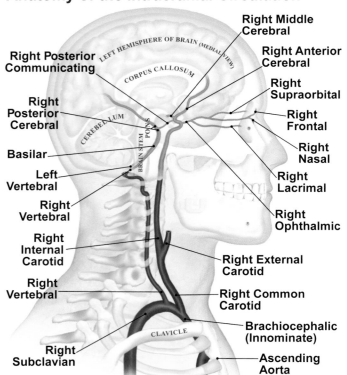

Ophthalmic Artery (OA)

- The ophthalmic artery is considered the first branch of the ICA and supplies the eye.

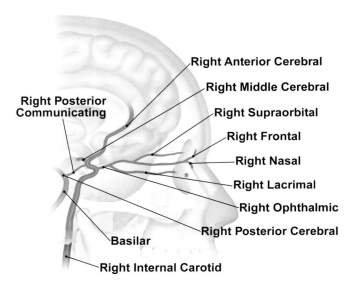

Anatomy of the Ophthalmic Artery (OA) with terminal branches

- Occurs at the level of the carotid siphon, and travels anterior through the optic canal to the orbit
- Can anastomose with the following branches of the ECA for collateral flow if the ICA becomes occluded:
  - Supraorbital artery
  - Frontal artery (supratrochlear artery)
  - Nasal artery
  - Laychrymal artery
- Collateral blood supply to the orbit is adequate to prevent blindness in the presence of an occluded ICA.[5]
- The OA is approximately 1.4 mm in diameter.

Vertebral Artery

- The cervical portion of the vertebral artery has several small branches to the spinal cord, vertebrae and adjacent muscles and are potential collateral channels in carotid or vertebral occlusive disease.

– Posterior meningeal	– Posterior inferior cerebellar
– Anterior spinal	– Bulbar
– Posterior spinal	

- The vertebral artery (VA) is the first branch of the subclavian artery and moves superiorly and posteriorly toward the cervical vertebrae through the foramina in the transverse process of the upper C6.[6]
- The right VA may arise as part of a trifurcation (vertebral, subclavian and common carotid arteries) of the brachiocephalic trunk.[7]
- The vertebral arteries are asymmetric in size with the left being dominant (larger) in approximately 50% of patients and the right being dominant in 25% of the patients. The remaining 25% are of equal size.[9]
- The VA can be divided into four segments:
  - Extracranial
  - Horizontal
  - Intravertebral
  - Intracranial

- The vertebrals carry approximately 25% of the blood to the brain.
- The right and left vertebral arteries enter the skull through the foramen magnum and join to form a singular basilar artery. Together these arteries form the vertebrobasilar circulation, which then supplies the Circle of Willis.
- The largest branch of the VA is the posterior inferior cerebellar artery (PICA).
- The vertebral arteries supply most of the posterior circulation.

Basilar Artery

- Formed by the joining of the right and left vertebral arteries.
- Approximately 4 mm in diameter and courses anteriorly and superiorly until its bifurcation into the right and left posterior cerebral arteries.
- Has many branches including the anterior inferior cerebellar, internal auditory and the superior cerebellar arteries.
- Can be tortuous, which is common in the elderly.

Anatomy of the Circle of Willis

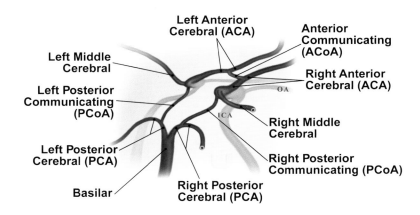

Circle of Willis

- Refers to the intracranial arteries which are in a polygonal shape.
- Located at the base of the brain and provides potential for collateral flow between the right and left cerebral hemispheres and the anterior (internal carotid) and posterior circulation (vertebrobasilar) to the brain.

- The anterior portion of the Circle of Willis includes the internal carotid arteries, middle cerebral arteries, anterior cerebral arteries and anterior communicating artery.

- The posterior portion of the Circle of Willis includes the vertebral arteries, basilar arteries, posterior cerebral arteries, and the posterior communicating arteries.

- A complete Circle of Willis is found in 20% of the populations.[9]

Anatomy of the Posterior Circulation

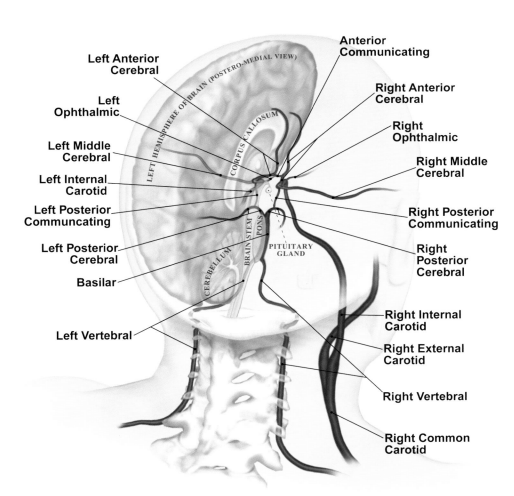

Anterior Cerebral Artery

- The anterior cerebral artery (ACA) originates off the internal carotid artery and is divided into several segments:
  - The A-1 segment of the ACA is the proximal, horizontal segment which connects to the contralateral A1 segment. This segment is sometimes referred to as the *precommunicating segment*.
  - The A-2 segment is distal to the junction with the anterior communicating artery and courses into the cerebral hemispheres. A2 segment joins branches of the PCA. This segment is sometimes referred to as the *postcommunicating segment*.
- Distal segments include segments A-3 to A-5. Approximately 25% of the time, the anterior cerebral artery is found to be hypoplastic.
- The anterior cerebral is approximately 2.6 mm in diameter and is the smaller of the two terminal branches of the internal carotid artery.
- The ACA (A-1) is absent in approximately 6% of patients.

Anterior Communicating Artery

- The anterior communicating artery (ACoA) is a short artery connecting the right and left A-1 segments of the anterior cerebral arteries.
- This artery runs medially and slightly anteriorly toward the middle of the brain.
- Tortuosity and kinking is noted in longer anterior communicating arteries.
- The ACoA is a potential collateral between the two sides of the anterior circulation.
- The ACoA is the most common site for intracranial aneurysm.
- The ACoA is approximately 1.5 mm in diameter and can be duplicated.

Middle Cerebral Artery

- The largest terminal branch of the ICA suppies much of the lateral surface of the brain.
- The MCA courses horizontally, laterally and slightly anteriorly.
- The MCA is approximately 3.9 mm in diameter and is the larger of the two terminal branches of the ICA. There are several perforators off the M1 segment.
- The most proximal segment is referred to as the M-1 segment and bifurcates or trifurcates into the M2 and M3 segments.
  - The M-2 segment is distal to the bifurcation and courses superior and posterior within the Sylvian fissure.
  - The terminal branches of the middle cerebral artery anastomose with the terminal branches of the anterior cerebral and posterior cerebral arteries.
  - Third most common site for congenital intracranial aneurysms and can account for about 25% of all intracranial aneurysms.

Posterior Cerebral Artery

- The right and left posterior cerebral arteries originate off the basilar artery.
- The proximal portion of the posterior cerebral artery joins with the PCoA and is referred to as the P-1 segment.
- The P-1 courses anteriorly and laterally. This segment is sometimes referred to as the *precommunicating segment*.
- The P-1 segment is approximately 2.6 mm in diameter.
- The P-2 segment begins distal to the junction with the posterior communicating artery (PCoA). The vessel then travels posteriorly around the lateral surface of the brain.
- The PCA (P-1) is absent in approximately 9% of patients.

Anatomical Variations of the Circle of Willis

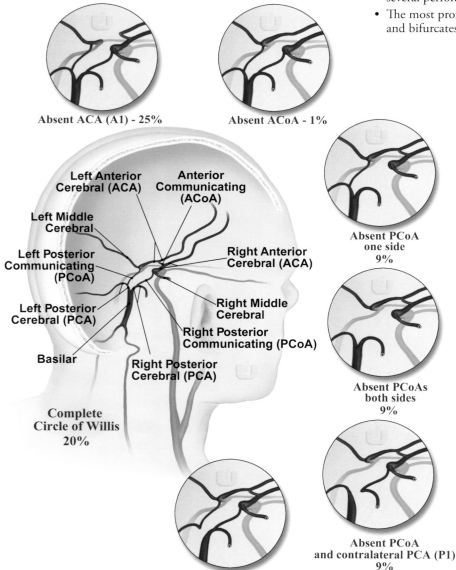

Absent ACA (A1) - 25%

Absent ACoA - 1%

Absent PCoA one side 9%

Absent PCoAs both sides 9%

Absent PCoA and contralateral PCA (P1) 9%

Absent PCA (P1) fetal origin - 9%

Left Anterior Cerebral (ACA)

Anterior Communicating (ACoA)

Left Middle Cerebral

Left Posterior Communicating (PCoA)

Left Posterior Cerebral (PCA)

Right Anterior Cerebral (ACA)

Right Middle Cerebral

Right Posterior Communicating (PCoA)

Basilar

Right Posterior Cerebral (PCA)

Complete Circle of Willis 20%

Posterior Communicating Artery

- Originates from the ICA and courses posteriorly to join the posterior cerebral artery.
- The size of the PCoA can be variable and blood flow through this segment can be in either direction, depending on the configuration of the Circle of Willis and if the blood supply is from the ICA or VA. [8]
- The PCoA anatomy is variable and is often hypoplastic. A complete segment is only found in a small percentage of the population.
- The posterior communicating artery is the second most common site for intracranial aneurysm.
- The PCoA is an important collateral in cases of extensive bilateral occlusive disease.
- PCoA and contralateral PCA are absent in 9% of patients.

Anatomic Variations of the Circle of Willis and Collateral Pathways

- Anatomical variations of the Circle of Willis are common. Only 20% of the population is thought to have a "normal" Circle of Willis.[8,9]
- The most common missing segments are the anterior communicating artery (ACoA), posterior communicating artery (PCoA), anterior cerebral artery (ACA) and the posterior cerebral artery (PCA). These vessels can be hypoplastic, aplastic or atretic.[8]
- The ACA has several possible variations:
  - The A1 segment of the ACA has variable courses; horizontal, ascending or descending and can be tortuous.[1]
  - Complete absence of the A1 segment is not uncommon. This condition is reported in the literature to occur in approximately 6% - 25% of patients and is also known as a "hypoplastic" or "atretic" A1 segment.[1,2]
  - The size of the A1 segment and the ACoA should be inversely proportionate, (e.g., a hypoplastic A1 segment exists with a larger ACoA).[3]
  - The Artery of Huebner is commonly a major branch of the A2 segment (80% of cases), but can also originate from the distal A1 segment. [9]
  - The ACoA may be duplicated or have multiple channels.
- The PCA can be supplied from the ICA, instead of the BA. This is known as a "fetal origin" of the PCA. The prevalence of this variation is approximately 15-22%. [9]
- The vertebral arteries vary in length. In approximately 90% of cases, one VA is larger than the other.[8] The left VA is often the larger or dominant vertebral artery.[10]

Collateral Pathways

- There are three categories of intracranial collateral circulation: the Circle of Willis, ICA-ECA network and the small interarterial communications.
- The primary collateral circulation is via the Circle of Willis and the meningeal anatomoses. (compensatory circulation)[8]
- The most common collateral connection between the left and right hemispheres is the ACoA.[8]
- The PCoA is a common collateral pathway, connecting the carotid and basilar vessels.[8]
- The second most common collateral pathway is the ICA-ECA network (prewillisian anastomoses), in which branches of the internal and external carotid arteries can join to provide blood flow.
- Examples of the ICA-ECA pathways are:
  - Back-front pathway would be vertebrobasilar arteries via the posterior cerebral and posterior communicating arteries (between basilar and right or left common carotid artery).
  - The ophthalmic artery is the common collateral pathway in the event of internal carotid artery obstruction via the ICA-ECA pathway.
  - Supraorbital and/or frontal arteries (ICA) to superficial temporal artery (ECA); usually on or across the forehead.
  - Nasal artery (ICA) to facial or angular artery (ECA).
  - Nasal artery (ICA) via the angular artery or infraorbital artery (ECA).
  - Ophthalmic artery (ICA) to middle meningeal artery (ECA).
- The third category of intracranial collateral circulation is the small interarterial communications called the Rete Mirabile or the "*wonderful net*". This network runs across the subdural space from the dural arteries to arteries on the surface of the brain.

References

1. Cronenwett J, Johnston, K., (2005) in Rutherford's Vascular Surgery Saunders; 7 edition. Philadelphia Saunders Elsevier.
2. Cronenwett J, Johnston, K., (2010) in Rutherford's Vascular Surgery Saunders; 7 edition. Philadelphia Saunders Elsevier.
3. Size, G, Laubach, M et al. Color Flow Imaging For Diagnosis Of Innominate And Carotid Artery Buckling, Video Journal of Color Flow Imaging; Vol 2, No. 3; pp 124-128, 1992.
4. Gerlock, A. et al. (1988) Applications of Non-invasive Vascular Techniques. Philadelphia Saunders p.126.
5. Uflacker, R. (1997) Arteries of the head and neck. In Atlas of Vascular Anatomy: An angiographic Approach P. 11. Baltimore Wolters Kluwer Lippincott Williams & Wilkins
6. Uflacker, R. (2007) Arteries of the head and neck. In Atlas of Vascular Anatomy: An angiographic Approach pp 18-19. Baltimore Wolters Kluwer Lippincott Williams & Wilkins.
7. Uflacker, R. (1997) Arteries of the head and neck. In Atlas of Vascular Anatomy: An angiographic Approach (5-79). Baltimore Wolters Kluwer Lippincott Williams & Wilkins
8. The Handbook of Transcranial Doppler McCartney JP, Lukes-Thomas KM, Gomez CR. (1997). Handbook of Transcranial Doppler. New York. Springer-Verlag
9. Naylor AR, Markose G. (2010) Cerebrovascular disease: diagnostic evaluation, In Cronenwett J, Johnston, K., (2005) in Rutherford's Vascular Surgery Saunders; (7 edition) (Chapter 93) Saunders Elsevier.
10. Cronenwett J, Johnston, K., (2010) in Rutherford's Vascular Surgery Saunders; 7th edition. Philadelphia Saunders Elsevier.

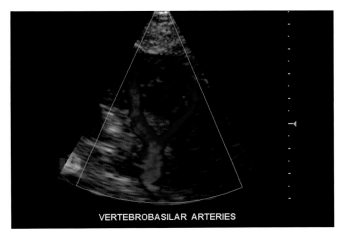

VERTEBROBASILAR ARTERIES

Abdominal Arterial System

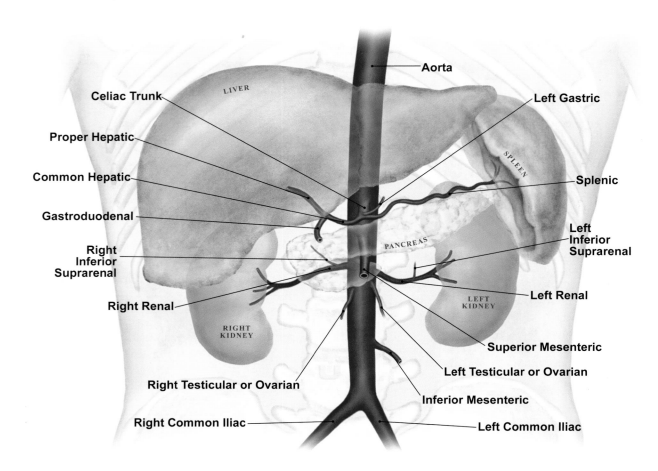

Abdominal Arterial Anatomy

- The abdominal aorta begins as the descending aorta and crosses the diaphragm.
- The abdominal aorta bifurcates into the right and left common iliac arteries at the level of the umbilicus.
- The abdominal aorta has five main branches:
  - **Celiac artery**: (also known as the celiac trunk or celiac axis) supplies the liver, gallbladder, stomach, intestines and pancreas.
    - There are three branches of the celiac artery:
      - Splenic artery
      - Common hepatic artery
      - Left gastric artery

> *In some cases, the SMA and celiac trunk have a common origin off the abdominal aorta.*

- **Superior mesenteric artery** (SMA): originates approximately 1 cm inferior to the celiac trunk. The SMA supplies the intestines and pancreas.
- **Renal arteries** (right and left): supplies the kidneys and adrenal glands.
- **Inferior mesenteric artery** (IMA): supplies the colon and rectum.
- For the purposes of the ultrasound examination, the abdominal aorta is divided into three regions:
  - Proximal aorta: diaphragm to the origin of the superior mesenteric artery
  - Mid aorta: superior mesenteric artery to the renal arteries
  - Distal aorta: renal arteries to the aortic bifurcation

> *Some labs use alternative terms, dividing the aorta into the suprarenal, juxtarenal and infrarenal aorta.*

- The average diameter of the abdominal aorta is 2.0 cm (range: 1.1-3.0 cm).
- The aorta normally decreases (tapers) in diameter from the diaphragm to the aortic bifurcation.

Arterial and Venous Systems at the Renal Level

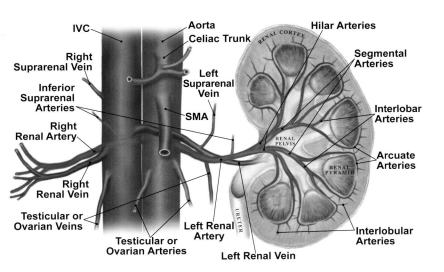

Abdominal Venous Anatomy

This anatomy is described from the pelvis to the abdomen.

- The external iliac vein (EIV) drains the inferior portion of the abdominal wall, as well as the legs.
- The internal iliac vein (IIV) drains the pelvis and joins the EIV to form the common iliac vein (CIV).
- The right and left CIV join to form the inferior vena cava (IVC).
- The IVC is the largest vein of the body; approximately 17.2 mm (infrarenal) during quiet respiration and drains blood flow from the lower extremities and abdomen back to the heart (right atrium).
- For the purposes of the ultrasound examination, the inferior vena cava is divided into three regions or thirds:
  - **Suprahepatic:** superior to the liver
  - **Intrahepatic:** includes tributaries from the liver
  - **Infrahepatic:** inferior to the liver and to the level to the iliac bifurcation

Renal Anatomy

- The right and left main renal arteries (RA) originate laterally from the abdominal aorta, immediately inferior to the superior mesenteric artery.

- The right and left renal veins (RV) originate from the inferior vena cava.

- The right RA is longer than the left and is posterior to the inferior vena cava and right RV.

- The left RV runs between the abdominal aorta and superior mesenteric artery.

- The left RA lies posterior to the left renal vein.

- The renal artery divides into the segmental arteries at the origin of the kidney.

- The segmental arteries give rise to the interlobar arteries in the kidney parenchyma.

- The parenchyma is divided into the *medulla and cortex*. The medulla is adjacent to the renal sinus and pyramids and the cortex is the most peripheral portion of the parenchyma, located between the medulla and renal capsule.

- Near the medulla and cortex junction, the arcuate arteries come off at right angles. As the arcuate arteries pass around the pyramids, they give rise to the interlobular arterioles.

> The right kidney is lower than the left kidney due to the R-lobe of the liver.

- The IVC has numerous tributaries including:
  - **Lumbar veins:** return blood flow from the posterior abdominal wall.
  - **Testicular or ovarian veins:** return blood from either the testes or the ovaries.
  - **Renal veins:** (right and left) return blood flow from the kidneys
  - **Suprarenal veins:** return blood from the adrenal glands (Note: the right suprarenal vein terminates in the IVC and the left suprarenal vein terminates in the left renal vein).
  - **Phrenic veins:** return blood flow from the diaphragm
  - **Hepatic veins:** return blood flow from the liver. Each hepatic vein drains different portions of the liver:
    - Right hepatic
    - Middle hepatic
    - Left hepatic
  - **Portal veins:** deliver deoxygenated blood from the stomach, pancreas, spleen, gallbladder and intestines to the hepatic venous system. There are several branches.
  - **Superior mesenteric vein:** returns blood flow from the intestines and stomach
  - **Inferior mesenteric vein:** drains blood flow from the colon
  - **Splenic vein:** returns blood flow from the spleen and receives blood from the stomach, pancreas and inferior mesenteric vein
  - **Gastric veins:** return blood flow from the stomach
  - **Main portal vein divides into the:**
    - Right portal vein
    - Left portal vein

> The splenic and superior mesenteric veins join to form the main portal vein.

Abdominal Venous System

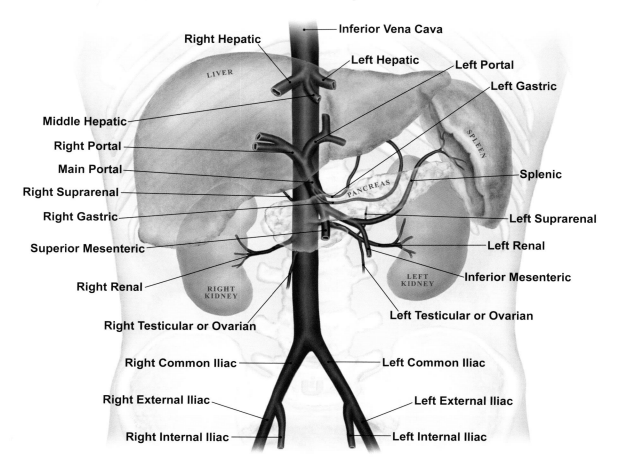

Labels (clockwise): Inferior Vena Cava, Right Hepatic, Left Hepatic, Left Portal, Left Gastric, Middle Hepatic, Right Portal, Main Portal, Right Suprarenal, Right Gastric, Superior Mesenteric, Right Renal, Right Testicular or Ovarian, Splenic, Left Suprarenal, Left Renal, Inferior Mesenteric, Left Testicular or Ovarian, Right Common Iliac, Left Common Iliac, Right External Iliac, Left External Iliac, Right Internal Iliac, Left Internal Iliac. Organs: LIVER, SPLEEN, PANCREAS, RIGHT KIDNEY, LEFT KIDNEY.

IVC-Iliac Venous Bifurcation

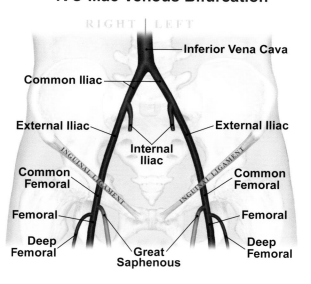

RIGHT | LEFT — Inferior Vena Cava, Common Iliac, External Iliac, External Iliac, Internal Iliac, Common Femoral, Common Femoral, Femoral, Femoral, Deep Femoral, Deep Femoral, Great Saphenous, INGUINAL LIGAMENT

Anatomy of the Iliac Bifurcation

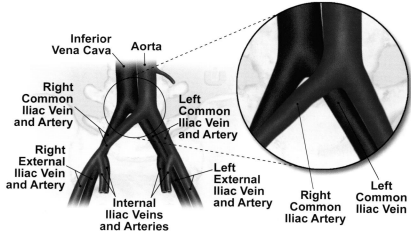

Inferior Vena Cava, Aorta, Right Common Iliac Vein and Artery, Left Common Iliac Vein and Artery, Right External Iliac Vein and Artery, Left External Iliac Vein and Artery, Internal Iliac Veins and Arteries, Right Common Iliac Artery, Left Common Iliac Vein

References

1. Gray, H. (1977). The portal system of veins. In Pick TP & Howden R. (Eds.), *Gray's Anatomy* (617-619). New York: Bounty Books

2. Netter FH. (2003). Abdomen. In *Atlas of Human Anatomy 3rd ed.* (239-338). Terterboro: Icon Learning Systems.

3. Netter FH. (2003). Pelvis and perineum. In *Atlas of Human Anatomy 3rd ed.* (339-400). Terterboro: Icon Learning Systems.

4. Tortora, G. J., & Anagnostakos, NP. (Eds.). (1990). The cardiovascular system: vessels and routes. In *Principles of Anatomy and Physiology, 6th ed.* (605-650) New York, NY: Harper & Row Publishers.

5. Uflacker R. (1997). Abdominal aorta and branches. In *Atlas of Vascular Anatomy: An Angiographic Approach.* (405-604). Baltimore: Wolters Kluwer Lippincott Williams & Wilkins.

6. Uflacker R. (1997). Arteries of the pelvis. In *Atlas of Vascular Anatomy: An Angiographic Approach.* (605-634). Baltimore: Wolters Kluwer Lippincott Williams & Wilkins.

7. Uflacker R. (1997). Veins of the abdomen and pelvis. In *Atlas of Vascular Anatomy: An Angiographic Approach.* (635-729). Baltimore: Wolters Kluwer Lippincott Williams & Wilkins.

Anatomy
Upper Extremity Venous

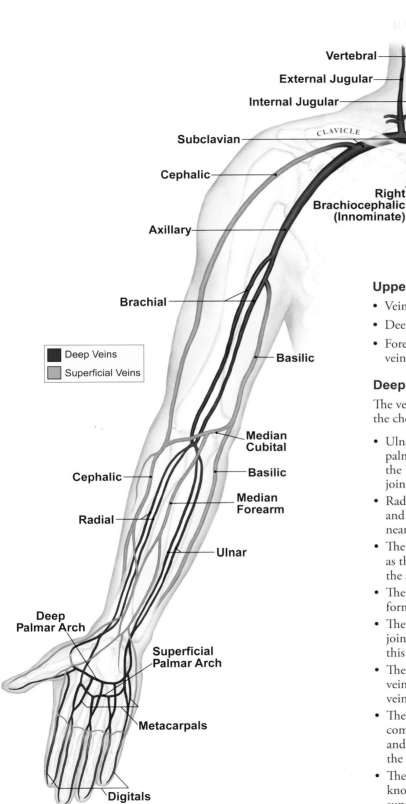

RIGHT | LEFT

Vertebral

External Jugular

Internal Jugular

Subclavian

CLAVICLE

CLAVICLE

Cephalic

Right Brachiocephalic (Innominate)

Left Brachiocephalic (Innominate)

Axillary

Superior Vena Cava

Brachial

Deep Veins

Superficial Veins

Basilic

Median Cubital

Cephalic

Basilic

Radial

Median Forearm

Ulnar

Deep Palmar Arch

Superficial Palmar Arch

Metacarpals

Digitals

Upper Extremity Venous System

- Veins return blood back to the heart.
- Deep veins have an accompanying artery.
- Forearm and brachial veins are duplicated. Axillary veins may also be duplicated.

Deep Veins

The vessel anatomy is described from the wrist to the chest:

- Ulnar veins (UV) arise from the tributaries of the palmar venous arch in the hand. With the palm up, the UV travel along the medial aspect of the forearm, joining near the elbow to form an ulnar trunk.
- Radial veins (RV) arise from the dorsal metacarpal veins and travel up the lateral aspect of the forearm, joining near the elbow to form the radial trunk.
- The radial and ulnar trunks may continue into the arm as the two brachial veins or the trunks may join before the split into a paired brachial system.
- The brachial veins (BRV) usually join near the axilla to form the axillary vein.
- The axillary vein (AXV) runs along the shoulder until joining the cephalic vein. The subclavian vein begins at this point, usually the upper border of the first rib.
- The subclavian vein (SCV) joins the internal jugular vein to form the brachiocephalic vein (or innominate vein) at the clavicular level.
- The internal jugular vein (IJV) runs adjacent to the common carotid artery and receives blood from the face and neck. As mentioned, the IJV joins the SCV to form the brachiocephalic (innominate) vein.
- The right and left brachiocephalic veins (BCV), also known as the innominate veins (INV), join to form the superior vena cava (SVC).
- The SVC enters the heart at the right atrium.

Typical Anatomic Variations of the Veins at the Antecubital Fossa

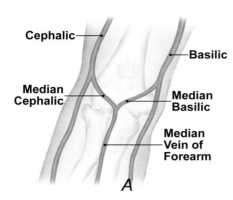

A

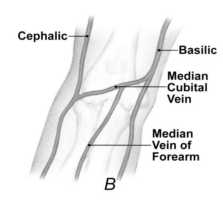

B

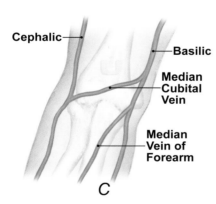

C

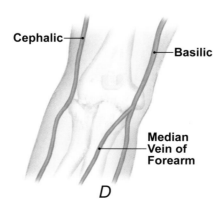

D

Anatomical variations of the superficial veins in the cubital fossa.(A) M-shaped configuration, (B and C) N-shaped configurations with the MCV terminating in CV and BSV, respectively, (D) no communication between the CV and BSV.

Superficial Veins

- The cephalic vein (CV) is the longest vein in the arm. The CV originates from the medial component of the dorsal venous arch in the hand and runs laterally along the arm. As it courses along the upper end of the deltoid muscle, it dives at the clavicular end of the pectoralis muscle to join the axillary-subclavian veins.

- The basilic vein (BSV) originates from the ulnar component of the dorsal venous arch in the hand and runs medially along the arm. The BSV joins the axillary vein near the medial border of the biceps muscle.

- The median cubital vein (MCV) crosses the antecubital fossa obliquely, connecting the cephalic and basilic veins. There are several anatomical variations to this connection.

> *Superficial veins run within the superficial compartment, above the deep fascia.*

Neck Veins

Additional veins of the neck (not already mentioned) are highlighted in this section.

- The vertebral vein drains the neck and terminates along the posterior aspect of the brachiocephalic (innominate) vein.

- Several other veins drain into the brachiocephalic (innominate) veins including the:
  - Internal thoracic veins
  - Inferior thyroid veins

- There is also an external jugular vein which drains blood from the cranium, face and neck into the SCV. Prior to entering the subclavian vein, the external jugular vein receives blood from the:
  - Suprascapular vein
  - Transverse cervical vein

- The anterior jugular vein is highly variable in both size and course. Typically there is a right and a left anterior jugular vein joined just above the sternum by a "trunk" called the jugular arch. The anterior jugular vein communicates with either the subclavian vein or distal portion of the external jugular vein. This vein also communicates with the internal jugular vein and is an important collateral channel, especially in the presence of subclavian venous thrombosis.

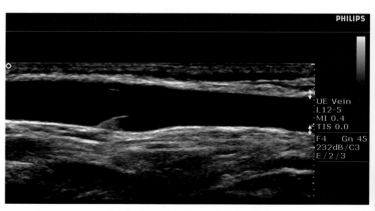

Cephalic vein with valve leaflets
Image courtesy of Philips Healthcare

Veins of the Neck

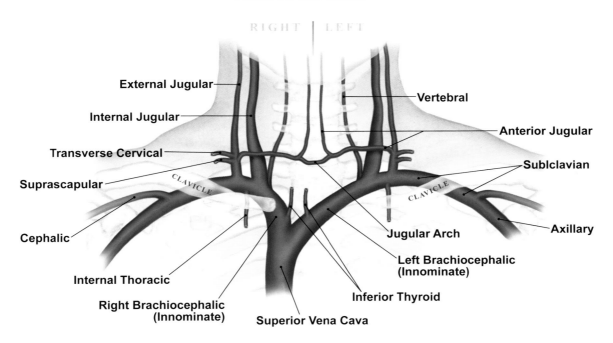

RIGHT | LEFT

External Jugular

Internal Jugular

Transverse Cervical

CLAVICLE

Suprascapular

Cephalic

Internal Thoracic

Right Brachiocephalic
(Innominate)

Superior Vena Cava

Vertebral

Anterior Jugular

Subclavian

CLAVICLE

Axillary

Jugular Arch

Left Brachiocephalic
(Innominate)

Inferior Thyroid

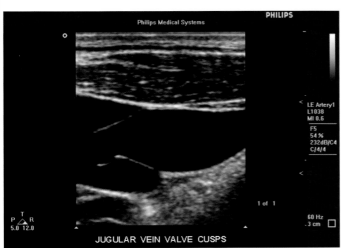

JUGULAR VEIN VALVE CUSPS

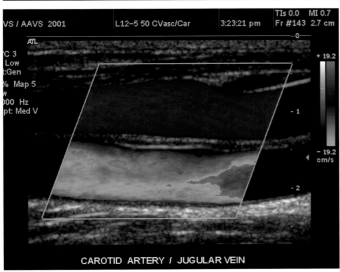

CAROTID ARTERY / JUGULAR VEIN

Images courtesy of Philips Healthcare

References:

1. Gray, H. (1977). The blood-vascular system. In Pick TP & Howden R. (Eds.), *Gray's Anatomy* (551-592). New York: Bounty Books.

2. Gray, H. (1977). The veins. In Pick TP & Howden R. (Eds.), *Gray's Anatomy* (593-614). New York: Bounty Books.

3. Netter FH. (2003). Head and neck. In Atlas of Human Anatomy 3rd ed. (1-144). Terterboro. Icon Learning Systems.

4. Netter FH. (2003). Thorax. In Atlas of Human Anatomy 3rd ed. (174-238). Terterboro. Icon Learning Systems.

5. Netter FH. (2003). Upper limb. In Atlas of Human Anatomy 3rd ed. (401-466). Terterboro. Icon Learning Systems.

6. Tortora, G. J., & Anagnostakos, NP. (Eds.). (1990). The cardiovascular system: vessels and routes. In *Principles of Anatomy and Physiology, 6th ed.* (605-650) New York, NY: Harper & Row Publishers.

7. Uflacker R. (1997). Veins of the head and neck. In Atlas of Vascular Anatomy: An Angiographic Approach. (81-112). Baltimore: Wolters Kluwer Lippincott Williams & Wilkins.

8. Uflacker R. (1997). Veins of the thorax. In Atlas of Vascular Anatomy: An Angiographic Approach. (189-212). Baltimore: Wolters Kluwer Lippincott Williams & Wilkins.

9. Uflacker R. (1997). Veins of the upper extremity. In Atlas of Vascular Anatomy: An Angiographic Approach. (389-399). Baltimore: Wolters Kluwer Lippincott Williams & Wilkins.

10. Zwiebel, WJ (2005). Extremity venous anatomy, terminology, and ultrasound features of normal veins. In Zwiebel WJ, Pellerito JS. (Eds) *Introduction to Vascular Ultrasonography 5th ed.* (415-429). Philadelphia: Elsevier Saunders.

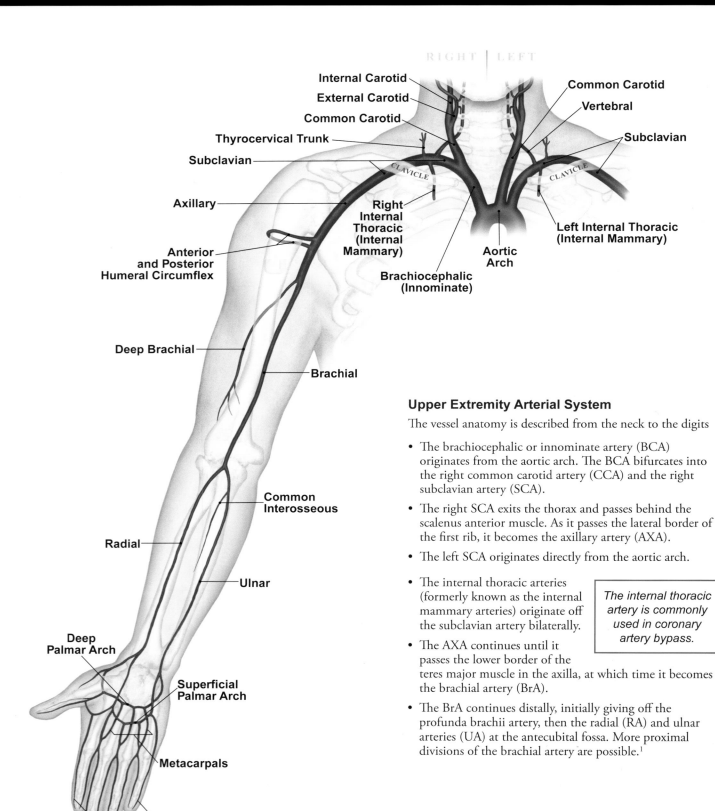

RIGHT | LEFT

Internal Carotid

External Carotid

Common Carotid

Thyrocervical Trunk

Subclavian

Axillary

Anterior
and Posterior
Humeral Circumflex

Deep Brachial

Brachial

Common
Interosseous

Radial

Ulnar

Deep
Palmar Arch

Superficial
Palmar Arch

Metacarpals

Digitals

Common Carotid

Vertebral

Subclavian

CLAVICLE

Right
Internal
Thoracic
(Internal
Mammary)

CLAVICLE

Left Internal Thoracic
(Internal Mammary)

Aortic
Arch

Brachiocephalic
(Innominate)

Upper Extremity Arterial System

The vessel anatomy is described from the neck to the digits

- The brachiocephalic or innominate artery (BCA) originates from the aortic arch. The BCA bifurcates into the right common carotid artery (CCA) and the right subclavian artery (SCA).

- The right SCA exits the thorax and passes behind the scalenus anterior muscle. As it passes the lateral border of the first rib, it becomes the axillary artery (AXA).

- The left SCA originates directly from the aortic arch.

- The internal thoracic arteries (formerly known as the internal mammary arteries) originate off the subclavian artery bilaterally.

- The AXA continues until it passes the lower border of the teres major muscle in the axilla, at which time it becomes the brachial artery (BrA).

The internal thoracic artery is commonly used in coronary artery bypass.

- The BrA continues distally, initially giving off the profunda brachii artery, then the radial (RA) and ulnar arteries (UA) at the antecubital fossa. More proximal divisions of the brachial artery are possible.[1]

- With the palm up, the RA passes along the lateral side of the forearm and the UA passes along the medial side.
- The RA and UA join in the palm of the hand to form the deep and superficial palmar arches. These arches may or may not communicate with each other.[1]
  - The RA becomes the deep palmar arch in the hand.
  - The UA becomes the superficial palmar arch in the hand and runs distal to the deep arch.
- The digital arteries arise from the palmar arches. There are often 4 palmar common digital arteries in the hand.[2]
- The common digital arteries branch into the proper digital arteries. These proper palmar digital arteries run along each side of the second through fifth fingers.[2]

> *An early bifurcation of the RA and UA (off the AXA) is possible in up to approximately 3% of the population.*[1]

- The thumb receives blood from the first palmar metacarpal artery, radial artery or the palmar arches (anatomy varies).[2]

Digital Arterial Anatomy

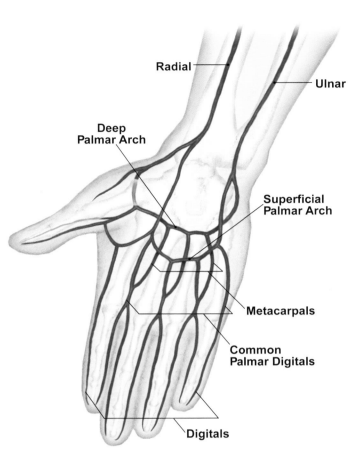

Radial

Ulnar

Deep Palmar Arch

Superficial Palmar Arch

Metacarpals

Common Palmar Digitals

Digitals

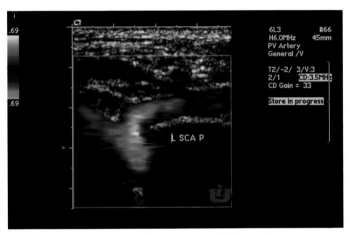

Left subclavian artery comes off the aortic arch

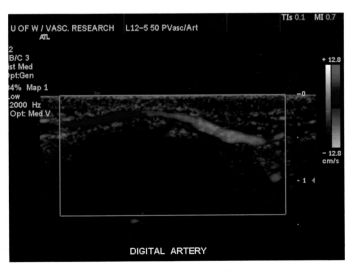

Image courtesy of Philips Healthcare

References

1. 1 Keck GM, Zwiebel, WJ (2005). Arterial anatomy of the extremities. In Zwiebel WJ, Pellerito JS. (Eds). *Introduction to Vascular Ultrasonography 5th ed.* (261-274). Philadelphia: Elsevier Saunders.

2. 2 Chloros, GD, et al. (2008). Non-invasive evaluation of upper extremity vascular perfusion. *J Hand Surg Am.* Apr; 33(4):(591-600).

3. Additional references:

4. Gray, H. (1977). The blood-vascular system. In Pick TP & Howden R. (Eds.), *Gray's Anatomy* (551-592). New York: Bounty Books.

5. Netter FH. (2003). Head and neck. In *Atlas of Human Anatomy 3rd ed.* (1-144). Terterboro. Icon Learning Systems.

6. Netter FH. (2003). Thorax. In *Atlas of Human Anatomy 3rd ed.* (174-238). Terterboro. Icon Learning Systems.

7. Netter FH. (2003). Upper limb. In *Atlas of Human Anatomy 3rd ed.* (401-466). Terterboro. Icon Learning Systems.

8. Uflacker R. (1997). Arteries of the head and neck. In *Atlas of Vascular Anatomy: An Angiographic Approach.* (3-79). Baltimore: Wolters Kluwer Lippincott Williams & Wilkins.

9. Uflacker R. (1997). Arteries of the upper extremity. In *Atlas of Vascular Anatomy: An Angiographic Approach.* (339-338). Baltimore: Wolters Kluwer Lippincott Williams & Wilkins.

10. Tortora, GJ, Anagnostakos NP. (Eds.). (1990). The cardiovascular system: vessels and routes. In Principles of Anatomy and Physiology, 6th ed. (605-650) New York, NY: Harper & Row Publishers.

Deep Veins

- Deep veins have an accompanying artery.
- Calf veins are duplicated.

The vessel anatomy is described from the foot to the IVC.

- The digital veins join to form the metatarsal veins and the plantar arch.
- Posterior tibial veins (PTV) arise from the confluence of the medial and lateral plantar veins and travel up the medial aspect of the calf.
- Peroneal veins (PerV) begin in the foot and travel up the lateral aspect of the calf (behind the fibula) to join the PTV and form the tibioperoneal trunk.
- Soleal sinuses are thick walled venous reservoirs within the soleal muscle. They do not contain venous valves and are a frequent site of thrombosis. They empty into the posterior tibial and peroneal veins.
- The tibioperoneal trunk is a short segment of vein in the upper calf, distal to the popliteal vein where the PTV and PerV join.
- Anterior tibial veins (ATV) originate from the pedal vein in the foot and travel upward, between the tibia and fibula to join the tibioperoneal trunk.
- The popliteal vein (PopV) begins as the ATV and the tibioperoneal trunk join.

Lower Extremity Venous System

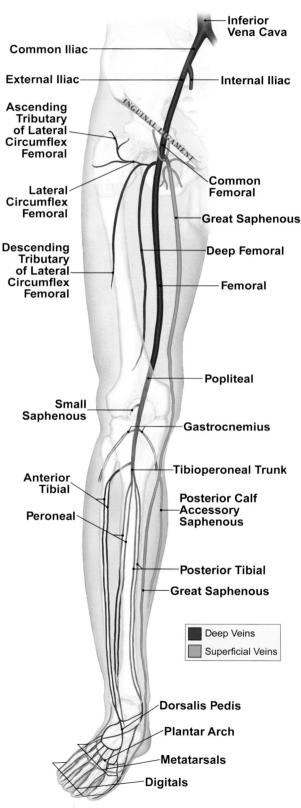

- Inferior Vena Cava
- Common Iliac
- External Iliac
- Internal Iliac
- Ascending Tributary of Lateral Circumflex Femoral
- INGUINAL LIGAMENT
- Lateral Circumflex Femoral
- Common Femoral
- Great Saphenous
- Descending Tributary of Lateral Circumflex Femoral
- Deep Femoral
- Femoral
- Popliteal
- Small Saphenous
- Gastrocnemius
- Tibioperoneal Trunk
- Anterior Tibial
- Posterior Calf Accessory Saphenous
- Peroneal
- Posterior Tibial
- Great Saphenous
- Dorsalis Pedis
- Plantar Arch
- Metatarsals
- Digitals

Deep Veins
Superficial Veins

Cross Section of Calf

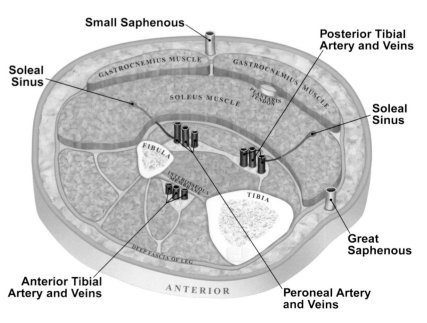

- Small Saphenous
- Posterior Tibial Artery and Veins
- Soleal Sinus
- GASTROCNEMIUS MUSCLE
- GASTROCNEMIUS MUSCLE
- PLANTARIS TENDON
- SOLEUS MUSCLE
- Soleal Sinus
- FIBULA
- INTEROSSEOUS MEMBRANE
- TIBIA
- Great Saphenous
- DEEP FASCIA OF LEG
- Anterior Tibial Artery and Veins
- ANTERIOR
- Peroneal Artery and Veins

Venous System of the Calf

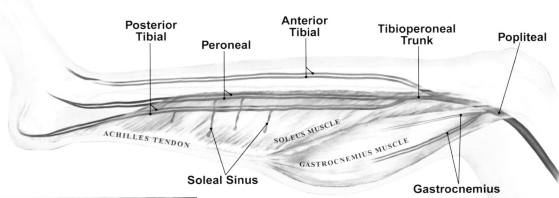

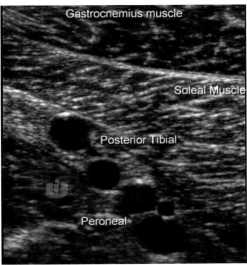

Gastrocnemius and soleal muscles along with the peroneal and posterior tibial veins

- The gastrocnemius veins, also referred to as the *sural veins*, are paired and may be seen in triplicate sets. These sets of vessels terminate in the PopV.
- As the PopV enters the adductor canal in the distal thigh, the vein becomes the femoral vein (FV).
- The femoral vein (FV) is a deep vein that travels the length of the thigh. The FV joins the deep femoral (DFV) to become the common femoral vein (CFV).
- The CFV travels upward towards the inguinal ligament, and is easily imaged at the groin crease. The great saphenous vein (GSV) joins the CFV in the groin (known as the saphenofemoral junction (SFJ).
- The CFV dives deep at the level of the proximal inguinal ligament where it becomes the external iliac vein (EIV). The EIV drains the inferior part of the abdominal wall, as well as the legs.
- The internal iliac vein (IIV) drains the pelvis, and joins the EIV to form the common iliac vein (CIV).
- The right and left CIV join to form the inferior vena cava (IVC).
- The IVC is the largest vein of the body and drains the lower extremities and the abdomen.

Superficial Veins

- The superficial veins do not have a corresponding artery, which makes them easy to distinguish from the deep veins.
- The great saphenous vein (GSV) is the longest vein in the body and originates on the dorsum of the foot. The GSV travels the medial aspect of the entire leg and ends at the common femoral vein. There are additional connections to the deep system via perforating veins.

> *The GSV has many tributaries and is commonly used as conduit for cardiac and vascular bypass surgery.*

- The small saphenous vein (SSV) begins posterior to the lateral malleolus and travels along the posterior calf often ending in the popliteal vein, (at the saphenopopliteal junction (SPJ)) though there are many terminal variations. The SSV has numerous tributaries connecting it to the GSV.
- The Giacomini vein is a continuation of the SSV above the SPJ along the back of the thigh. Termination of the Giacomini vein varies.
  - The Giacomini vein can terminate at the GSV somewhere in thigh or in the groin via the posteriomedial thigh vein.
  - Another possible course is up the back of thigh, terminating in the femoral vein or tributaries of the internal iliac vein (inferior gluteal vein).

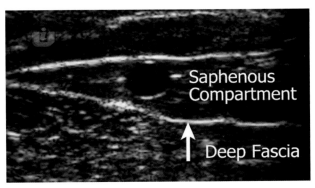

Superficial veins run within the saphenous compartment, above the deep fascia.

Lower Extremity Superficial Venous System

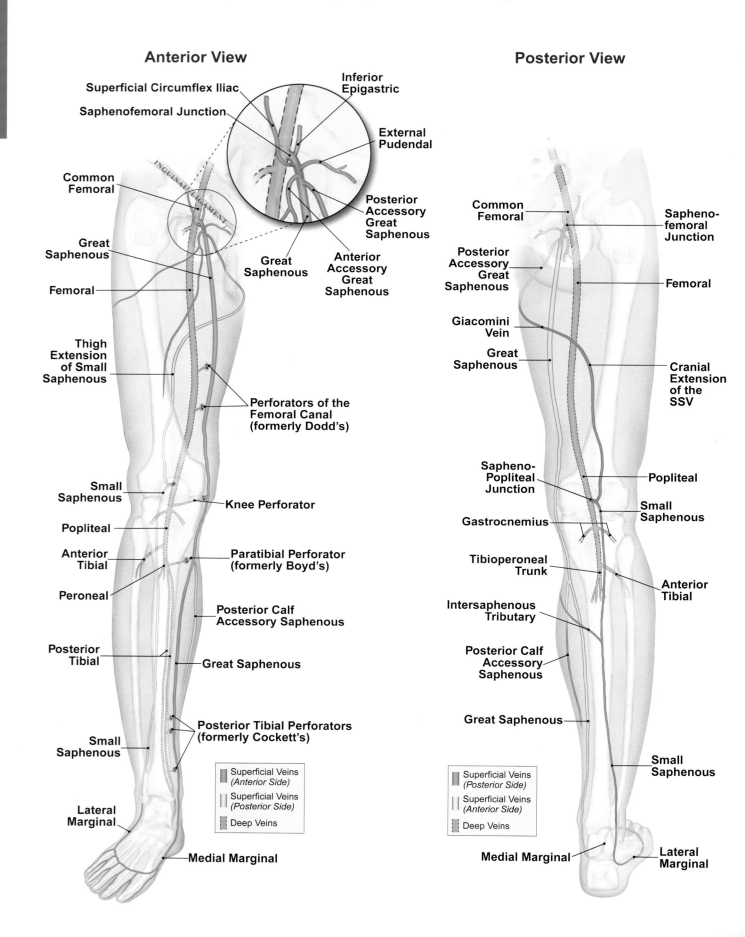

Anterior View

Superficial Circumflex Iliac

Saphenofemoral Junction

Inferior Epigastric

External Pudendal

INGUINAL LIGAMENT

Common Femoral

Great Saphenous

Posterior Accessory Great Saphenous

Great Saphenous

Anterior Accessory Great Saphenous

Femoral

Thigh Extension of Small Saphenous

Perforators of the Femoral Canal (formerly Dodd's)

Small Saphenous

Knee Perforator

Popliteal

Anterior Tibial

Paratibial Perforator (formerly Boyd's)

Peroneal

Posterior Calf Accessory Saphenous

Posterior Tibial

Great Saphenous

Posterior Tibial Perforators (formerly Cockett's)

Small Saphenous

Lateral Marginal

Medial Marginal

Superficial Veins *(Anterior Side)*
Superficial Veins *(Posterior Side)*
Deep Veins

Posterior View

Common Femoral

Sapheno-femoral Junction

Posterior Accessory Great Saphenous

Femoral

Giacomini Vein

Great Saphenous

Cranial Extension of the SSV

Sapheno-Popliteal Junction

Popliteal

Gastrocnemius

Small Saphenous

Tibioperoneal Trunk

Anterior Tibial

Intersaphenous Tributary

Posterior Calf Accessory Saphenous

Great Saphenous

Small Saphenous

Medial Marginal

Lateral Marginal

Superficial Veins *(Posterior Side)*
Superficial Veins *(Anterior Side)*
Deep Veins

Anatomy of the Saphenofemoral Junction

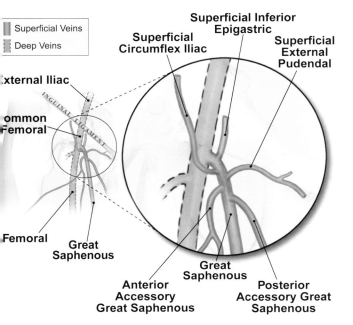

- Superficial Veins
- Deep Veins

External Iliac

Common Femoral

Femoral

Great Saphenous

Superficial Circumflex Iliac

Superficial Inferior Epigastric

Superficial External Pudendal

Anterior Accessory Great Saphenous

Great Saphenous

Posterior Accessory Great Saphenous

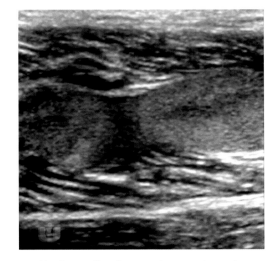

Rouleaux flow in a gastrocnemius vein.

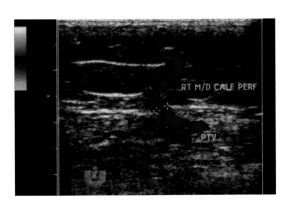

Perforator vein shown communicating with the posterior tibial vein.

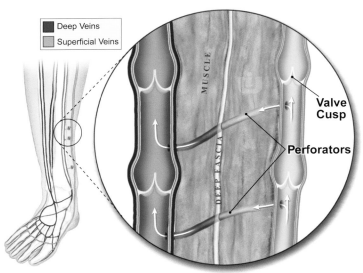

- Deep Veins
- Superficial Veins

Valve Cusp

Perforators

Perforator Venous System

Blood flows from the superficial to the deep system under normal circumstances.

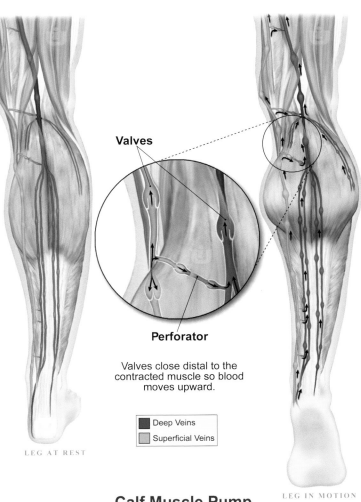

Valves

Perforator

Valves close distal to the contracted muscle so blood moves upward.

- Deep Veins
- Superficial Veins

LEG AT REST

LEG IN MOTION

Calf Muscle Pump

When the leg is in motion (walking), muscle contractions squeeze the veins, forcing blood past the open valves of the deep, superficial and perforating veins upward towards the heart. After the muscle relaxes, valves close to prevent backflow (reflux).

Venous Valves

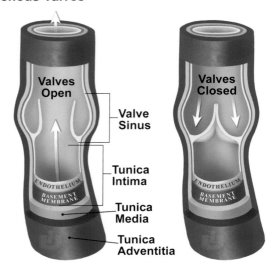

Vein wall anatomy

- The venous valves are comprised of two leaflets (bicuspid valves) that are formed from folds of the intimal lining with a layer of connective tissue.
- The venous valve sinus is wider than the vein segment above and below the valve cusps and will expand with increased pressure.

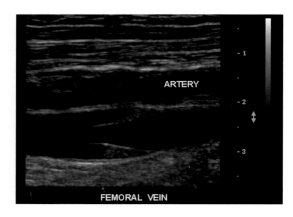

Femoral vein leaflets with cell aggregates behind valves, superficial femoral artery is above the femoral vein

Image courtesy of Philips Healthcare

Points to Remember

- The Union Internationale de Phlébologie (UIP) is a group dedicated to scientific research and the development of initiatives to improve venous practice. In recent years, the UIP published a consensus paper regrading the nomenclature of the lower extremity veins.[1]
  - The femoral vein (FV) was formerly known as the superficial femoral vein (SFV). The term "superficial" caused confusion that the SFV was not a deep vein.
  - The deep femoral vein (DFV) was formerly known as the profunda femoral vein (PFV).
  - The great saphenous vein (GSV) was formerly known as either the greater saphenous vein or the long saphenous vein.
  - The small saphenous vein (SSV) was formerly known as either the lesser saphenous vein (LSV) or the short saphenous vein.
- Compression of the left common iliac vein (CIV), by the right common iliac artery (CIA), increases the risk for deep vein thrombosis and can result in left CIV stenosis and left leg swelling.

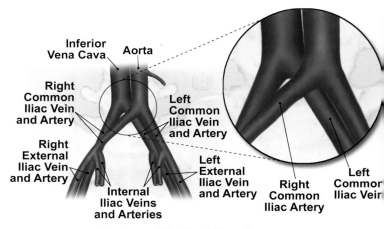

Anatomy of the iliac bifurcation

References

1. Coleridge-Smith P, Labropoulos N, Partsch H, Myers K, Nicolaides A, Cavezzi A. (2006). Duplex ultrasound investigation of the veins in chronic venous disease of the lower limbs: UIP consensus document. Part I. Basic principles. *Eur J Vasc Endovasc Surg* .31, 83–92.

2. Cavezzi A, Labropoulos N, Partsch H, Ricci S, Caggiati A, Myers K. Nicolaides A. Smith PC. (2006). Duplex ultrasound investigation of the veins in chronic venous disease of the lower limbs: UIP consensus document. Part II. Anatomy. *Eur J Vasc Endovasc Surg* 31, 288–299.

3. Gray, H. (1977). The blood-vascular system. In Pick TP & Howden R. (Eds.), *Gray's Anatomy.* (551-592). New York: Bounty Books.

4. Gray, H. (1977). The veins. In Pick TP & Howden R. (Eds.), *Gray's Anatomy.* (593-614). New York: Bounty Books.

5. Netter FH. (2003). Pelvis and perineum. In *Atlas of Human Anatomy 3rd ed.* (339-400). Terterboro. Icon Learning Systems.

6. Netter FH. (2003). Lower limb. In *Atlas of Human Anatomy 3rd ed.* (467-528). Terterboro. Icon Learning Systems.

7. Tortora, G. J., & Anagnostakos, NP. (Eds.). (1990). The cardiovascular system: vessels and routes. In *Principles of Anatomy and Physiology, 6th ed.* (605-650) New York, NY: Harper & Row Publishers.

8. Uflacker R. (1997). Veins of the abdomen and pelvis. In *Atlas of Vascular Anatomy: An Angiographic Approach.* (635-729). Baltimore: Wolters Kluwer Lippincott Williams & Wilkins.

9. Uflacker R. (1997). Veins of the lower extremity. In *Atlas of Vascular Anatomy: An Angiographic Approach.* (779-789). Baltimore: Wolters Kluwer Lippincott Williams & Wilkins.

10. Zwiebel, WJ (2005). Extremity venous anatomy, terminology, and ultrasound features of normal veins. In Zwiebel WJ, Pellerito JS. (Eds) *Introduction to Vascular Ultrasonography 5th ed.* (415-429). Philadelphia: Elsevier Saunders

Lower Extremity Arterial System

The vessel anatomy is described from the pelvis to the foot:

- The abdominal aorta bifurcates into the right and left common iliac arteries (CIA) at the level of the umbilicus.
- The common iliac arteries travel distally and bifurcate into the internal iliac artery (IIA) and external iliac artery (EIA).
- The EIA travels laterally and enters the thigh at the inguinal ligament where it becomes the common femoral artery (CFA).

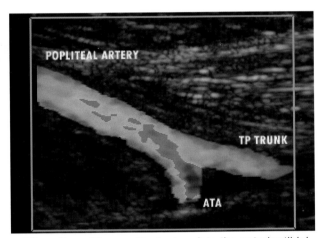

Bifurcation of the popliteal artery into the anterior tibial artery and tibioperoneal trunk

Image courtesy of Philips Healthcare

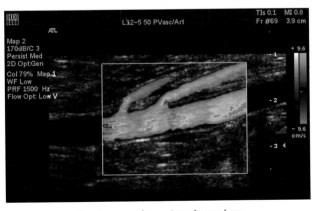

Gastrocnemius artery branches

Image courtesy of Philips Healthcare

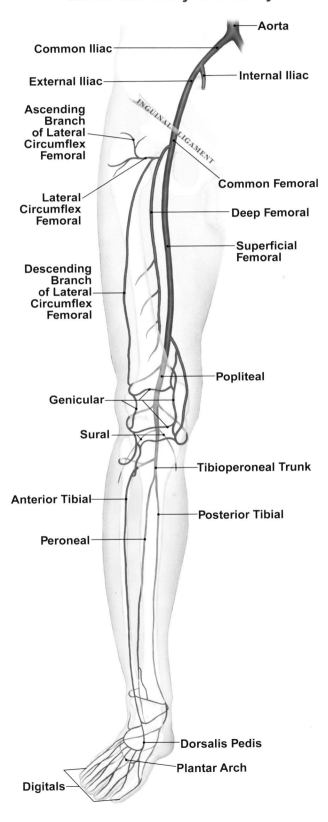

Lower Extremity Arterial System

- The CFA travels for approximately 4 cm and bifurcates into the superficial femoral artery (SFA) and the deep femoral artery (DFA). The profunda femoral artery (PFA) is an older, alternative term for the DFA.
- The DFA travels laterally and medially to supply the deep muscles of the thigh. Distal branches of the DFA communicate with popliteal artery tributaries.
- The SFA travels distally in the thigh entering the adductor canal (Hunter's Canal) then into the popliteal fossa behind the knee to become the popliteal artery (POPA).
- The POPA has numerous branches including the gastrocnemius, medial and lateral superior genicular, medial and lateral inferior genicular and middle genicular arteries.
- The POPA bifurcates into the anterior tibial artery (ATA) and the tibioperoneal trunk (TPT).
- The ATA travels anteriorly and laterally between the tibia and fibula. The vessel name changes to the dorsalis pedis artery (DPA) as it travels across the foot.
- The DPA crosses the dorsal aspect of the foot and bifurcates into the metatarsal arteries.
- The TPT bifurcates into the posterior tibial artery (PTA) and the peroneal artery (Per A).
- The PTA travels posterior to the medial malleolus and the Per A travels down the mid line of the calf.
- The PTA bifurcates into the medial plantar and lateral plantar arteries in the foot.
- The lateral plantar artery and four plantar metatarsal arteries join to form the plantar arch.
- The plantar digital arteries run along the sides of the second through fourth toes. The fifth toe receives blood on its medial side from a plantar digital branch and on its lateral side from the lateral plantar artery.
- The great toe receives blood on its medial side from the first dorsal metatarsal artery.

Lower Extremity Digital Arterial Anatomy

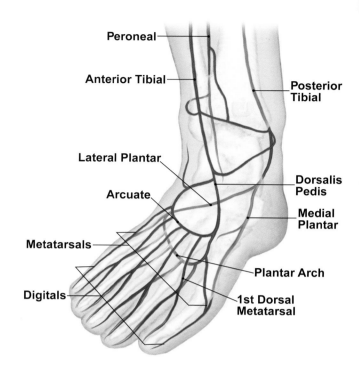

References:

1. Gray, H. (1977). The blood-vascular system. In Pick TP & Howden R. (Eds.), Gray's Anatomy (551-592). New York: Bounty Books.
2. Keck GM, Zwiebel, WJ (2005). Arterial anatomy of the extremities. In Zwiebel WJ, Pellerito JS (Eds.), *Introduction to Vascular Ultrasonography 5th ed.* (261-274). Philadelphia: Elsevier Saunders.
3. Netter FH. (2003). Lower limb. In Atlas of Human Anatomy 3rd ed. (467-528). Terterboro. Icon Learning Systems.
4. Thrush A, Hartshorne, (2005). "Duplex assessment of lower limb arterial disease" in Peripheral Vascular Ultrasound, How Why and When, 2nd ed. (112-131). Edinburgh. Elsevier Churchill Livingstone.
5. Tortora, G. J., & Anagnostakos, NP. (Eds.). (1990). The cardiovascular system: vessels and routes. In *Principles of Anatomy and Physiology*, 6th ed. (605-650) New York, NY: Harper & Row Publishers.
6. Uflacker R. (1997). Arteries of the lower extremity. In Atlas of Vascular Anatomy: An Angiographic Approach. (743-778). Baltimore: Wolters Kluwer Lippincott Williams & Wilkins.

Cross Section of Calf

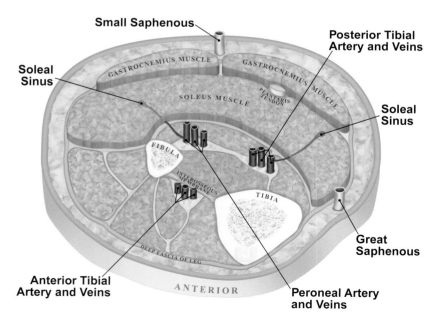

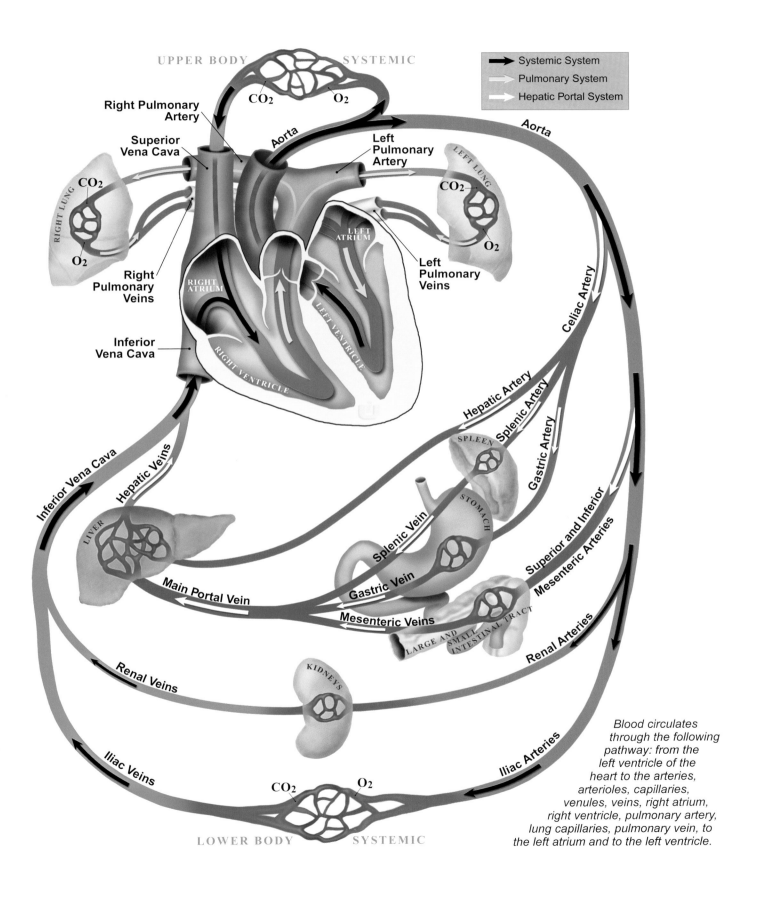

UPPER BODY SYSTEMIC

CO_2 O_2

Systemic System
Pulmonary System
Hepatic Portal System

Right Pulmonary Artery

Superior Vena Cava

Aorta

Left Pulmonary Artery

Aorta

LEFT LUNG

RIGHT LUNG

CO_2

O_2

CO_2

O_2

LEFT ATRIUM

Left Pulmonary Veins

Right Pulmonary Veins

RIGHT ATRIUM

LEFT VENTRICLE

Inferior Vena Cava

RIGHT VENTRICLE

Celiac Artery

Hepatic Artery

Splenic Artery

SPLEEN

Gastric Artery

Inferior Vena Cava

Hepatic Veins

STOMACH

LIVER

Splenic Vein

Superior and Inferior

Main Portal Vein

Gastric Vein

Mesenteric Arteries

Mesenteric Veins

LARGE AND SMALL INTESTINAL TRACT

Renal Arteries

Renal Veins

KIDNEYS

Iliac Veins

Iliac Arteries

CO_2 O_2

LOWER BODY SYSTEMIC

Blood circulates through the following pathway: from the left ventricle of the heart to the arteries, arterioles, capillaries, venules, veins, right atrium, right ventricle, pulmonary artery, lung capillaries, pulmonary vein, to the left atrium and to the left ventricle.

Blood Composition

The average human body contains approximately 5 liters of blood circulating through the body about once every minute.

> *Time in minutes for blood volume to circulate once throughout the body*
> $= (0.07 * wt\ in\ kg) / (3 * body\ surface\ area\ in\ m^2)$

Blood consists of approximately 55% plasma and 45% formed particles (hematocrit)

- *Plasma*, the liquid component of the blood:
  - Composed of a mixture of water (90%), sugar, fat, proteins, enzymes nutrients, hormones, gases and salts.
  - Transports blood cells and nutrients, waste products, antibodies, clotting proteins, hormones, and proteins.
  - Maintains the body's fluid balance.
- *Hematocrit* contains three type of blood cells: **red blood cells**, **white blood cells** and **platelets**. The hematocrit level is higher in males than females.

Red blood cells (RBC) or "erythrocytes"

- RBC's function is specifically to transport oxygen to body tissues and transfer carbon dioxide to the lungs.
- RBC's are shaped like biconcave disks with a flattened surface.
- The RBC does not contain a nucleus and can easily change its shape for passage through small capillaries.
- RBCs measure about 7μ in diameter. Since this is much smaller than the wavelength of an ultrasound beam, the RBC causes the beam to scatter in every direction, creating a very weak reflection. This reflection pattern is known as "Rayleigh scattering".[1]

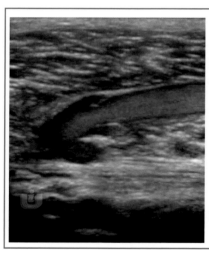

"Rouleaux flow" (moving smoke-like echoes sometimes noted within the vessel) are really red blood cells (RBCs) which aggregate to form a larger reflector so they can be seen, whereas a single RBC is too small to be seen on B-mode.

- The RBC survives 120 days on average.
- An increase or decrease in RBC size is usually characteristic of one of the many types of anemia. [2] *Anemia* is a condition when there are not enough healthy red blood cells to carry a sufficient amount of oxygen to the tissues.

- A common RBC disorder found in the African-American population is *sickle-cell anemia*. [1]
  - RBCs become malformed and elongated.
  - Clumping and thrombosis commonly occurs in branch vessels causing ischemia and infarction.
  - Stroke is a major concern and occurs in over 10% of children with homozygous sickle cell anemia (HbSS) [2].
- Blood appears red because of the large number of red blood cells, which get their color from the hemoglobin.

> *TCD studies can help identify children at higher risk for stroke.*

White blood cells or "leukocytes"[2]:

- White blood cells are the largest cells, followed by RBCs.
- Although white blood cells (WBC) are larger in size, they are fewer in number than RBCs, approximately 1% of blood.
- WBCs protect the body from infection and can move in and out of capillaries to fight disease, infections or injuries.
- The most common type of WBC is the *neutrophil*, accounting for 55 to 70% of the total white blood cell count.
- Another type of WBC:
  - Lymphocytes
    - T-lymphocytes regulate the function of other immune cells and directly attack infected cells and tumors.
    - B-lymphocytes make antibodies, that specifically target bacteria, viruses, and other foreign materials.

Platelets, also called "thrombocytes"[2]:

- Platelets are small fragments of cells.
- Platelets help the blood clotting process (coagulation) by adhering to the intimal lining of the injured vessel so that blood coagulation can begin.
- A decrease in platelets can cause extensive bleeding.
- *Thrombocytopenia* can result from a decrease in thrombocytes during heparin therapy.
- Some patients receiving heparin experience *heparin-induced thrombocytopenia* or HIT, which is a >50% drop in their baseline platelet count following administration of heparin. This is a serious complication of heparin therapy which can be limb/life-threatening. Patient symptoms range from chills, fever, chest pain to skin lesions and venous gangrene. Direct thrombin inhibitors can be used as alternative anticoagulants in such cases.
- An increase in platelets can cause unnecessary clotting, leading to stroke or heart attack. (See *Antiplatelet Therapy* in *Pharmacology* section)
- Platelets are associated with early stages of atherosclerosis. The interruption of the intima attracts platelets to the site of injury, causing potential embolic material or further obstruction of the vessel at the site. (See *Atherosclerosis* in *Mechanisms of Disease* section)

Blood Circulation [2,3]

The systems involved in blood circulation include:

- Coronary
- Systemic: blood vessels
- Pulmonary
- Hepatoportal

Coronary

The heart muscle itself is fed by the right and left coronary arteries, which arise from the aorta just outside the aortic valve. The coronary arteries supply the branches of the outer surface of the heart, the smaller arteries, capillaries and finally the coronary sinus, which is a large vein that collects deoxygenated blood from the coronary veins and feeds it into the right atrium for oxygen/carbon dioxide exchange in the lungs.

- Note that blood does not pass from the chambers of the heart to the heart muscle.
- Flow in the coronary arteries is greater during diastole because systolic contractions compress the vessels in the heart wall. Coronary flow is determined by the diastolic level of arterial pressure.
- Significant aortic regurgitation is back flow of blood through the aortic valve during ventricular diastole into the ventricle. (See *Cardiac Effects on Spectral Doppler* section).

Systemic

The heart muscle is essentially a pump that pushes blood out of the heart. Blood flows from the left ventricle to the arteries, arterioles, capillaries, venules, veins, and back to the right atrium of the heart.

- Arterioles are responsible for controlling flow and resistance in the vascular system.
- At the capillary level, oxygen is delivered to the tissues and waste materials are picked up for later discharge.
- Deoxygenated blood flow returns to the heart via the veins to the right atrium for distribution to the lungs.

Pulmonary

Blood flows from the right atrium to the right ventricle, pulmonary artery, lung capillaries, pulmonary vein and back to the left atrium.

- The right ventricle pumps blood into the pulmonary artery.
- Deoxygenated blood moves from the pulmonary artery through the pulmonary capillaries where carbon dioxide is excreted and oxygen is absorbed in the lung alveoli .
- The oxygenated blood leaves the alveoli and enters the pulmonary veins. These are the only veins in the body that contain oxygenated blood; all other veins contain deoxygenated blood.
- From the pulmonary veins, the oxygenated blood flows into the left atrium and is then pumped into the left ventricle for redistribution to the systemic circulation via the aorta.

Hepatoportal

Blood flow to the liver is unusual because it is delivered in two forms, 1) as oxygenated blood from the celiac artery and 2) as deoxygenated blood from the portal vein.

- The portal vein collects blood from the veins of the spleen, stomach, intestines, gallbladder and pancreas and actually feeds blood INTO the liver, even though it is a vein.
- Blood is cleansed in the liver before it enters the general circulation.
- Blood is drained from the liver by the hepatic veins that enter the inferior vena cava.

TABLE 1: **Average Distribution And Blood Volumes**		
Region	**Absolute Volume (ml)**	**Relative Volume (%)**
Systemic Circulation		
Aorta and Large Arteries	300	6
Small Arteries	400	8
Capillaries	300	6
Small Veins	2300	46
Large Veins	900	18
TOTAL	4200	84
Pulmonary Circulation		
Arteries	130	2.6
Capillaries	110	2.2
Veins	200	4.0
Heart (End Diastole)	360	7.2
TOTAL	800	16
Overall Volume	**5000**	**100**

Adapted from Medical Physiology, A Cellular and Molecular Approach. Boron, WF and Boulpaep, EL. Elsevier, 2005, p. 450.

Arterial Hemodynamics

Energy [3,4,5,6]

Pressure is the amount of force placed on an artery at any given point in time and is measured in millimeters of mercury (mmHg).

- For the blood to flow from the left ventricle through the entire circulatory system and back to the right atrium, there has to be a pressure gradient.
- A *pressure gradient* is a reduction in pressure from one point to the next. There must be a pressure gradient present for flow to move.
- To maintain flow in the body, if the resistance increases, the pressure gradient must increase as well.

$$Q = \frac{(P_1 - P_2)}{R}$$

Q = Flow
P$_1$ & **P$_2$** = Pressure gradient
R = Resistance

> *If the flow increases and the resistance stays the same, the gradient will increase too. If the resistance increases, the pressure gradient must increase as well to maintain flow.*

- There is an increase in the systolic pressure as the blood moves from the heart to the ankles. The diastolic pressure simultaneously decreases, so there is a decrease in the *mean* pressure from the aorta to the ankles causing the blood to flow from high pressure to low pressure
- Systolic pressure slightly increases in the distal arteries compared to the aorta due to the reflection of waves from the high resistance distal arterioles.

- Energy for flow is a combination of kinetic energy (KE) and potential energy (PE). Kinetic energy decreases as potential energy increases and vice versa.
  - **Kinetic energy** is the energy of motion and represents approximately 2% of the energy in the circulatory system. Kinetic energy occurs when blood flows and results from density and velocity squared.
  - **Potential energy** is "stored" energy and represents approximately 98% of the energy in the circulatory system. The vast majority of this stored or potential energy is in the form of pressure pushing against the arterial wall and is measured in mmHg. There are two other components to potential energy – hydrostatic pressure and gravitational potential energy.
  - **Total energy = potential energy + kinetic energy**

Flow, Pressure and Resistance [2,3,4]

Flow is the amount of a liquid moving past a point in a given amount of time, Flow units are "volume per time" e.g., pouring 5 gallons of milk down the drain in a minute (gal/min).

Pressure is the amount of force placed on an artery at any given point in time and is measured in *millimeters of mercury* (mmHg).

Resistance is a force that must be overcome for flow to occur. The relationship between these three is shown in this equation

$$Q = \frac{(P_1 - P_2)}{R}$$

Q = Flow
P = Pressure, $(P_1 - P_2)$ is also known as the pressure gradient (ΔP)
R = Resistance

- A *pressure gradient* is a change in pressure (ΔP) from point 1 to point 2. There must be a pressure gradient present for flow (Q) to occur from the left ventricle through the entire circulatory system and back to the right atrium. The pressure gradient is needed to overcome resistance to flow(R).
- In order to maintain flow in the body, if the resistance increases, the pressure gradient must increase as well or flow will decrease

Poiseuille's Law and Equation

Poiseuille's Law describes the relationship of pressure, flow, and resistance with steady flow in a straight tube. This is obviously not the case in the circulatory system where pulsatile and sometimes turbulent flow is found in curved vessels. However, the law helps us to understand the relationship between pressure and blood flow. The following is a variation of the equation discussed above:

$$Q = \frac{\Delta P}{R}$$

This equation can also be seen as $\Delta P = Q \times R$

> Flow should not be confused with velocity (speed in a particular direction).

- Resistance (R) can be further described in the following equation, using the factors that affect resistance; length, viscosity, and most importantly, radius:

$$R = \frac{8 L \eta}{\pi r^4}$$

R = Resistance
L = Length of the vessel
η = Viscosity of blood
π = pi (constant), 3.14
r^4 = radius to the 4th power

- As length or viscosity increase, so does resistance, but as radius decreases, resistance increases to the 4th power making radius the most powerful component of resistance. If a vessel size decreases, resistance increases dramatically. (See later section for more on resistance).

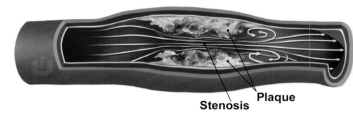

Stenosis Plaque

Flow through a stenosis: elevated flow velocities throughout narrowing followed by turbulent flow beyond plaque. Laminar flow resumes distally.

Pressure Gradients Through the Circulation

- The primary source of pressure is the systolic contraction of the heart. The contraction creates an energy gradient to move blood through the circulatory system.
- The amount of blood that leaves the heart is dependent upon the arterial pressure and peripheral resistance.
- In systole, a certain amount of blood is expelled from the left ventricle, known as "stroke volume," into the aorta. The walls of the arteries expand in response to the pressure that is placed on the artery walls from the increased blood volume and creates potential energy in the form of an expanded artery. This pressure is called the *systolic pressure*.
- As blood volume decreases in the artery during the resting phase (diastole), the artery decreases in size, pressure is reduced and blood flows on its own momentum since the heart is resting. This pressure is called the *diastolic pressure*.
- The blood flows because of a pressure gradient from the left ventricle which is typically 120 mmHg and returns to the right atrium where the typical pressure is 2–6 mmHg.
- There is an increase in the systolic pressure as the blood moves from the heart to the ankles. The diastolic pressure simultaneously decreases, resulting in a decrease in the *mean pressure* from the aorta to the ankles causing the blood to flow from high pressure to low pressure.
- Systolic pressure slightly increases in the distal arteries compared to the aorta due to the reflection of waves from the high resistance distal arterioles.

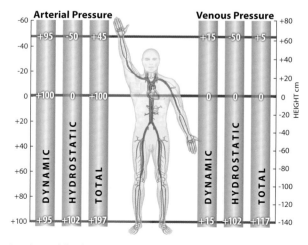

Systemic and hydrostatic pressure within the vascular system [6]

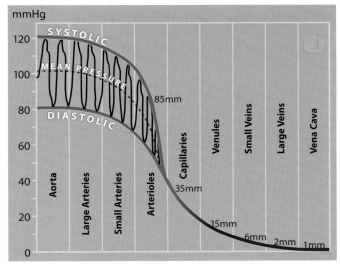

Pressure drop across different levels of the circulation

Effects of Gravity on Pressure

Other types of pressure affect blood flow in the body.

- **Hydrostatic pressure:** The force of gravity on a column of fluid. The pressure is highest in the lower portion of the body. A patient with arterial rest pain often dangle their legs over the bedside to ease their pain. This maneuver increases hydrostatic pressure and creates an increase in blood flow, which may relieve some of the discomfort. Hydrostatic pressure is also important in the venous system. (See *Venous Hemodynamics*).

> *Lower extremity arterial pressure exams are performed in the supine position to negate hydrostatic pressure, because for every 10 inches the heart is elevated above the ankle level, pressure increases 18.67 mmHg. If the supine position is not possible, place the foot on a chair to get the leg closer to the heart. The exact position of the leg should be documented for interpretation and follow up exams.*

- **Gravitational potential energy** is highest at the upper portion of the body, which is usually the right atrium. If an arm is raised above the level of the heart, hydrostatic pressure is negative in that arm. This negative pressure causes the pressure in the arteries and veins to be lower. That is why veins collapse when the arm is raised.

> *Hydrostatic pressure is highest in the lower part of the body, gravitational potential energy is highest in the upper part of the body. Usually the two pressures cancel each other out.*

Resistance to Flow [3,4,7]

- In order for blood to flow throughout the vascular system, the pressure created by the heart must overcome many forms of resistance.
- Resistance to blood flow is created by the friction of the blood against the arterial wall.
- Resistance to flow is influenced by the length of the tube, the viscosity of the fluid and the radius. Resistance increases to the 4th power, making the radius the most powerful component of resistance.

- The resistance equation relates these features:

$$R = \frac{8\,\eta\,L}{\pi\,r^4}$$

R = Resistance
η = Viscosity of blood
L = Length of the vessel
π = pi (constant), 3.14
r^4 = radius to the 4th power

- **Length**: A longer tube will cause more friction and therefore more resistance to flow than a short tube. As length increase, so does resistance.
- **Viscosity**: Resistance to flow depends on the "stickiness" of the fluid, called *viscosity*. An example of a highly viscous fluid is syrup, while water has a low viscosity. The most important factor affecting viscosity is the concentration of RBCs (hematocrit) and plasma protein. Friction is caused by the RBCs dragging against each other in the layers of flow.
- **Radius**: Resistance is highly affected by the radius of the arterioles. If a vessel size decreases, resistance increases dramatically (to the 4th power). Arterioles have sphincters, that may dilate or constrict, thus regulating the amount of flow entering the tissue. For instance, when the calf muscles are at rest the arterioles are typically constricted because little flow is needed, causing higher resistance. However, if the calf muscles are in the middle of exercise, the arterioles open to reduce resistance to flow and allow more blood to enter the muscle bringing the oxygen and nutrients needed to continue the work of exercise.
- If the resistance variables are included in the flow equation

$$Q = \frac{\Delta P}{R} \quad \text{then} \quad Q = \frac{\Delta P\,\pi\,r^4}{8\,\eta\,L}$$

So if the radius decreases and everything else stays the same, there is an decrease in flow

TABLE 2: **Flow, Pressure and Resistance Relationships**	
↑ Vessel diameter	↓ Velocity
↓ Vessel diameter	↑ Velocity
↑ Length	↑ Resistance
↓ Width	↑ Resistance
↑ Viscosity	↑ Resistance
↑ Velocity produces	↓ Pressure
↓ Velocity produces	↑ Pressure

Flow Characterization: High and Low Resistance Flow Patterns [1,2,3,4,5,6]

- Absolute measured velocities vary throughout the circulatory system, from patient to patient, and depend on the hemodynamic conditions of the patient at the time.

- Doppler derived velocity waveform patterns can give information regarding the proximal, focal, and distal conditions of flow at any given location.

- In its normal resting state, each artery has a velocity waveform pattern that is typically broadly characterized as being either high resistance or low resistance. A low resistance pattern for one artery may be normal and for another artery may be abnormal. In addition, there are many other characterizations of velocity flow patterns in disease states. Each chapter will describe these.

  - **Low Resistance** flow is characterized by a constant forward flow in systole and diastole with elevated diastolic component and can be described as a more consistent appearing waveform. The increased diastolic component indicates the vessel supplies a low resistance (highly-vascular) distal vascular bed with more constant flow.

  - Examples of low resistant vessels:

  - Internal carotid artery
  - Post-prandial mesenteric artery
  - Vertebral arteries
  - Celiac artery
  - Renal arteries
  - Hepatic artery
  - Splenic artery

  - **High Resistance** flow is characterized by a sharp upstroke, with low to no diastolic flow and can be described as having more "pulsatility" in the waveform pattern. The decreased diastolic component indicates the vessel supplies a distal bed that has higher resistance to flow since constant forward flow is not necessary (i.e., peripheral arteries, at rest).

  - Examples of high resistance vessels:

  - External carotid artery
  - Aorta
  - Pre-prandial mesenteric artery
  - Upper/Lower extremity peripheral vasculature

- 90% of total vascular resistance results from flow through the arteries and capillaries and 10% results from venous flow.

- The arterioles and capillaries are responsible for over 60% of the total resistance.

- The large and medium sized arteries are responsible for 15% of the total resistance.

- Stenoses can occur in series or parallel:

  - **Series**: multiple stenoses within the same blood vessel will increase total resistance.

  - **Parallel**: Stenoses in parallel vessels (e.g., collateral vessels) have a less profound effect on flow than those in series.

> Arteries with atherosclerotic disease usually have low resistance waveforms because the distal ischemia causes the distal arterioles to open widely, reducing the normal resistance to flow.

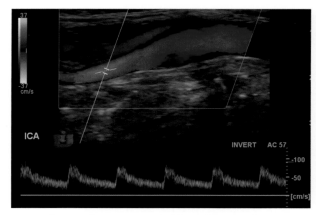

Low resistance spectral Doppler waveform

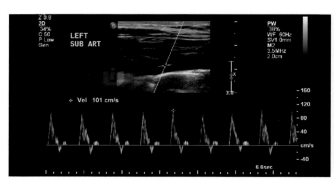

High resistance spectral Doppler waveform
Image courtesy of Philips Healthcare

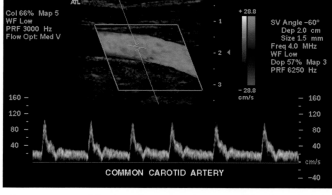

Common carotid artery demonstrates a combination of high and low resistance characteristics
Image courtesy of Philips Healthcare

Normal Velocity Changes and Flow Patterns [1,3,5,7]

Flow is related to velocity and the area of the conduit in which it flows. In order to maintain flow, as the tube size increases the velocity must decrease and if the area decreases the velocity must increase to maintain flow and the width of the vessel.

$$Q = v \times A$$

Q = flow
v = average velocity of fluid
A = area of the conduit

↑ Vessel radius	↓ Velocity
↓ Vessel radius	↑ Velocity

Laminar (Parabolic) Flow

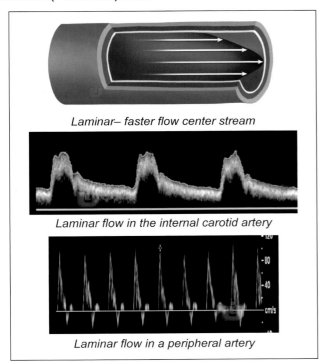

Laminar– faster flow center stream

Laminar flow in the internal carotid artery

Laminar flow in a peripheral artery

*Both spectral Doppler waveforms
are examples of laminar flow.*

- **Laminar Flow (Parabolic)** is normal flow traveling through a vessel where the slower flow can be located near the vessel wall, while the faster flow can be found in the center of the vessel.
- Laminar means "in layers" Blood layers slide smoothly over each other in concentric layers.
- Each layer travels a different velocity with the fastest in the center of the stream, creating a normal spectral Doppler with a clear spectral window.
- Laminar flow is referred to as "parabolic flow" because of the velocity profile; in the shape of a parabola.

Blunt Flow (plug flow)

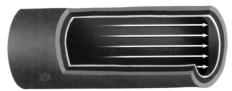

Blunt: uniform flow across vessel

- Blunt flow is also referred to as "plug flow."
- Flow travels at the same speed across a tube.
- Blunt flow occurs during systole in larger vessels, e.g., aorta.
- Blunt flow can also occur at arterial branch origins and just proximal to a stenosis.

Flow Separation. When there is a sudden widening of a tube or vessel (e.g., at carotid bulb or reopening of lumen past a stenosis), flow separation can occur. Flow separation describes the fact that the fluid layers separate to fill the newly open area, causing a reversal of the flow direction along the wall. This is considered a normal variation in flow.

Bifurcations and Branches

- **Flow at a branch.** When a branch is encountered, the layers must become disrupted at the branch point, causing a disturbed flow pattern.
- The flow patterns may differ depending on the angulation and size of the vessel. The angle and anatomy of the curves and bifurcations determine the flow changes, disturbances and loss of energy. The greater the angle, the greater the flow disturbance.
- There is a small pressure drop at bifurcations of normal vessels.
- In branching or arterial vessels with significant disease, there is usually disturbed flow.

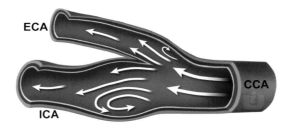

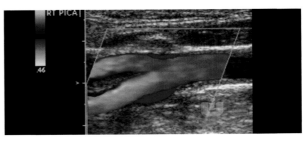

The configuration of the bifurcation determines the flow changes, vortices and stagnant flow. The reversed flow component is usually seen opposite the flow divider.

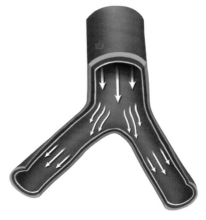

Disturbed flow occurs at branching/bifurcations and at bypass anastomotic sites. The disturbed flow can predispose the artery to new or recurrent disease.

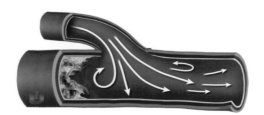

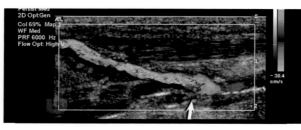

Reversed flow direction proximal to the anastomosis.

Curved Vessels

As blood flows around a curve, fluid in the center of the vessel flows outward and is replaced by the slower flow located near the arterial wall, resulting in a type of helical flow pattern.

- **Flow on a curve**: Fluids flow faster on the outside of curve and the flow pattern on the inside of the curve may appear reversed as the fluid fills the inner void from this shift outward.

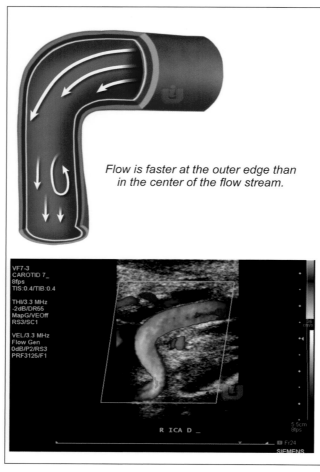

Flow is faster at the outer edge than in the center of the flow stream.

Note the brighter color on the curve of the vessel indicating faster flow.

Bernoulli Principle [1,3,4,7]

The Bernoulli Principle describes the relationship between area, velocity, and pressure at a stenosis.

Kinetic E + Potential E = Total E

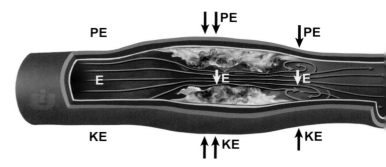

PE = potential energy
KE = kinetic energy
E = energy

- Since energy must remain the same; an increase in velocity creates a corresponding decrease of pressure energy. When fluid flows from one point to another, its total energy remains constant; assuming that flow is steady with no frictional energy losses.

- Velocity and pressure are inversely related within a stenosis.

- **Proximal to a stenosis**, the velocity and pressure are used as the baseline.

- **Within the stenosis**, the velocity is high and the pressure is low. The area becomes smaller so the velocity must increase to maintain flow. However, the pressure at this location has lowered since the total energy must remain the same.

- **Immediately distal to the stenosis**, the velocity will begin to decrease again and the pressure will rise higher than in the stenosis.

↑ Velocity	↓ Pressure at the point of stenosis
↓ Velocity	↑ Pressure distal to stenosis compared to in-stenosis value

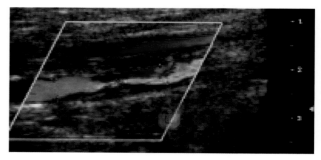

Blood flowing at a higher velocity has a higher ratio of kinetic to potential energy. Due to the resistance of the stenosis and post-stenotic turbulence, the post-stenosis potential energy and overall energy will fall.

Abnormal Flow Characteristics [1,3,4,5,6]

(See *Identifying and Analyzing Atypical Spectral Doppler Waveforms* in *Measurements* section)

Stenosis

When a stenosis occurs, the velocity of blood flow increases due to the narrowing of the tube. When the stenosis reaches 50% diameter reduction (mathematically equivalent to a 75% reduction in area) the velocity increases significantly, usually at least two times the pre-stenosis velocity.

Spectral Broadening

- Laminar flow is disrupted at the end of the tightest point of stenosis causing a broadening of the measured velocities, filling in the typical spectral "window" below the systolic peak. This is called *spectral broadening*.
- Spectral broadening indicates disrupted laminar flow.
- At this point there is often reversed flow under the systolic peak that is associated with a stenosis.

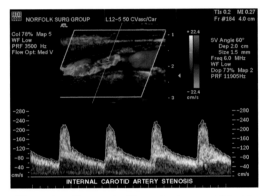

Stenosis with spectral broadening and filled in spectral window due to a stenosis or an obstruction.
Image courtesy of Philips Healthcare

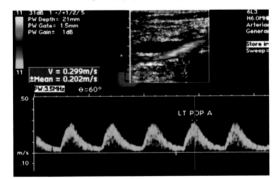

Broad peaked waveform distal to a peripheral obstruction

Turbulence

Turbulence is characterized as chaotic flow where the fluid is coming out of a tight spot into a widened area which must be filled by fluid moving in eddies and whirls of flow. This is much more chaotic than disturbed flow.

- Most energy is lost due to disturbed flow and turbulence at the entrance and exit of a stenosis.

- Turbulence can develop more readily in larger vessels with high flow.

- The turbulent velocity pattern typically has a "feathered" appearance which makes the upper border of the waveform difficult to trace, unlike the normal laminar or disturbed pattern, which is typically smooth.

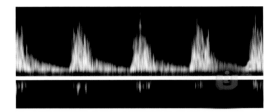

Feathered spectral waveform

- Turbulent flow is associated with spectral broadening, e.g., multiple spectral frequencies are displayed.
- Turbulence increases distal to the stenosis and is known as *post-stenotic turbulence*. In addition to the velocity increase and spectral broadening, post-stenotic turbulence is a marker of a stenosis.
- The highest velocity will be associated with the narrowest point or segment.
- The Reynolds' number predicts when turbulence will occur. The number increases as velocity increases and decreases as viscosity increases (e.g., sickle cell anemia), usually causing turbulent flow.

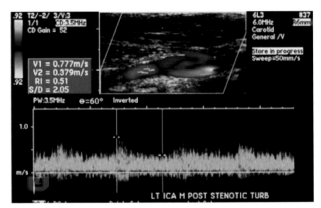

Post stenotic turbulence

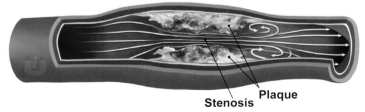

Stenosis   **Plaque**
Turbulent flow occurs beyond the stenosis. Laminar flow resumes distally.

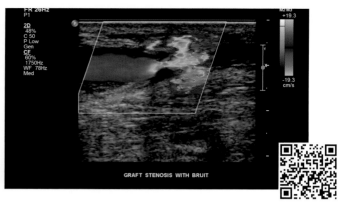

Turbulence creates a color Doppler bruit here by causing vibrations that radiate into the tissues surrounding the stenosis. Doppler picks up motion so it displays these vibrations as pulsatile color in the tissue.

Image courtesy of Philips Healthcare

Reynolds' Number (disturbed and turbulent flow) [5,8]

Reynolds' Number (Re) describes the variables in blood flow that will cause the flow to become disrupted and disturbed. Turbulence occurs when a critical Reynolds number (Re) is exceeded.

$$Re = \frac{Vq2r}{\eta}$$

Re = Reynolds's Number
V = Velocity
q = Fluid Density
r = Radius
η = Viscosity

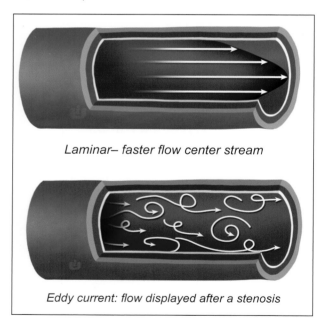

Laminar– faster flow center stream

Eddy current: flow displayed after a stenosis

Laminar flow occurs at a low Re and is characterized by smooth, constant fluid motion. Turbulent flow occurs at a high Re producing flow instabilities, e.g., flow eddies and vortices

- The Reynolds number is dimensionless.
- Re increases as velocity increases and decreases as viscosity increases (e.g., sickle cell anemia).

- Turbulence occurs when the flow velocity is so high that laminar flow is disrupted. Blood flow becomes chaotic and energy and pressure losses occur. The point where flow breaks up is defined as the *Reynolds' number*.

- Turbulence can develop more readily in larger vessels with high flow.

- Turbulence can create vessel vibrations called *bruits*.

- When the Re <2000, flow is laminar. Re between 2000-3500 usually displays *transitional flow*, or a mixture of both laminar and turbulent flow. Re >3500 creates turbulent flow. Some references refer to transitional flow as 2000-4000 and turbulence >4000.

- In the circulatory system, flow disturbances and turbulence can occur at lower Re values because of body movement, pulsatile flow, vessel diameter changes and diseased endothelium.

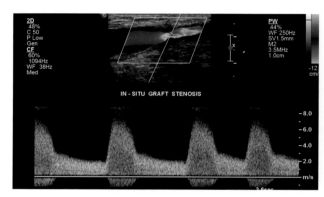

Spectral broadening in a graft stenosis. Note the reversed flow direction under the peak.

Image courtesy Philips Healthcare

Tandem Lesions

Given the effect of energy loss across a single stenosis, the occurrence of tandem lesions has an even greater loss of energy and volume. This can underestimate the degree of stenosis within the second lesion if based off of velocity criteria alone.

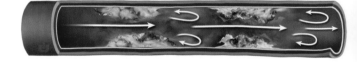

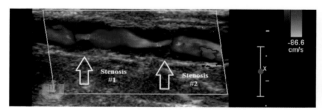

Velocities in stenosis #1 will have greater incoming energy, typically producing higher velocities than stenosis #2 which is approximately the same percent stenosis but has less energy coming in, so velocities will be lower.

Exercise [5]

Normal Response

Exercising muscles demand more blood flow due to the need for more oxygen and nutrients for the muscles to work.

- Upon exercise, arterioles normally open, decreasing resistance and increasing flow.
- Blood flow increases 3-5 times over the resting flow in normal vessels.
- Post-exercise pressures should remain the same as the pre-exercise pressures or increase slightly due to decreased peripheral resistance.

$$\text{Poiseuille's Law } (Q = \Delta P / R)$$

Abnormal Response

- When arterial obstruction is present, resting pressures are often already decreased and arterioles are frequently already dilated to maintain adequate resting flow to the tissues according to Poiseuille's Law $(Q = \Delta P / R)$.
- When obstructions are present, during exercise the body cannot reduce the resistance any further, so the pressures decrease even more to expand the pressure gradient and increase flow. This explains why a drop in post-exercise pressure is an abnormal response and indicates a significant obstruction.
- When adequate flow cannot be reached during exercise, the patient experiences pain in the muscle area.
- At times, proximal obstruction does not decrease ankle pressures at rest because it is of borderline hemodynamic significance or there is excellent compensation of flow from collaterals.
- Exercise increases blood flow, which will exaggerate a pressure gradient according to Poiseuille's Law $(Q = \Delta P / R)$ and decrease post-exercise pressures, uncovering the flow blockage unable to be appreciated at rest.

Collateral Blood Flow

- Mechanism that compensates for the hemodynamic effect of the stenosis or obstruction.
- Collateral vessels are pre-existing pathways that enlarge in the presence of stenosis or obstruction.
- Collateral formation becomes the new pathway for blood to re-route itself and perfuse the extremity in significant obstruction and are typically of lower resistance.
- The collateral takes over the supply of blood when needed during exertion and strenuous activity.
- Collateral vessels are smaller, longer and numerous compared to the native artery.
- There is very little vasodilation in response to vasodilator drugs in collateral vessels which have a relatively fixed vasomotor tone and the vessels do not respond to exercise as native arteries.

- A collateral alongside a main vessel is much like a parallel-resistor electrical circuit.
- Collateral systems have three components:
  - **Stem arteries:** large branches
  - **Mid zone:** smaller intramuscular channels
  - **Re-entry vessels:** join main artery distal to the disease.

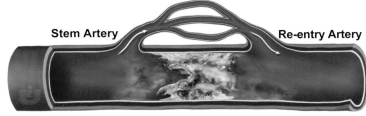

Mid Zone Collateral Arteries

Stem Artery   **Re-entry Artery**

- The total resistance in the circuit takes into account the collective resistance beds:
  - Flow, like current, always takes the path of "least resistance".
  - In a diseased patient, the flow would predominantly pass through the "lowest resistance" bed available.
  - Collaterals are generally less efficient. They would by definition be higher resistance than an efficient, non-diseased main vessel; but may be lower compared to a diseased main vessel.

> *Careful evaluation of tortuous segments and branches is extremely beneficial, as a Doppler sample taken very near or within the origin of these branches can result in increased velocities without the presence of stenosis.*

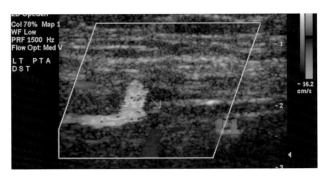

The collateral formation proximal to an occluded segment.

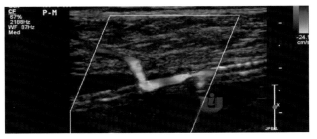

The collateral re-supplying the patent segment of the artery, also known as "re-entry artery"

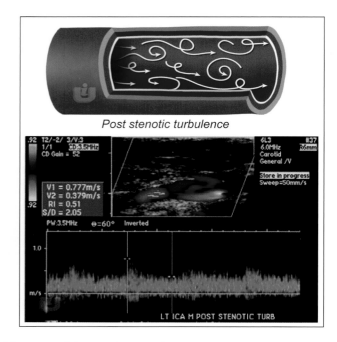

Post stenotic turbulence

Venous Hemodynamics [2,4,5,6,8,9,10]

The primary function of the venous system is to return blood back to heart from the capillaries and act as a reservoir to maintain homeostasis. Veins rely on a series of mechanisms to prevent bidirectional flow and assist in the return of the blood through the veins against gravitational force. These mechanisms include: skeletal muscle contraction, venous valves, compliance, respiratory function, pressure gradients, motor tone and cardiac function.

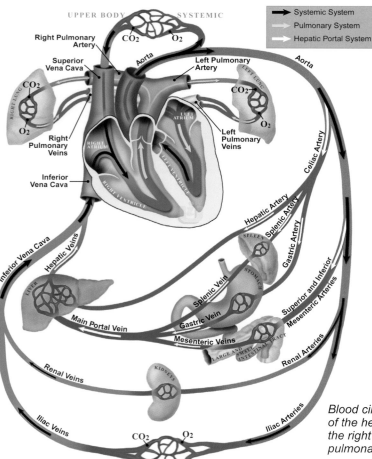

As the left ventricle contracts, it sends the blood on its way through the arteries as a high pressure, pulsatile stream. As the blood flows through the high resistance arterioles and capillaries, it loses pressure. By the time the blood leaves the capillaries and enters the venules, its pressure has been reduced to about 15 mmHg.

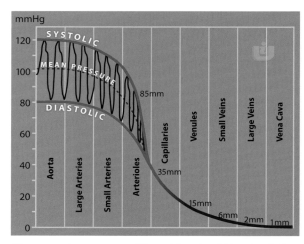

Pressure drop across different levels of the circulation

Hydrostatic Pressure

The hydrostatic pressure caused by gravity upon standing increases venous pressure which must be overcome for blood to flow in the LE veins. Other physiologic forces facilitate venous return to the heart and reduce the high venous pressure at the ankle including: respiratory changes, skeletal muscle contraction, venous valves, temperature control and motor tone.

- All fluids need a pressure gradient to flow. Since the pressure in the capillaries is about 15 mmHg and the central venous pressure in the right atrium of the heart is much lower, a pressure gradient does exist.

- However, when a person stands upright, gravity resists the flow of blood from the ankle and wrist to the heart. In fact, a 6 foot tall individual who is standing has a venous pressure of approximately 117 mmHg.

- The additional 102 mmHg pressure is called hydrostatic pressure, which is caused by the weight of the column of blood from the ankle to the heart, where the hydrostatic pressure is zero.

> *The vein wall stiffens with standing.*

- The pressure is highest in the lower portion of the body

- The further the distance from the right atrium, the greater the force of gravity.

- In an arm that is lifted, the dependent wrist is closer to the heart than the ankle, making the column shorter, and the hydrostatic pressure lower. Capillary pressure increases in the arm so vessels do not collapse.

Blood circulates through the following pathway; from the left ventricle of the heart to the arteries, arterioles, capillaries, venules, veins, to the right atrium, right ventricle, pulmonary artery, lung capillaries, pulmonary vein, back to the left atrium and to the left ventricle.

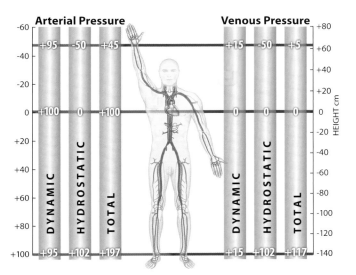

Arterial Pressure | Venous Pressure

+95	-50	+45		+15	-50	+5
+100	0	+100		0	0	0
DYNAMIC	HYDROSTATIC	TOTAL		DYNAMIC	HYDROSTATIC	TOTAL
+95	+102	+197		+15	+102	+117

Systemic and hydrostatic pressure within the vascular system

Compliance and Capacitance [5,6]

- Approximately 2/3 of systemic blood is located in the veins. The vein walls are very compliant and collapse or expand depending on the internal (intramural) and external pressures (tissue pressure) placed on the vein.
- The shape of the venous wall depends upon the pressure, volume and flow.
- This ability to collapse and expand is referred to as the *capacitance* and allows the venous system to easily adapt to variations in blood volumes. Extra fluids can be stored or adjusted to blood loss.
- This compliance allows for a large increase in venous flow without a significant increase in venous pressure. A wide range of venous volume changes can occur without changing the central venous pressure.
- Veins are less elastic than arteries, but more compliant.
- This variable amount of blood capacitance is dependent upon the position of the limb, muscle pump activity, integrity of the venous valves and blood volume.

> *Veins act similarly to a rubber band and can be stretched and collapsed in a wide range of sizes.*

- Extremes of fluid overload or severe blood loss will affect the central venous pressure.

> *Compliance decreases at higher pressures and volumes.*

- By changing the cross sectional area, the vein can change its resistance. Veins can distend 3-4 times that of the corresponding artery [2]
- The greatest resistance occurs when the vein is elliptical and the least resistance exists when the vein is distended.

Flow/Pressure/Volume Relationships

- As venous flow increases, pressure and volume decrease and as venous flow decreases, pressure and volume increase.
- The shape of the vein wall is dependant upon the pressure, volume and flow.

↑ Blood back to the heart ↓ Venous pressure ↓Blood volume

↓ Blood back to the heart ↑ Venous pressure ↑ Blood volume

Transmural Pressure

- Different pressure forces surround blood vessels. The force occurring from outside the vein is the *tissue pressure*. The force occurring within the walls of a vessel is called *intraluminal pressure*. The pressure difference between the forces pushing on the inside and outside of the vessel wall is called *transmural pressure*.
  - Low transmural pressure: as volume and pressure decrease, the vein wall collapses and becomes elliptical in shape.
  - High transmural pressure: as volume and pressure increase, the vein wall becomes circular and may even distend at higher venous pressures.

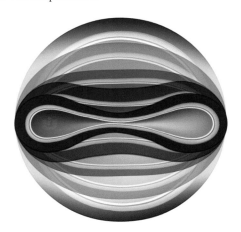

Transmural pressure (intraluminal vs. tissue pressure)

> *The more blood a vein contains, the more pressure within the vein, making the vein more circular in shape.*

- A high volume of blood may be stored in the vein with only a small change in pressure.

$$c = \frac{\Delta V}{\Delta P}$$

c = Vessel compliance

(ΔV) = Change in volume

(ΔP) = Change in pressure

Pressure While Supine [4,5,6,9]

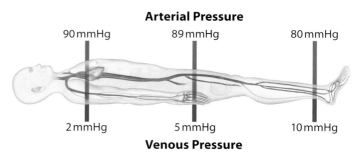

Arterial Pressure

90 mmHg   89 mmHg   80 mmHg

2 mmHg   5 mmHg   10 mmHg

Venous Pressure

*When supine the venous pressures is
approximately 10-15 mmHg*

- During inspiration, the intrathoracic cavity pressure is less than the abdominal cavity pressure; this causes the pressure gradient in the inferior vena cava. The intrathoracic pressure decreases, the intra abdominal pressure increases, blood moves from the abdomen into the chest, but the outflow from the peripheral veins stops. During inspiration, inflow is allowed from the upper extremities.

TABLE 3: **Pressure and Flow Relationships of Inspiration and Expiration**	
Inspiration	Expiration
Intrathoracic pressure decreases ↓	Intrathoracic pressure increases ↑
Diaphragm moves down ↓	Diaphragm moves up ↑
Intra abdominal pressure increases ↑	Intra abdominal pressure decreases ↓
Outflow from peripheral veins decreases ↓	Outflow from peripheral veins increases ↑

Venous Return

Respiratory function at rest

- Respiration creates large changes in intrathoracic and intra-abdominal pressures. [4]
- During inspiration, intra-abdominal pressure increases by the lowering of the diaphragm which causes the vena cava to collapse and reduces or stops the venous flow from the lower extremities.
- During expiration, intra abdominal pressure decreases by the lifting of the diaphragm, the vena cava opens and flow resumes in a phasic pattern from the lower extremities.
- During expiration there is a decrease in venous flow into the thorax.
- The presence of respiratory variation is a major indicator of normal venous flow.
- Respiratory function has a lesser effect on the upper extremity veins than the lower extremities:

- During inspiration the intra-thoracic pressure decreases, resulting in increased flow from the upper extremity veins, increasing venous flow. Sometimes we ask the patient to perform a quick sniff, which results in a drop in pressure and an increase of venous flow.
- During expiration the intra-thoracic pressure increases in the upper extremity veins decreasing venous flow.
- Augmentation is less and sometimes not seen because of the smaller vein size and lower blood volume.
- Venous flow in the upper extremities is more pulsatile because of the close proximity to the heart.
- Respiration has a small effect on venous flow when standing.

TABLE 4: **Inspiration/Expiration Changes**	
Upper Extremities	**Lower Extremities**
↑ **Increases** with Inspiration	↓ **Decreases** with Inspiration
↓ **Decreases** with Expiration	↑ **Increases** with Expiration

Skeletal Muscle Contraction [9]

- During muscle contraction, venous flow in the deep and superficial veins is toward the heart. On relaxation of the muscles, a small amount of flow occurs in the perforators, from the superficial to the deep veins.
- The foot pump (plantar pump) assists with filling the calf with venous flow.
- **Calf pump:** contraction of the gastrocnemius and soleus muscles is the most efficient of the pumps. The calf has a high capacitance and generates great pressure; about 200 mmHg during contraction, while 40-60% of the venous volume is ejected with a single contraction.
  - The calf muscles act as a venous "heart" when contracted and squeezes the calf veins, propelling the blood in the calf veins toward the heart. The venous valves are very important for the effective working of the calf muscle pump, stopping the blood from flowing toward the foot rather than the heart.
  - The calf muscle pump lowers venous pressure, reduces venous volume in the leg and facilitates venous return to the heart.
  - The thigh veins are extramuscular and the thigh pump has an ejection fraction of approximately 15%. [8]
  - Chronic venous insufficiency occurs from venous hypertension or the failure to reduce venous pressure with exercise.
  - There is abnormally high venous pressure on standing with ambulatory venous hypertension. When the calf muscle pumps the blood, it is expelled in any direction due to dysfunction of the valves. Subsequently, venous pressures do not decrease normally.[42] (See *Chronic Venous Insufficiency* in *Vascular Diseases*)

TABLE 5: Calf Muscle Pump Dynamics

High venous pressure on standing

↓

Muscles squeeze veins on walking

↓

Blood is expelled toward heart due to valve direction

↓

Venous pressure and volume are lowered in the legs

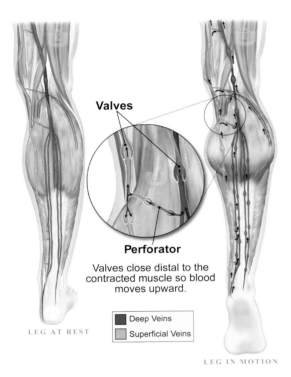

Valves

Perforator

Valves close distal to the contracted muscle so blood moves upward.

LEG AT REST

LEG IN MOTION

| Deep Veins |
| Superficial Veins |

When the leg is in motion (walking), muscle contractions squeeze the veins, forcing blood past the open valves of the deep, superficial and perforating veins upward towards the heart. After the muscle relaxes, valves close to prevent backflow (reflux).

The valves are forced open by pressure from below the valve (i.e. during walking) and are closed by pressure from above (i.e. standing or inspiration).

Venous valves

- Venous valves serve to propagate blood flow back toward the heart and prevent retrograde flow (*reflux*) back down the venous segment. [42]
- The valves are bicuspid and function to divide the column of blood into segments.
- There are more venous valves in the calf veins, which may be due to high hydrostatic pressure in the distal limb. The calf has a valve approximately every 2-5 centimeters.
- Valves in the perforating veins prevent deep to superficial venous flow.

- Valves can withstand retrograde pressures >300 mmHg.
- UE veins have fewer valves than LE veins. Gravity has a lesser effect in UE flow due to the shorter column of blood and the closer proximity to the heart.
- Valvular damage and dysfunction (*valvular incompetence*) results in venous reflux and subsequent venous hypertension. Ambulatory venous pressure (AVP) is the "gold standard" test for evaluation for efficiency of the calf pump and is performed by placing a small needle into one of the foot veins and connecting a needle to a blood pressure unit.
- Air Plethysmography (APG)® has widely replaced the AVP exam by measuring changes of the calf in response to positional changes and exercise by measuring absolute volume changes. (See *APG* section).

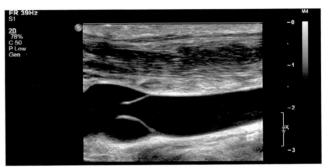

The venous valve sinus is always wider than the vein segment above and below the valve cusps, and will expand with increased pressure. Image courtesy of Philips Healthcare

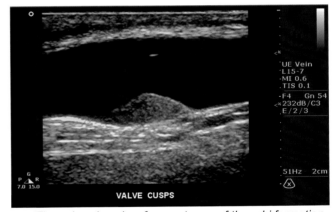

VALVE CUSPS

The valve sinus is a frequent area of thrombi formation because of stagnant venous flow. Image courtesy of Philips Healthcare

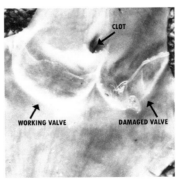

CLOT

WORKING VALVE   DAMAGED VALVE

Normal and abnormal venous valves
Image courtesy of Joseph A. Caprini, MD, Original author unknown

Vasomotor Tone

- Veins contain sympathetic-androgenic constrictor nerves, which control contraction of smooth muscle. [10]
- Vasodilatation increases venous blood volume at a lower pressure so cardiac output can be reduced. [10]
- Veins react to physical and emotional stress, creating vasoconstriction.
- Vasoconstriction increases blood flow to the heart, increasing cardiac output.

Effect Of Cardiac Contraction

- With cardiac contraction and relaxation, there is a suction effect on venous blood flow.
- Because of the strong respiratory variation in the legs, cardiac contraction does not affect the blood flow from the lower extremities.
- In the presence of congestive heart failure, central venous pressure increases creating pulsatile waveforms in the lower extremities.

Thermal Regulation

- Thermal regulation is controlled by the sympathetic nerves.
- Vasoconstriction occurs in response to cold and vasodilatation occurs in response to heat.
- Superficial veins are sensitive to cold and vasoconstriction.
- Venous blood flow in the superficial veins is slow, allowing for heat to be transferred from the body to the skin.

Normal Flow Characteristics

Phasicity with Respiration: cyclical increase and decrease in the venous Doppler waveform is directly associated with respiration and movement of the diaphragm.

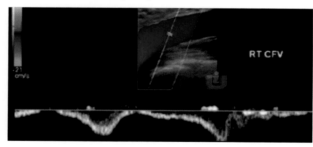

Normal spectral waveform in a common femoral vein

Distal Augmentation: Augmentation is a distinct pattern in the spectral Doppler that is produced by a sudden surge and increase in flow through the vein. The augmentation is directly related to the patency of the vein, usually when the limb veins are manually compressed distal to the probe or upon muscle contraction. Less augmentation is seen in the upper extremities.

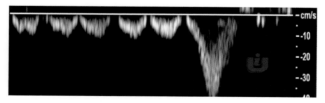

Distal compression producing augmentation

Valsalva maneuver: Proximal compression or a Valsalva maneuver demonstrates competency of the venous valves. Normal flow will stop on proximal compression of veins or a Valsalva maneuver, returning on release of the maneuver.

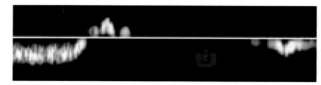

Normal venous Doppler waveform from a valsalva maneuver

Pulsatility: An expected finding in the upper extremity veins due to their central proximity to the heart.

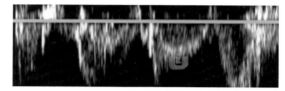

Pulsatile venous Doppler signal in the subclavian vein

Abnormal Flow Characteristics

Venous Incompetence can increase venous pressure essentially due to the lack of unidirectional flow back to the heart. While distal augmentation also helps in confirming patency of the vein of interest, this maneuver can also elicit venous incompetence and demonstrate the inability of the venous valves to function properly.

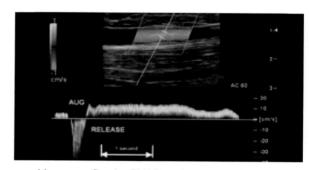

Venous reflux by PW Doppler upon release of distal compression Image courtesy of GE Healthcare

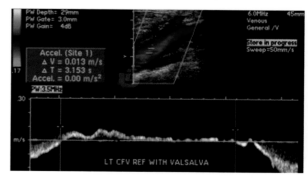

Venous reflux with a valsalva maneuver

Continuous flow takes on a steady and consistent appearance with little to no variability during normal respiration. It is suggestive of significant proximal obstruction, impeding the venous outflow causing the continuous appearance in the spectral Doppler.

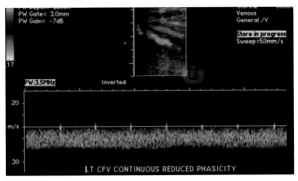

Continuous venous Doppler flow

Augmentation: reduced augmentation indicating an obstruction distal to the probe.

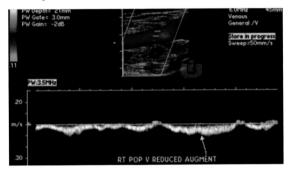

No flow augmentation (increase) with compression of the distal limb

Pulsatility: This finding is abnormal in the lower extremity veins and could be suggestive of congestive heart failure.

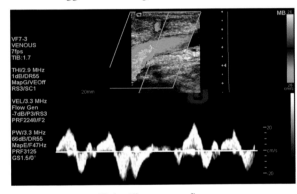

Pulsatile venous flow

Soft Tissue Edema [5,6]

- Edema is a common cause of limb swelling and is usually associated by elevated venous pressures. [5]

- Causes of edema include: congestive heart failure (CHF), tricuspid valvular disease, venous congestion, venous compression, and deep vein thrombosis (DVT).

- Venous hypertension increases pressures within the venules and capillaries. Local edema results in a decrease in fluid and protein reabsorption. Fibrinogen and red blood cells (RBC) escape into the tissues. Proteins organize and form tissue fibrosis. The RBCs break down and cause hyperpigmentation. This fibrotic, hyperpigmented condition is known as *lipodermatosclerosis*. Oxygen intake is decreased in the tissues causing tissue malnutrition/hypoxia. Ulceration may follow. [5,8,11,12]

- The swelling that results is from excessive accumulation of fluid within the tissue. Fluids are exchanged in the different compartments:
  - Intravascular compartments: contain fluid within the cardiac chambers and vascular system of the body.
  - Extravascular compartments: contains the cellular, interstitial, and lymphatic sub compartments, and cerebrospinal fluid in the central nervous system.

- Factors associated with edema include:
  - Increased capillary pressure result from gravitational forces (standing), heart failure and venous obstruction. Upon standing, capillary pressure increases due to hydrostatic pressure and the balance of re-absorption and fluid lost is compromised.

  > *The forces between the pressures are usually balanced with little fluid if remaining, being absorbed by the lymphatics.*

  - Increased capillary permeability (leaking) caused by damaged capillaries is usually associated with burns and severe inflammation.
  - Decreased plasma pressures is seen in hypoproteinemia (malnutrition).

- Elevating the legs causes a drop in hydrostatic pressure which will reduce the intracapillary pressure, thus decreasing the swelling.

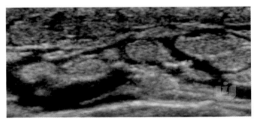

Soft tissue edema in the lower extremity

Ambulatory Venous Pressure (AVP)

Ambulatory venous pressure is the lowest pressure reached during exercise. [10] The AVP is a function of a calf muscle pump venous capacitance, amount of reflux and outflow resistance. The normal AVP equals 30 mmHg and the pressure is greater when venous reflux is present. Pressures of >40 mmHg are associated with venous ulceration. (See *APG* section)

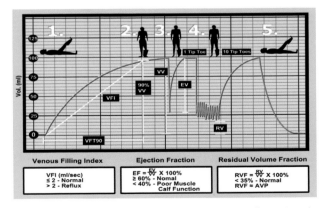

Reflux, calf muscle pump function and venous hypertension

Arteriovenous Fistula/Grafts

An Arteriovenous fistula (AVF) is a direct connection between an artery and vein. The AVF can be:

- Congenital
- Iatrogenic
- Traumatic
- Surgically created

- A surgical creation that connects a high pressure artery and a vein together so that a high flow situation is created in order to produce an access site that can be used for dialysis.
- Flow is increased in the proximal portion of the artery feeding the AVF.
- Low resistance waveforms are found in the proximal artery before the AVF.
- Increased flow velocity and volume is dependent on the size of the AVF, venous out-flow resistance, collaterals and the overall resistance of the distal peripheral bed.
- In distal arteries, the flow pattern is dependent on the fistula's resistance, proximal artery, collaterals and the distal vascular bed.
- A lower pressure is noted in the artery beyond the fistula.
- Flow beyond the connect is usually turbulent and disturbed.

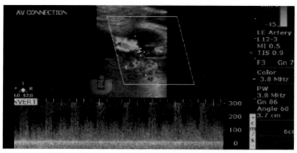

Disturbed and turbulent flow in a AVF

- Flow into the proximal venous segment is from the artery and has high pressure which jets into the low pressure vein.
- High pressure gradients increase flow volume and velocities in the vein.
- Venous pressure at and beyond the AVF site is low and has a more pulsatile waveform.

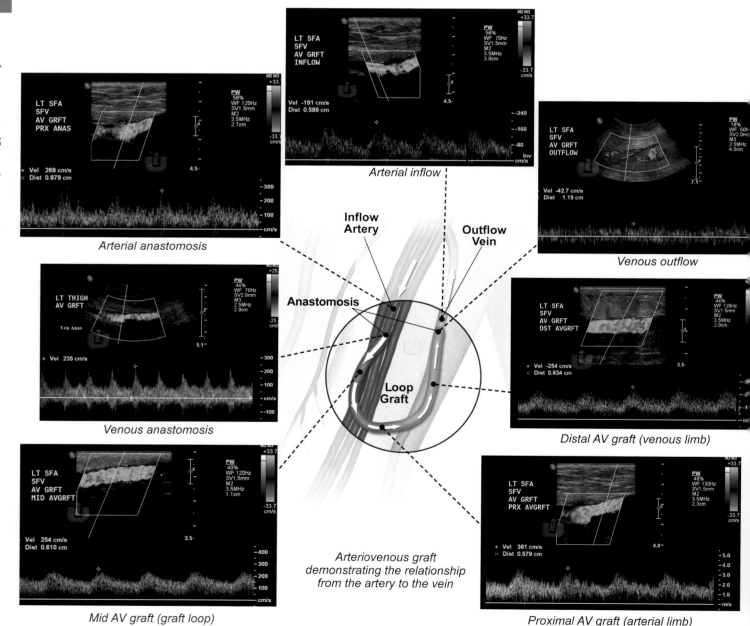

Arterial inflow

Arterial anastomosis

Venous anastomosis

Venous outflow

Distal AV graft (venous limb)

Mid AV graft (graft loop)

Arteriovenous graft demonstrating the relationship from the artery to the vein

Proximal AV graft (arterial limb)

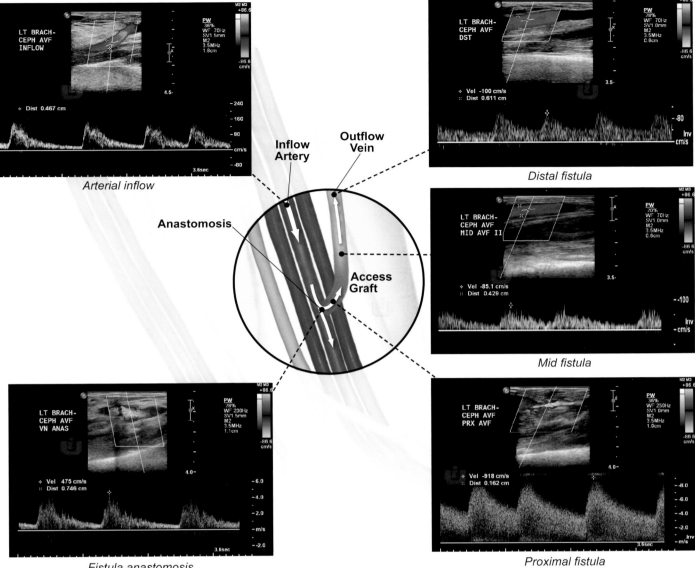

Arterial inflow

Distal fistula

Mid fistula

Fistula anastomosis

Proximal fistula

Points to Remember

- Two-thirds of the blood is within the venous system.
- As we age, the arteries becomes stiffer increasing systolic pressure.
- Circulation is controlled by the nervous system and the state of the tissue bed.
- The amount of volume moving past a point at a given time (volume per unit of time) is measured in units of flow, e.g., L/min, ml/min or cc/hour.
- Blood flow moves from one point to another in response to differences in the energy across the system. Blood will move from an area of high pressure to an area of lower pressure (energy).
- Small changes in the radius of the vessel can result in large changes in flow volume.

- During exercise, the flow increases and the pressure gradient also increases.
- After eating, the superior mesenteric artery (SMA) changes from high to a low resistance flow pattern because of the increased metabolic demand.
- Flow resistance is higher in smaller vessels.
- A longer vessel has more wall surface for flow to drag on, which can create higher resistance.
- Vein diameter varies with muscle contraction (vasomotor tone).
- The normal venous system is a compliant, low pressure, non-pulsatile flow system which is responsive to positional changes, cold, respiratory variation and muscle contraction.

References

1. Owen, C, Robers, M. Arterial Vascular Hemodynamics .Journal of Diagnostic Medical Ultrasound 23:129-140, May/June 2007.

2. M Boron,WF and Boulpaep, EL Medical Physiology, A Cellular and Molecular Approach. Elsevier, 2005.

3. Cardiovascular Physiology Concepts, Richard E. Klabunde, PhD, Lippincott, Williams and Wilkins 2011 Chapters 5,7,& 8.

4. Needham, T, Needham, A. Characteristics of Pressure and Flow in Arteries and Veins: The Application to Noninvasive Peripheral Vascular Testing. The journal for Vascular Ultrasound 35(4):229-236, 2011.

5. Sumner DS, Zierler RE. (2005). Vascular physiology: essential hemodynamic principles. In Rutherford Vascular Surgery 6th edition. Philadelphia. Elsevier Saunders.

6. Kupinski, Anne Marie (2013) In The Vascular System 1st edition (p 66, 81), Philadelphia. Wolters Kluwer/

7. Miele, FR: Ultrasound Physics and Instrumentation. 4th edition,. Forney, TX, Miele enterprises, 2006

8. Meissner MH. (2010). Chronic venous disorders. In Zierler RE (Ed.), Strandess's duplex scanning. disorders in vascular diagnosis 4th ed. (223-229). Philadelphia Wolters Kluwer Lippincott Williams & Wilkins.

9. Size, Gail, Introduction to Venous testing, Inside Ultrasound, Pearce, AZ, Inside Ultrasound 1995.

10. Gianni Belcaro, Andrew N. Nicolaides, M. Veller, A Manual of Diagnosis and Treatment W.B. Saunders, 1995.

Adventitial Cystic Disease

Presence of a cyst within the wall of the artery that extends into the arterial lumen causing focal stenosis or occlusion. Adventitial cystic disease (ACD) often occurs in the popliteal fossa.

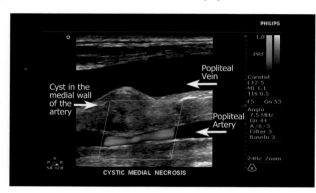

Arterial cyst narrows arterial lumen
Image courtesy of Philips Healthcare

Etiology
- Developmental
- Trauma
- Occupational arterial injury
- Unknown

Risk Factors
- Young males
- Certain occupations (involving heavy manual leg work or repetitive kneeling)

Mechanism of Disease

There are several theories on how this disease develops:[50]

- **Repetitive trauma theory**: The adventitial layer of the popliteal artery is thought to degenerate due to repetitive stretch injuries. Small tears between the adventitial and medial layers result in the formation of mucinous cyst(s) within the vessel wall. Joint capsule degeneration may also contribute to cyst development.
- **Embryonic (developmental) theory**: Cells which would normally synthesize connective tissue in the knee joint migrate into the adventitial layer of the artery during limb bud development. These cells secrete mucin which eventually forms a cyst within the vessel wall.
- **Ganglion theory**: Cysts which form due to joint capsule degeneration extend and invade the adventitia of the adjacent artery where they grow and coalesce. This theory stems from the finding that adventitial cysts closely resemble ganglion cysts in chemical composition.

Location of Disease
- Popliteal artery (most common)
- Femoral artery
- External iliac artery
- Upper extremity: ulnar, radial, brachial axillary artery (rare)[44]

Differential Diagnosis
- Atherosclerosis
- Aneurysm
- Extrinsic compression
- Deep vein thrombosis
- Venous entrapment
- Compartment syndrome
- Muscle strain/tendonitis
- Arterial embolism

Diagnostic Modalities
- Duplex ultrasonography
- CT angiography
- Arteriography

Medical Treatment
- Ultrasound guided cyst aspiration

Surgical Treatment
- Resection with vein or prosthetic bypass (end-to-end anastomosis)
- Intraoperative aspiration/evacuation
- Venous patch angioplasty

Points to Remember
- Duplex findings of ACD include: focal stenosis or occlusion of the popliteal artery and observance of compression on the arterial lumen by the cyst (Scimitar sign).[44,50]
- ACD is a rare condition. When it does occur, popliteal cystic disease is the most common type of ACD.
- Males are affected by ACD 15:1 more than females. [44]

Aneurysm

Localized dilatation of a blood vessel to at least 1.5 times the normal diameter.

Etiology
- Atherosclerosis
- Trauma
- Dissection
- Infection
- Inflammation
- Congenital abnormalities
- Connective tissue disorders (e.g., Marfan's syndrome, Ehler-Danlos syndrome)

Risk Factors
- Smoking
- Male
- Hypertension
- Age
- Atherosclerosis
- Caucasian
- Immediate relative with an abdominal aortic aneurysm (AAA) history
- Family history (other than an immediate relative)
- Dyslipidemia
- COPD

Types of Aneurysm

> *Multiple aneurysms can be present. The terms "bilobed" (two aneurysms) or "multilobed" are sometimes used for multiple dilatations in the same area.*

- **True aneurysm**: wall is made up of all arterial layers
  - **Fusiform**: shaped like a spindle
  - **Saccular**: round, berry-like or shaped like a sac
- **Pseudoaneurysm**: a hole in the arterial wall which allows blood to escape into the surrounding tissue (essentially a hematoma, in which blood continues to circulate). Because the wall of a pseudoaneurysm does not contain all three layers of a blood vessel, they are not true aneurysms. [34]

Mechanism of Disease

- Aneurysms are most commonly caused by atherosclerotic or inflammatory processes. Inflammatory aneurysms are diagnosed 5-10 years earlier than atherosclerotic. [16] Average age at diagnosis is 66 years for inflammatory and 71 years for atherosclerotic aneurysms.

- The exact cause of degenerative (atherosclerotic) aneurysms, which comprise 90-95% of aneurysms and contain atherosclerotic plaques, is unknown.

- A variant of the common degenerative (atherosclerotic) aneurysm is the inflammatory aneurysm which accounts for 5-10% of all abdominal aortic aneurysms. [16]

- Whether atherosclerosis has an active role in the formation of aneurysms, simply co-exists or if it develops as a result of aneurysms is still debated. [3] The factors that determine if a vessel will proceed towards occlusion or dilatation in the presence of atherosclerosis have yet to be identified. However, several of the processes that contribute to aneurysm formation have been identified and hypotheses for the development of this disease have been proposed.

- Aneurysms are caused by the breakdown of the vessel wall by a multifactorial process involving: connective tissue metabolism, nutrient and oxygen levels, chronic inflammation and biomechanical wall stress.
  - Connective tissue metabolism: Elastin and collagen are important structural components of the vascular wall. Elastin is a regulator of smooth muscle cell function. [9]
    - There is increased degradation of elastin and collagen in aneurysmal arteries. An increase in enzymes, such as matrix metalloproteinases (MMPs) is one cause. Inflammatory and smooth muscle cells are responsible for the increase in protease levels. [10, 11]
    - Elastin degradation plays a key role in aneurysmal dilatation whereas the degradation of collagen leads to rupture.
    - It has been suggested that the infrarenal abdominal aorta is at greater risk for aneurysm compared to the thoracic aorta because the infrarenal abdominal aorta has fewer vasa vasorum per medial lamellar unit. Vasa vasorum are the primary source of nutrients and oxygen for media smooth muscle cells. [46]
  - Reduced nutrient and oxygen levels: The thickened intima could significantly decrease the diffusion of nutrients and oxygen from the lumen to the media. This would presumably cause smooth muscle cells to become dysfunctional and a significant number to undergo *apoptosis*, programmed cell death. [2, 34]

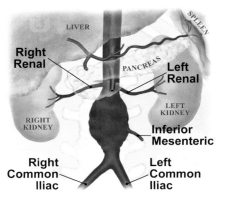

Fusiform aneurysm of the abdominal aorta

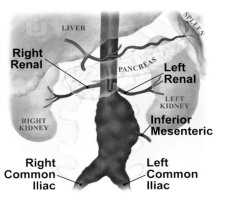

Fusiform aneurysm of the abdominal aorta with iliac artery involvement

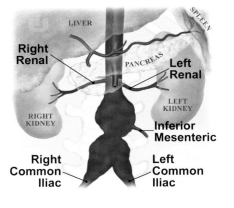

Bilobed aneurysm involving the aortoiliac arteries

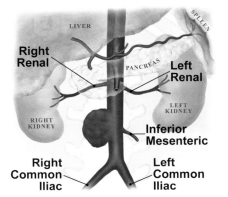

Saccular aneurysm of the infrarenal abdominal aorta

– Chronic inflammation: Aneurysms are characterized as a chronic inflammatory condition.

– There is an increase in inflammatory cells (neutrophils, macrophages and lymphocytes) especially in the media and adventitial layers of the blood vessels. [5]

– There is significant degradation and thinning of the media during the progression of aneurysms which mediate connective tissue destruction. Smooth muscle cell apoptosis increases and may be mediated by inflammatory cells which secrete death-promoting proteins in aneurysms. [7] Smooth muscle cell density is 74% less in the media of aneurysm tissue than in healthy vessels. [6]

– Biomechanical wall stress: Tangential stress is directly proportional to vessel radius and lumenal pressure, and inversely proportional to wall thickness.

– Loss of elastin and especially collagen fibers decreases the tensile strength of the arterial wall.

– The tension applied to the vessel by the luminal pressure is first resisted by elastin. As elastin breaks down the force is transferred to the collagen fibers. When the collagen fibers no longer have the strength to resist the wall tension, the vessel bursts. Large aneurysms are more likely to rupture than small aneurysms. [13, 14, 15]

- Inflammatory aneurysms are differentiated from atherosclerotic aneurysm by three gross pathological differences. [17] Inflammatory aneurysms have:

> *Hypertension: high luminal pressure correlates more with rupture than initial aneurysm formation.*

– A thickened aneurysm wall measuring approximately 0.5-3.0 cm (primarily the adventitia, but some thickening of the intima will occur).

– Perianeurysmal and retroperitoneal fibrosis.

– Extensive adhesion of adjacent abdominal organs.

- *Ehler-Danlos syndrome*-is a group of over 10 distinct diseases in which genetic mutations cause the inhibition of collagen synthesis and fiber formation, as well as a decrease in its stability. [48]

- Destruction of the arterial wall may also be caused by virulent gram-negative organisms or fungal infections resulting in atypical aneurysms. [36]

Location of Disease

- *Note*: Although aneurysmal disease can occur anywhere in the body, typical locations are:

– Infrarenal abdominal aorta (most common)

– Thoracoabdominal

– Iliac artery

– Femoral artery

– Popliteal artery

– Mesenteric artery

– Cerebral artery

– Subclavian artery

– Superficial or deep venous segments (rare)

Diagnostic Modalities

- Duplex ultrasonography
- CT angiography
- MR angiography with or without contrast

Aneurysms Identified by Duplex Ultrasound Scans

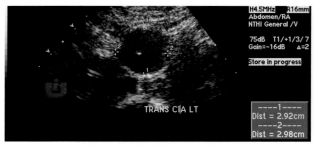

B-mode image of a common iliac artery aneurysm

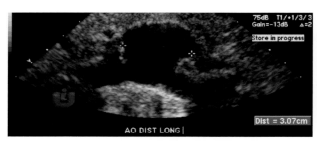

B-mode image of a saccular aneurysm off the distal aorta-longitudinal view

Saccular Aneurysm Identified by CT Angiogram

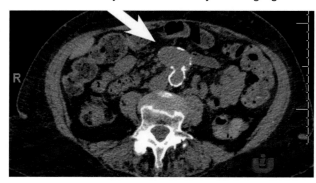

CT angiogram image of the same saccular aneurysm detected by duplex exam in previous figure

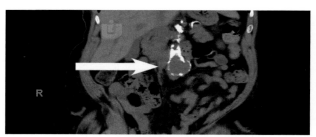

CT angiogram- coronal multiplanar reconstruction (MPR) of the saccular aneurysm in previous two figures

Points to Remember

- The aorta is considered one of the three pumps of the circulatory system (heart, calves, and aorta).

- The primary disease sites in aneurysms are the media and adventitia, whereas in occlusive atherosclerosis it is the intima.

- Incidence of AAA in the general population is 5-7%. [1]

- Family history of AAA increases risk 4-fold. The risk increases to 12-fold if an immediate family member develops an AAA. [34]

- Many AAA cases present without symptoms (asymptomatic). [34]
- The majority of AAA are degenerative (atherosclerotic) and occur below the renal arteries (infrarenal). [2, 34]
- The anterior-posterior diameter measurement taken perpendicular to the flow channel is more reliable than the transverse diameter. [12]
- The predicted expansion rate of AAA is 0.2-0.5 cm per year. [34]
- An AAA >5.5 cm in diameter is generally an indication for intervention
- Smaller aneurysms may require intervention. Rapidly expanding aneurysms in symptomatic patients is another indication for intervention.
- Rupture, regardless of aneurysm size is always an indication for intervention. [38]
- The primary complication of aneurysms is rupture. Ruptured abdominal and thoracic aortic aneurysms have mortality rates of 50 and 94%, respectively. [40]
- Predicted rates of rupture for aneurysms double for every 1 cm increase in size: 5% for 5 cm, 10% for 6 cm and 20% for 7 cm.
- 62% of individuals with a popliteal artery aneurysm will have an AAA and between 36-38% will have an iliofemoral arterial aneurysm. [41]
- Aortic and peripheral aneurysms are associated with mural thrombosis. [15]
- Patients may present with "blue toe syndrome" due to an embolization secondary to a peripheral or abdominal aortic aneurysm. [16]
- Multiple pregnancies can induce degenerative changes in specific arterial segments and increase the risk of rupture of any pre-existing visceral artery aneurysms. [44]
- The infrarenal abdominal aorta is at greater risk for an aneurysm than the thoracic aorta with an annual rupture incidence of 9.2 and 2.7 per 100,000 persons, respectively. [45]
- The "Screening Abdominal Aortic Aneurysms Very Efficiently (SAAAVE) Act" as part of the Deficit Reduction ACT (DRA) of 2005 calls for CMS to cover a one-time abdominal aortic aneurysm ultrasound screening test for men ages 65-75 with a history of smoking, and men and women ages 65-75 with a family history of AAA. Reimbursement began January 1,2007. [47]

Aortic Coarctation

A segmental narrowing of the aorta which increases blood flow resistance. This leads to hypertension and the left ventricle must pump harder to overcome this resistance and maintain adequate blood flow.

Etiology

- Congenital
- Takayasu's arteritis
- Neurofibromatosis

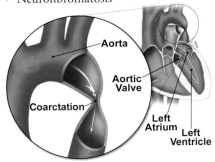

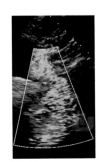

Aortic coarctation
Image courtesy of
Brad Roberts, RDCS, RCS

Risk Factors

- Hypertension
- Turner's syndrome (females)
- Heart defects
- Bicuspid aortic valve
- Ventricular septal defect
- Patent ductus arteriosus
- Valvular aortic stenosis
- Subaortic stenosis
- Family history

Mechanism of Disease

- During fetal development, the *ductus arteriosus* is a shunt between the pulmonary artery and aortic arch, allowing blood from the right ventricle to bypass the fetus' fluid-filled lungs. The ductus arteriosus functionally closes during the first three hours after birth.
- Aortic coarctations are classified based on their position relative to the ductus arteriosus and can occur preductal, postductal or at the ductus arteriosus (juxtaductal).
- Aortic coarctations are caused by congenital defect or abnormality that occurs during fetal development of the aortic arch. According to one theory, the abnormality is caused by migration of smooth muscle cells from the ductus arteriosus to the periductal aorta. There they synthesize an extensive amount of extracellular matrix narrowing the lumen. Another theory credits diminished left ventricular and aortic isthmus fetal blood flow for the development of coarctation. [75]

Location of Disease

- Thoracic aorta (most common)
- Abdominal aorta (rare; 2% of cases) [65]

Differential Diagnosis

- Takayasu's arteritis
- Neurofibromatosis
- Fibromuscular dysplasia

Diagnostic Modalities

- Electrocardiogram (EKG)
- Chest x-ray
- MRI
- Transesophageal echocardiography
- Angiography
- Cardiac catheterization

Medical Treatment

- Treatment for heart failure
- Antihypertensive medication

Surgical Treatment

- Synthetic graft insertion (Dacron)
- Dacron patch
- Bypass
- Resection of the coarctation site with end-to-end anastomosis
- Subclavian arterial flap angioplasty

Endovascular Treatment

- Angioplasty
- Stent

Points to Remember

- Symptoms vary according to the severity of the narrowing. [76]
- Aortic coarctation typically occurs with other heart defects. [76]
- Coarctation of the aorta may occur at the level of the abdominal aorta and present with symptom of claudication. [77]
- Coarctation is a part of *Shone's complex* (supravalvular mitral valve ring, parachute mitral valve, discrete subaortic stenosis, bicuspid aortic valve and coarctation). [78]

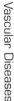

Arterial Dissection

A tear in the intimal lining of an artery, with or without outer medial wall involvement. Blood enters the media of the vessel through this tear creating a "false lumen". Simultaneously, blood is also flowing through the original or "true lumen."

The false lumen may have one or more "*fenestrations*" which are additional openings to the true lumen allowing blood to flow through the false lumen and back to the true lumen (*fenestrated dissection*).

Etiology

- Iatrogenic (caused by medical exam or treatment)
- Collagen vascular diseases (such as Marfan's and Ehlers-Danlos syndromes)
- Trauma
- Atherosclerosis
- Uncontrolled hypertension
- Fibromuscular dysplasia

Risk Factors

- Abdominal aortic aneurysm
- Age (40-70 years)
- Connective tissue disorders (e.g., Marfan's syndrome)
- Hypertension
- Smoking
- Pregnancy
- Drug abuse

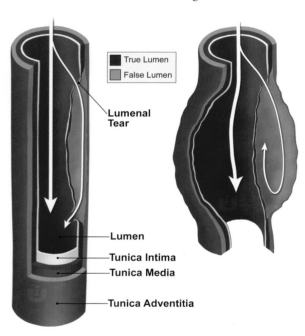

A fenestrated arterial dissection (left) and a non-fenestrated dissection within an aneurysmal artery (right)

Mechanism of Disease

- The breakdown of collagen and elastin fibers within the arterial wall (cystic medial necrosis) due to aging or connective tissue disorders, such as Marfan's syndrome causes degenerative changes, rendering the arterial wall weak and at risk for tears. [54, 56]
- Tears in the intimal layer of the arterial wall allow blood flow to access the media.
- Pulsatile flow and high blood pressure cause propagation of a dissection. [54]

- Blood flows through the tear in the intimal layer and sometimes clots.
- Dissection between the medial layers may result in a false lumen. [54] A false lumen can progressively dilate into a pseudoaneurysm. [56]
- Expansion of the false lumen that develops during dissection can narrow the carotid lumen. [57]
- Malperfusion or end organ ischemia can be caused by occlusion or transient occlusion of a branch vessel or the aortic lumen due to the motion of the dissection flap.
- Arterial dissection can result in rupture of the aorta.

Location of Disease

- Left subclavian artery (most common site for origin of aortic dissection)
- Ascending aorta or arch (2nd most common site for origin of aortic dissection)
- Extracranial carotid arteries
- Intracranial carotid arteries
- Vertebral arteries
- Renal arteries
- Brachiocephalic vessels
- Infrarenal abdominal aorta (rare)

Types of Dissection

- **"Stanford Classification"**[56]
  - **Type A**: dissections involve the area from the heart (aortic valve) up to the left subclavian artery
  - **Type B**: dissections from the left subclavian artery and beyond, not involving the ascending aorta

Differential Diagnosis

- Myocardial infarction
- Acute abdominal conditions (e.g., appendicitis, diverticulitis, pancreatitis, perforated ulcer of the stomach)
- Chronic diseases of the digestive tract
- Urinary tract infections

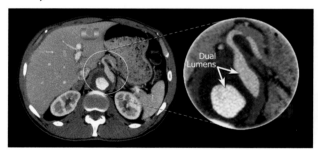

Dissecting aneurysm at the celiac axis level imaged by CT angiogram

Diagnostic Modalities

- Duplex ultrasonography
- Echocardiography
- CT angiography
- MR angiography with contrast
- Angiography
- Aortography
- Intravascular ultrasound (IVUS)

Medical Treatment

- Serial imaging exams to monitor changes

Surgical Treatment

- Resection and bypass grafting

Endovascular Treatment

- Stenting

Points to Remember

- Dissections can occur spontaneously without a clear cause. [57]
- The mortality rate of an acute aortic dissection within the first week is high when left untreated. [54]
- Carotid artery dissection is a significant cause of ischemic stroke. [57]
- Extracranial internal carotid artery (ICA) dissection is more common than intracranial ICA dissection. [58]

Atherosclerosis

Process involving accumulation of fatty substances (cholesterol, triglycerides, oxidized lipids) extracellular matrix, inflammatory cells and calcific regions in the intima of medium and large sized arteries.

- **Atheroma**: derived from the Greek word for porridge or gruel.
- **Sclerosis:** hardening

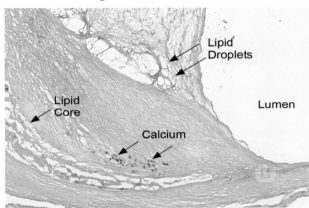

Calcium deposits develop within atherosclerotic plaques

Etiology

- Endothelial cell dysfunction
- Hemodynamic forces (oscillatory flow, turbulent flow, low shear stress)
- Inflammation

Risk Factors

- Hypertension
- Diabetes
- Hypercholesterolemia
- Smoking
- Obesity
- Physical inactivity
- Renal failure
- Genetic predisposition
- Homocystinaemia

Mechanism of Disease:
Plaque Evolution

- An artery consists of three layers: the intima, media and adventitia.

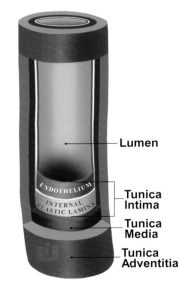

Lumen

Tunica Intima

Tunica Media

Tunica Adventitia

- The intimal layer (tunica intima) consists of a confluent monolayer of endothelial cells residing on a thin basement membrane. The endothelial cells, by their regulation of smooth muscle cells, regulate vascular tone (degree of vessel constriction) and the intima plays a role in platelet aggregation and formation of surface thrombi. [1] The intimal and medial layers are separated by a thin layer of elastic fibers known as the *internal elastic lamina.*

- The medial layer (tunica media) is composed of smooth muscle cells, surround by extracellular matrix consisting primarily of elastin, collagen and proteoglycans. The collagen and elastin fibers provide structural support for the artery. The smooth muscle cells constrict and dilate the vessel to maintain vascular tone and blood flow rates. [1, 2, 20]

- The adventitial layer (tunica adventitia) consists primarily of fibroblast cells and collagen. Vasa vasorum (small arteries, capillaries and venous channels) enter the vascular wall through the adventitia and may extend into the outer layers of the media. They are usually present in vessels with more than 29 layers of cells and lumens greater than 0.5 mm in diameter. They provide nutrients and oxygen to cells in the adventitia and outer layers of the media in large vessels, as these regions are too distant for diffusion from the luminal surface. Vasa vasorum are also present in the plaques of atherosclerotic vessels and it has been postulated that they play a role in atherogenesis. [19]

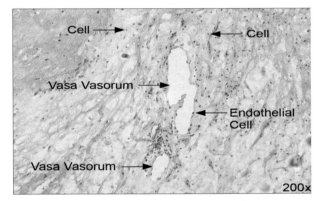

The function of the vasa vasorum is to provide nutrients and oxygen to the cells [1]

- Damage to the endothelium is caused by various risk factors such as those listed, resulting in dysfunctional endothelial cells. As a result, there is an increase in the adhesion of *monocytes* (a white blood cell) to endothelial cells, which is required for their migration across the endothelial cell barrier, into the intima and medial layers of the artery. In the medial layer and in the "neointima," which forms below the endothelial cells, the monocytes will differentiate into macrophages. [1, 20]

- Macrophages take up cholesterol and oxidized lipids that have accumulated in the vessel wall, and become macrophage foam cells. This is one of the initial microscopically detectable cellular events in the formation of lesions. Later, smooth muscle cells will also contain lipid droplets and a "fatty streak", the precursor to atherosclerotic plaque, will form. [1, 21]

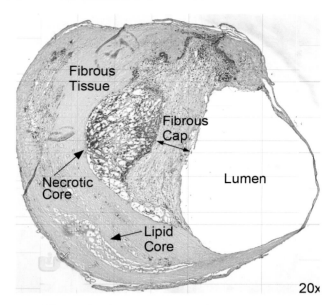

Plaque development narrows the arterial lumen

- Initially, arteries dilate and the arterial wall remodels to increase the diameter of the lumen (**Glagovian remodeling**). This is in response to an increase in wall *shear stress* (frictional force due to blood flow) acting on the endothelial cells, as the arterial lumen narrows due to plaque growth. Eventually, the artery will reach a threshold and will no longer be able to increase in lumenal diameter. Additional plaque growth will cause significant stenosis, defined as a greater than 50% reduction in lumenal area. [1, 22]

- **Early lesions**: consists of lipid-laden macrophages or "foam cells" that go from being dispersed to forming organized layers. Also present are smooth muscle cells with lipid droplets, although at a lower density and a "fatty streak" may be visible. [21] Early lesions can be reversed by exercise and risk factor modification. These lesions can also progress depending on an individual's risk factors.

- **Atheroma**: characterized by a lipid core, with displacement of smooth muscle cells and extracellular matrix by lipid particles and a proteoglycan matrix between the core and luminal surface of the intima. This is the first stage of the disease at which the lesion has the potential to become clinically significant. Ischemic events may occur as a result of the formation of fissures or tears, which expose thrombogenic surfaces to the blood.

- **Fibrous plaques** (or *fibroatheromas*): typically appear after 40 years of age. They are characterized by a lipid core that is separated from the lumenal surface by the "fibrous cap", a layer of fibrous connective tissue, consisting primarily of collagen and elastin. [1, 23]

- **Fibrous cap**: organized layers of smooth muscle cells and connective tissue fibers which provides a barrier between the necrotic core and the blood. Once the fibrous cap forms, the lesion is called a "fibroatheroma" which can project into the intima and cause lumenal reduction. Disruption of the fibrous cap can cause thrombosis, which can lead to vessel occlusion or embolization. [1]

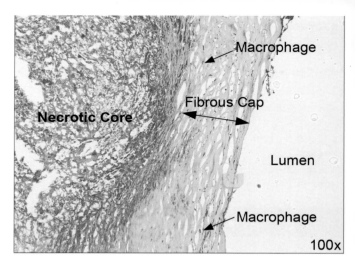

Macrophages in the fibrous cap increase the probability of plaque rupture

- **Necrotic core**: deep region of a plaque containing primarily dead, macrophage foam cells. [1]

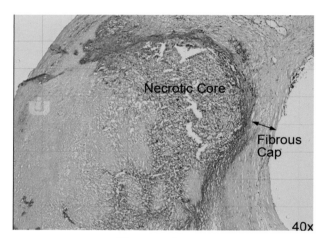

The necrotic core

- **Complicated lesions**: complex plaques that contain areas of hemorrhage, necrosis, ulceration and/or thrombosis. [33]
  - **Hemorrhage:** bleeding into or within a plaque. Occurs either due to the breakdown or tearing of the fibrous cap ("plaque hemorrhage") or the breakdown of defective microvessels within the plaque ("intraplaque hemorrhage").

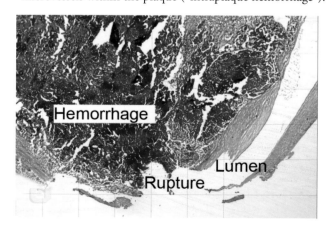

Hemorrhage within a plaque

- **Necrosis:** dead cells
- **Ulceration:** loss of the non-thrombogenic intimal surface, plus a portion of the plaque, which results in the exposure of a thrombogenic substrate and thus a risk of thrombosis.
- **Embolization/Thrombosis:** due to disruption of the fibrous cap and endothelium, plaque content are shed into the bloodstream leaving behind a thrombogenic surface. A blood clot (thrombosis) then forms on this surface.
  - After a thrombus forms, part may break off (embolus) and travel through the blood stream. This is carried distally where it may occlude an artery (embolization) resulting in an ischemic event (e.g., stroke, myocardial infarction, etc.).

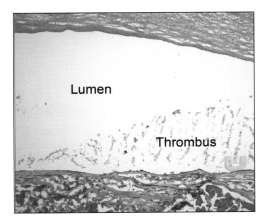

Thrombus on the surface of an ulcerated plaque

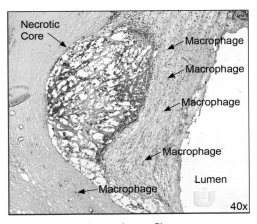

Macrophage dense fibrous cap

Location of Disease

- Disease can be focal or diffuse and affect any level or multiple levels of the vasculature.
- Atherosclerosis primarily occurs in regions where the endothelial cells are dysfunctional due to shear stress exposure. Pathological shear stresses, (low, oscillatory or turbulent) occur at the outer wall of arterial bifurcations, the inner wall of curved arteries and at the ostia.
- Typical locations for disease include:
  - Carotid arteries
  - Coronary arteries
  - Infrarenal abdominal aorta and the iliac bifurcation
  - Distal femoral/popliteal arterial segment
  - Tibial arteries

Diagnostic Modalities

- Non-invasive vascular testing, including physiological exams and duplex ultrasonography
- CT angiography
- MR angiography
- Arteriography

Please refer to individual disease/testing sections for "Differential Diagnosis, Medical, Surgical and Endovascular Treatments" on this topic.

Points to Remember

- Atherosclerosis is a type of "arteriosclerosis," though the terms are often used incorrectly and in place of each other.
- Fatty streaks can appear in infants, although many of these may regress. They will continue to form during childhood and early adulthood.

Cerebrovascular Events (Transient Ischemic Attack, Stroke)

Brain tissue damage due to disruption of blood flow.

Traditionally a cerebrovascular event is considered a transient ischemic attack (**TIA**) if the neurological deficit (motor, sensory, speech deficit, etc.) lasts less than 24 hours. However, neuroimaging informed operational definitions, which state that there should be no evidence of an acute infarction, have been proposed. [24]

Deficits lasting longer than 24 hours are considered a completed stroke (**CVA**).

Previously, an episode where symptoms lasted longer than 24 hours, but eventually completely resolved, was classified as a reversible ischemic neurological deficit (**RIND**). However, this is now considered obsolete as it was realized that events lasting between 24 hours and 7 days are associated with infarctions. [24]

The two types of stroke are *ischemic* and *hemorrhagic*: [25,26]

- **Ischemic stroke** (most common, approximately 85% of all strokes): due to a decrease in blood flow to the brain caused by an arterial narrowing or blockage. The five widely accepted sub classifications of ischemic stroke based on etiology are:
  - **Cardioembolic (embolic):** an embolus from a cardiac or pericardiac source causes a territorial infarction. Most common cause is atrial fibrillation, where there is pooling of the blood in the heart which can lead to the formation of blood clots. *Note: Some classifications will include emboli that originate from peripheral arteries, (such as the carotid arteries) under this sub-category and then use the term embolic stroke for this sub-classification. Others will place them under the classification large vessel atherosclerosis.*
  - **Large vessel atherosclerosis:** (atherothrombotic), Occlusion or stenosis greater than 50% of the major intra- and extracranial arteries supplying the vascular territory of the stroke (internal carotid, common carotid, vertebral, basilar, middle cerebral, anterior cerebral or posterior cerebral). Decrease in lumen area due to atherosclerosis and/or thrombosis.

- **Lacunar:** (Small vessel disease) account for approximately 25% of all acute ischemic strokes. [25, 26] Lacunar infarcts are small infarcts (3 - 20 mm in diameter) in the deeper noncortical parts of the cerebrum and brainstem. They result from occlusion or stenosis of penetrating branches of the large cerebral arteries.

- **Stroke of other determined etiology:** these rare cases normally occur in the young who have no stroke risk factors. They include coagulopathies, vasculopathies, genetic disorders and metabolic disorders.

- **Stroke of undetermined etiology**: in a significant number of cases (≤40%), no clear explanation can be found for an ischemic stroke despite an extensive diagnostic evaluation.

- **Hemorrhagic stroke:** (approximately 15% of all strokes) due to arterial rupture or venous malformation in the brain. Blood accumulates and compresses the surrounding brain tissue. In addition there is no or little blood flow distal to the rupture site. Hemorrhagic strokes are classified as either subarachnoid hemorrhage or intracerebral hemorrhage.

  - **Subarachnoid hemorrhage:** most commonly due to trauma, but also occur due to rupture of a cerebral aneurysm. In 10-20% of spontaneous, nontraumatic cases, no cause is found.

  - **Intracerebral hemorrhage:** (*parenchymatous*) Rupture of a blood vessel within the parenchyma, often the result of chronic hypertension or an intrinsic vessel problem such as amyloid angiopathy or other vascular malformation. May also be caused by a brain tumor.

- An enormous amount of research is conducted on what makes a plaque vulnerable to rupture or stable and how to identify these plaques, as a plaque's vulnerability is a major determinant in whether or not it should be removed. There are many theories on what makes a plaque vulnerable to rupture and thus likely to cause a TIA or stroke. Both the plaque's hemodynamic environment and composition need to be considered. Considerations include:

  - **Active plaques:** plaques with a large number of macrophages. Their presence is thought to increase the likelihood of plaque rupture as they degrade the fibers in the extracellular matrix decreasing the structural integrity of the plaque, increasing its susceptibility to rupture. The destruction caused by macrophages in the fibrous cap is especially harmful, as it increases the risk of plaque rupture the most.

  - **Fibrous cap thickness:** the thinner the fibrous cap, the more vulnerable the plaque. The thicker the cap, the more stable the plaque is thought to be. Smooth muscle cells are important for the maintenance of fibrous caps as they synthesize collagen and elastin. Macrophages are detrimental to fibrous caps as they secrete enzymes, such as metallomatrix proteases which degrade the fibrous cap.

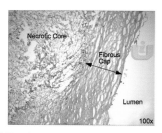 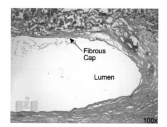

Histological images of a thick (right) and thin (left) fibrous cap.

  - **Calcium:** its effect depends upon size, location and type of artery. In carotid arteries calcium is believed to stabilize the plaque, with stability increasing as the percentage of calcium increases. The effect of calcium in coronary arteries is debated with many studies showing a negative effect on plaque stability. Micro-deposits of calcium near the surface of the plaque have been suggested to increase the vulnerability of plaques. Calcium is used as an indication of plaque stability clinically as it can be detected by both ultrasound and CT angiography.

Etiology

- Atherosclerosis
- Embolism
- Thrombus
- Fibromuscular dysplasia
- Arterial kinking
- Arterial dissection
- Traumatic occlusion
- Extrinsic compression
- Radiation-therapy induced carotid stenosis

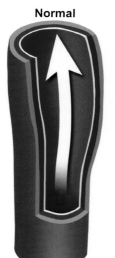 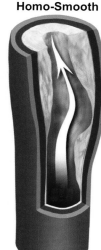 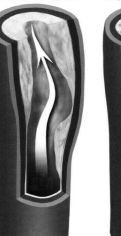 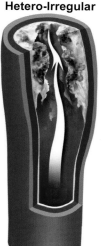 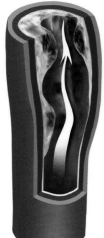 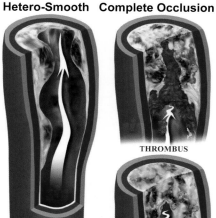 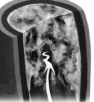

Normal **Homo-Irregular** **Homo-Smooth** **Hetero-Irregular** **Hetero-Smooth** **Complete Occlusion**

THROMBUS

ATHEROSCLEROTIC

Presentations of atherosclerosis within an artery

Risk Factors

- Age
- Hypertension
- Smoking
- Hypercholesteremia
- Diabetes
- Obesity
- Hypercoaguable state
- Cardiac disease (e.g., arrhythmia, heart failure, infection)
- Patent foramen ovale
- Mechanical heart valve
- Family history
- Sedentary lifestyle
- Previous TIA or stroke
- Radiation-therapy
- Hormone therapy or use of birth control pills
- Alcohol abuse

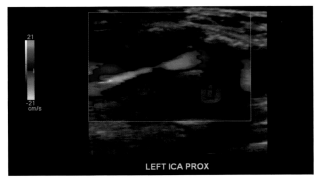

Duplex scan of a symptomatic ICA stenosis (50-79%)

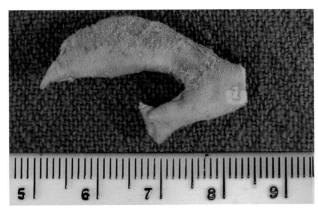

Atherosclerotic plaque removed from the carotid arteries using the semi-eversion method

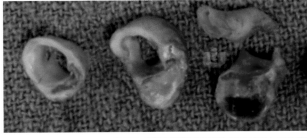

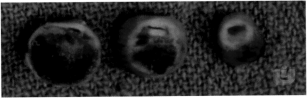

Sectioned atherosclerotic carotid plaque (same plaque shown above intact).

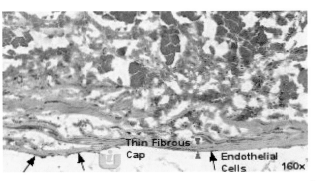

Histological image of a thin fibrous cap (between red arrows).

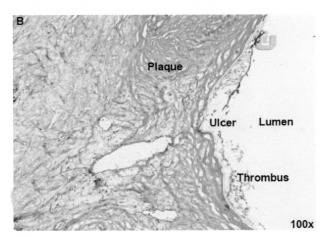

Plaque ulceration

Mechanisms of Disease

Ischemic infarcts

Ischemic infarcts can be separated into three categories based on their pathophysiological mechanism: lacunar, territorial and border zone.

- **Lacunar strokes:** are caused by the occlusion of a single small perforating cerebral artery.
  - Due to the stenosis or occlusion of the penetrating arteries of the middle cerebral artery, anterior choroidal artery, anterior cerebral artery, posterior cerebral artery, posterior communicating artery, basilar artery, vertebral artery and the cerebellar arteries. Lacunar strokes result in small infarcts, 3-20 mm in diameter in the putamen, caudate, thalamus, pons, internal capsule, and convolutional white matter.
  - Occlusion is most commonly due to a microatheroma, with or without a superimposed thrombus in an artery that ranges from 400-900 µm in diameter resulting in infarcts 5 mm in diameter or larger.
  - Small lacunar infarcts, 2-5 mm in diameter are usually the result of occlusion by *lipohyalinosis* (small vessel disease in the brain). This is a hypertensive vasculopathy in which the lumen of arteries 40-200 µm in diameter are occluded. There is a loss of normal arterial architecture and the presence of macrophage foam cells.
  - Rarely will lacunar infarcts be caused by emboli from the heart or atherosclerotic lesions in the carotid artery or aortic arch.
  - Lacunar infarcts 3 mm or less in diameter are usually asymptomatic. Larger lacunar infarcts are normally symptomatic.

– Although it is debatable, there is evidence linking hypertension and diabetes with lacunar infarctions, especially with those caused by lipohyalinosis.

– The mechanisms described above for lacunar stroke has become known as the "lacunar hypothesis". Currently, this hypothesis is debated. The lacunar hypothesis was formed when hypertension was not as well controlled as it its today. Later studies have suggested that a significant number of lacunar infarcts occur in the absence of hypertension or diabetes. It has been proposed that emboli (cardiac or arterial origin) may be a major cause of these lacunar infarcts.

- **Territorial or embolic infarcts** are most frequently due to an embolus, which originates from a proximal thrombus and occludes a cerebral vessel. The embolus circulates through the vasculature until the vessel becomes too narrow for its passage. It occludes the artery, which blocks blood flow causing ischemia leading to infarction. Territorial infarcts are restricted to territories supplied by major intracerebral arteries, their branches or pial arteries.

– If the embolus originates from the heart it is classified as a *cardioembolic infarction*. However, they may originate elsewhere, particularly the carotid arteries.

- **Border zone infarcts** (*watershed infarcts*) 10% of all cerebral infarcts [27] occur in an area between two "neighboring" vascular territories (distal fields of two non-anastomizing arterial systems).[28, 29] The two subtypes, based on location are cortical (external) border zones (**cortical watershed areas**) or subcortical (internal) border zones (**internal watershed areas**).

– Cortical watershed areas are located between:

– Anterior and middle cerebral arteries

– Posterior and middle cerebral arteries.

– Internal watershed areas are located between:

– Lenticulostriate and middle cerebral arteries

– Lenticulostriate and anterior cerebral arteries

– Heubner and anterior cerebral arteries

– Anterior chorodial and middle cerebral arteries

– Anterior choroidal and posterior cerebral arteries

– The pathophysiology of these infarcts is still unclear and debated.

– The classical theory states that a change in hemodynamics, caused by repeated systemic hypotension in conjunction with occlusion or severe arterial stenosis, primarily of the internal carotid artery, leads to infarction. Hypotension causes a decrease in perfusion pressure, which significantly decreases blood flow within the border zones. Since border zone perfusion pressures are already low at the distal ends of the arterial tree, these areas are highly susceptible to ischemia and infarcts during repeated episodes of hypotension.

– A recent hypothesis states that microemboli (50-300μm), which may originate from the heart or carotid arteries, occlude the terminal vascular field causing border zone infarcts, rather than the slowing of the cerebral blood flow. This is observed primarily in cortical border zone infarcts that occur in the absence of subcortical border zone infarcts. Since microemboli are small, they tend to circulate to cortical border zones, where the low perfusion rate limits their wash out. Isolated cortical border infarcts have occurred without hemodynamic compromise.

– Another hypothesis combines the previous two; microemboli and hypoperfusion together have a greater chance of causing border zone infarcts since the microemboli would be more likely to cause micro-infarcts in the presence of chronic hypoperfusion. The hypoperfusion would reduce the clearance of the microemboli and the microemboli, due to their blockage of the vessels, would increase the local hypoperfusion.

Carotid Artery Stenosis Mechanisms

- **Atherosclerosis** [1] is the most common arterial disease. Atherosclerotic plaque forms in the arterial wall and decreases or stops blood flow by either narrowing the lumen (*arterial stenosis*) or completely blocking the artery (*arterial occlusion*). The term "*hemodynamically significant obstruction*" refers to either a stenosis or an occlusion that results in a significant decrease in blood pressure or flow distal to the obstruction. A stenosis is considered clinically significant, with measurable decreases in pressure and flow velocities distally, when the area is decreased 50% or more. An arterial occlusion is typically seen from one major branch to the next.

- **Kinks**: Blood flow is compromised in kinked arteries and kinks are often associated with plaque and arterial stenosis. Congenital kinks are a result of faulty descent of the vessels during embryonic development. Kinks can be acquired with age; arteries can elongate and at the same time, the medial layer degenerates. [57]

- **Fibromuscular dysplasia** (FMD): The internal carotid is a long segment artery without branches that lacks vasa vasorum (which supplies nutrients and oxygen to vessel walls) typically found at branch points. Arterial wall ischemia may result, which is one theory for the development of FMD. [113] This long arterial segment is also thought to be subject to unique mechanical forces (greater axial stress).

Location of Disease

- Brain tissue
- Contributing atherosclerotic or emboli origination sites, include:

– Intracranial vessels

– Proximal internal carotid artery (ICA)

– Origin of the vertebral artery

– Basilar artery

– Middle cerebral artery

– Anterior or posterior cerebral arteries

– Aortic arch

– Heart

Differential Diagnosis for CVA/TIA

- Vasculitis (e.g. arteritis)
- Fibromuscular dysplasia
- Moyamoya disease
- Cerebral hemorrhage
- Carotid artery dissection
- Seizure
- Lupus
- Metabolic problems (e.g., glucose derangement)
- Migraines
- Cardiac embolization
- Nonatherosclerotic vasculopathy
- Systemic infections
- Mass lesions
- Intracranial tumor
- Primary central nervous system (CNS)
- Metastatic
- Subdural hematoma
- Cerebral abscess
- Multiple sclerosis
- Alcohol or drug abuse
- Cardiac failure
- Syncope
- Positional vertigo

Diagnostic Modalities

- Duplex ultrasonography
- TEE (transesophageal echocardiography)
- CT angiography
- Brain CT
- MR angiography
- MRI
- Cerebral angiography

Medical Treatment

- Modify risk factors (e.g., smoking cessation, lower cholesterol, etc.)
- Statin therapy
- Antithrombotics
- Tissue plasminogen activator (TPA) therapy: to treat ischemic stroke, within three hours of onset of symptoms
- Intra-arterial thrombolysis - within six hours of onset of symptoms

Surgical Treatment

- Carotid endarterectomy
- ICA resection and reanastomosis (for kinking)
- Carotid thrombectomy
- Bypass (subclavian-carotid or carotid-carotid)
- Vertebral artery transposition (to CCA)
- Vertebral artery reconstruction

Endovascular Treatment

- Carotid angioplasty and stenting

Points to Remember

- Approximately 795,000 cases of new or recurrent stroke occur each year. About 610,000 of these are new events, while 185,000 are recurrent attacks. [114]
- NASCET (North American Symptomatic Carotid Endarterectomy Trial) demonstrated that the long term benefit of carotid endarterectomy was significantly greater than medical treatment in symptomatic patients with >70% stenosis. [90] ACAS (Asymptomatic Carotid Atherosclerosis Study) demonstrated marginal benefit of carotid endarterectomy in asymptomatic male patients with >60% stenosis. [116]
- For occluded ICAs it is important to clearly demonstrate that there is no "trickle" flow present during the duplex scan since carotid endarterectomy is not usually performed on completely occluded ICAs.

- The ICA may be coiled or tortuous; creating an "S" or "C" shape or it can be elongated or curved. Either may produce a bruit. Double, complete loops have also been reported. The patient is usually asymptomatic. [57]
- The ICA may be "kinked," which is a sharp angulation of the vessel, usually resulting in stenosis. The kink is typically located 2-3 cm from the bifurcation. These patients may present with cerebrovascular symptoms.
- Carotid artery kinks occur four times more often in women than men. [57]

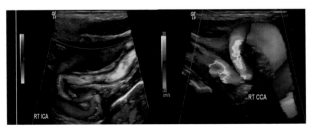

*Duplex image of a tortuous artery-ICA (left)
and kinked artery-CCA (right)*

Images courtesy of Patrick Washko, BS RT RDMS RVT

- The mechanisms leading to cortical and subcortical infarcts are likely to be different. Subcortical infarcts have a strong hemodynamic mechanism. Micro-emboli may have more of a causal relationship with isolated cortical border zone infarcts than hemodynamic compromise (low flow). Cortical infarcts in the presence of subcortical infarcts appear to be a result of hemodynamic compromise. [28]
- The prognosis for patients with subcortical infarcts is poor with increased risk for morbidity and a future stroke compared to patients with cortical infarcts. [28]
- Systemic reasons for low flow states include: hypotension, arrhythmia, heart failure, anemia or pacemaker malfunction.
- Dementia and cognitive decline are associated with silent lacunar infarcts, infarcts that are not associated with obvious acute clinical stroke symptoms. [30]
- Treatments for ischemic and hemorrhagic strokes are very different. [31,32]

Carotid Body Tumor

A highly vascularized tumor of the carotid body. The carotid body is a chemoreceptive organ located in the adventitia of the common carotid artery at the bifurcation.

The carotid body normally measures 5 x 3 x 2 mm in size. [57]

Within the carotid body are the peripheral arterial chemoreceptors that sense arterial partial pressures of oxygen and carbon dioxide as well as blood pH. Through the release of neurotransmitters they are primarily responsible for hyperventilation during hypoxia and contribute significantly to the hyperventilation associated with respiratory or metabolic acidosis.

The tumor can widen the bifurcation by separating the internal and external carotid arteries.

- Types (Shamblin classification)
  - **Group 1:** small tumors, minimally attached to the carotid vessels.
  - **Group 2:** moderately-sized tumors, partially encircling the carotid vessels.
  - **Group 3:** large tumors which encase both carotid arteries and the vagus nerve.

Etiology

- Genetic mutations: approximately 10-30% of carotid body tumors (CBTs) are inherited. [58]
- Sporadic etiology: (70-90% of cases) not predisposed to CBT formation by an inherited genetic mutation.
- Environmental factors

Risk Factors

- Middle age (occurring during the 5th decade of life on average)
- Female (more common)
- Individuals born/living at high altitudes [58]

Mechanism of Disease

- The carotid body is a parasympathetic, extra-adrenal paraganglion, which is a neuroendocrine organ. [60] Parasympathetic paraganglia are clusters of two cell types, chemoreceptive cells (type I cells, chief cells) and supporting cells (type II cells, sustentacular cells) that arise embryologically from neural crest cells. The chemoreceptive cells form nests. Each nest is surrounded by supporting cells and an extensive capillary network making CBTs highly vascularized. [58] CBTs are driven by genetically mutated chemoreceptive cells.

- Inherited CBTs result from a genetic mutation from one generation to the next. Inherited CBTs follow the "two-hit model", first was the inherited genetic mutation in one of the alleles and second hit was the mutation that the second allele acquired in the somatic cell. [58]

- Hereditary CBTs are caused by mutations in the genes encoding subunits and related proteins of the mitochondria enzyme complex *succinate dehydrogenase* (SDH). [61, 62, 63, 64]

  - SDH, also known as complex II, is a component of the Krebs cycle as well as the mitochondrial electron transport chain.

  - Only offspring who inherit a mutated SDHD gene from their father are predisposed to CBTs. Tissue specific epigenetic methylation causes maternal genomic imprinting (suppression) of SDHD alleles in certain tissues. [65] Thus, the expression of mutated SDHD genes is suppressed when they are inherited from the mother. No CBTs have been histopathologically proven in offspring who inherited SDHD mutations from their mother. [66] This results in CBTs skipping a generation making it difficult to assess familial history. The mutated gene continues to be passed down through the generations and when a child inherits it from their father they are genetically predisposed to develop CBTs. Maternal genomic imprinting also occurs for the SDHAF2 gene. [64, 67]

- In paternal SDHD hereditary cases of CBT, there is a mutation in the germline cells, which results in the somatic cells being heterozygous (paternal allele is inactive but the maternal allele is active) for SDHD. In the tumor, cells there is a loss of heterozygosity (the maternal allele is completely lost). [61] The germline loss of function mutation in the paternal allele combined with the loss of the maternal allele in the tumor cells classifies SDHD as a tumor suppressor gene. Furthermore it shows that SDHD needs *two-hits* for inactivation. The chemoreceptive cells in the carotid body have been identified as the cells containing the required *two-hits*, germline mutation and somatic cell mutation. They are considered the neoplastic proliferating cells of CBTs. [68]

- The mechanisms by which mutations in the genes lead to tumorigenesis are unknown. However, it has been postulated that mutations in the genes create a "pseudo-hypoxic" microenvironment that leads to an increase in cell number. [64] For both hypoxia and a lack of SDH activity result in an increase in succinate levels. Plus there is evidence that suggests SDH mutations activate the same signaling pathways as hypoxia. [70] And hypoxic conditions due to high altitudes or chronic hypoxemia cause hyperplasia (an increase in cell number) of the carotid body. [71,72,73,74]

> *Sporadic CBTs are associated with high altitude.* [59]

- There is also an environmental factor in the etiology of CBTs as individuals living at high altitudes in Peru develop CBTs at a frequency ten times greater than individuals living at sea level. [58] It has been postulated that this is due to chronic hypoxia and resulting hyperplasia in carotid bodies. [71,72,73,74]

- In most cases, the external carotid artery supplies blood to the tumor. [57,117] As the tumor grows, blood flow can also be supplied by the internal carotid, vertebral artery or thyrocervical trunk. [57]

Location of Disease

- Common carotid artery bifurcation between the internal and external carotid arteries.

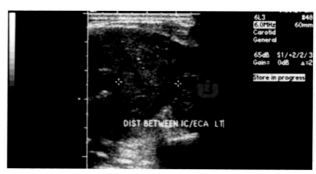

B-mode ultrasound image with distance measured between the carotid arteries

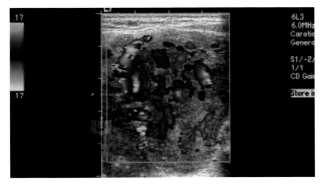

Color flow duplex ultrasound image of a CBT showing the extensive vascularization

Differential Diagnosis

- Lymphomas
- Metastatic tumors
- Aneurysms of the carotid arteries
- Thyroid lesions
- Brachial cleft cysts
- Salivary gland tumors

Diagnostic Modalities

- Color duplex ultrasonography
- CT scan (with contrast)
- MRI
- MR angiography
- Angiography

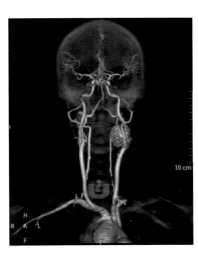

CT angiogram multiplanar reconstruction of a CBT

Conservative Treatment

- Monitor for changes

Medical Treatment

- Radiation therapy

Surgical Treatment

- Surgical excision with and without prior transcatheter embolization to decrease vascularity

Endovascular Treatment

- Some tumors are treated with pre-operative transcatheter embolization to reduce blood loss during the surgical excision.

Points to Remember

- CBTs are bilateral in 26-33% of hereditary cases and 3-5% of sporadic cases. [75,76,77]
- CBTs are benign tumors in 90-95% of all cases. [78]
- CBTs are more frequent in people living at higher altitudes. [117,118]
- CBTs are also referred to as "Glomus" tumors. [57,78]
- The percent of men and women with hereditary CBTs are similar, whereas women are more likely to have sporadic CBTs. [77]
- There is evidence that genes other than SDHB, SDHC, SDHD and SDHAF2 have a significant role in the tumorigenesis of a subset of CBTs. [78, 80]

Fibromuscular Dysplasia (FMD)

Non-atherosclerotic arterial disease which affects medium and large sized vessels, especially the renal and internal carotid arteries. Multiple, focal stenoses present in an arterial segment, resemble a "string of beads" on imaging studies.

Etiology

- Hormonal
- Mechanical stressors
- Arterial wall ischemia
- Genetics
- Younger than 60 years of age (pre-menopausal)
- Family history
- Tobacco use
- Certain medications causing irritation of arterial walls

Risk Factors

- Female

Mechanism of Disease

- Since the renal, internal and external iliac are long segment arteries without branches, they lack vasa vasorum typically found at these branch points which supply nutrients and oxygen to vessel walls. Arterial wall ischemia results and is one theory for the development of arterial dysplasia. [119]
- According to another theory, long arterial segments, such as the renal and internal carotid arteries, are subject to unique mechanical forces (i.e., greater axial stress) which cause stretching of vessels. [119]
- Although the exact mechanism remains unclear, hormonal influences on smooth muscle cells are suspected due to the prevalence of FMD in women during their reproductive years. [119]

Location of Disease *(can be unilateral or bilateral)*

- Distal renal artery (most common)
- Mid-distal internal carotid artery
- External iliac artery
- Brachial artery
- Abdominal arteries, including the mesenteric

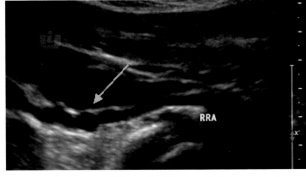

B-mode image of "beading" in the distal renal artery

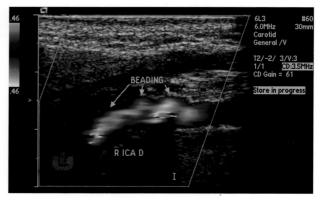

Detection of FMD in the distal ICA at the level of the mandible by color duplex

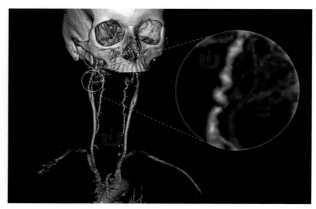

FMD by CT angiogram: 3-D reconstruction

Differential Diagnosis

- Atherosclerotic stenosis
- Takayasu's arteritis
- Vasospasm
- Neurofibromatosis
- Moyamoya disease
- Vasculitis
- Neurosyphillis
- Varicella zoster virus

Diagnostic Modalities

- Duplex ultrasonography
- CT angiography
- MRI
- MR angiography
- Angiography

Medical Treatment

- Antiplatelet medication (e.g., aspirin)
- Serial imaging studies to check for disease progression

Surgical Treatment

- Open arterial dilation
- Bypass grafting

Endovascular Treatment

- Balloon angioplasty
- Stenting

Points to Remember

- Fibromuscular dysplasia (FMD) usually occurs in females in the mid section of the internal carotid artery. [113,120]
- On duplex ultrasound, FMD is characterized by a series of tandem stenoses and dilatations accompanied by a moderate-significant increase in peak-systolic velocity. [117] A "string of beads" is a term commonly used to describe the FMD image in a duplex ultrasound image. [56,119,120]
- Although much less common, FMD also occurs in young children and infants. [119]

- Coexisting FMD in the renal and carotid arteries is a common occurrence. [113]
- Approximately 25% of individuals with FMD have more than one narrowed artery. [113]

Lymphedema

An accumulation of interstitial fluid which develops due to obstruction or abnormal development of the lymphatic system (vessels or lymph nodes). There are two types of lymphedema:

- **Primary lymphedema**: occurs independently (less common)
- **Secondary lymphedema**: secondary to a disease or another condition (most common)

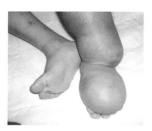

Physical presentation of primary lymphedema

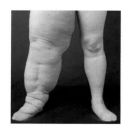

Physical presentation of secondary lymphedema

Images courtesy of Byung-Boong Lee MD PhD FACS

Etiology

- Congenital
- Surgery (post-op complication)
- Infection
- Cancer
- Radiation
- Trauma

Risk Factors

- Family history
- Female
- Cancer, with history of surgery or radiation for the condition (e.g., breast cancer with mastectomy)
- History of lymph node dissection
- Exposure to infectious bacteria, especially in tropical regions
- Trauma

Mechanism of Disease

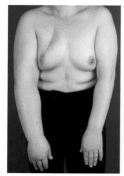

- Primary lymphedema is an inherited condition which affects development of the lymph vessels. During the embryonic stage, there is a malformation of lymph nodes or absence of valves in the lymph vessels. Affects can occur during infancy (Milroy disease), in childhood or puberty (Meige disease) or later, after the age of 35 (lymphedema tarda). [137]

- Certain conditions or interventions can damage your lymph vessels and cause lymphedema (secondary lymphedema). Lymph nodes are often removed during surgery in order to biopsy and assess for the spread of cancer. [137, 138] If the remaining lymph nodes/ vessels do not compensate for this loss, the limb will swell. [138]

Physical presentation of secondary lymphedema after breast surgery

Image courtesy of Byung-Boong Lee MD PhD FACS

- Scarring and inflammation of the lymph nodes/vessels after radiation treatment can restrict flow in the lymphatic system. [138]
- Cancerous tumors can block lymphatic pathways and prevent flow. [137]
- Infections and parasites can gain access to the lymphatic system and restrict lymphatic flow. [137]

Location of Disease

- Lower and upper extremities

Differential Diagnosis

- Vascular conditions such as venous insufficiency, congenital malformation or arteriovenous fistula
- Infection
- Cardiac failure (edema is usually bilateral)
- Renal failure
- Liver failure
- Rheumatoid arthritis
- Side effects of certain drugs, hormones
- Insect bites

Diagnostic Modalities

- Duplex ultrasonography
- CT angiogram
- MR angiography
- Contrast lymphangiography
- Lymphoscintigraphy

Medical Treatment

- Leg elevation
- Compression stockings
- Manual lymph drainage
- Intermittent pneumatic compression
- Prompt treatment of cellulitis
- Exercise

Surgical Treatment

- Microsurgical lymphatic reconstruction (lymphatic grafting)
- Liposuction (reduce edema)

Points to Remember

- The lymphatic system serves to balance intracellular and extracellular environments. Some of the components of this system include: lymph nodes, spleen, thymus, nasopharyngeal tonsils, lymphocytes and macrophages. This unidirectional system transports fluid throughout the tissues and collects bacteria, viruses and waste products. There are numerous communications between the blood and lymph streams. For example, lymph from the upper extremities enters the blood stream at the junction of the subclavian and jugular veins. [139]
- **Lymphedema** is a common differential diagnosis for lower extremity edema and is aggravated by repetitive attacks of cellulitis which scar the existing lymphatic channels.[137]
- **Elephantitis** is a complication of lymphedema where the skin becomes extremely hard and thick. These patients are at risk for chronic ulcers and infection. [138]
- **Lymphangiosarcoma** is a rare soft tissue cancer resulting from severe cases of untreated lymphedema that originate in the lymph nodes and vessels. [139]

May-Thurner Syndrome

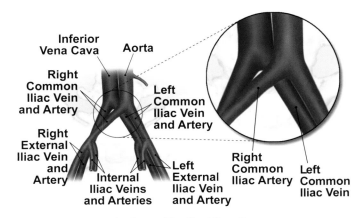

Anatomy of the iliac bifurcation

Compression of the left common iliac vein (CIV) by the right common iliac artery (CIA), which increases the risk for deep vein thrombosis and can result in left CIV stenosis and left leg swelling.

Etiology

- Congenital
- Trauma

Risk Factors

- Female >Male
- Middle aged
- Postpartum females

Mechanism of Disease

- The left common iliac vein is compressed against the fifth lumbar vertebra by the right iliac artery. [142]
- There is thought to be constant intermittent extrinsic compression of adjacent vessel walls (right CIA compresses the left CIV). Development of spurs or webs which obstruct the venous lumen have been described at the termination of the common iliac vein. Histological studies indicate the webs consist of connective tissue and endothelium, but lack elastic fibers and smooth muscle cells. [142]

Location of Disease

- Left common iliac vein, at the point the right common iliac artery crosses over

Differential Diagnosis

- Unilateral deep venous thrombosis not caused by iliac compression

Diagnostic Modalities

- Duplex ultrasonography
- CT angiography
- Venography
- Intravascular ultrasound (IVUS)

Medical Treatment

- Anticoagulation

Surgical Treatment

- Iliocaval bypass
- Transposition of the right common iliac artery
- Iliac vein disobliteration (opened to remove webs/spurs)

Endovascular Treatment

- Balloon angioplasty and stenting of the CIV
- Vena caval filters (in cases of thrombus and risk for PE)

Points to Remember

- "Iliac compression syndrome" is another term for May-Thurner's syndrome.

Mesenteric Ischemia

Mesenteric ischemia is caused by a significant decrease in blood flow to the small intestines or colon due to the blockage of the mesenteric arteries (celiac, superior and inferior mesenteric arteries), with two out of the three usually being effected.[154, 155, 156]

- **Chronic mesenteric ischemia**–progressive condition with symptoms developing over a long period of time (e.g., involuntary weight loss).[155]
- **Acute mesenteric ischemia**–symptoms present abruptly and progress quickly over a short period of time.

Etiology

- Embolic
- Thrombosis of pre-existing arterial stenosis
- Atherosclerosis
- Intestinal hypoperfusion (caused by small vessel insufficiency)
- Vasospasm
- Venous thrombosis
- Takayasu's arteritis

Risk Factors

- Atherosclerosis
- Age (>50 years)
- Female >Male
- Young-female (should consider median arcuate ligament syndrome as a cause)
- Hypertension
- Diabetes
- Hypercholesteremia
- Smoking
- Gastrointestinal disease
- Coronary disease (e.g., arrhythmia, congestive heart failure, etc.)
- Mesenteric venous thrombosis
- Risk factors for mesenteric venous thrombosis: obesity, cancer, oral contraceptives
- History of abdominal surgery
- Hernia
- Genetic prothrombotic conditions (e.g., clotting disorders, such as Factor V Leiden)
- Aortic dissection
- Arteritis

Mechanism of Disease

- Mesenteric blood flow is regulated by several mechanisms; intrinsic (metabolic) and extrinsic (neural and hormonal).[154]
  - Atherosclerosis or vasospasm can significantly narrow the arterial vessels supplying the intestinal organs.[95] Emboli are a common cause of acute ischemia.[156]
  - A lack of oxygen to the mesenteric organs causes cellular injury and mucosal ischemia within the intestines. Tissue necrosis and metabolic acidosis are significant consequences.
  - Extracellular volume decreases. The renin-angiotensin system is activated, releasing renin which increases angiotensin II levels, causing vasoconstriction.[154]

- Plasma volume decreases and fluid concentrations increase abnormally resulting in the release of vasopressin (antidiuretic hormone) from the pituitary gland, causing mesenteric vasoconstriction and venorelaxation.[154]
- A low cardiac output state can cause a non-occlusive form of acute mesenteric ischemia.[156] This is commonly seen in ICU patients who are in heart failure or who are on multiple pressors (medication) to help support blood pressure.
- Compression of the celiac trunk by the median arcuate ligament of the diaphragm is another mechanism for mesenteric ischemia.[154] Lumenal stenosis is thought to be caused by intimal fibrosis resulting from the compression. Compression is increased during expiration.[157]

- Mesenteric ischemia is categorized as chronic or acute
  - **Chronic Mesenteric Ischemia**
    - Most commonly caused by progression of atherosclerotic disease (stenosis or occlusion) in the aorta, celiac or proximal mesenteric arteries.
    - Less common causes include arteritis, aneurysm, mesenteric artery dissection and hypercoaguable conditions.

> *Acute mesenteric ischemia has a high mortality rate.*[155]

  - **Acute Mesenteric Ischemia**[154, 155, 156]
    - Caused by arterial occlusion, usually due to a cardiac embolism, occurring most frequently in the SMA due to its smaller size.[171]
    - Caused by arterial occlusion due to thrombosis most commonly in the SMA
    - Caused by small vessel insufficiency (e.g., poor collateral circulation)

Location of Disease

- Superior mesenteric artery (most common site of embolic occlusion)
- Celiac artery (CA)
- Inferior mesenteric artery

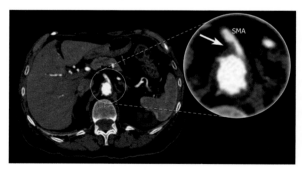

Mesenteric artery stenosis detected by CT angiography

Differential Diagnosis

- Cholecystitis
- Diverticulitis
- Appendicitis
- Intestinal obstruction
- Cancer

Diagnostic Modalities

- Duplex ultrasonography
- CT angiography
- MR angiography
- Endoscopy–upper/lower GI
- Colonoscopy/sigmoidoscopy
- Angiography

Explorative surgery

Medical Treatment

- Serial imaging exams to monitor changes
- Risk factor management
- Systemic heparinization (acute cases)
- Treatment of contributing conditions (e.g., cardiac, hypovolemia or sepsis)

Surgical Treatment

- Mesenteric bypass (e.g., aorto-celiac-SMA, Ileo-SMA)
- Thromboendarterectomy
- Laparotomy
- Resection of dead bowel
- Decompression of the median arcuate ligament with bypass grafting

Endovascular Treatment

- Angioplasty
- Stenting

Points to Remember

- The SMA is almost always one of the "two out of three" arteries involved in cases of chronic ischemia. [154, 155, 157]
- Usually an isolated celiac or inferior mesenteric artery obstruction does not cause symptoms. [154]
- In acute ischemia, intestinal collaterals are able to partially compensate for the blocked mesenteric arteries, delaying substantial injury for approximately 12 hours. [155]
- Extrinsic compression of the CA (median arcuate ligament syndrome) can lead to mesenteric ischemia. [154]
- Emergent surgical/endovascular treatment is often required for acute mesenteric ischemia. [154]

Neointimal and Intimal Hyperplasia

Many use the terms intimal hyperplasia and neointimal hyperplasia interchangeably. This sections discusses both.

From the ancient Greek language, *neointimal hyperplasia* translates to "over-formation of a *young* intima".

Neointimal hyperplasia is often used in connection with the growth of an existing intima. This is similar to the definition for intimal hyperplasia. It is used many to mean either an increase in the thickness of the intima, as occurs in vein grafts, or the formation of a new intima due to an increase in smooth muscle cell number.

> *Many exclude atherosclerosis and use intimal hyperplasia to mean an increase in intimal thickness due to an increase in smooth muscle cell number in the intima and their synthesis of extracellular matrix.*

Intimal hyperplasia (IH) strictly means an increase in cell number in the intima. This would include atherosclerosis, where there is a large increase in the number of macrophages and a smaller increase in smooth muscle cell number.

Neointimal hyperplasia could also be defined as *pathologic* intimal hyperplasia that occurs in response to blood vessel injury.

Etiology

- Endovascular trauma
- Surgical intervention
- Other injury or trauma

Risk Factors

- Surgical or endovascular procedures including:
  - Angioplasty
  - Vein grafting
  - Arteriovenous fistula creation
  - Arteriovenous graft
  - Stenting

Mechanism of Disease [123]

- Intimal hyperplasia (IH) occurs in arteries exposed to abnormal mechanical forces, low wall fluid shear stress and/or high mural tensile stress. [163] IH will reduce lumen diameter and/or increase wall thickness depending upon vessel remodeling. [22] A reduction in lumen diameter, which causes an increase blood flow velocity will increase wall shear stress, as wall shear stress is directly proportional to velocity and inversely proportional to the radius cubed. An increase in the thickness will decrease mural tensile stress as it is inversely proportional to wall thickness. IH tends to be concentric in straight vessels as wall shear stress is constant around the circumference of the vessel. In vessels such as branches, bifurcations, and bends, the growth is asymmetric occurring in regions of low shear stress.

> *Note that these are the same locations that favor atherosclerosis and atherosclerosis can develop on top of intimal hyperplasia*

- There are slight differences in IH mechanisms, especially the initial stimulus. However, it always involves a change in the regulation of the smooth muscle cells by the endothelial cells. The endothelial cells are either lost or become dysfunctional. In contrast to early hypotheses, inflammatory cells are being discovered to be a key component of IH.
- IH is characterized by the proliferation of smooth muscle cells in the media, followed by their migration to the intima where proliferation continues and then their synthesis of an abundance of extracellular matrix. [161, 162, 164] IH lesions that reach a steady state are approximately 80-90% extracellular matrix and 10-20% cells, mainly smooth muscle cells. [165]
- Mechanical injury causes IH after procedures such as percutaneous transluminal angioplasty, stenting, etc.
- *Pathological intimal hyperplasia* occurs most often after a surgical or endovascular procedure that results in the loss or dysfunctionality of endothelial cells, which plays an important role in the development of intimal hyperplasia.
  - Endothelial cell dysfunction also occurs with exposure to a dramatically different hemodynamic environment. Such a change occurs when veins are used as grafts.
    - This results in the endothelial cells being exposed to arterial level shear stresses, which are significantly greater than those in the venous circulation.
    - The creation of an arterio-venous fistula or graft for dialysis access also exposes venous endothelial cells to sudden increases in shear stress levels. In this case, the venous flow pattern also becomes nonlaminar, which is pathological for endothelial cells.

- Endothelial cells are primary regulators of smooth muscle cells.
  - In a healthy vessel, smooth muscle cells contract and relax to maintain vascular tone. There is low proliferation, migration and extracellular matrix synthesis rates at this stage. Functional endothelial cells secrete factors such as nitric oxide and prostacyclin to control normal function.
  - In pathological conditions, like intimal hyperplasia, the cells increase their rates of proliferation, migration and protein synthesis. Dysfunctional endothelial cells secrete nitric oxide and prostacyclin, as well as other factors at a significantly lower level.
- Endothelial cells also regulate the adherence of monocytes and platelets to the vessel wall. Monocytes and activated platelets secrete smooth muscle cell mitogens and chemoattractants required for the migration of the smooth muscle cells from the media to the intima in intimal hyperplasia. Monocytes adhere directly to endothelial cells by binding specific proteins (receptors) on the endothelial cell surface.
  - In a healthy vessel, these receptors are absent or present at a very low level.
  - In intimal hyperplasia there is an increase in receptors, which increases the number of adhered monocytes.
  - Endothelial cells prevent platelet adhesion and activation by maintaining a nonthrombogenic surface at the interface of the blood and vessel wall, and by secreting factors such as nitric oxide and prostacyclin, to inhibit platelet activation and adhesion. In addition, they cover thrombogenic factors in the subendothelial matrix such as collagen and platelet activating factor.[164] When the endothelial cells detach, these factors are exposed and platelet adhesion and activation ensue.
- The extracellular matrix must also be modified for the smooth muscle cells to be able to migrate through as they move from the media to the intima. This is done by proteolysis in which enzymes break down the proteins that comprise the extracellular matrix.[166,162]

Location of Disease

- The location of disease can be focal or diffuse throughout a vessel and affect any level or multiple levels.
- Most commonly occurs in vessels that have had surgical or endovascular intervention, especially procedures which remove or damage the endothelial cells.

Differential Diagnosis

- Atherosclerosis

Diagnostic Modalities

- Duplex ultrasonography
- CT angiography
- MR angiography
- Angiography

Medical Treatment

- Supervised exercise programs

Surgical Treatment

- Bypass grafting

Endovascular Treatment

- Angioplasty
- Drug coated stents
- Atherectomy
- Laser-assisted angioplasty
- Endovascular irradiation

Points to Remember

- Intimal hyperplasia (IH) is the principle cause for graft failure and occlusion of stented arteries.[123]
- Over distension of the lumen during graft preparation causes IH in vein grafts.[160]
- Mis-sizing of stents causes continual physical trauma resulting in IH.
- IH occurs pathologically and during normal development, e.g. the closure of the ductus arteriosus shortly after birth.
- The reader is cautioned to consider what they mean to convey when using the terms *intimal hyperplasia* and *neointimal hyperplasia* and to define their use of the terms when necessary for clarity.

Phlegmasia Alba Dolens

Decreased venous drainage due to thrombosis of extremity deep veins, without collateral vein involvement.

Etiology

- Hypercoaguable state
- Massive venous thrombosis

Risk Factors

- Female >Male
- Middle aged
- Pregnancy (esp. during last trimester)

Mechanism of Disease [147, 148]

- Extensive edema (usually as a result of iliofemoral thrombosis) obscures capillary circulation causing a "white" discoloration to the skin.
- Arterial spasms similar to those in phlegmasia cerulea dolens may also be a contributing factor.

Location of Disease

- Iliofemoral deep veins; iliac, common femoral, deep femoral and femoral veins
- Upper extremity deep veins (rare)

Differential Diagnosis

- Arterial embolism
- Aortic dissection
- Lymphedema

Diagnostic Modalities

- Duplex ultrasonography
- Arteriography
- Venography

Medical Treatment

- IV heparin and coumadinization
- Graduated compression stockings

Surgical Treatment

- Venous thrombectomy
- Compartment fasciotomy
- Cross pubic vein-vein reconstruction with PTFE
- Creation of an arteriovenous fistula between the femoral artery and great saphenous vein
- Amputation

Endovascular Treatment

- Thrombolytic therapy

Points to Remember

- Phlegmasia alba dolens can progress to phlegmasia cerulea dolens

Phlegmasia Cerulea Dolens

Massive venous occlusion due to multi-segment thrombosis of extremity deep veins; iliofemoral, lower leg veins and their collaterals.

Etiology

- Malignancy
- Hypercoaguable state
- Trauma

Risk Factors

- Female >Male
- Middle aged
- Post-operative
- Vena caval insertion
- Ulcerative colitis
- Gastroenteritis
- Heart failure
- Mitral valve stenosis
- May-Thurner syndrome

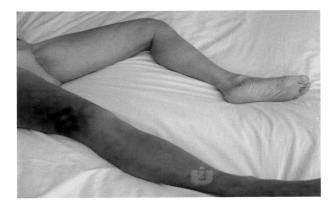

Mechanism of Disease

- Massive obstruction of venous outflow reduces arterial inflow to the limb and causes arterial vasoconstriction and may cause arteriolar thrombosis. [42, 147]
- Venous congestion results from significant iliac vein thrombosis and causes a "blue" discoloration to the skin. [42]

Location of Disease

- Iliofemoral deep veins; iliac, common femoral, deep femoral and femoral veins (along with their collaterals).
- Upper extremity deep veins (only 2-5% of cases)[147]

Differential Diagnosis

- Arterial ischemia/thrombosis
- Aortic dissection
- Toxic shock syndrome
- Superficial phlebitis of the upper extremity

Diagnostic Modalities

- Duplex ultrasonography
- Arteriography
- Venography

Medical Treatment

- Maximize limb elevation
- Correct any hypovolemia
- Aggressive anticoagulation
- Graduated compression stockings

Surgical Treatment

- Venous thrombectomy
- Compartment fasciotomy
- Cross pubic vein-vein reconstruction with PTFE
- Creation of an arteriovenous fistula between the femoral artery and great saphenous vein
- Amputation

Endovascular Treatment

- Thrombolytic therapy

Points to Remember

- *Venous gangrene* can occur with phlegmasia cerulea dolens as a result of substantial venous outflow and arterial inflow obstructions. [42] All toes and part of the foot will be gangrenous, instead of only one or two toes which typically occurs in cases of gangrene caused by arterial disease.

Portal Hypertension

Increased blood pressure within the portal venous system. The normal portal venous pressure is 5 mmHg. Portal hypertension is defined as pressures >12 mmHg. [135] Complications from portal hypertension include varices and ascites. [159]

Etiology

- Cirrhosis (scarring of the liver)
- Hepatitis
- Alcohol abuse
- Portal splenic vein thrombosis
- Schistosomiasis

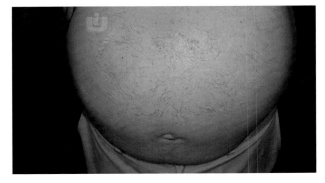

Typical presentation of portal hypertension with abdominal varices

Risk Factors

The theory of Virchow's triad explains portal splenic thrombosis; venous thrombosis is caused by venous stasis, vein wall (intimal) injury or a hypercoaguable state.

Additional risk factors for portal hypertension include:

- Hepatocellular disease (acute or chronic)
- Liver disease (e.g., cirrhosis)
- Tricuspid regurgitation–backflow of blood through the tricuspid valve resulting in increased pressures within the IVC and hepatic circulation.
- Heart disease causing increased right-heart pressures (e.g., congestive heart failure)
- Schistosomiasis-parasitic disease found in Asia, Africa and South America
- Constrictive pericarditis
- Trauma
- Family history
- Cancer
- Appendicitis
- Diverticulitis

Mechanism of Disease

- Pressure is affected by changes in volume or resistance. Portal hypertension refers to the elevation of portal pressure within the portal circulation caused by an increased resistance to flow, usually within the hepatic parenchyma. [159]
- Changes in resistance are affected by the radius of the blood vessel which can be significantly decreased when liver disease, liver fibrosis, thrombosis or tumor are present. A decrease in vessel radius increases hepatic resistance. [159,160]
- Nitric oxide (NO) levels are believed to affect portal hypertension in cirrhosis cases. An increase in NO levels causes vasodilatation and increased portomesenteric blood flow. Decreased NO causes vasoconstriction and increased portal pressure. [158]
- In response to increased pressure within the portohepatic system, the body attempts to reduce pressure by diverting blood away from the liver through collaterals, varices or shunts. This dilatation of veins may progress to causes esophageal, gastric, and anal varices. [159] Rupture of these varices can result in life threatening hemorrhage. [159, 160]
- Other consequences of portal hypertension are encephalopathy [158] and *splenomegaly* (enlarged spleen).[160]

Location of Disease

- Portal veins
- Main portal vein
- Right portal vein
- Left portal vein

Differential Diagnosis

- Budd-Chiari syndrome
- Tuberculosis
- Polycystic kidney disease
- Cirrhosis
- Pericarditis
- Congestive heart failure
- Tricuspid regurgitation
- Sarcoidosis
- Vitamin A toxicity

Diagnostic Modalities

- Duplex ultrasonography
- Upper GI series
- CT angiography
- MRI or MRA
- Endoscopy
- Angiography

Medical Treatment

- Managing complications of portal hypertension (e.g., variceal hemorrhage, ascites)
- Managing the cause of portal hypertension (e.g., anticoagulation for hepatic vein thrombosis, treating any identified cause of liver disease).
- Beta-blockers can reduce portal pressure
- Dietary changes

Surgical Treatment

- Paracentesis
- Liver transplant
- Splenectomy
- Transjugular intrahepatic portosystemic shunt (TIPS)
- Distal splenorenal shunt (DSRS)
- Portocaval shunt (main portal blood shunted to the IVC)
- Mesocaval shunt (blood from the superior mesenteric vein shunted to the IVC)

Endovascular Treatment

Endoscopic treatments/banding/sclerotherapy all are treatment modalities for esophageal varices not direct treatment of portal hypertension.

Points to Remember

- The portal vein receives blood from the stomach, intestines, spleen, gallbladder and pancreas.
- TIPS involves placing a stent to connect the hepatic vein to the portal vein (usually right portal to right hepatic).[158]
- Distal splenorenal shunting connects the splenic vein to the left renal vein in order to reduce varices and bleeding. [158]
- A serious complication associated with varices is the risk of rupture which may be fatal due to internal bleeding. [159,160]
- Budd-Chiari syndrome results from obstruction to hepatic venous outflow. The syndrome presents with ascites, abdominal pain and can result in liver necrosis. [158]

Pseudoaneurysm

A pseudoaneurysm (PA) or "false aneurysm" forms due to trauma to all three layers of the arterial wall. The "false aneurysm" is actually a hematoma, receiving its blood supply from the communication with an adjacent artery via a small channel or patent "neck". These "necks" vary in size and length.

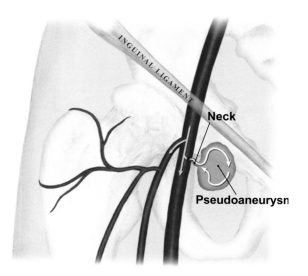

Arterial pseudoaneurysm off the superficial femoral artery

Etiology

- Trauma
- Penetrating trauma (e.g., gunshot wound, blunt trauma, iatrogenic arterial puncture)
- Infection

Risk Factors

- Post-cardiac catheterization
- Post-angiography
- Post-operative arterial intervention (bypass graft)
- Post-endarterectomy
- Renal dialysis; PA commonly develop in synthetic grafts
- Intravascular drug abuse

Mechanism of disease

- Insertion of a needle for diagnostic, therapeutic or recreational purposes is a trauma to the arterial wall and may cause a pseudoaneurysm.
- Reasons for pseudoaneurysm at an anastomotic site include; infection, tension at the anastomosis, thin-walled arteries, suture deterioration or improper suture technique. [49]
- Repeated puncture of hemodialysis grafts leads to formation of subcutaneous hematomas. [50]
- A reduction in tensile strength post-endarterectomy may weaken the arterial wall, increasing the risk of a pseudoaneurysm. [42]

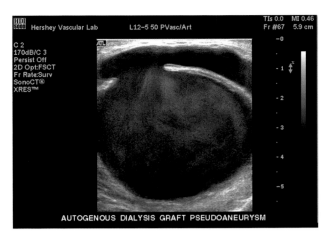

Duplex ultrasound image of a pseudoaneurysm off a dialysis graft Image courtesy of Philips Healthcare

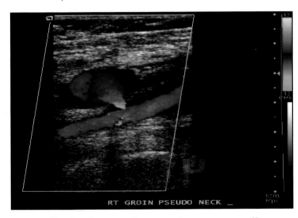

Duplex image of a pseudoaneurysm off the superficial femoral artery

Location of Disease

- Common femoral artery
- Superficial femoral artery
- External iliac artery
- Deep femoral artery
- Brachial artery
- Axillary artery
- Radial artery
- Carotid artery
- Anastomotic sites
- Hemodialysis grafts or AV fistulas
- Thoracic aorta (due to trauma)

Diagnostic Modalities

- Duplex ultrasonography
- CT angiography
- Angiography

Medical Treatment

- Follow-up observation for pseudoaneurysms <2 cm in diameter
- Thrombin injection under duplex ultrasound guidance
  - Can be performed electively
  - Performed if pseudoaneurysm:
    - Persists beyond 2 weeks
    - Causes significant compression and associated symptoms
    - Enlarges
- Duplex guided compression repair

Surgical Treatment

- Open repair to evacuate the hematoma and repair the arterial wall.
- Resection of the pseudoaneurysm site and surrounding graft in hemodialysis conduits.
- Interposition graft placement or bypass around the affected section.

Endovascular Treatment

- Covered stent graft placed within existing dialysis access.

Points to Remember

- The sizes of pseudoaneurysms vary.
- In dialysis conduits, there are risks of graft thrombosis, infection and bleeding associated with pseudoaneurysms. [50] Difficulty with graft access during a hemodialysis session can also be an issue.
- Pseudoaneurysm formation is less common in AV fistulas compared to prosthetic grafts. [50]
- Pseudoaneurysms may spontaneously thrombose. [51, 53]
- Document patency of the native peripheral arteries, pre-treatment/repair. [52]
- After a repair, observe the patient for distal symptoms (e.g., toe discoloration) which may result from a micro-thrombotic embolization that may have occurred as a result of the procedure. [52, 53]

Popliteal Artery Entrapment Syndrome

Dynamic compression of the popliteal artery by surrounding muscles or tendons which may result in intermittent reduction of blood flow to the tibial arteries. If untreated, a thrombus may form in the artery. The resulting abnormal hemodynamics can also lead to atherosclerosis.

Etiology

- Anatomic variations in the popliteal fossa

Risk Factors

- Middle-aged, sedentary males (anatomic entrapment)
- Young male (functional entrapment)

Mechanism of Disease

- The popliteal artery courses between the medial and lateral heads of the gastrocnemius muscles in the popliteal fossa. Variations during embryonic development result in an entrapment of the popliteal artery by neighboring muscles/tendons. [104, 105]
- In one type of entrapment known as "functional", symptoms occur without evidence of anatomic variant. [105]
- In certain leg positions, the gastrocnemius muscle compresses the popliteal artery resulting in loss of distal pulses. [105]

Types of Entrapment [105, 106]

- **Type I (classic):** occurs when the distal popliteal artery forms before the medial head of the gastrocnemius muscle is able to get into position. As a result, the popliteal artery will lay more medial than it normally does when the gastrocnemius muscle is in place to properly position the artery.
- **Type II:** the popliteal artery displaces the medial head of the gastrocnemius muscle laterally.
- **Type III:** abnormal muscle bundles surround the popliteal artery due to the persistence of mesodermal tissue or embryonic cells in the popliteal fossa.
- **Type IV:** atypical development of the popliteal artery, deeper than usual within the popliteal fossa which leads to entrapment by the popliteal muscle or a fibrous band.
- **Type V:** both the popliteal artery and vein are compressed.
- **Type VI (type F):** the popliteal artery is compressed by certain maneuvers of the leg but the reason for the compression is unknown. This type is also referred to as *functional entrapment.*

Location of Disease

- Popliteal artery (often bilateral)

Differential Diagnosis

- Popliteal adventitial cystic disease (ACD)
- Synovial cyst
- Popliteal artery occlusive disease
- Extrinsic compression (from hematoma, cyst or tumor)

Diagnostic Modalities

- Duplex ultrasonography (while performing active plantarflexion)
- MRI
- MR angiography
- CT angiography
- Angiography

Medical Treatment

- None

Surgical Treatment

- Division of the muscle and replacement of the damaged artery with a bypass graft if needed

Endovascular Treatment

- Balloon angioplasty (most successful if source of entrapment is also addressed)

Points to Remember

- Duplex findings include obliteration of the popliteal artery waveform with plantarflexion of the knee. [105]
- Post-stenotic aneurysm or dilatations are not uncommon findings in popliteal entrapment cases. [43, 106]
- An acquired form of entrapment is possible after infragenicular bypass surgery.
- Popliteal entrapment can also occur due to muscle hypertrophy induced by exercise.
- Males are twice as likely to suffer from popliteal entrapment than females. [105]

Pulmonary Embolism

Definition

The occlusion of a pulmonary artery by a thromboembolus.

Etiology

- Venous sites that may thrombose and be the source of the embolus include:
  - Lower extremity deep veins (90%)[34]
  - Pelvic deep veins
  - Upper extremity deep veins

Risk Factors

- Age (greater with advanced age)
- Immobilization (e.g., long distance air travel, paraplegia)
- Genetic prothrombotic conditions (clotting disorders, such as Factor V Leiden)
- Post-operative phase (especially after orthopedic surgery)
- Central venous or femoral catheters
- Cancer/malignancy
- Pregnancy
- Medications (e.g., oral contraceptives)
- Estrogen replacement therapy
- Previous DVT
- Heart complications
- Obesity
- Family history
- Smoking
- Chronic obstructive pulmonary disease (COPD)
- Blood type (highest risk with type-A, lowest risk with type-O)
- Trauma
- Antiphospholipid antibodies (lupus, etc.)
- Varicose veins
- Inflammatory bowel disease

Mechanism of Disease

- Embolization occurs when a piece of a blood clot (embolus) breaks free from a venous wall thrombus and travels centrally to the pulmonary arterial circulation.
- An embolus can pass through the right side of the heart to the lungs, where it obstructs one of the pulmonary arteries. As a result, lung tissue is deprived of blood, which can be fatal. [143]

Location of Disease

- Pulmonary artery
- Pulmonary artery branches

Differential Diagnosis

- Bronchitis pneumonia
- Pleurisy
- Myocardial ischemia (MI)

Diagnostic Modalities

- CT angiography
- Ventilation-perfusion (VQ) Scan
- Chest X-ray
- Pulmonary angiogram

Medical Treatment

- Heparinization
- Long-term anticoagulation

Surgical Treatment

- Caval filter placement
- Pulmonary embolectomy

Endovascular Treatment

- Thrombolytic therapy
- Pulmonary suction embolectomy

Points to Remember

- Pulmonary embolism (PE) is a complication of venous thrombosis. [144]
- PE is the third most common cause of death in the US, with approximately 630,000 cases/year. [127] It is one of the top causes of "unexpected death" in any age group. [144]
- Venous duplex exams do not rule out a pulmonary event, they can only suggest a source of emboli for an episode of PE. [144, 145]
- A normal, negative VQ scan excludes PE. False positive results may occur in patients for other reasons, such as lung disease. [146]
- Studies have indicated that approximately one-third of PE cases are asymptomatic. [127, 145]
- The source of emboli is usually iliofemoral thrombus. Calf thrombi rarely result in pulmonary emboli, though they often propagate above the knee where they become a greater risk for embolus. [127]
- To decrease the risk of a pulmonary embolism, an inferior vena cava (IVC) filter is placed via catheter (typically using CFV, EIV or jugular access). The aim of this procedure is to "catch" any thrombi floating in the blood stream, lowering the risk of a PE

Raynaud's Syndrome: Raynaud's Disease and Raynaud's Phenomenon

In Raynaud's syndromes, digits display episodes of cyanosis or pallor due to vasoconstriction of the small, digital arteries or arterioles during times of cold or emotional stress.

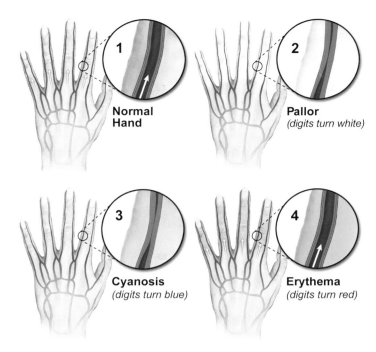

Raynaud's Syndrome

1. Normal Hand
2. Pallor *(digits turn white)*
3. Cyanosis *(digits turn blue)*
4. Erythema *(digits turn red)*

Etiology

Patients exhibiting digital ischemia are divided into two categories:[98]

- **Raynaud's disease:** primary vasospastic disorder without an identifiable underlying cause
- **Raynaud's phenomenon:** vasospasm is secondary to some underlying condition (e.g., lupus, scleroderma, etc.)

Risk Factors

- Young females
- Age (between 11- 45 years)
- History of autoimmune disease
- Cooler climates (including England, Denmark, France)
- Diabetes
- Patients on hormone therapy
- Certain occupations at risk for "occupational arterial disease" (e.g., hammer syndrome, vibration white finger, thermal damage)
- Drug use
- Smoking
- Heart disease/ myocardial infarction
- Family history of Raynaud's syndrome

Mechanism of Disease [98]

- The majority of blood flow to the digits is for thermoregulation of the body. The skin contains nerve fibers which sense temperature.
- The hypothalamus in the brain controls body temperature by varying the sympathetic outflow to the digital vessels using the medulla, spinal chord, sympathetic ganglion and local nerves. Sympathetic nerves stimulate smooth muscle cells in the digits to constrict the vessel. Vessel dilatation cools the body while constriction serves to warm/conserve body heat.

- Alpha-2 adrenoceptors are located in and on the smooth muscle cells in the thermoregulatory blood vessels, which help control body temperature. As the body is cooled additional alpha-2c adrenoceptors move from inside the cell to the surface. Here they are activated by the sympathetic nerves causing the smooth muscle cell to contract and thus the vessel to constrict. Constriction increases as the number of receptors on the cell surface increases. It has been suggested that in individuals with Raynaud's phenomenon, the receptors may abnormally accumulate on smooth muscle cell surfaces under certain circumstances, causing pathological vessel constriction.[173,174]
- Static blood in the capillaries becomes deoxygenated causing the digits to appear bluish in color.
- Post-ischemic vasodilatation causes hyperemia and rubor or *erythema* (redness) of the digit once the vasospastic episode is over.
- When there is an underlying cause for vasospasm, rewarming of the finger oftentimes results in pain, since the blood flow can not return fast enough to meet the metabolic need of the digit.
- Individuals with low blood pressure have a decreased ability to dilate their arteries. Contraction of smooth muscle cells can result in vessel closure.
- An episode of vasospasm can be triggered by cold or emotionally stressful situations.
- Sympathetic nerves respond to stress by releasing neurotransmitters that cause smooth muscle cell contraction.
- Endothelial cells release vasoactive factors (e.g., nitric oxide, angiotensin II) which control smooth muscle cell contraction and relaxation and hence vasodilation/vasoconstriction. Dysfunctional endothelial cells may not release these factors appropriately resulting in abnormal regulation of vessel constriction/relaxation.
- Endothelial damage caused by repetitive movements or use of vibrational tools (e.g., jack hammers) can lead to intralumenal thrombosis and embolism.
- Connective tissue disorders, such as scleroderma, cause fibrosis and disease of small arteries, arterioles and capillaries resulting in tissue ischemia from vasoconstriction.

Location of Disease

- Fingers (most common)
- Toes
- Nose (rare)
- Ear (rare)
- Nipples (rare)

Differential Diagnosis

- Atherosclerosis
- Buerger's disease (thromboangiitis obliterans)
- Giant cell arteritis
- Trauma
- Vasculitis (such as Wegener's granulomatosis)
- Scleroderma (or other connective tissue disorders such as lupus, rheumatoid arthritis, etc.)
- Myeloma
- Hematological cancers
- Malignancy
- Prinzmetal's angina
- Infection (hepatitis B and C, parovirus)
- Embolic (arterial or cardiac)
- Thoracic outlet syndrome
- Toxin induced vasospasm
- Hepatitis antigenemia Cryoglobulinemia
- Carpal tunnel syndrome
- Frostbite
- Neurological disorders

Diagnostic Modalities

- Non-invasive vascular testing:
  - Upper extremity arterial testing, including digital plethysmography
  - Cold immersion
  - Digital temperature recovery testing
  - Duplex ultrasonography
- Laser Doppler
- Laboratory blood tests (for Raynaud's phenomenon only)
- Platelet count, sedimentation rate, etc.

Medical Treatment

- Vasodilators (calcium channel blockers)
- Treatment of underlying condition
- Nerve block injection
- Risk factor management (smoking cessation, avoidance of cold)
- Thermal biofeedback

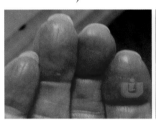 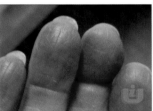

Typical presentation of Raynaud's (with cyanotic episode-right)

Surgical Treatment

- Open digital sympathectomy
- Amputation

Endovascular Treatment

- None

Points to Remember

- Approximately 28 million (5-10%) of people in the U.S. suffer from Raynaud's phenomenon.[99]
- Raynaud's affects women nine times more than men.[74]
- Only one or two digits may be affected by a Raynaud's attack. Attacks can last anywhere from a few minutes to several hours.
- Raynaud's attacks do not always affect the same digits.
- Holding an iced-drink or taking something out of a freezer can be enough to trigger a Raynaud's attack.
- In some Raynaud's patients, there may be underlying fixed digital occlusive disease that is complicated by digital vasospasm (both disease and phenomenon can exist simultaneously).

Renovascular Hypertension

Elevated blood pressure caused by decreased kidney perfusion due to stenosis or occlusion of the renal arteries.

Etiology

- Atherosclerosis
- Acute arterial thrombosis
- Embolism
- Fibromuscular dysplasia
- Renal artery trauma
- Aneurysm
- Aortic dissection
- Renal artery malformation
- Polyarteritis nodosa
- Neurofibromatosis
- Fibrosis, post-radiation
- Inadequate immune system or poor diet during pregnancy

Risk Factors

- Any risk factors for atherosclerosis
- Ethnicity (with Caucasians having a higher risk)
- Younger female (due to FMD, pregnancy)
- Elderly male (due to atherosclerosis)
- Younger than 20 years of age and older than 50 years of age
- Smoking
- Malignant or accelerated hypertension
- Radiation therapy
- Renal arterial intimal dysplasia in children

Mechanism of Disease [151, 152]

- The kidney maintains blood pressure by regulating the balance of sodium and water retention.
- Renal arterial stenotic/occlusive disease results in decreased renal blood flow to the kidney.
- When *baroreceptors* (pressure sensors in the arterial wall) detect a decrease in renal blood flow, the enzyme renin is released.
- The renin-angiotensin system is activated which increases angiotensin II levels. Angiotensin II increases blood pressure and causes peripheral vasoconstriction.
- Angiotension II increases the synthesis of aldosterone by the adrenal gland. Aldosterone increases sodium and water retention, which increases blood pressure. If the contralateral kidney is healthy, increased renal perfusion causes a decrease in sodium reabsorption and increase sodium excretion. Blood pressure will decrease, which will decrease perfusion pressure of the stenotic kidney and increase the release of renin.
- When there is only a single functioning kidney and that renal artery is obstructed, the kidney can not rely on increased urine output from the contralateral kidney to prevent sodium and water retention. The volume expansion which results causes elevated blood pressure and suppresses renin production by the stenotic kidney.
- In fibromuscular dysplasia, the lack of vasa vasorum in the long renal arterial segment may result in vessel wall ischemia and dysplasia. [119]

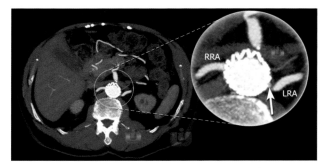

CT illustrating left renal artery stenosis

Location of Disease

- Renal ostia or proximal renal arterial segment (atherosclerosis as etiology)
- Middle-distal renal arterial segments (FMD as etiology)

Renovascular hypertension is the most common type of secondary hypertension (HTN). A "secondary condition" is a condition caused by another medical condition (e.g. HTN due to atherosclerosis or FMD).

Differential Diagnosis

- Other forms of hypertension
- Pheochromocytoma
- Primary hyperaldosteronism

Diagnostic Modalities

- Duplex ultrasonography
- Renal vein renin assay
- CT angiography
- MR angiography
- Renal arteriography

Medical Treatment

- Serial renal artery duplex exams to monitor for change
- Drug therapy
- Smoking cessation

Surgical Treatment

- Endarterectomy
- Bypass grafting (e.g., aorto-renal, splachno-renal)
- Renal artery reimplantation
- Ex-vivo reconstruction

Endovascular Treatment

- Angioplasty
- Stenting
- Endovascular neuro-ablation in trials

Points to Remember

- Stenosis of the renal artery may be unilateral, although bilateral renal stenosis is possible, especially when caused by atherosclerosis. [152]

Subclavian Steal Syndrome

Vertebral artery flow reverses (flows away from the brain, in a retrograde direction) in an attempt to provide circulation to the upper extremity when the subclavian or right innominate artery is severely stenosed or occluded.

Bidirectional flow may occur in the vertebral artery if there is a hemodynamically significant stenosis in the ipsilateral subclavian artery at its ostia. The patient may complain of dizziness with use of the arm.

"Subclavian steal phenomenon" is diagnosed when there is retrograde vertebral flow without neurological symptoms related to cerebral ischemia. [122]

Etiology

- Atherosclerosis
- Takayasu's arteritis

Risk Factors

- Caucasian
- Males
- Females with Takayasu's arteritis
- Age
- Diabetes
- Smoking
- Hypercholesteremia
- Hypertension

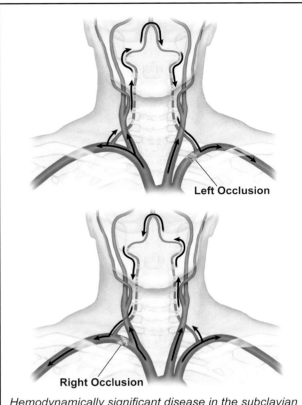

Hemodynamically significant disease in the subclavian creates subclavian steal syndrome. Flow reverses in the vertebral artery to supply the brachial artery and the upper extremity. Flow in the CCA is uneffected.

Mechanism of Disease

- The subclavian artery is typically a low resistant pathway. Blood normally flows from the aorta to the subclavian (via the innominate on the right) to the vertebral artery, which is a branch of the subclavian.
- Hemodynamics change when there is an obstruction between the aorta and the vertebral artery. This path becomes high resistant, but fluids prefer to flow along the path of least resistance. The blood flows around the obstruction by going up the carotids and/or contralateral vertebral artery and then down the ipsilateral vertebral artery (retrograde direction) to the subclavian artery in order to supply the ipsilateral upper extremity.
- For some individuals, the flow rate down the vertebral artery is too great and blood is stolen from the cerebrum resulting in ischemia.

Location of Disease

- Origin of the left subclavian artery
- Subclavian artery (either side)
- Right innominate artery

Differential Diagnosis

- Arteritis
- Tumor
- Multiple sclerosis
- Cerebellar degeneration or neoplasm
- Neurologic

Diagnostic Modalities

- Duplex ultrasonography
- CT angiography
- MR angiography
- Angiography

Medical Treatment

None

Surgical Treatment

- Carotid-subclavian artery bypass
- Endarterectomy
- Subclavian transposition
- Vertebral transposition
- Subclavian endarterectomy
- Brachiocephalic endarterectomy
- Aorto-subclavian bypass

Endovascular Treatment

- Angioplasty
- Stenting

Points to Remember

- The majority of subclavian steal cases occur on the left side (3 times more than the right side).[121]
- Most cases of physiologic steal are neurologically asymptomatic. [122]

Superior Vena Cava (SVC) Syndrome

Obstruction of the superior vena cava due to thrombosis or extrinsic compression.

Etiology

- Central venous interventions (e.g., central catheters, pacemakers)
- Malignancy, with or without lymphadenopathy (esp. of lung and thorax)
- Histoplasmosis (fungal disease)
- Genetic prothrombotic conditions (clotting disorders, such as Factor V Leiden)
- Radiation therapy to the thorax

Risk Factors

- Cancers/lymphoma of the head, neck, thorax regions
- Central catheterization
- Cardiac pacemaker

Mechanism of Disease

- Decreased venous return from the head, neck and upper extremities can result in extremity edema, headaches, facial swelling, dilated torso veins and in extreme cases, respiratory embarrassment. [149]

Location of Disease

- Superior vena cava

Differential Diagnosis

- Acute respiratory distress
- COPD/emphysema
- Aortic dissection
- Mediastinitis
- Pericarditis
- Pneumonia
- Syphilis
- Tuberculosis

Diagnostic Modalities

- X-ray
- Duplex ultrasonography
- CT angiography
- MRI
- Venography
- IVUS

Medical Treatment

- Elevation of head during nighttime hours
- Limit daily episodes of bending over
- Clothing: loose collars
- Diuretics to reduce edema
- Anticoagulation

Surgical Treatment

- SVC reconstruction (using femoral vein, spiral saphenous, PTFE, allograft or cryopreserved homografts)
- Removal of external compression (e.g., tumor resection)

Endovascular Treatment

- Thrombolysis
- Angioplasty and stenting

Points to Remember

- Malignancies are the chief cause of SVC syndrome. [149]
- The severity of symptoms depends on the degree of collateral circulation.[150]
- Chemotherapy and radiotherapy may relieve symptoms in patients suffering from SVC syndrome caused by malignancies (extrinsic compression).[150]

Thoracic Outlet Compression Syndrome

Compression of the brachial plexus, subclavian artery or subclavian vein in the *thoracic outlet* or space between the collarbone and first rib of the upper extremity, resulting in symptoms of pain or neurologic deficit.

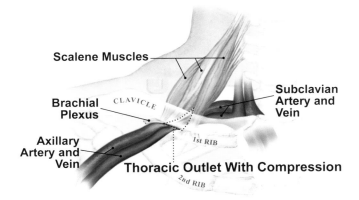

Thoracic Outlet With Compression

Etiology

- Congenital (cervical rib, costoclavicular tendon)
- Trauma
- Occupational related injury
- Sports related injury
- Vasculitis
- Atherosclerosis
- Thrombus
- Embolization from the subclavian or axillary arteries
- Aneurysm
- Pseudoaneurysm
- Intimal hyperplasia
- Traumatic occlusion
- Extrinsic compression
- Radiation arteritis

Risk Factors

- Age (young)
- Males > females
- Athletic, active lifestyle
- Family history
- Obesity
- History of radiation

Mechanism of Disease

- There are three types of thoracic outlet syndrome (TOS): neurogenic, venous and arterial. [46] All result from mechanical compression of the subclavian vein, artery or brachial plexus in the thoracic outlet region. One cause may be an anatomical defect such as congenital abnormalities of the first rib or fracture of the clavicle, which would be a source of compression.
- Types of thoracic outlet syndrome [107, 108]
  - **Neurogenic** (most common): compression of the brachial plexus from the cervical ribs, first rib, anterior scalene muscles, congenital myofascial bands and ligaments.
  - **Venous:** also known as ***effort thrombosis*** or ***Paget-Schroetter syndrome*** results from repetitive trauma to the subclavian vein (SCV). Arm abduction causes the SCV to be compressed against the first rib and scalenus anticus muscle, resulting in this trauma. Venous trauma may result in venous thrombosis. [109]
  - **Arterial** (least common): The head of the humerus can cause arterial compression when the arm is abducted and externally rotated. Due to such repetitive extrinsic compression of the SCA, post-stenotic dilatation or frank aneurysm develops. The typical pathogenesis then is focal compression, dilation, ulceration, and thrombus formation. [1]
    - Most of these patients will present with thromboembolic symptoms.
    - Patients also present with ischemic complications secondary to repeated episodes of embolization.

- Venous or arterial compression results in:
  - **Stenosis:** significant narrowing of the artery or vein decreasing the vessel lumen and possibly resulting in decreased blood flow.
  - **Occlusion:** plaque, thrombus, or external compression of the artery completely blocking blood flow in that arterial segment.
  - **Embolization:** contents of a plaque and/or fragments of an organized thrombus become lodged in a distant blood vessel.
  - **Swelling:** significant compression of the subclavian vein causes limb swelling.

Location of Disease

- Subclavian vein
- Subclavian or axillary artery
- Brachial plexus

Differential Diagnosis

- Spinal stenosis
- Carpal tunnel syndrome
- Nerve impingement (herniated disc)
- Raynaud's disease
- Venous thrombosis
- Neuropathy
- Muscle/tendon strains or tears
- Arthritis
- Tumors, including Pancoast's tumors (lung tumor which grows in the thoracic area)
- Degenerative spinal chord diseases (MS)
- Orthopedic shoulder problems
- Angina pectoris

Diagnostic Modalities

- Non-invasive arterial vascular testing
  - UE including volume pulse recording and digital testing
  - Duplex ultrasonography
- X-ray (chest, cervical spine)
- Electromyography
- Nerve conductivity testing
- CT angiography
- MRI
- MR angiography
- Arteriography
- Positional venography

Medical Treatment

- Modify risk factors
- Anti-inflammatory medication (e.g., aspirin)
- Muscle relaxants
- Physical therapy
- Nerve block treatments
- Anticoagulation (warfarin)
- Thrombolytic therapy (acute blockage)

Surgical Treatment

- Thoracic outlet decompression
- Removal of the first rib or cervical rib
- Dividing scalene muscle attachments and fibromuscular bands
- Cervical sympathectomy
- Resection of aneurysmal disease with bypass grafting
- Embolectomy
- Bypass grafting

Endovascular Treatment

- Thrombolysis
- Angioplasty
- Stent

Points to Remember

- The cause of TOS is neurogenic in 93% of cases. A venous cause is present in 5%, while an arterial cause is present in only 1% of cases. [108]
- In cases of venous compression, the severity of symptoms relates to the length of the thrombosed segment and activity level of the patient.
- "White-finger syndrome" resulting in small artery vasospasm can occur with the repetitive use of vibrating tools. [110]
- Weight training can result in muscle enlargement significant enough to cause compression in the thoracic outlet. [86]

Varicose Veins

Elongated, dilated, tortuous veins which are most commonly found in the lower extremities.

- **Primary varicosities** occur without deep venous incompetence
- **Secondary varicosities** caused by vein thrombosis or deep valvular incompetence

Etiology

- Genetic
- History of venous thrombosis

Risk Factors

- Age (greater with advanced age)
- Female
- Pregnancy
- Obesity
- Occupations requiring long periods of standing
- Family history
- Congenital abnormalities (e.g., Klippel-Trenaunay)
- Arteriovenous fistula (acquired or congenital)

Mechanism of Disease

The pathogenesis of primary varicose veins remains unclear. Initially it was thought that varicose veins are due to valvular incompetence. [172] However, a current hypothesis states that alterations in vein wall structure (cells and extracellular matrix) cause weakness and altered tone, leading to valvular dysfunction.

There is a decrease in the elastin content of varicose vein walls. There is also a change in the ratio of type I to type III collagen, with an increase in type I (rigid, provides tensile strength) and a decrease in type III (compliant, increases elasticity). These changes undoubtedly contribute to the weakening of the varicose vein wall.

The degradation of the extracellular matrix (ECM) is a function of matrix metalloproteinases and their inhibitors. An increase in matrix degradation would weaken the wall, while a decrease could promote ECM accumulation. Reports have varied on whether their levels remain the same, increase or decrease in varicose veins. [172]

Interspersed in varicose veins are thick (2-fold thicker than normal veins) and thin regions (2-fold thinner than normal veins). [173] In the thick regions, smooth muscle cells are no longer organized in circumferential and longitudinal bundles but disrupted by an increased amount of fibrous tissue. The intima is thickened with an increase in smooth muscle cells. In the thin regions, there is a decrease in cell number. The adventitia is thin and lacks vasa vasorum. These regions correspond to areas of dilatation.

Varicose veins demonstrate decreased ability to contract normally [136] and the valves of varicosed veins become stretched. [42]

Branches of the great saphenous vein (GSV) are thought to varicose before the main trunk of the GSV [42] because they contain fewer smooth muscle cells in their vessel walls and lack support in the subcutaneous fat layer under the skin, where they are commonly located. [137]

Pregnancy increases the amount blood circulating in the cardiovascular system and causes veins to enlarge. The pressure of the gravid uterus on veins decreases the blood flow back through the pelvic venous system. [42,127,138]

Location of Disease (in order of typical occurrence)

- Below-knee great saphenous vein and its tributaries
- Above-knee great saphenous vein
- Saphenofemoral junction
- Any other superficial or deep venous segment

Differential Diagnosis

- Nerve compression
- Arthritis
- Deep venous thrombosis
- Peripheral neuritis
- Stasis dermatitis
- Klippel-Trenaunay
- Lymphatic obstruction

Diagnostic Modalities

- Duplex ultrasonography
- Continuous-wave Doppler
- Plethysmography
- Venography

Medical Treatment

- Compression stockings
- Injection sclerotherapy
- Ultrasound-guided sclerotherapy

Endovascular Treatment

- Radiofrequency ablation
- Laser ablation
- Transilluminated power phlebectomy

Surgical Treatment

- Ligation/stripping (of saphenofemoral junction, for example)
- Stab avulsion phlebectomy
- Valve transplant

Points to Remember

- Varicose veins can occur anywhere in the body, though they are usually located in the leg.

- Approximately 20-25% of American women and 10-15% of American men suffer from some type of varicose veins (VV). Higher estimates have been reported. [139, 140]

- Approximately 50% of those over 50 years of age have VV. [138]

- If both parents had VV, there are estimates that there is a 90% chance of developing them. If you are male and only one parent had VV, the chances of developing VV is 25%. If you are female the chances of developing VV is 62%. Even if neither parent had VV, there is still a 20% chance of developing VV. [136]

- Spiders veins are not true varicose veins and are oftentimes thought to be related to hormonal changes.[138]

- Varicose veins may return after treatment.

- **Klippel-Trenaunay syndrome** is a congenital condition characterized by port-wine stains on the skin, varicosed veins and excessive limb growth. Either one limb or multiple limbs may be affected. In some cases, deep veins are abnormal (absent segments, smaller diameters or dilated veins and/or lack of venous valves).[133, 141]

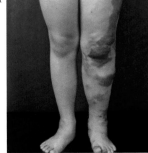

Klippel-Trenaunay syndrome exhibiting port-wine stains and varicosities of the left leg
Image courtesy of
Byung-Boong Lee MD PhD FACS

- Varicose veins can improve post-partum. The number and severity of varicose veins can increase with each additional pregnancy. [42, 138]

- Birth control pills can increase the risk of varicose/spider veins. [138]

Vasculitis

Inflammation of the vessel wall resulting in damage to the blood vessel. This can occur in all blood vessels and is classified based on vessel size: large, medium or small vessel vasculitis.

Etiology

- Autoimmune
- Infection
- Radiation therapy
- Drug abuse

Risk Factors

- Age (young, for some types of arteritis)
- Female
- Arthritic conditions (e.g. polymyalgia rheumatica, which is often seen with temporal arteritis)
- Far Eastern, Asian or Middle Eastern descent
- Young, Japanese and Korean males (Kawasaki disease)
- HIV positive

Mechanism of Disease

- Relatively little is known about the causes of vasculitis. Genetics, infectious and toxic factors are suspected. Since there are wide variations in patient demographics and histopathological findings for vasculitis, they likely have significant differences as well as similarities in their pathogenic pathways.

- Giant cell arteritis, a large vessel vasculitis is the most common type of vasculitis and the most studied. The following is a brief description of the pathogenic mechanisms:[83,84,85,86]

  - Giant cell arteritis, is a T-cell dependent disease. Next to the external elastic lamina are resident dendritic cells. *Dendritic cells* are antigen-presenting cells required for the activation of T-cells in vessel walls.

  - In a healthy vessel, dendritic cells are characterized as immature and unactivated.

  - Mature dendritic cells are required for the activation of T-cells. The maturation and activation of dendritic cells is considered to be the first step in the pathogenesis of giant cell arteritis. There is a significant increase in the number of dendritic cells in the adventitia during giant cell arteritis.

  - Circulating T-cells exit the blood only if endothelial cells have been activated. T-cells bind activated endothelial cells and then migrate into the vessel wall. In giant cell arteritis, this occurs in the vasa vasorum, not in the macrolumen.

  - The other requirement for the departure of T-cells is the synthesis of chemokines in the tissue. *Chemokines* are chemotactic cytokines, which induce directed chemotaxis. *Chemotaxis* is the migration of cells along a chemical concentration gradient. Activated dendritic cells synthesize chemokines, which attract T-cells.

  - *Granulomas* are small delineated collections of immune cells, primarily macrophages that are highly activated. The formation of granulomas in the media is dependent upon T-cells. The T-cells in the adventitia release interferon-gamma, which recruits and activates macrophages. These interferon-gamma stimulated macrophages are responsible for the granulomatous reaction.

- Macrophages synthesize *matrix metalloproteinases (MMPs)* which are thought to be responsible for the fragmentation of the internal elastic lamina. Macrophages also mediate oxidative stress which causes smooth muscle cell injury and *apoptosis*, programmed cell death.

- Macrophages join together to form giant cells, which may be present along the fragmented internal elastic lamina. In the adventitia, they optimize T-cell stimulation by the release of pro-inflammatory cytokines.

- Giant cell arteritis can lead to ischemia if there is occlusion of the lumen. This is caused by rapid concentric intimal hyperplasia. Rarely does thrombotic occlusion contribute to the blockage of blood flow.

- The critical growth factor for intimal hyperplasia is most likely *platelet derived growth factor* (PDGF), as it correlates with the degree of luminal stenosis. Smooth muscle cells synthesize PDGF, but the predominate sources are macrophages and giant cells.

- In healthy vessels, the vasa vasorum is limited to the adventitia. In giant cell arteritis neovascularization of the media and hyperplastic intima occurs through the formation of microvessels. The number of neocapillaries correlates with the level of *vascular endothelial growth factor (VEGF)*, a stimulator of angiogenesis. Macrophages and giant cells are the primary producers of the VEGF.

- In Takayasu's arteritis, another large vessel vasculitis, T-cells may contribute to the weakening of the wall by secreting *perforin*, a pore-forming protein.

- Radiation therapy causes injury to the vasa vasorum and necrosis of the vessel wall. Endothelial cells lining the arterial walls of vessels in the irradiated field are susceptible to damage. Lipid-containing plaques can then form in the intimal layer of the artery. [87]

Location of Disease

- Superficial temporal artery
- Aortic artery
- Renal artery
- External iliac artery
- Mesenteric artery
- Subclavian artery
- Axillary artery
- Innominate artery
- Carotid arteries

Types [63, 64, 651]

Large Vessel

- **Takayasu's arteritis**: predominately affects the aorta and its branches, usually causing a dilatation and an aneurysm, stenosis rarely occurs.
- **Giant cell arteritis** (temporal arteritis): affects medium and large size vessels. The extracranial branches of the carotid, especially the temporal artery, are susceptible. Affects persons older than 50 years of age, especially those who are 75 - 85 years of age.

Medium Vessel

- **Kawasaki disease**: affects small and medium sized arteries (including coronary) in young children between the ages of 2-5 years of age.
- **Behcet's disease**: results in mouth/genital sores, inflammation of the eyes.

- **Churg-Strauss angiitis**: affects the nose, sinuses, lungs, nerves and intestines.
- **Polyarteritis nodosa**: occurs in any organ, resulting in aneurysm, thrombosis, hemorrhage or tissue infarction.

Small Vessel

- **Wegener's granulomatosis**: necrotizing vasculitis involving the kidney or upper/lower respiratory tracts
- **Henoch-Schonlein purpura**: affects kidneys
- **Essential cryoglobulinemia**: caused by abnormal proteins in the blood which affect the spleen, skin, nerves and kidneys
- **Arteritis of connective tissue** (e.g., systemic lupus erythematosus, rheumatoid arthritis)
- **Microscopic polyangiitis**: affects kidneys, lung, nerves, skin, and joints

Differential Diagnosis

- Childhood diseases (e.g., scarlet fever)
- Juvenile rheumatoid arthritis
- Toxic shock syndrome
- Measles
- Epstein-Barr syndrome
- Crohn's disease
- Marfan's syndrome
- Ehlers-Danlos syndrome
- Sarcoidosis
- Aortic dissection
- Appendicitis
- Cholecystitis
- Intestinal perforation

Diagnostic Modalities

- Duplex ultrasonography
- MRI
- MR angiography
- CT angiography
- Angiography

Medical Treatment

- Aspirin therapy
- Corticosteroids

Surgical Treatment

- Biopsy of affected tissue (e.g., of temporal arteries to confirm diagnosis of giant cell arteritis)
- Bypass

Endovascular Treatment

- Angioplasty (percutaneous or coronary)
- Stenting

Points to Remember

- Arteritis is a type of "vasculitis" or "angiitis."
- The American College of Rheumatology in 1990 and the Chapel Hill Consensus Conference in 1994 developed definitions for classification. However, these classifications of vasculitis are limited and controversial. Efforts are underway to improve the criteria used in the diagnosis and classification of vasculitis. [91,92]
- Giant cell arteritis is typically seen in Caucasian women >50 years of age. The mean age is 72 years. [93]
- Women develop temporal arteritis 2-3 times more than men. [93]
- Takayasu's arteritis primarily affects females (80-90%) under the age of 50 years, especially those between 20-40 years of age. [94]
  - Takayasu's arteritis is more frequent in Asia and India than in Western Europe or North America. [95]

– Japanese with Takayasu's arteritis have a higher incidence of aortic arch involvement. The arteries most commonly involved in US patients suffering from Takayasu's arteritis are the left subclavian, superior mesenteric and abdominal aorta. [94]

- Kawasaki's disease most commonly affects the Japanese-American population. Outside of the US, the disease most frequently occurs in Japan. [96]

   – Japanese children exhibit the disease at a younger age (6-12 months) than American children (18-24 months).[96]

   – In the US, Kawasaki disease patients are most commonly middle and upper-middle class children.[96]

   – Kawasaki's disease is 1.5 times more common in males than females. [96]

- Behcet's disease is uncommon in the US. It is common in the Mediterranean, Middle and Far Eastern regions. [87,97]

   – Men are affected more often than women by Behcet's disease (in some regions 24:1). The disease also seems to be more severe in men. [97]

- Aneurysms will form in the aorta but not in medium size arteries.

Venous Insufficiency (Postphlebitic Syndrome)

Inadequate venous return resulting in an increase in ambulatory venous pressure. Symptoms range from varicose veins to swelling and ulceration.

Etiology

- Venous hypertension, caused by valve damage or dysfunction
- History of venous thrombosis
- Genetic factors

Risk Factors

- History of venous thrombosis
- Occupations requiring long periods of standing or sitting
- Female
- Family history
- Pregnancy
- Obesity
- Smoking
- Age (greater with advanced age)

When the leg is in motion, (walking) muscle contractions squeeze the veins, forcing blood past the open valves of the deep, superficial and perforating veins upward towards the heart. After the muscle relaxes, valves close to prevent backflow (reflux).

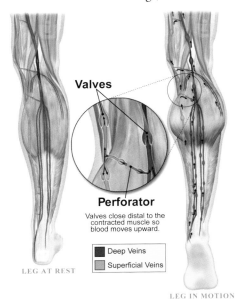

Valves

Perforator

Valves close distal to the contracted muscle so blood moves upward.

■ Deep Veins
■ Superficial Veins

LEG AT REST

LEG IN MOTION

Mechanism of Disease

- The calf muscle pump functions to move blood from the superficial to the deep venous system through *perforators* or communicating veins. [42]
- Venous valves serve to propagate blood flow back toward the heart and prevent retrograde flow (*reflux*) back down the venous segment. [42]
- Valvular damage and dysfunction (*valvular incompetence*) results in venous reflux and subsequent venous hypertension. [130] When one suffers from *ambulatory venous hypertension*, there is an abnormally high venous pressure on standing. When the calf muscle pumps the blood, it is expelled in any direction due to dysfunction of the valves. Subsequently, venous pressures do not decrease normally.[42]
- Venous hypertension increases pressures within the venules and capillaries. Local edema results in a decrease in fluid and protein reabsorption. Fibrinogen and red blood cells (RBC) escape into the tissues. Proteins organize and form tissue fibrosis. The RBCs break down and cause hyperpigmentation. This fibrotic, hyperpigmented condition is known as *lipodermatosclerosis*. Oxygen intake is decreased in the tissues causing tissue malnutrition/hypoxia. Ulceration may follow. [42, 131]

Location of Disease

- Gaiter area (most common): medial aspect of the leg, just above the medial malleolus
- Lateral or posterior calf

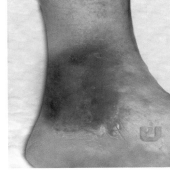

Venous ulcerations in the gaiter area can result from venous insufficiency

Differential Diagnosis

- Arterial disease
- Lymphedema
- Cellulitis
- Collagen vasculitis
- Skin cancer

Diagnostic Modalities

- Duplex ultrasonography
- Plethysmography
- Continuous-wave Doppler
- Descending venography

Medical Treatment

- Compression stockings
- Periods of leg elevation
- Proper skin care
- Compression bandaging (ulceration)
- Sclerotherapy

Surgical Treatment

- GSV or SSV stripping/ ligation
- Subfascial ligation of perforators
- Subfascial endoscopic perforator vein surgery
- Transverse repair of incompetent valves
- Ambulatory phlebectomy

Endovascular Treatment

- Radiofrequency ablation of GSV, SSV, or perforators

Points to Remember

- Approximately 2 - 5% of Americans suffer from venous insufficiency. [132]
- Approximately 500,000 Americans suffer from venous ulceration. [127, 132]
- A congenital absence of valves (as in Klippel Trenaunay syndrome) is extremely rare. When it does occur, it can affect the entire body or just the extremities (legs >arms). [133]
- Studies estimate than 80% of patients with a history of DVT will develop chronic venous insufficiency. [127]
- The American Venous Forum has developed a classification system for chronic venous disease called CEAP which categorizes; clinical class (C), etiology (E), anatomic location (A) and pathological mechanism (P). Classification examples include: [134,135]
  - Category "C1" relates to telangectasias
  - Category "C2" relates to varicose veins
  - Categories "C3" and "C4" relate to edema and skin changes, such as eczema
  - Category "C5" relates to healed ulceration
  - Category "C6" relates to active ulceration

Venous Thrombosis

The obstruction of venous outflow within a deep or superficial vein by thrombus.

Etiology

- The theory of Virchow's Triad states that venous thrombosis is caused by: venous stasis, vein wall (intimal) injury or a hypercoaguable state.
- Varicose veins
- Extrinsic compression (e.g., Paget-Schroetter, May-Thurner syndromes)

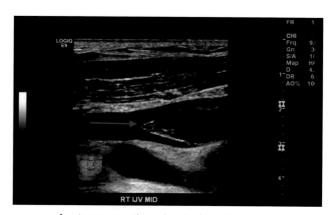

Acute venous thrombosis; free-floating tail located in the internal jugular vein

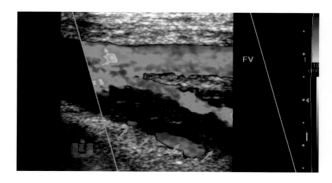

Acute thrombus: free-floating tail in the deep femoral vein

Risk Factors

- Age (greater with advanced age)
- Immobilization
- Genetic prothrombotic conditions (clotting disorders, such as Factor V Leiden)
- Post-operative phase (especially after orthopedic surgery)
- Central venous or femoral catheters
- Female
- Pregnancy
- Oral contraceptives
- Estrogen replacement
- Cancer/malignancy
- Previous DVT
- Heart complications (MI, CHF, etc.)
- Obesity
- Family history
- Smoking
- COPD
- Blood type (highest risk with type-A lowest risk with type-O)
- Trauma
- Antiphospholipid antibodies (lupus, etc.)
- Occupations requiring long period of standing or sitting
- Varicose veins
- Congenital abnormalities (Klippel-Trenaunay)
- Inflammatory bowel disease
- Drug abuse
- Cerebrovascular events (stroke, TIA)
- May-Thurner syndrome

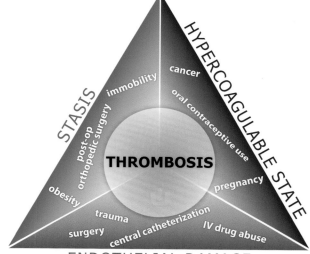

Virchow's Triad with examples of risk factors that can lead to thrombosis

Mechanism of Disease

- There are three factors responsible for the formation of venous thrombosis, as outlined in Virchow's Triad: vein wall injury, hypercoagulability and stasis of blood flow. A combination of any of these events may result in venous thrombosis. [125]

- There is a balance in normal blood flow between *coagulation* (the process to prevent excessive bleeding after injury) and *anticoagulation* (the process to prevent spontaneous intravascular clotting).

- The venous endothelial layer is normally antithrombotic. In response to endothelial injury, leukocytes (white blood cells) attach to the vessel wall. A plasma protein known as *prothrombin* is activated. Prothrombin activator, (activated Factor X (Xa)) catalyzes conversion of prothrombin into thrombin. Thrombin is an enzyme that converts fibrinogen into fibrin threads, forming a clot. [125]

- Hypercoaguable states result from genetic mutation or acquired deficiencies that accompany certain diseases (e.g., liver disease). In such cases, naturally occurring anticoagulants (antithrombin, protein C, protein S, etc.) are deficient. [124]

- One genetic mutation, factor V Leiden, causes resistance to the natural anticoagulant protein C. [126]

- Non-movement of blood flow (stasis) permits coagulation. Platelets are thought to become trapped due to flow recirculation behind the valve cusps. Platelets adhere to the subendothelial (or collagen) layer of the venous wall and may aggregate depending on the amount of coagulation and thrombolysis occurring in the body at the time. [127]

- Increased activation of coagulation factors in cancer is thought to lead to formation of venous thrombosis. In addition, the levels of coagulation inhibitors (e.g., proteins C or S) in the blood are thought to be reduced. [127]

- Thrombosis in pregnancy is attributed to a prothrombotic state [124] along with decreased venous outflow due to the weight of the fetus. [127]

- The use of estrogen (in replacement therapy or contraceptives) alters coagulation and may predispose an individual to thrombosis. [127]

- Once a thrombus is formed, it can remain stable, propagate or shed/embolize:

  - *Stabilize*: Stabilization includes adherence of the thrombus to the vessel wall without changing location or propagating. If a thrombus has formed, the most favorable occurrence would be stabilization. This reduces the risk to the individual.

  - *Propagate*: Propagation includes "growth of thrombus" in size or location. The most notable importance of propagation is the possibility that a superficial thrombus might propagate into the deep system.

  - *Shed/Embolize*: A portion of a thrombus breaks free and travels elsewhere within the vascular system. The greatest risk is that the thrombus travels to the lungs and causes a pulmonary embolism.

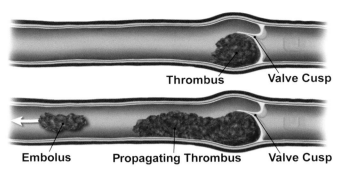

Thrombosis of a vein; Should a piece of the thrombus break off or "shed", an embolism may occur upstream

Location of Disease

- Muscular veins (gastrocnemius and soleal sinus)
- Behind venous valves
- Venous confluences
- Deep venous system (common femoral, deep femoral, femoral, popliteal, peroneal, posterior tibial, anterior tibial, jugular, innominate, subclavian, axillary, brachial, radial, ulnar, inferior vena cava and iliac veins)
- Superficial venous system (great saphenous, small saphenous, basilic, cephalic, median cubital veins)

Differential Diagnosis

- Arterial disease
- Lymphedema
- Cellulitis
- Cysts (popliteal, Baker's, etc.)
- Extrinsic compression
- Hematoma
- Muscle tear
- Joint effusion
- Adenopathy
- Arteriovenous fistula
- Heart failure (edema)
- Direct injury to extremity
- Vascularized mass
- Collagen vasculitis
- Abscess

Diagnostic Modalities

- Duplex ultrasonography
- Venogram
- MRI
- CT angiography

Medical Treatment

- Serial venous duplex exams to monitor for change
- Anticoagulation therapy (e.g., heparin, low-molecular weight heparin or warfarin)
- DVT prophylaxis (e.g., intermittent pneumatic cuff)
- Limit long periods of inactivity
- Promote venous drainage (e.g., elevate legs, wear elastic stocking/support hose)

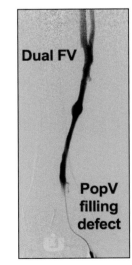

Venogram showing partial popliteal vein thrombosis

Surgical Treatment

- IVC filter
- Iliofemoral venous thrombectomy
- Bypass grafting (caval occlusion)
- SVC reconstruction (using femoral vein, spiral saphenous, PTFE or cryopreserved grafts)

Endovascular Treatment

- Catheter-directed thrombolysis with Urokinase, etc. (acute DVT)
- Balloon venoplasty and stenting (chronic iliofemoral DVT)
- Mechanical catheter directed thrombectomy (acute DVT)
- Percutaneous transluminal angioplasty and stenting (SVC syndrome)

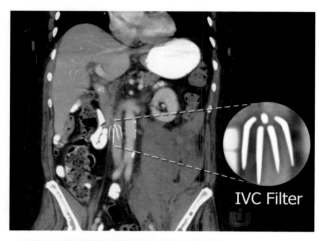

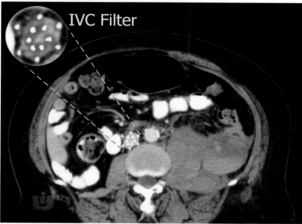

IVC filter on CT angiogram

Points to Remember

- Clinical diagnosis of DVT based on patient's symptoms and history is not very reliable (<50%).[128]
- A thrombus frequently originates at a valve cusp site or in the soleal veins. [103]
- The length of the thrombosed segment, the number of veins involved and the degree of collateralization all effect the presentation of venous symptoms. [42]
- "Economy class syndrome," where travel passengers have been exposed to cramped positions for extended periods of time, can result in venous thrombosis. Venous stasis during travel may increase the incidents of clot formation for those already at risk for venous thrombosis due to other risk factors. [103]
- Von Willebrand factor (vWF) is a blood protein activated by thrombin early in the coagulation process to help promote clotting by binding with platelets. [100,129] Patients with vWF deficiency or dysfunction (Von Willebrand Disease) have bleeding complications, (GI bleeds, nosebleeds, etc). This disease can be inherited or acquired and occurs in approximately 1 - 2% of the population. [129]

- A pulmonary embolism can occur when a portion or an entire thrombus breaks loose and travels to the lungs.
- Differentiation of chronic DVT versus acute DVT may be difficult.

References

1. Zarins CK, Xu C, Glagov S. (2005). Artery wall pathology in atherosclerosis. In Rutherford Vascular Surgery 6th edition. (123-148). Philadelphia. Elsevier Saunders.
2. Curci JA, Baxter TB, Thompson RW. (2005). Artery aneurysms. In Rutherford Vascular Surgery 6th edition. (475-492). Philadelphia. Elsevier Saunders.
3. Wassef M, Upchurch Jr GR, et al. (2007). "Challenges and opportunities in abdominal aortic aneurysm research." Journal of Vascular Surgery 45(1): 192-198.
4. Zarins CK, Xu C., et al. (2001). "Atherosclerotic enlargement of the human abdominal aorta." Atherosclerosis 155(1): 157-164.
5. Lindeman JH, Ashcroft BA, Beenakker JW, van Es M, Koekkoek NB, Prins FA, Tielemans JF, Abdul-Hussien H, Bank RA, Oosterkamp TH. Distinct defects in collagen microarchitecture underlie vessel-wall failure in advanced abdominal aneurysms and aneurysms in Marfan syndrome. (2010). Proc Natl Acad Sci U S A. Jan 12;107(2):862-5.
6. López-Candales A, Holmes DR, Liao S, Scott MJ, Wickline SA, Thompson RW. Decreased vascular smooth muscle cell density in medial degeneration of human abdominal aortic aneurysms. (1997). Am J Pathol. March; 150(3): 993–1007.
7. Henderson, E. L., Y.-J. Geng, et al. (1999). "Death of Smooth Muscle Cells and Expression of Mediators of Apoptosis by T Lymphocytes in Human Abdominal Aortic Aneurysms." Circulation 99(1): 96-104.
8. Allaire E, Muscatelli-Groux B., et al. (2002). "Paracrine effect of vascular smooth muscle cells in the prevention of aortic aneurysm formation." Journal of Vascular Surgery 36(5): 1018-1026.
9. Karnik, S. K., B. S. Brooke, et al. (2003). "A critical role for elastin signaling in vascular morphogenesis and disease." Development 130(2): 411-423.
10. Patel, M. I., J. Melrose, et al. (1996). "Increased synthesis of matrix metalloproteinases by aortic smooth muscle cells is implicated in the etiopathogenesis of abdominal aortic aneurysms." Journal of Vascular Surgery 24(1): 82-92.
11. Abdul-Hussien, H., R. G. V. Soekhoe, et al. (2007). "Collagen Degradation in the Abdominal Aneurysm: A Conspiracy of Matrix Metalloproteinase and Cysteine Collagenases." The American Journal of Pathology 170(3): 809-817.
12. Krettek, A., G. K. Sukhova, et al. (2003). "Elastogenesis in human arterial disease: a role for macrophages in disordered elastin synthesis." Arteriosclerosis, thrombosis, and vascular biology 23(4): 582-587.
13. Szilagyi, D. E., R. F. Smith, et al. (1966). "Contribution of abdominal aortic aneurysmectomy to prolongation of life." Annals of Surgery 164(4): 678-699.
14. Sterpetti, A. V., A. Cavallaro, et al. (1991). "Factors influencing the rupture of abdominal aortic aneurysms." Surgery, Gynecology & Obstetrics 173(3): 1750178.
15. Darling, R. C., C. R. Messina, et al. (1977). "Autopsy study of unoperated abdominal aortic aneurysms. The case for early resection." Circulation 56(3 Suppl): II161-164.
16. Hellmann, D. B., D. J. Grand, et al. (2007). "Inflammatory Abdominal Aortic Aneurysm." JAMA: The Journal of the American Medical Association 297(4): 395-400.
17. Walker, D. I., K. Bloor, et al. (1972). "Inflammatory aneurysms of the abdominal aorta." British Journal of Surgery 59(8): 609-614.
18. Abdul-Hussien, H., R. Hanemaaijer, et al. (2010). "The pathophysiology of abdominal aortic aneurysm growth: corresponding and discordant inflammatory and proteolytic processes in abdominal aortic and popliteal artery aneurysms." Journal of vascular surgery: official publication, the Society for Vascular Surgery [and] International Society for Cardiovascular Surgery, North American Chapter 51(6): 1479-1487.
19. Ritman, E. L. and A. Lerman (2007). "The dynamic vasa vasorum." Cardiovascular research 75(4): 649-658.
20. Halka AT, Turner NJ, Carter A, Ghosh J, Murphy MO, Kirton JP, Kielty CM, Walker MG. (2008). The effects of stretch on vascular smooth muscle cell phenotype in vitro. Cardiovascular Pathology. (98-102). March-April;17(3).
21. Stary HC, Chandler AB, Glagov S, Guyton JR, Insull W, Rosenfeld ME, Schaffer SA, Schwartz CJ, Wagner WD, Wissler RW. A definition of intimal, fatty streak and intermediate lesions of atherosclerosis. (2462-2478). Circulation 1994; 89.
22. Glagov S, Weisenberd E, Zarins C, et al. (1987). Compensatory enlargement of human atherosclerotic coronary arteries. (1371-5). N Engl J Med; 316.
23. Stary HC, Chandler AB, Dinsmore RE, Fuster V, Glagov S, Insull W, Rosenfeld ME, Schwartz CJ, Wagner WD, Wissler RW. A definition of advanced types of atherosclerotic lesions and histological classification of atherosclerosis. Atherosclerosis, Thrombosis and Vascular Biology. 1995; 15; 1521-1531.
24. Easton JD, Saver JL., et al. (2009). "Definition and Evaluation of Transient Ischemic Attack." Stroke 40(6): 2276-2293.
25. Bamford J, Sandercock P., et al. (1987). "The natural history of lacunar infarction: the Oxfordshire Community Stroke Project." Stroke 18(3): 545-551.
26. Petty GW, Brown RD, et al. (2000). "Ischemic Stroke Subtypes: A Population-Based Study of Functional Outcome, Survival, and Recurrence." Stroke 31(5): 1062-1068.
27. Torvik, A. (1984). "The pathogenesis of watershed infarcts in the brain." Stroke 15(2): 221-223.
28. Mangla R, Kolar B., et al. (2011). "Border Zone Infarcts: Pathophysiologic and Imaging Characteristics." Radiographics 31(5): 1201-1214.
29. Momjian-Mayor I, and Baron JC., (2005). "The Pathophysiology of Watershed Infarction in Internal Carotid Artery Disease." Stroke 36(3): 567-577.
30. Vermeer SE, Longstreth Jr WT., et al. (2007). "Silent brain infarcts: a systematic review." The Lancet Neurology 6(7): 611-619.
31. Morgenstern LB, Hemphill JC, et al. (2010). "Guidelines for the Management of Spontaneous Intracerebral Hemorrhage." Stroke 41(9): 2108-2129.
32. Adams HP, del Zoppo G, et al. (2007). "Guidelines for the Early Management of Adults With Ischemic Stroke." Stroke 38(5): 1655-1711.
33. Mitchell ME, Sidaway AN. (2005). Basic considerations of the arterial wall in health and disease. In Rutherford Vascular Surgery 6th edition. (62-75). Philadelphia. Elsevier Saunders.
34. Schermerhorn ML, Cronenwett JL. (2005). Abdominal aortic and iliac aneurysms. In Rutherford Vascular Surgery 6th edition. (1408-1452). Philadelphia. Elsevier Saunders.
35. Shepard RJ, Rooke T. (2005). Uncommon arteriopathies. In Rutherford Vascular Surgery 6th edition. (453-474). Philadelphia. Elsevier Saunders.

36. Reddy DJ, Weaver MR. (2005). Infected aneurysms. In Rutherford Vascular Surgery 6th edition. (1581-1596). Philadelphia. Elsevier Saunders.
37. Gerhard-Herman M, Gardin JM, Jaff M, Mohler E, Roman M, Naqvi TZ. (2006). Guidelines for non-invasive vascular laboratory testing: a report from the American society of echocardiography and the society of vascular medicine and biology. J Am Soc Echocardiogr 19:955-972.
38. Hallett JW, Brewster DC, Rasmussen TE. (2001). Non-invasive vascular testing. In: Handbook of Patient Care in Vascular Diseases. (29-49), Philadelphia Lippincott Williams & Wilkins
39. Nordon IM, Hinchliffe RJ, Loftus IM, Thompson MM. (2010). Pathophysiology and epidemiology of abdominal aortic aneurysms Nat Rev Cardiol. Nov 16.
40. Bickerstaff LK, Pairolero PC, Hollier LH, Melton LJ, Van Peenen HJ, Cherry KJ, Joyce JW, Lie JT. Thoracic aortic aneurysms: a population-based study. (1982). Surgery. Dec;92(6):1103-8.
41. Lawrence PF, Rigberg D. (2010). Arterial aneurysms: general considerations. In Rutherford Vascular Surgery 7th edition. (Chapter 126). Philadelphia. Elsevier Saunders.
42. Sumner DS, Zierler RE. (2005). Vascular physiology: essential hemodynamic principles. In Rutherford Vascular Surgery 6th edition. (75-123). Philadelphia. Elsevier Saunders.
43. Van Bockel JH, Hamming JF. (2005). Lower extremity aneurysm. In Rutherford Vascular Surgery 6th edition. (1534-1551). Philadelphia. Elsevier Saunders.
44. Upchurch GR, Zelenock GB, Stanley JC. (2005). Splanchnic artery aneurysms. In Rutherford Vascular Surgery 6th edition. (1565-1581). Philadelphia. Elsevier Saunders.
45. Isselbacher EM, 2005, "Thoracic and Abdominal Aortic Aneurysms," Circulation, 111(6), pp. 816-828.
46. Clouse WD, Hallett JW Jr., Schaff HV, Spittell PC, Rowland CM, Ilstrup DM, and Melton LJ 3rd, 2004, "Acute Aortic Dissection: Population-Based Incidence Compared with Degenerative Aortic Aneurysm Rupture," Mayo Clinic proceedings. Mayo Clinic, 79(2), pp. 176-80.
47. Centers for medicare and medicaid services. (09/20/2010 1:09:09 PM). Retrieved from https://www.cms.gov/deficitreductionact.
48. Beridze, N. and W. H. Frishman (2012) Byers, P. H. (1994) Nataatmadja, M., M. West, et al. (2003
49. Casey PJ, LaMuraglia GM. (2005). Anastomotic aneurysms. In Rutherford Vascular Surgery 6th edition. (894-902). Philadelphia. Elsevier Saunders.
50. Adams ED, Sidway AN. (2005). Nonthrombotic complications of arteriovenous access for hemodialysis. In Rutherford Vascular Surgery 6th edition. (1692-1706). Philadelphia. Elsevier Saunders.
51. Lumsden AB, Peden E, Bush RL, Lin PH. (2005). Complications of endovascular procedures. In Rutherford Vascular Surgery 6th edition. (809-820). Philadelphia. Elsevier Saunders.
52. Kang, SS, (2005). Pseudoaneurysm: diagnosis and treatment. In Mansour MA, Labropoulos N. (Eds.), Vascular Diagnosis, (319-323). Philadelphia: Elsevier Saunders.
53. Rowe VL, Yellin AE, Weaver FA. (2005). Vascular injuries of the extremities. In Rutherford Vascular Surgery 6th edition. (1044-1058). Philadelphia. Elsevier Saunders.
54. Black JH, Cambria RP. (2005). Aortic dissection: perspectives for the vascular/endovascular surgeon. In Rutherford Vascular Surgery 6th edition. (1512-1533). Philadelphia. Elsevier Saunders.
55. Bickerstaff LK, Pairolero PC, et al. (1982). "Thoracic aortic aneurysms: a population-based study." Surgery 92(6): 1103-1108.
56. Zwiebel, WJ. Pellerito JS. (2005). Carotid occlusion, unusual carotid pathology, and tricky carotid cases. In Zwiebel WJ, Pellerito JS (Eds.), In Introduction to Vascular Ultrasonography 5th ed, (192-210). Philadelphia: Elsevier Saunders.
57. Krupski WC. (2005). Uncommon disorders affecting the carotid arteries. In Rutherford Vascular Surgery 6th edition. (2064-2092). Philadelphia. Elsevier Saunders.
58. Saldana, M. J., L. E. Salem, et al. (1973). "High altitude hypoxia and chemodectomas." Human Pathology 4(2): 251-263.
59. Jech M, Alvarado-Cabrero L, et al. (2006). "Genetic analysis of high altitude paragangliomas." Endocrine Pathology 17(2): 201-202.
60. McNicol A.M. (2010). Adrenal Medulla and Paraganglia in Endocrine Pathology: Differential Diagnosis and Molecular Advances. R.V. Lloyd (Ed). Springer Science + Business Media LLC.
61. Baysal, BE, Ferrell RE, et al. (2000). "Mutations in SDHD, a mitochondrial complex II gene, in hereditary paraganglioma." Science 287(5454): 848-851.
62. Niemann S. and Muller U. (2000). "Mutations in SDHC cause autosomal dominant paraganglioma, type 3." Nature genetics 26(3): 268-270.
63. Astuti, D, Latif F, et al. (2001). "Gene mutations in the succinate dehydrogenase subunit SDHB cause susceptibility to familial pheochromocytoma and to familial paraganglioma." American journal of human genetics 69(1): 49-54.
64. Hao,HX, Khalimonchuk O, et al. (2009). "SDH5, a Gene Required for Flavination of Succinate Dehydrogenase, Is Mutated in Paraganglioma." Science 325(5944): 1139-1142.
65. Baysal B E, McKay SE, et al. (2011). "Genomic imprinting at a boundary element flanking the SDHD locus." Human molecular genetics 20(22): 4452-4461.
66. Neumann, H. P. and Z. Erlic (2008). "Maternal transmission of symptomatic disease with SDHD mutation: fact or fiction?" The Journal of clinical endocrinology and metabolism 93(5): 1573-1575.
67. Mariman EC, van Beersum, SE. et al. (1995). "Fine mapping of a putatively imprinted genefor familial non-chromaffin paragangliomas to chromosome 11q13.1: evidence for genetic heterogeneity." Human Genetics 95(1): 56-62.
68. Van Schothorst, EM, Beekman M, et al. (1998). "Paragangliomas of the head and neck region show complete loss of heterozygosity at 11 q22-q23 in chief cells and the flow-sorted dna aneuploid fraction." Human Pathology. 29(10): 1045-1049.
69. Favier J. Gimenez-Roqueplo AP. (2010). "Pheochromocytomas: the (pseudo)-hypoxia hypothesis." Best practice & research. Clinical endocrinology & metabolism 24(6): 957-968.
70. Baysal BE. (2008). "Clinical and molecular progress in hereditary paraganglioma." Journal of Medical Genetics 45(11): 689-694.
71. Arias-Stella J, Human carotid bodies at high altitutdes. (Abstract) American Journal of Pathology 1969; 55: 82a. (not in endnotes library)
72. Arias-Stella, J. and J. Valcarcel (1973). "The human carotid body at high altitudes." Pathologia et microbiologia 39(3): 292-297.
73. Lack, E. E. (1977). "Carotid body hypertrophy in patients with cystic fibrosis and cyanotic congenital heart disease." Human Pathology 8(1): 39-51.
74. Heath, D., C. Edwards, et al. (1970). "Post-mortem size and structure of the human carotid body." Thorax 25(2): 129-140.
75. Rush BF. Jr. (1963). "Familial bilateral carotid body tumors." Annals of Surgery 157: 633-636.
76. Pratt, LW. (1973). "Familial Carotid Body Tumors." Arch Otolaryngol 97(4): 334-336.
77. Grufferman S, Gillman MW et al. (1980). "Familial carotid body tumors: Case report and epidemiologic review." Cancer 46(9): 2116-2122.
78. Koenigsberg RA, Dastur BS. (1-29-2008). "Imaging of Head and Neck Glomus Tumors" Emedicine. medscape.com Retrieved from http://www.emedicine.medscape.com/article/382908 (12-4-2010).
79. Bayley JP, van Minderhout I, et al. (2006). "Mutation analysis of SDHB and SDHC: novel germline mutations in sporadic head and neck paraganglioma and familial paraganglioma and/or pheochromocytoma." BMC medical genetics 7: 1.
80. Sevilla, MA, Hermsen MA, et al. (2009). "Chromosomal changes in sporadic and familial head and neck paragangliomas." Otolaryngology--head and neck surgery: official journal of American Academy of Otolaryngology-Head and Neck Surgery 140(5): 724-729.
81. Kidwell CS, Burgess RE. (5-25-2010). "Dissection syndromes" Emedicine.medscape.com. http://emedicine.medscape.com/article/1160482 (12-4-2010).
82. Watts, RA and Scott, DGI. (2010). Classification and Epidemiology of Vasculitis in Clinical Practice. RA Watts and DGI Scott, Springer London: 7-11.
83. Weyand, CM and Goronzy, JJ. (2003). "Medium- and Large-Vessel Vasculitis." New England Journal of Medicine 349(2): 160-169.
84. Michael B Gravanis. (2000). "Giant cell arteritis and Takayasu aortitis: morphologic, pathogenetic and etiologic factors." International Journal of Cardiology 75, Supplement 1(0): S21-S33.
85. Yilmaz, A and Arditi M. (2009). "Giant Cell Arteritis." Circulation Research 104(4): 425-427.
86. Weyand, CM, Ma-Krupa W., et al. (2004). "Immunopathways in giant cell arteritis and polymyalgia rheumatica." Autoimmunity Reviews 3(1): 46-53.
87. Shepard RJ, Rooke T. (2005). Uncommon arteriopathies. In *Rutherford Vascular Surgery 6th edition.* (453-474). Philadelphia. Elsevier Saunders.
88. Young JR, Graor RA, Olin JW, Bartholomew JR. (1991*). "Systemic vasculitis" in Peripheral Vascular Diseases.* (339-360). St Louis: Mosby Elsevier Health Science.
89. Young JR, Graor RA, Olin JW, Bartholomew JR. (1991). *"Vasospastic disease" in Peripheral Vascular Diseases.* (361-378). St Louis: Mosby Elsevier Health Science.
90. Young JR, Graor RA, Olin JW, Bartholomew JR. (1991). *Miscellaneous arterial disease" in Peripheral Vascular Diseases.* (379-394). St Louis:Mosby Elsevier Health Science.
91. Basu N, Watts R., et al. (2010). "EULAR points to consider in the development of classification and diagnostic criteria in systemic vasculitis." Annals of the Rheumatic Diseases 69(10): 1744-1750.
92. Watts RA, and Scott DGI., (2010). Classification and Epidemiology of Vasculitis in Clinical Practice. R. A. Watts and D. G. I. Scott, Springer London: 7-11.
93. Johns Hopkins Vasculitis Clinic "Giant cell arteritis" Johns Hopkins Medicine (2009). http://vasculitis.med.jhu.edu/types of/giantcell.html (12-4-2010).
94. Hom C. (8-25-2010). "Takayasu's arteritis" Emedicine.medscape.com. http://emedicine.medscape.com/article/1007566-overview (12-4-2010).
95. Hajj-Ali RA, Mandell B. (2005). Approach to and management of inflammatory vasculitis. In Rajagopalan S, Mukherjee D, Mohler E. (Eds). Manual of Vascular Diseases. (353-375). Philadelphia. Lippinott Williams & Wilkins.
96. Parrillo SJ, Parrillo CV. (3-18-2010). "Pediatrics, Kawasaki disease" Emedicine.medscape.com. http://emedicine.medscape.com/article/804960-overview (12-4-2010).
97. Yousefi M, Ferringer T, Lee S, Bang, D. (6-19-2009). "Bechet disease" Emedicine.medscape.com. http://emedicine.medscape.com/article/1122381-overview (12-4-2010).
98. Shepherd RFJ. (2005). Raynaud's syndrome: vasospastic and occlusive arterial disease involving the distal upper extremity. In *Rutherford Vascular Surgery 6th edition.* (1319-1346). Philadelphia. Elsevier Saunders.
99. "What is Raynaud's" (2010). Raynaud's Association. www.raynauds.org (12-4-2010).
100. Shah SN. (10-2-2008). Aortic Coarctation. Emedicine.medscape.com. Retrieved from http://www.emedicine.medscape.com/article/150369 (12-4-2010).
101. "Coarctation of the aorta" (3-2-2010). Mayo Clinic. Retrieved from http://www.mayoclinic.com/health/coarctation-of-the-aorta/DS00616. (12-4-2010).
102. "Coarctation of the aorta" (11-15-2010). U.S. Department of Health and Human Services National Institutes of Health, http://www.nlm.nih.gov/medlineplus/ency/article/000191.htm (12-4-2010).
103. 42 Narvencar K PS, Jaques e Costa AK, Patil VR. "Shones complex" May 2009 Journal of Association of Physicians of India, 57: 415-416. http://www.japi.org/may_2009/article_12.pdf. (12-4-2010).
104. Giordano JM. (2005). Embryology of the vascular system. In Rutherford Vascular Surgery 6th edition. (53-62). Philadelphia. Elsevier Saunders.
105. Levien LJ. (2005). Nonatheromatous causes of popliteal artery disease. In Rutherford Vascular Surgery 6th edition. (1236-1255). Philadelphia. Elsevier Saunders.
106. Myers K, Clogh A, (2004). Disease of arteries to the lower limbs. In Making Sense of Vascular Ultrasound, (141-180). London: Hodder Arnold.
107. Kreienberg PB, Shah, DM, Darling III, RC, Change BB, Paty SK, Roddy SP, Ozsvath KJ, Manish,, (2005). Thoracic Outlet Syndrome: In Mansour MA, Labropoulos N. (Eds.), Vascular Diagnosis, (517-522). Philadelphia,: Elsevier Saunders.
108. Thompson RW, Bartoli MA. (2005). Neurogenic thoracic outlet syndrome. In Rutherford Vascular Surgery 6th edition. (1347-1365). Philadelphia. Elsevier Saunders.
109. Green RM. (2005). Subclavian-axillary vein thrombosis. In Rutherford Vascular Surgery 6th edition. (1371-1392). Philadelphia. Elsevier Saunders.
110. Eskandari MK, Yao JST. (2005). Occupational vascular problems. In Rutherford Vascular Surgery 6th edition. (1393-1401). Philadelphia. Elsevier Saunders.
111. Flanigan DP, Burnham SJ, Goodreau JJ, Bergan JJ. Summary of cases of adventitial cystic disease of the popliteal artery. Ann Surgery 1979 Feb: 189 (2): 165-75.
112. Morasch MD, Berguer R. (2005). Vertebrobasilar ischemia. In Rutherford Vascular Surgery 6th edition. (2030-2051). Philadelphia. Elsevier Saunders.
113. Stanley JC, Wakefield TW. (2005). Arterial fibrodysplagia. In Rutherford Vascular Surgery 6th edition. (431-452). Philadelphia. Elsevier Saunders.
114. "Heart disease and stroke statistics; 2010 updates at-a-glance". American Heart Association, http://www.americanheart.org (12-4-2010).
115. Paciaroni M, Eliasziw M, Kappelle LJ, Finan JW, Ferguson GG, Barnett HJ. Medical complications associated with carotid endarterectomy. North American Symptomatic Carotid Endarterectomy Trial (NASCET). Stroke. 1999 Sep;30(9):1759-63.
116. Walker, MD, Marler JR, Goldstein M, Grady PA, Toole JF, Baker WH, Castaldo JE, Chambless LE, Moore WS, Robertson JT, Young B, Howard VJ, Marler JR, Ourvis S, Vernon D, Needham K, Beck P, Celani VJ, Sauebeck L, von Rajcs JA, Atkins D. Endarterectomy for Asymptomatic Carotid Artery Stenosis JAMA 1995; 273: 1421-1428.
117. Labropoulos N, Erzurum V, Sheehan MK, Maker WH. (2005). Cerebral vascular color-flow scanning techniques and applications. In Mansour MA, Labropoulos N. (Eds.), Vascular Diagnosis, (91-104). Philadelphia: Elsevier Saunders.
118. Chaaban M, Stenson KM. (5-5-2009). "carotid body tumors. Emedicine.medscape.com. Retrieved from http://www.emedicine.medscape.com/article/1575155. (12-4-2010).
119. Schneider DB, Stanley JC, Messina LM. (2005). Renal artery fibrodysplagia and renovascular hypertension. In Rutherford Vascular Surgery 6th edition. (1789-2371). Philadelphia. El sevier Saunders.

Vascular Diseases

Vascular Diseases

Vascular Diseases

Vascular Diseases

Vascular Diseases

120. Schneider PA. (2005). Endovascular and surgical management of extracranial carotid fibromuscular arterial dysplagia. In Rutherford Vascular Surgery 6th edition. (2044-2051). Philadelphia. El sevier Saunders.

121. D'Souza D. (11-16-2008). "Subclavian steal syndrome". Radiopaedia.org. Retrieved from http://radiopaedia.org/articles/subclavian-steal-syndrome (12-5-2010).

122. Hallett JW, Brewster DC, Rasmussen TE. (2001). Cerebrovascular diseases. In: Handbook of Patient Care in Vascular Diseases. (131-149), Philadelphia Lippincott Williams & Wilkins.

123. Davies MG. (2005). Intimal hyperplasia: basic response to arterial and vein graft injury and reconstruction. In *Rutherford Vascular Surgery 6th edition*. (149-172). Philadelphia. Elsevier Saunders.

124. Fareed J, Hoppensteadt DA, Iqbal O, Florian-Kujowski, M, Tobu M, Bick RL, Sheikh T, Jeske W. (2005). Normal and abnormal coagulation. In Rutherford Vascular Surgery 6th edition. (493-511). Philadelphia. Elsevier Saunders.

125. Gloviczki P. (2005). Introduction and general consideration. In Rutherford Vascular Surgery 6th edition. (2111-2123). Philadelphia. Elsevier Saunders.

126. Henke PK, Schmaie A, Wakefield TW. (2005). Vascular thrombosis due to hypercoaguable states. In Rutherford Vascular Surgery 6th edition. (568-578). Philadelphia. Elsevier Saunders.

127. Meissner MH, Strandess DE. (2005). Pathophysiology and natural history of acute deep venous thrombosis. In Rutherford Vascular Surgery 6th edition. (2124-2142). Philadelphia. Elsevier Saunders.

128. Cook J, Meissner MH. (2005). Clinical and diagnostic evaluation of the patient with deep venous thrombosis. In Rutherford Vascular Surgery 6th edition. (2143-2156). Philadelphia. Elsevier Saunders.

129. Eagleton M, Ouriel K. (2005). Perioperative considerations: coagulation and hemorrhage. In Rutherford Vascular Surgery 6th edition. (545-567). Philadelphia. Elsevier Saunders.

130. Cantwell-Gab, K. (2010). Diagnostic approach to the vascular patient. In Zierler RE (Ed.), Strandess's duplex scanning disorders in vascular diagnosis 4th ed. (3-12).Philadelphia Wolters Kluwer Lippincott Williams & Wilkins.

131. Meissner MH. (2010). Chronic venous disorders. In Zierler RE (Ed.), Strandess's duplex scanning disorders in vascular diagnosis 4th ed. (223-229).Philadelphia Wolters Kluwer Lippincott Williams & Wilkins.

132. Tessier DJ, Williams RA. (2008). Chronic Venous Insufficiency. eMedicine. Retrieved from http://www.emedicine.medscape.com/article/461449.

133. Janniger CK. (3-17-2010). Klippel-Trenaunay-Weber Syndrome. eMedicine. Retrieved from http://www.emedicine.com/article/1084257-overview. (12-5-2010).

134. Porter JM , Moneta GL . (1995) International Consensus Committee on Chronic Venous Disease (Reporting standards in venous disease: an update). J Vasc Surg. 21:635–645.

135. Eklöf B, Rutherford RB, Bergan JJ, Carpentier PH, Gloviczki P, Kistner RL, Meissner MH, Moneta GL, Myers K, Padberg FT, Perrin M, Ruckley CV, Smith PC, Wakefield TW; American Venous Forum International Ad Hoc Committee for Revision of the CEAP Classification. (2004). Revision of the CEAP classification for chronic venous disorders: consensus statement. J Vasc Surg. Dec;40(6):1248-52.

136. Pappas PJ, Lal BK, Cerveira JJ, Duran WN. (2005). The pathophysiology of chronic venous insufficiency. In Rutherford Vascular Surgery 6th edition. (2220-2229). Philadelphia. Elsevier Saunders.

137. Caggiati A. (2000). Fascial relations and structure of the tributaries of the saphenous veins. Surg Radiol Anat. 22(3-4):191-6.

138. Min RJ, Rosenblatt M. US Department of Health and Human Services, Office on Women's Health (2010). Varicose Veins and Spider Veins. Retrieved from http://www.womenshealth.gov/faq/varicose-spider-veins.cfm. (7-7-2010).

139. Varicose veins and venous insufficiency: Interventional radiology nonsurgical outpatient procedure treats varicose veins. (2010). Society of Interventional Radiologists. http://www.scvir.org/patients/varicose-veins/. (12-9-2010).

140. Callam MJ. (1994). Epidemiology of varicose veins. British Journal of Surgery, 81:167-173.

141. Connors JP, Mulliken JB. (2005). Vascular tumors and malformations in childhood. In Rutherford Vascular Surgery 6th edition. (1626-1645). Philadelphia. El sevier Saunders.

142. Gloviczki P, Cho JS. (2005). Surgical treatment of chronic occlusion of the iliac veins and the inferior vena cava. In Rutherford Vascular Surgery 6th edition. (2303-2320). Philadelphia. El sevier Saunders.

143. Tortora GJ, Anagnostakos NP. (1990). The respiratory system. In principles of Anatomy and Physiology 6th edition. (689-730). New York. Harper Row Publishers.

144. 84 Feied CF. Handler JA. (12-23-2004). Pulmonary Embolism. eMedicine. Retrieved from http://www.blueguitar.org/new/misc/pe_copd.pdf. (12-10-2010).

145. Stein PD, Matta F, Musani MH, Diaczok B. Silent pulmonary embolism in patients with deep venous thrombosis: a systematic review. Am J Med. 2010 May;123(5):426-31.

146. Torbicki A, van Beek EJR, Charbonnier B, Meyer G. (2000). Guidelines on diagnosis and management of acute pulmonary embolism. European Heart Journal. 21, 1301–1336.

147. Dardik A, Rahhal D. (9-10-2009). Phlegmasia alba and cerulea dolens. eMedicine. Retrieved from http://emedicine.medscape.com/article/461809-overview. (12-10-2010),

148. Browse NL, Burnand, KG, Thomas, ML. Disease of the Veins; Pathology, Diagnosis and Treatment, Edward Arnold, a division of Hodder & Stoughton 1988.

149. Gloviczki P, Kalra M, Andrews JC. (2005). Surgical treatment of superior vena cava syndrome. In Rutherford Vascular Surgery 6th edition. (2357-2371). Philadelphia. El sevier Saunders.

150. Dake, MD. (2005). Endovascular treatment of vena caval occlusions. In Rutherford Vascular Surgery 6th edition. (2352-2344). Philadelphia. Elsevier Saunders.

151. Murherjee D, Rajagopalan S, Olin JW. (2005). Approach to and management of renovascular disease. In Rajagopalan S, Mukherjee D, Mohler E. (Eds). Manual of Vascular Diseases. (120-134). Philadelphia. Lippincott Williams & Wilkins.

152. Hansen KJ. (2005). Renovascular disease: an overview. In Rutherford Vascular Surgery 6th edition. (1763-1772). Philadelphia. El sevier Saunders.

153. About Preeclampsia. (2010). Preeclampsia Foundation. Retrieved from http://www.preeclampsia.org. (12-10-2010).

154. Wyers MC, Zwolak RM. (2005). Physiology and diagnosis of splanchnic arterial occlusion. In Rutherford Vascular Surgery 6th edition. (1707-1717). Philadelphia. Elsevier Saunders.

155. Stamatakos M, Stefanaki C, Mastrokalos D, Arampatzi H, Safioleas P, Chatziconstantinou C, Xiromeritis C, Safioleas M. (2008). Mesenteric ischemia: still a deadly puzzle for the medical community. Tohoku J Exp Med. 216: 197-204.

156. Hallett, JW, Brewster DC, Rasmussen TE, (2001) Intestinal ischemia. In Handbook of Patient Care in Vascular Diseases, (231-237), Philadelphia: Lippincott Williams & Wilkins.

157. Aziz F, Comerota AJ. (12-3-2009). Abdominal Angina. eMedicine. Retrieved from http://emedicine.medscape.com/article/188618-overview. (12-11-2010).

158. Johansen K. (2005). Portal hypertension. In Rutherford Vascular Surgery 6th edition. (1752-1761). Philadelphia. Elsevier Saunders.

159. Carale J, Murherjee S. (9-24-2010). Portal Hypertension. eMedicine. Retrieved from http://emedicine.medscape.com/article/182098-overview. (12-10-2010).

160. Raja SG, Haider Z, Ahmad M, Zaman H. Saphenous vein grafts: Heart Lung Circ. 2004;13:403-409.

161. Bauters, C., Meurice, T., Hamon, M., Mcfadden, E., Lablanche, J. M., and Bertrand, M. E., 1996, "Mechanisms and Prevention of Restenosis: From Experimental Models to Clinical Practice," Cardiovascular research, 31(6), pp. 835-46.

162. Newby, A. C., and Zaltsman, A. B., 2000, "Molecular Mechanisms in Intimal Hyperplasia," The Journal of pathology, 190(3), pp. 300-9.

163. Glagov, S., Zarins, C. K., Masawa, N., Xu, C. P., Bassiouny, H., and Giddens, D. P., 1993, "Mechanical Functional Role of Non-Atherosclerotic Intimal Thickening," Frontiers of medical and biological engineering: the international journal of the Japan Society of Medical Electronics and Biological Engineering, 5(1), pp. 37-43.

164. Zargham, R., 2008, "Preventing Restenosis after Angioplasty: A Multistage Approach," Clinical science, 114(4), pp. 257-64.

165. Allaire, E., and Clowes, A. W., 1997, "Endothelial Cell Injury in Cardiovascular Surgery: The Intimal Hyperplastic Response," The Annals of thoracic surgery, 63(2), pp. 582-91.

166. Fay, W. P., Garg, N., and Sunkar, M., 2007, "Vascular Functions of the Plasminogen Activation System," Arteriosclerosis, thrombosis, and vascular biology, 27(6), pp. 1231-7.

167. Zwiebel, WJ (2005). Ultrasound assessment of the hepatic vasculature. In Zwiebel WJ, Pellerito JS (Eds.), Introduction to Vascular Ultrasonography 5th ed, (586-609). Philadelphia: Elsevier Saunders.

168. Gloviczki P, Wahner HW. (2005). Clinical diagnosis and evaluation of lymphedema. In Rutherford Vascular Surgery 6th edition. (2396-2415). Philadelphia. Elsevier Saunders.

169. Jobst Publication. (9-2002). Lymphedema; its cause and how to manage it. (3-22).Charlotte. BSN-Jobst, Inc.

170. Witte CL, Witte MH. Lymph circulatory dynamics, lymphangiogenesis and pathophysiology of the lymphovascular system. In Rutherford Vascular Surgery 6th edition. (2379-2396). Philadelphia. Elsevier Saunders

171. McKinsey JF, Gewertz BL. (1077) Acute mesenteric ischemia. Clin North Am; 77:301-318.

172. Oklu et al. J Vasc Interv Radiol 2012; 23:33–39, Lim and Davies 2009 Pathogenesis of primary varicose veins British Journal of Surgery 2009; 96: 1231–1242

173. Jeyaraj SC, Chotani MA, Mitra S, Gregg HE, Flavahan NA, Morrison KJ. Cooling evokes redistribution of ⍺2C-adrenoceptors from golgi to plasma membrane in transfected HEK293 cells. Mol Pharmacol. 2001;60:1195–1200. [HYPERLINK "/pubmed/11723226"PubMed]

174. Nicholas A. Flavahan, PhD Rheumatic Disease Clinics of North America; "Regulation of Vascular Reactivity in Scleroderma: New Insights into Raynaud's Phenomenon" Volume 34, Issue 1, February 2008, Pages 81–87

Definition

The combination of real-time B-mode imaging with pulsed wave and color Doppler to evaluate the extracranial vessels.

Etiology

- Atherosclerosis (90%)
- Intimal hyperplasia
- Dissection
- Traumatic occlusion
- Extrinsic compression
- External radiation
- Carotid body tumor
- Fibromuscular dysplasia
- Post-traumatic pseudoaneurysm

Risk Factors

- Age
- Hypertension
- Diabetes
- Hypercholesterolemia
- Smoking
- Obesity
- Patent foramen ovale
- Physical inactivity
- Genetic predisposition
- Homocystinaemia
- Cardiac disease
- Previous TIA or stroke

Indications for Exam

- Carotid bruit
- Follow-up of known carotid stenosis
- Syncope
- Abnormality of gait
- Hemiparesis/hemiplegia
- Paresthesia
- Aphasia
- Positional vertigo
- Visual symptoms (e.g., amaurosis fugax, retinal ischemia, transient visual loss, etc.)
- Transient ischemic attack (TIA)
- Stroke: Cerebrovascular Accident (CVA)
- Follow-up (carotid endarterectomy, stent, bypass)
- Infarction (previously known as RIND - reversible ischemic neurologic deficit)
- Neck trauma
- Pulsatile mass in the neck
- Fibromuscular dysplagia
- Moyamoya disease
- Carotid artery dissection
- Seizure

Contraindications/Limitations

- Patients with extensive bandages or cervical collars
- Patients with neck IV
- Poor visualization due to vessel depth
- Diffuse arterial wall calcification may interfere with acquisition of duplex information
- Patients who cannot be adequately positioned.

Location of Disease

- First 1-2 cm of the internal carotid artery (most common)
- Common carotid artery
- Subclavian artery
- Origin of the vertebral artery
- External carotid artery

Mechanism of Disease for Carotid Artery Stenosis

Atherosclerosis

- Atherosclerosis is the most common arterial disease.
- Atherosclerotic plaque forms in the arterial wall and decreases or stops blood flow by either narrowing the lumen (stenosis) or completely blocking the artery (occlusion).
- Hemodynamically significant obstruction refers to either a stenosis or an occlusion that results in a significant decrease of blood pressure or flow distal to the obstruction. This term is typically used to describe an obstruction >50% diameter reduction. [1]
- Typically, a stenosis must narrow the diameter of the artery by at least 50% to increase the peak systolic velocity significantly.

Emboli

- An embolus is typically a piece of plaque or thrombus that moves from a proximal point and stops at a point in the artery that is too narrow for it to pass. This causes an *infarction*, a sudden reduction of flow to a part.
- A cerebral embolus is frequently a piece of carotid plaque or thrombus from a plaque in the heart, but it may originate elsewhere.
- If the embolus originates from the heart, it is classified as a *cardioembolic infarction.*
- *Territorial infarcts* are restricted to territories supplied by major intracerebral arteries, their branches or the *pial arteries* that surrounding the brain and spinal cord.

Normal   **Homo-Irregular**   **Homo-Smooth**   **Hetero-Irregular**   **Hetero-Smooth**   **Complete Occlusion**

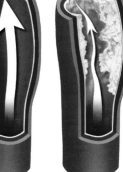
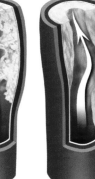
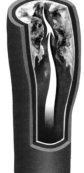
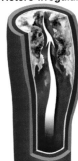
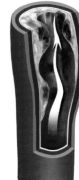
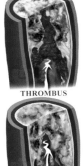
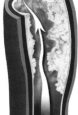

THROMBUS

ATHEROSCLEROTIC

Presentations of atherosclerosis within an artery

Dissection

- A tear in the intimal lining of an artery, with or without outer medial wall involvement. Blood enters the media of the vessel through this tear creating a "false lumen." Simultaneously, blood is also flowing through the original or "true lumen."
- Blood flows through the tear in the intimal layer and sometimes clots.
- Can be spontaneous or result from trauma or an iatrogenic complication.
- ICA dissection typically starts in the first 2-4 cm of the ICA
- Expansion of the false lumen that develops during dissection can narrow the true carotid lumen. [57]
- CCA dissection may be an extension of an aortic dissection or blunt trauma.
- The false lumen can progressively dilate into a pseudoaneurysm. [2]

Kinking and tortuosity

- Kinking or tortuosity refers to a sharp angle of 90° or less usually located 2-4 cm above the bifurcation
- Blood flow is compromised in kinked arteries and is often associated with plaque and arterial stenosis.
- The most important difference between a tortuous, coiled and kinked vessel is that the kinked vessel is most often associated with symptoms of cerebral ischemia.
- Congenital kinks are a result of faulty descent of the vessels during embryonic development.
- Kinks can be acquired with age; arteries can elongate and at the same time, the medial layer degenerates. [3]
- Approximately 25% of the population are affected by this condition which is often bilateral. [4]

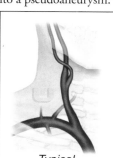

Typical

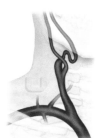

Tortuous

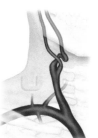

Kinked

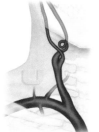

Coiled

Common shape distortions found at the extracranial internal carotid artery

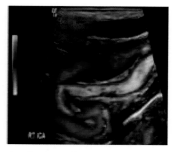

Duplex image of a tortuous artery-ICA

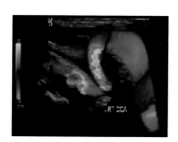

Duplex image of and kinked-CCA

Images courtesy of Patrick Washko, BS RT RDMS RVT

Fibromuscular dysplagia (FMD)

- Non-atherosclerotic arterial disease; multiple, focal stenoses, followed by widening in an arterial segment, resemble a "string of beads" on imaging studies. [7,8,9]
- FMD affects medium and large sized vessels, especially the renal and internal carotid arteries.
- Usually occurs in females in the mid section of the internal carotid artery. [5,6]
- The carotid bulb area typically has no evidence of disease.
- Characterized on duplex ultrasound by a series of tandem stenoses and dilatations accompanied by a moderate-significant increase in peak systolic velocity with extensive turbulence. [1,9]
- Coexisting FMD in the renal and carotid arteries is not an uncommon occurrence. [10]

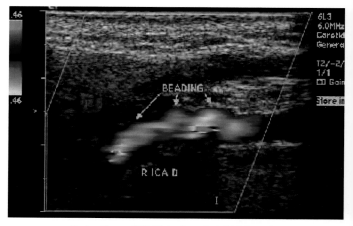

Detection of FMD in the distal ICA at the level of the mandible by color duplex

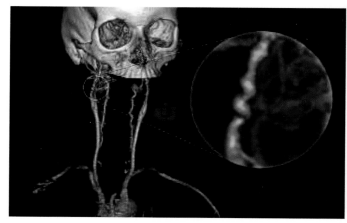

FMD detected by CT scan

Carotid Body Tumor

- The carotid body is a small cluster of primarily chemoreceptor cells located at the split of the carotid bifurcation.
- A carotid body tumor (CBT) is a *paraganglioma* (tumor or ganglioma comprised of chromaffin). They arise off the ganglion of the glossopharyngeal nerve.
- In most cases, the external carotid artery supplies blood to the tumor. [3, 10] Flow will be low resistance. As the tumor grows, blood flow can also be supplied by the internal carotid, vertebral artery or thyrocervical trunk. [54]

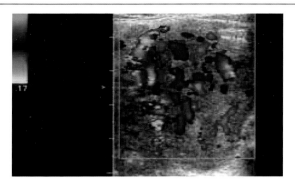

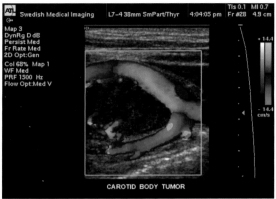

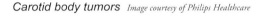

Carotid body tumors *Image courtesy of Philips Healthcare*

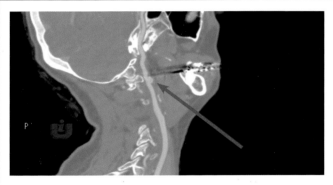

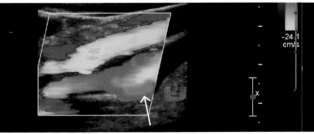

CT and color flow of a carotid aneurysm

Carotid Aneurysm

- Carotid aneurysms and pseudoaneurysms are very rare
- A reduction in tensile strength of the wall post-endarterectomy may weaken the arterial wall, increasing the risk of a pseudoaneurysm. [13]
- Reasons for pseudoaneurysm at a carotid bypass anastomotic site include; infection, tension at the anastomosis, thin-walled arteries, suture deterioration or improper suture technique. [14]

Radiation injury

- Radiation therapy causes injury to the vasa vasorum and necrosis of the vessel wall. Endothelial cells lining the arterial walls of vessels in the irradiated field are susceptible to damage. Lipid-containing plaques can then form in the intimal layer of the artery. [15]

Vasculitis

- Inflammation of the vessel wall results in damage to the blood vessel.
- Relatively little is known about the causes of vasculitis, Genetics, infectious and toxic factors are suspected.
- *Giant cell* or *temporal arteritis* affect the extracranial branches of the carotid. The temporal artery is especially susceptible.

Patient History

Anterior Circulation (Internal Carotid Artery)

- Transient ischemic attack (TIA resolves within 24 hours)
- Cerebral vascular accident (CVA – permanent deficit)
- Amaurosis fugax—partial or complete loss of vision (often described as a "window shade being pulled down")
- Hemiparesis/hemiplegia: weakness or complete loss of function to one limb or one side of the body
- Paresthesia (tingling, numb or burning sensation)
- Aphasia: inability to speak or comprehend language
- Homonomous hemianopia (blindness or visual defect in half of the field of vision)

Posterior Circulation (Vertebrobasilar Artery)

- Ataxia (lack of muscle coordination which can affect walking, swallowing, eye movements, speech, etc.)
- Confusion
- Diplopia (double vision)
- Dizziness
- Dysarthria (abnormal speech or difficulty with speech)
- Drop attacks (sudden fall while walking or standing that is recovered from quickly)
- Dysphagia (difficulty swallowing)
- Headache
- Motor/sensory disturbances (unilateral, bilateral, alternating)
- Syncope (fainting)
- Vertigo ("spinning" or sensation that your surroundings are moving around you)
- Subclavian steal syndrome

Physical Examination

- Carotid auscultation for bruits.
- Bilateral blood pressure (>20 mmHg difference between right and left arm may indicate pathology, e.g., subclavian obstruction on the side with the lower pressure may have resulted in a subclavian steal)

TABLE 6: Identification of ICA vs ECA Vessels

Characteristic	Internal Carotid Artery	External Carotid Artery
Anatomical location	Posterolateral	Anteromedial
Branch vessels in neck	Extremely rare	Yes
Luminal size	Larger diameter	Smaller diameter
Responds to temporal tap*	No	Yes
Doppler flow pattern	Low resistance	High resistance
Normal PSV	<125 cm/s	Varies, <200 cm/s

* tapping too hard can cause reverberation in the ICA. Best to tap STA while listening to each vessel and compare the waveforms for the strongest response.

Carotid Artery Examination Protocol

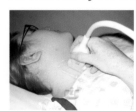

- Obtain a patient history to include symptoms and risk factors, past vascular interventions and general dates of surgery.
- Obtain bilateral brachial blood pressures.

- Patient is examined in the supine position with the head supported by a small pillow or towel, turning the head approximately 45° toward the opposite side.
- Some patients may require the use of a range of transducers, including high-frequency (5-7 MHz), (8-15 MHz) transducers and a lower frequency (1-4 MHz) transducer to assist with large, short necks.
- Locate the common carotid artery (CCA) at the base of the neck in the transverse (short axis) plane.
- Obtain and record grayscale images in transverse view of the following:
  - Common carotid artery
  - Carotid bifurcation; distal CCA before the complete split of the proximal internal and external carotid arteries.
  - Internal carotid artery (ICA); can be in same view with ECA.
  - These images can be repeated with color flow Doppler.
- Obtain and record grayscale images in the longitudinal (sagittal) view of the following:
  - Common carotid artery
  - Carotid bifurcation, distal CCA into the ICA, this is the most diagnostic view.
  - Carotid bifurcation; distal CCA into the ECA
  - Proximal, mid and distal ICA
  - ECA
- These images can be repeated with color flow Doppler.
- Use a 60° PW Doppler angle or less with the angle cursor set parallel to the vessel wall or to flow and the sample volume placed center stream. It is VITAL to do this to obtain accurate velocity measurements. Document the peak systolic (PSV) and end diastolic velocity (EDV) for the following:
  - Proximal, mid and distal CCA
  - Proximal ECA (PSV only)
  - Proximal, mid and distal ICA
  - Vertebral artery

TABLE 7: Normal Values for Extracranial Vessels

Vessel	Normal PSV	Normal EDV	Flow Pattern	Abnormal Flow	Area Supplied
Subclavian	Varies	Reversal of flow with high diastolic component	High resistance triphasic flow	High PSV may indicate stenosis; biphasic or monophasic waveform associated with obstruction	Vertebral artery and arm
Common carotid	Varies	Between ECA and ICA EDV	Low resistance	Low or zero EDV may indicate distal CCA, bifurcation and/or proximal ICA high grade stenosis or occlusion	ICA and ECA
External carotid	Typically higher than normal ICA	Low diastolic flow; may have reversal of flow	High resistance	>50% = roughly > 200 cm/sec with post-stenotic turbulence and plaque in the image	Face and scalp
Internal carotid	<125 cm/s with no or minimal spectral broadening	High diastolic flow with normal velocities <40 cm/s flow beyond the bulb	Low resistance	Increased PSV and EDV with spectral broadening	Intracranial vessels
Vertebral	20-60 cm/s but can vary from side to side	Flow above the baseline; high diastolic flow, but not as great as the ICA	Low resistance	Reversed flow pattern may indicate subclavian steal syndrome	Intracranial vessels

- Subclavian artery when clinically indicated (PSV only), this can be optional view for some labs.
- It is extremely important to "walk" the PW Doppler sample volume through an area of stenosis to obtain the maximum peak systolic velocity and end-diastolic velocities.
- Take additional spectral Doppler measurements as appropriate. Areas of stenosis should include pre, at and post stenosis waveform measurements. Use color Doppler as needed to define anatomy and areas of stenosis.
- Document additional grayscale and color images in areas of suspected stenosis. Measure lumenal reduction, especially when lesions cause a hemodynamically significant velocity increase. This provides backup information for the velocity data.
  - Measure in multiple planes to get full effect of plaque:
    - Transverse
    - Longitudinal-anterior/posterior
    - Longitudinal-lateral
  - Calculate and report the average of 2-3 measurements from these different planes
    - Oblique plane as needed to follow tortuous vessels
    - STAY ON AXIS of vessel in long view
    - Use color only if needed to clearly define edges of plaque, and update with B-mode frequently to avoid color overgain
    - Most difficult point to define is the true lumen. Look for black line separating wall from plaque.
- Determine classification of stenosis according to laboratory diagnostic criteria. *(See diagnostic criteria tables)*.
- Document any additional abnormal findings with grayscale and color imaging (e.g., aneurysmal formation, thrombus, wall irregularity, aneurysm, etc).
- When arterial occlusion is suspected, document the lack of flow with PW Doppler. Decrease the color and velocity scales to detect low flow and confirm occlusion.
- A suspected occlusion must be examined and documented in both longitudinal and transverse planes.
- Optimize exam; sample volume, gain and scales may all need to be adjusted
- Repeat on the opposite side.

Duplex Exam After Carotid Endarterectomy or Carotid Bypass Graft

- First exam is usually within 30 days of the procedure.
- Exams performed within the first few days may encounter shadowing from air entrapment associated with a synthetic patch or graft, multiple views may be required to view the vessel.
- In addition to standard duplex, the following conditions should be noted. [3]

- Restenosis
- Residual plaque
- Tissue flaps
- Vessel narrowing

- Neointimal hyperplasia
- Hematoma
- Extravascular leak
- Pseudoaneurysm (associated with a synthetic patch)

- The length of the surgical area is dependent on the extent and level of disease.
- With patch angioplasty closure, a wider vessel will be noted and sutures may be visible as small echoes regularly spaced on the wall of the vessel.

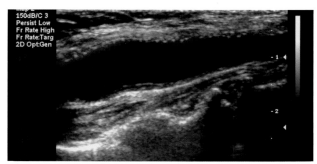

B-mode image of a carotid patch *Image courtesy of Philips Healthcare*

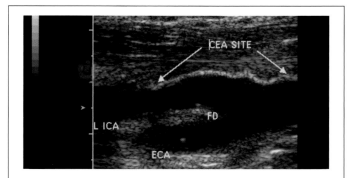

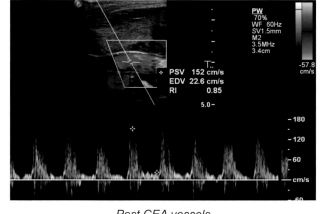

Post CEA vessels

Duplex Evaluation for Carotid Stents

- First exam is usually within 30 days of the procedure.
- In addition to standard duplex, the following additional views are to be documented.
  - Proximal native artery
  - Proximal stent attachment
  - Proximal, mid and distal stent
  - Distal attachment site
  - Native artery beyond the stent
- In-stent restenosis is infrequent [16], stents borders are the most common site of restenosis. Stents can overlap.
- Walk the Doppler through areas of hyperplasia for stent fractures which can cause elevated velocities.
- Follow flow changes over time.
- When scanning post-stent placement, the proximal and distal ends of the stent should not reveal any major flow abnormalities. Make comparisons over serial studies and observe for any flow changes over time.

> HINT: Color Doppler may be helpful to evaluate residual lumens.

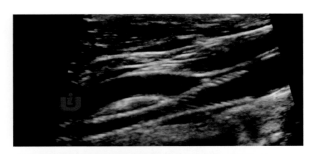

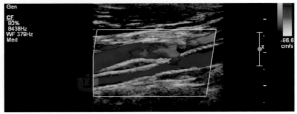

The proximal end of this stent is in the distal CCA with the distal end in the ICA

Hint: Color flow can obscure the true lumenal reduction if the color gain is set too high. Measure luminal reduction in grayscale whenever possible.

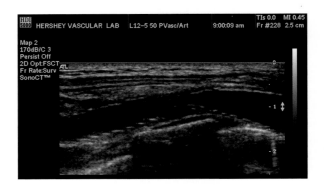

Using power Doppler to find residual lumen within a stent

Image courtesy of Philips Healthcare

Most labs use the patient's first duplex exam post CAS values as their baseline for subsequent duplex exams

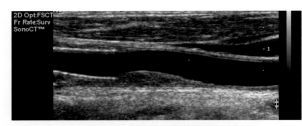

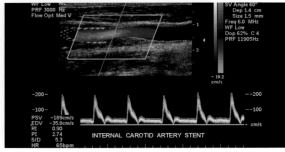

Intimal hyperplasia proximal to the stent

Image courtesy of Philips Healthcare

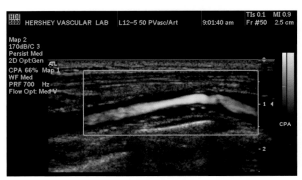

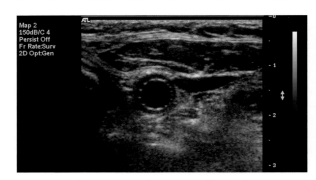

Transverse view of carotid stent

Image courtesy of Philips Healthcare

TABLE 8: Velocity Criteria Defining Stenoses in the Stented Carotid Artery Compared to Criteria for the Native Carotid Artery

Stenosis %	Stented carotid artery	Native carotid artery
0-19%	PSV* <150 cm/s and ICA/CCA ratio <2.15	PSV <130 cm/s
20-49%	PSV 150-219 cm/s	PSV 130-189 cm/s
50-79%	PSV 220-339 cm/s and ICA/CCA ratio ≥2.7	PSV 190-249 cm/s and EDV <120 cm/s
80-99%	PSV ≥340 cm/s and ICA/CCA ratio ≥4.15	PSV ≥250 cm/s and EDV <120 cm/s, or ICA/CCA ratio ≥3.2

PSV: Peak systolic velocity; EDV: end diastolic velocity; ICA: Internal carotid artery; CCA: common carotid artery.
*PSV and EDV measurements for stented carotid arteries are performed within the stented segments.

Lal BK, Hobson II RW, Tofighi B, Kapadia I, Cuadra S, and Jamil Z. Duplex ultrasound velocity criteria for the stented carotid artery. 2007. JOURNAL OF VASCULAR SURGERY Volume 47, Number 1. pp 63-73.[17]

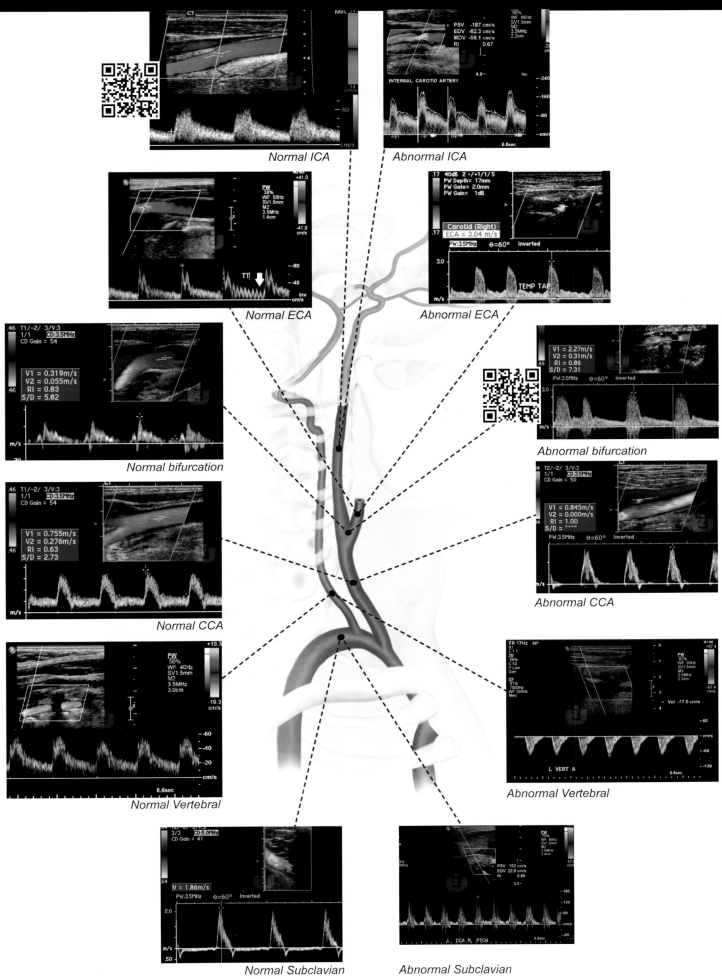

Normal ICA

Abnormal ICA

Normal ECA

Abnormal ECA

Normal bifurcation

Abnormal bifurcation

Normal CCA

Abnormal CCA

Normal Vertebral

Abnormal Vertebral

Normal Subclavian

Abnormal Subclavian

Cerebrovascular Testing

Carotid Artery Duplex Ultrasound

TABLE 9: Grayscale and Plaque Morphology

Echogenicity	Composition	Texture	Surface
Reflections determined by plaque's composition of lipids, collagen, hemorrhage and calcification	Determined by levels of lipid, hemorrhage, collagen and calcification		

Echogenicity

Anechoic
- No echogenicity (lipids, intraplaque hemorrhage)

Hypoechoic
- Low echogenicity (fibrofatty plaque)

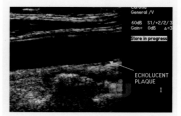

Hyperechoic
- Moderate echogenicity (fibrous plaque) acoustic shadowing may or may not be present

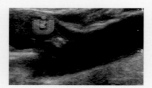

Calcific
- Highly reflective plaque(s) with acoustic shadowing

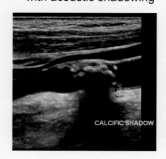

CALCIFIC SHADOW

Composition

Fibrofatty plaque
- Contains lipid material
- Lightly echogenic
- Acoustics similar to blood: uniform echo distribution

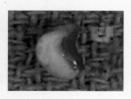

Fibrous plaque
- Moderate to strong echogenicity
- Lipid or thrombus may create hypoechoic regions

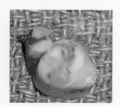

Complex plaque
- Multiple levels of echogenicity
- Acoustic calcific shadowing may or may not be present.

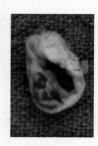

Texture

Homogeneous
- Uniform echo pattern and composition
- May be echogenic or echolucent

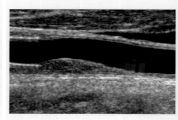

Heterogeneous
- Non-uniform echo pattern, multiple echo densities of anechoic and hyperechoic areas.
- May be classified as primarily echolucent if greater than 50% of the plaque is dark.

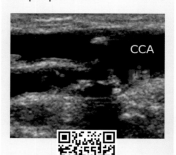

CCA

- May be classified as primarily echogenic if greater than 50% of the plaque demonstrates brighter echoes

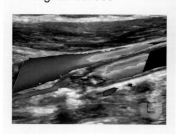

Surface

Smooth
- Surface plaque appears continuous with no irregularities

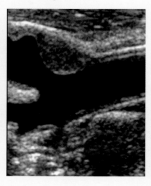

Irregular
- Plaque surface is discontinuous, may have multiple echoes present
- Possibility of ulceration on such surfaces. However, presence of ulcer cannot be determined by duplex ultrasound

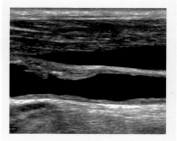

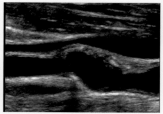

Images courtesy of Philips Healthcare

TABLE 10: University of Washington Diagnostic Criteria for Classification of Internal Carotid Artery Disease

Category	Peak Systolic Velocity	End Diastolic Velocity	Spectral waveform characteristics
Normal (0%)	<125 cm/s	–	Minimal or no spectral broadening; boundary layer separation present in the carotid bulb
Mild (1-15%)	<125 cm/s	–	Spectral broadening during deceleration phase of systole only
Moderate (16-49%)	<125 cm/s	–	Spectral broadening throughout systole
Severe (50-79%)	>125 cm/s	<140 cm/s	Marked spectral broadening
Critical (80-99%)		≥140 cm/s	Marked spectral broadening
Occlusion	No Flow	No Flow	No flow signal in the internal carotid artery; decreased diastolic flow in the ipsilateral common carotid artery

ICA/CCA Ratio: >60% >3.2
>70% = >4.0

Moneta GH, Edwards JM, Chitwood RW, et al. Correlation of North American Symptomatic Carotid Endarterectomy Trial (NASCET) angiographic definition of 70-99% internal carotid artery stenosis with duplex scanning. J Vasc Surg. 17:152-159, 1995

Moneta GH, Edwards JM, Papanicolaou G, et al. Screening for asymptomatic internal carotid artery stenosis; duplex criteria for discriminating 60-99% stenosis, J Vasc Surg, 21(6): 989-994, 1995

TABLE 11: New Consensus Diagnostic Criteria for Classification of Internal Carotid Artery Disease

Degree of stenosis (%)	ICA PSV (cm/s)	Plaque Estimate (%)*	ICA/CCA PSV Ratio	ICA EDV (cm/s)
Normal	<125	None	<2.0	<40
<50	<125	<50	<2.0	<40
50-69	125-230	>50	2.0-4.0	40-100
>70 but < near occlusion	>230	>50	>4.0	>100
Near occlusion	High, low or undetectable	Visible	Variable	Variable
Total occlusion	Undetectable	Visible, no detectable lumen	N/A	N/A

*Plaque estimate (diameter reduction) with grayscale and color Doppler US

Grant, E., Benson, C., et al, Carotid Artery Stenosis: Gray-Scale and Doppler US Diagnosis: Society of Radiologists in Ultrasound Consensus Conference, Radiology 229 (2): 340-346, 2003 [18]

TABLE 12: University of Chicago Diagnostic Criteria for Classification of Internal Carotid Artery Disease

Category of Disease	Peak Systolic Velocity	End Diastolic Velocity	ICA/CCA Ratio
0-49 %	<155 cm/s		<2.0
50-79%	>155 cm/s	<140 cm/s	>2.0
80-99%	>370 cm/s	>140 cm/s	>6.0
Occluded	N/A	N/A	N/A

TABLE 13: Bluth Diagnostic Criteria for Classification of Internal Carotid Artery Disease

Category	PSV	EDV	Systolic Velocity Ratio ICA/CCA	Diastolic Velocity Ratio ICA/CCA	Spectral Broadening (cm/s)
Normal 0%				<2.4	<30
Mild 1-39%	<110	<40	<1.8	<2.4	<40
Moderate 40-59%	<130	<40	<1.8	<2.4	<40
Severe 60-79%	>130	>40	>1.8	>2.4	>40
Critical 80-99%	>250	>100	>3.7	>5.5	>80
Occluded	N/A	N/A	N/A	N/A	N/A

Bluth, EI, Wetzner, SM, Baker, JD, et al: Carotid duplex sonography: a multicenter recommendation for standardized imaging and Doppler criteria. Radiographics 8:487-506, 1988. [19]

TABLE 14: **Carotid Artery Examination Protocol Summary**	
Scan transverse (short-axis) with grayscale and color flow Doppler	**Scan longitudinal (sagittal) with grayscale, color flow and PW Doppler**
• Proximal CCA	• Proximal CCA
• Mid CCA	• Mid CCA
• Distal CCA	• Distal CCA
• Carotid bifurcation	• Proximal ECA*
• Proximal ECA	• Proximal ICA
• Proximal ICA	• Mid ICA
• Mid ICA	• Distal ICA
• Distal ICA	• Vertebral
	• Subclavian*

- Determine plaque location, plaque surface characteristics, plaque texture
- Measure highest peak systolic velocity (PSV) and end-diastolic velocity (EDV)
- At areas of stenosis measure PSV and EDV proximal, within and distal to the stenosis
- Calculate systolic ICA/CCA ratio bilaterally using the highest PSV of the ICA and the mid/distal CCA just proximal to the bulb where the CCA walls are parallel
- Determine vertebral flow direction (normally antegrade)
- Determine classification of internal carotid artery disease using the velocity criteria chosen by the laboratory

Measure only the PSV

Carotid Interpretation

- Check CCA for inflow/outflow obstruction and compare right and left sides
- Categorize ICA disease by PSV, EDV ratio and image according to the diagnostic criteria. Make sure these measurements support each other and give a possible explanation if they do not correlate (e.g., compensatory flow, inflow obstruction).
- Check ECA for stenosis
- Assess vertebral flow direction and check for obstruction
- Assess SCA for obstruction
- Observe for other pathology
- Repeat on the contralateral side
- Compare results to previous exam
- Consider whether symptoms and results match

Normal Carotid Velocities (absence of a hemodynamically significant stenosis, <50%)

Doppler waveforms and flow velocities:

- Normal carotid artery waveforms demonstrate low-resistance in the CCA, ICA and vertebral. Waveforms demonstrate high-resistance in the ECA.
- PSV should be relatively uniform throughout the carotid arteries.
- Velocities are higher in younger people

- The EDV is generally above the zero baseline except:
  – CCA or ECA may have a short duration of reversed flow at end systole
  – Areas of the bulb have reversed flow
  – Long duration reversed flow may be due to aortic regurgitation if noted bilaterally in the CCA
- General grayscale and color characteristics:
  – The arteries are free of intraluminal echoes.
  – When utilized, color Doppler fills the entire arterial lumen.

Abnormal Doppler Waveforms and Flow Velocities

Common Carotid Artery (CCA)

- No particular velocity value is considered abnormal.
- Low or zero end-diastolic velocity may indicate distal common carotid artery, carotid bifurcation and/or proximal internal carotid artery high grade stenosis or occlusion.
- A hemodynamically significant lesion (>50%) will result in a focal velocity increase (at least double the velocity in the proximal arterial segment) and post-stenotic turbulence.
- Compare right and left CCA velocities, if there is about 30 cm/s or more difference between CCAs at multiple levels, consider the following
  – Proximal CCA with slow upstroke and lower velocity waveform indicates proximal obstruction.
  – Higher proximal CCA velocities can result from vessel tortuosity.
  – Proximal CCA waveforms with a quick upstroke but low velocities may indicate a tight distal CCA stenosis. A tight distal CCA stenosis is sometimes labeled mistakenly for a stenosis at the origin of the ICA, so watching for the low proximal and mid CCA velocities will help.
  – CCA velocities which are much higher compared to the other side may be a sign of compensatory flow due to a contralateral occlusion.

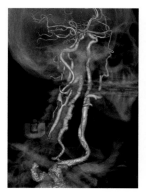
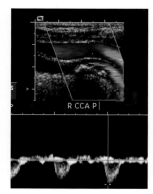

Reversal of flow in the right CCA due to occlusion of the brachiocephalic artery

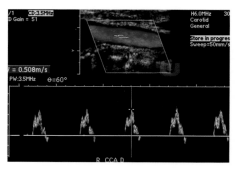

Loss of diastolic flow in the CCA due to ICA occlusion

Internal Carotid Artery (ICA)

> The criterion for abnormal carotid artery duplex varies across institutions.

- Peak systolic velocity >125 cm/s with spectral broadening as the higher velocities are reached
- End-diastolic velocity >40 cm/s
- Use the highest PSV and EDV from the pre-bulb CCA and first 3 cm of the ICA to calculate the ICA/CCA ratio. Refer to criteria options in this chapter.
- Check that the ICA/CCA ratio and image measurement agree with the category of disease suspected.
- Exact location and plaque characteristics should be described:
  - Homogeneous, echolucent
  - Homogeneous, echodense
  - Heterogeneous, primarily echolucent
  - Heterogeneous, primarily echodense
  - Smooth vs irregular

- Modest flow disturbances seen early after CEA may disappear on subsequent studies due to natural vessel remodeling.

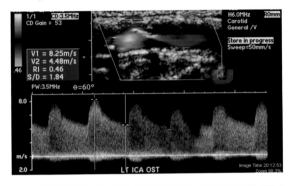

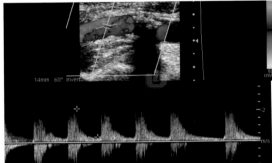

Post stenotic turbulence after a high grade obstruction

External Carotid Artery (ECA)

- High resistance waveform pattern. Branches are noted.
- Peak systolic velocity >150-200cm/sec with evidence of plaque and post stenotic turbulence indicates >50% stenosis [16]
- Some labs define a hemodynamically significant ECA lesion (>50%) by a focal velocity increase (at least double the velocity in the proximal ECA segment), with post-stenotic turbulence and a possible color bruit.
- Low resistance flow pattern may occur due to severe ICA stenosis/occlusion resulting in the ECA acting as a collateral to feed the low resistance vessels of the brain. In this case it is important to look for branches to identify this vessel as the ECA.
- In cases of CCA occlusion, ECA flow direction will often reverse in order perfuse the ICA and the brain (ECA flow will be retrograde to the bifurcation to give antegrade flow to the ICA).

- Performing a temporal tap helps identify the ECA. The spectral trace should "oscillate" when you tap on the superfical temporal artery (STA).

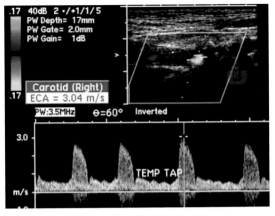

Internalized ECA signal

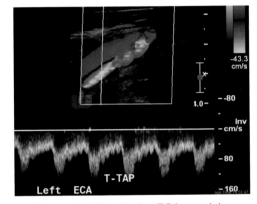

Reversal of flow in the ECA supplying the ICA due to CCA occlusion

Vertebral Artery (VA)

- The vertebral artery is assessed for normalcy, occlusion and flow direction. Flow direction is normally antegrade with a low resistance signal.
- Vertebral artery stenoses occur most frequently in the proximal VA which is often not directly assessed. Some labs define a hemodynamically significant VA lesion (>50%) by a focal velocity increase (at least double the velocity in the proximal VA segment), with post-stenotic turbulence and a possible color bruit.
- Flow velocities can vary from side to side due to one vertebral artery being dominant, this is commonly seen on the left side.
- Flow direction is usually antegrade, reversed flow pattern may indicate subclavian steal syndrome and should be confirmed with abnormal subclavian artery waveform documentation or brachial pressure decrease of >20 mmHg on the same side.
- Loss of EDV may indicate a distal occlusion
- No flow despite low scales and higher gains in PW and color along with a well visualized artery below the vein indicates vertebral occlusion.
- Pendulum waveforms (a.k.a. bunny ears) suggests subacute subclavian steal syndrome.

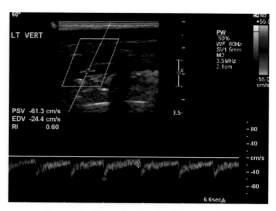

Reversed flow in the vertebral artery suggesting subclavian steal syndrome

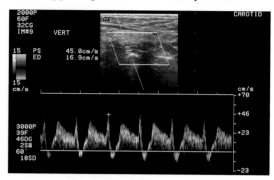

Early systolic deceleration in the vertebral waveform suggestive of subclavian artery stenosis

Image courtesy of Robert Scissions, RVT

Subclavian Artery (SA)

- Waveform configuration is normally triphasic.

- There is no absolute abnormal velocity, but velocities are typically higher than the carotid arteries.

- Compare waveforms and brachial pressures from side to side.

- A hemodynamically significant SA lesion (>50%) is indicated by a focal velocity increase (at least double the velocity in the proximal SA segment), with post-stenotic turbulence and a possible color bruit.

- Biphasic or monophasic signals may be observed when significant stenosis or occlusion is present in the SA.

  - Biphasic arterial signals are characterized by strong forward flow in arterial systole (sharp upstroke) with a loss of flow reversal in early diastole (no flow below the baseline) and either forward flow or no flow in the late diastolic component.

  - Monophasic arterial signals are characterized by reduced pulsatility or forward flow in late systole (blunted upstroke). A diastolic flow component may or may not be apparent. Continuous forward flow and a slow, blunted systolic component is another way to describe monophasic flow.

Occlusion

- An occlusion of the artery is present when no flow is detected by color or spectral Doppler. Determine the extent of the occlusion when possible.

- To confirm occlusions:
  - Decrease scales
  - Increase color and PW gain
  - Decrease filter
  - Increase sample volume but avoid ECA branches and veins

- Investigate with PW and color Doppler distal to the bulb in the transverse and longitudinal views. Check for flow with PW Doppler in transverse view, but do not measure the velocity in transverse since the angle to flow direction cannot be measured accurately.

- ICA occlusions may result in loss of diastolic flow in the CCA.

- ICA may be filled in with plaque and horizontal motion with each pulse may be noted in grayscale.

- A "staccato" waveform often indicates that there is downstream occlusion.

- Intracranial ICA occlusion demonstrates no EDV in distal ICA

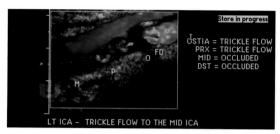

Trickle flow noted in the ICA These images represent a functionally occluded ICA or a "string sign"

Compensatory Flow

- With occlusion or very high grade stenosis on one side, the opposite carotid artery may be feeding both sides of the brain which increases flow, including velocities throughout the CCA, ECA and ICA.

- Sometimes there is no compensatory flow due to other contributions from other collateral systems.

- When compensatory flow is present contralateral to an occlusion, a stenosis may be placed in a higher category based on the absolute velocities alone, e.g., although the stenosis would normally fall into the 50-79% category, the velocities in the stenosis may reach the 80-99% range because the incoming velocities are higher from the compensatory flow state.

- Multiple points of evidence identify when a stenosis appears higher due to compensatory flow and should used in the interpretation:

  - ICA/CCA ratio is in a lower category than the absolute velocity criteria

  - Image measurement is in a lower category than the absolute velocity criteria

  - PSV throughout the CCA is generally higher than normal and higher than the contralateral side

  - The interpretation should indicate which velocities are suspected to be falsely elevated and it should be explained that compensatory flow is the likely cause.

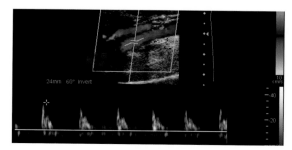

Staccato arterial waveform (pre-occlusive)

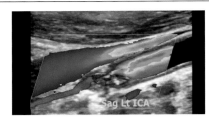

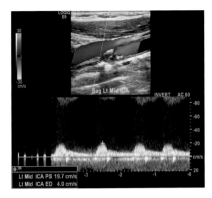

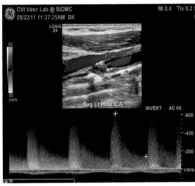

This series of images represent a high grade stenosis

Image courtesy of Steve Knight, BSc, RVT, RDMS

Use color flow as a guide to identify an occluded artery. But always confirm flow by placing the Doppler sample volume in the vessel lumen.

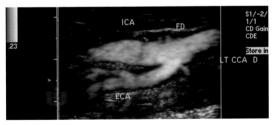

Power Doppler of the carotid system

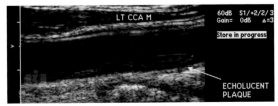

Echolucent plaque

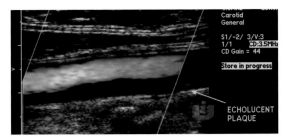

Color flow demonstrates the true lumen especially in images with echolucent plaque as seen in the above image

Other Pathology

- **Aneurysm:** An aneurysm is defined as a focal enlargement of an artery at least twice the diameter of the proximal segment. Intraluminal thrombus may be observed and is a possible source of distal emboli. [12] PSV are typically reduced with abnormal flow patterns within an aneurysm. [22]

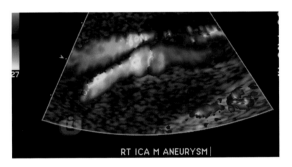

- **Arterial dissection:** A dissection of the arterial lumen is recognized by two distinct flow channels by B-mode and/or color Doppler separated by the dissected intima seen as a white line within the lumen. One lumen is known as the "true lumen" while the other is referred to as the "false lumen. Each lumen has a distinctly different flow pattern or one lumen may be occluded. [23]

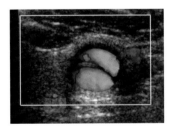 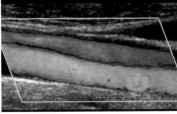

- **Fibromuscular dysplasia:** When a series of hemodynamically significant velocity increases are noted in the mid/distal segment of the ICA accompanied by significant turbulence, FMD is suspected. [20] A "string of beads" is the classic appearance on B-mode and color Doppler images (where segments of the artery can be seen narrowing and then widening in series). [24, 25]

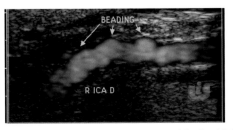

Typical "string of pearls" sign noted in the ICA

Differential Diagnosis for CVA/TIA

- Vasculitis (e.g. arteritis)
- Fibromuscular dysplagia
- Moyamoya disease
- Cerebral hemorrhage
- Carotid artery dissection
- Seizure
- Lupus
- Metabolic problems (e.g., glucose derangement)
- Migraines
- Cardiac embolization
- Nonatherosclerotic vasculopathy

- Systemic infections
- Mass lesions
- Intracranial tumor
  - Primary central nervous system (CNS)
  - Metastatic subdural hematoma
- Cerebral abscess
- Multiple sclerosis
- Alcohol or drug abuse
- Cardiac failure
- Syncope
- Positional vertigo

Correlation

- Spiral CT scan
- MRA

- MRI
- Cerebral arteriography

Medical Treatment

- Modify risk factors (e.g., smoking cessation, lower cholesterol, etc.)
- Statin therapy
- Antithrombotics

- Tissue plasminogen activator (TPA) therapy: to treat ischemic stroke, within three hours of onset of symptoms
- Anticoagulation (e.g., warfarin)

Surgical Treatment

- Carotid endarterectomy
- ICA resection and reanastomosis (for kinking)
- Carotid thrombectomy
- Bypass (subclavian-carotid or carotid-carotid)

- Vertebral artery transposition to CCA
- Vertebral artery reconstruction
- Direct focal repairs (e.g., subclavian artery, vertebral)

Endovascular Treatment

- Carotid angioplasty
- Carotid stent

Points to Remember

- Always compare flow velocities from side to side.
- NASCET (North American Symptomatic Carotid Endarterectomy Trial) demonstrated that the long term benefit of CEA was significantly greater than medical treatment in symptomatic patients with >70% stenosis. [26]
- ACAS (Asymptomatic Carotid Atherosclerosis Study) demonstrated marginal benefit of carotid endarterectomy in asymptomatic male patients with >60% stenosis. [27]
- CREST was the largest randomized clinical trial for patients at risk for stroke from carotid artery disease to either CEA or carotid stent placement with embolic protection.
- It is important to clearly demonstrate that the ICA is occluded and that there is no "trickle" flow present during the duplex scan since carotid endarterectomy is not usually performed on completely occluded ICAs.
- The ICA may be coiled or tortuous; creating an "S" or "C" shape or can be curved, typically located in the first 2-3 cm of the ICA and may produce a bruit. The patient is usually asymptomatic. [11] Carotid artery kinks occur four times more often in women than men. [11]

- The carotid body is a chemoreceptor which is part of the autonomic nervous system. It regulates arterial blood levels of oxygen, carbon dioxide and hydrogen ions and can signal vasoconstriction when necessary.
- CBT are unilateral in 95% of reported cases [3] and females suffer from carotid body tumors 3-5 more times than men. [54] The tumors are benign in 90-95% of all cases. [28] CBTs are more frequent in people living at higher altitudes. [29, 30]
- There are two different methods for measuring a carotid stenosis: NASCET versus a duplex derived measurement.
  - The NASCET derived measurement tends to be about 10% less than a duplex derived measurement for stenoses < 80%. (e.g., 65% reduction by duplex will only measure about 55% by NASCET).
  - In a large bulb, a 50% duplex reduction may be only 10% by NASCET.
  - Duplex % diameter stenosis $= 1 - \dfrac{\text{residual lumen}}{\text{true lumen}} \times 100$

    (NASCET method uses the lumen beyond the bulb where the walls are parallel for the denominator in this calculation.)

References

1. Zarins CK, Xu C, Glagov, S. (2005). Artery wall pathology in atherosclerosis. In Rutherford Vascular Surgery 6th edition. (123-148). Philadelphia. Elsevier Saunders.
2. Henderson, E. L., Y.-J. Geng, et al. (1999). "Death of Smooth Muscle Cells and Expression of Mediators of Apoptosis by T Lymphocytes in Human Abdominal Aortic Aneurysms." Circulation 99(1): 96-104.
3. Black JH, Cambria RP. (2005). Aortic dissection: perspectives for the vascular/endovascular surgeon. In Rutherford Vascular Surgery 6th edition. (1512-1533). Philadelphia. Elsevier Saunders.
4. Kupinski, Anne Marie (2013) In The Vascular System 1st edition (p 66, 81), Philadelphia. Wolters Kluwer.
5. Shepard RJ, Rooke T. (2005). Uncommon arteriopathies. In Rutherford Vascular Surgery 6th edition. (453-474). Philadelphia. Elsevier Saunders.
6. Young JR, Graor RA, Olin JW, Bartholomew JR. (1991). "Vasospastic disease" in Peripheral Vascular Diseases. (361-378). St Louis : Mosby Elsevier Health Science.
7. Rowe VL, Yellin AE, Weaver FA. (2005). Vascular injuries of the extremities. In Rutherford Vascular Surgery 6th edition. (1044-1058). Philadelphia. Elsevier Saunders.
8. Hom C. (8-25-2010). "Takayasu's arteritis" Emedicine.medscape.com. http://emedicine.medscape.com/article/1007566-overview (12-4-2010).
9. Hajj-Ali RA, Mandell B. (2005). Approach to and management of inflammatory vasculitis. In Rajagopalan S, Mukherjee D, Mohler E. (Eds). Manual of Vascular Diseases. (353-375). Philadelphia. Lippinott Williams & Wilkins.
10. Basu N, Watts R., et al. (2010). "EULAR points to consider in the development of classification and diagnostic criteria in systemic vasculitis." Annals of the Rheumatic Diseases 69(10): 1744-1750.
11. Krupski WC. (2005). Uncommon disorders affecting the carotid arteries. In Rutherford Vascular Surgery 6th edition. (2064-2092). Philadelphia. Elsevier Saunders.
12. Saldana, M. J., L. E. Salem, et al. (1973). "High altitude hypoxia and chemodectomas." Human Pathology 4(2): 251-263.
13. Sumner DS, Zierler RE. (2005). Vascular physiology: essential hemodynamic principles. In Rutherford Vascular Surgery 6th edition. (75-123). Philadelphia. Elsevier Saunders.
14. Casey PJ, LaMuraglia GM. (2005). Anastomotic aneurysms. In Rutherford Vascular Surgery 6th edition. (894-902). Philadelphia. Elsevier Saunders.
15. Shepard RJ, Rooke T. (2005). Uncommon arteriopathies. In Rutherford Vascular Surgery 6th edition. (453-474). Philadelphia. Elsevier Saunders.
16. Zieler, R. Eugene (2010) In Strandness's Duplex Scanning in Vascular Disorders. 4th edition (93, 100, 117-121), Philadelphia. Wolters Kluwer.
17. Lal BK, Hobson II RW, Tofighi B, Kapadia I, Cuadra S, and Jamil Z. Duplex ultrasound velocity criteria for the stented carotid artery. 2007. Journal of vascular surgery Volume 47, Number 1. pp 63-73.
18. Grant, E., Benson, C., et al, Carotid Artery Stenosis: Gray-Scale and Doppler US Diagnosis—Society of Radiologists in Ultrasound Consensus Conference, Radiology 229 (2): 340-346, 2003.
19. Bluth, EI, Wetzner, SM, Baker, JD, et al: Carotid duplex sonography: a multicenter recommendation for standardized imaging and Doppler criteria. Radiographics 8:487-506, 1988.
20. Karnik, S. K., B. S. Brooke, et al. (2003). "A critical role for elastin signaling in vascular morphogenesis and disease." Development 130(2): 411-423.
21. Krettek, A., G. K. Sukhova, et al. (2003). "Elastogenesis in human arterial disease: a role for macrophages in disordered elastin synthesis." Arteriosclerosis, thrombosis, and vascular biology 23(4):582-587.
22. Patel, M. I., J. Melrose, et al. (1996). "Increased synthesis of matrix metalloproteinases by aortic smooth muscle cells is implicated in the etiopathogenesis of abdominal aortic aneurysms." Journal of Vascular Surgery 24(1): 82-92.
23. Henderson, E. L., Y.-J. Geng, et al. (1999). "Death of Smooth Muscle Cells and Expression of Mediators of Apoptosis by T Lymphocytes in Human Abdominal Aortic Aneurysms." Circulation 99(1): 96-104.
24. López-Candales A, Holmes DR, Liao S, Scott MJ, Wickline SA, Thompson RW. Decreased vascular smooth muscle cell density in medial degeneration of human abdominal aortic aneurysms. (1997). Am J Pathol. March; 150(3): 993–1007.
25. Hellmann, D. B., D. J. Grand, et al. (2007). "Inflammatory Abdominal Aortic Aneurysm." JAMA: The Journal of the American Medical Association 297(4): 395-400.
26. Young JR, Graor RA, Olin JW, Bartholomew JR. (1991). Miscellaneous arterial disease" in Peripheral Vascular Diseases. (379-394). St Louis :Mosby Elsevier Health Science.
27. Walker, MD, Marler JR, Goldstein M, Grady PA, Toole JF, Baker WH, Castaldo JE, Chambless LE, Moore WS, Robertson JT, Young B, Howard VJ, Marler JR, Ourvis S, Vernon D, Needham K, Beck P, Celani VJ, Sauebeck L, von Rajcs JA, Atkins D. Endarterectomy for Asymptomatic Carotid Artery Stenosis JAMA 1995; 273: 1421-1428.
28. Watts RA, and Scott DGI., (2010). Classification and Epidemiology of Vasculitis in Clinical Practice. R. A. Watts and D. G. I. Scott, Springer London: 7-11.
29. Basu N, Watts R., et al. (2010). "EULAR points to consider in the development of classification and diagnostic criteria in systemic vasculitis." Annals of the Rheumatic Diseases 69(10): 1744-1750.
30. Johns Hopkins Vasculitis Clinic "Giant cell arteritis" Johns Hopkins Medicine (2009).http://vasculitis.med.jhu.edu/types of/giantcell.html (12-4-2010).

Definition

The use of real time B-mode ultrasonography to identify areas of increased thickness along the lumen-intima and media-adventitia interfaces of an extracranial carotid artery in order to predict early atherosclerosis or classify patients with cardiovascular disease (CVD).

The common carotid artery is typically used for this evaluation since it is often free of plaque. The clear interface between the anechoic arterial lumen and the echoic intima makes definition of these interfaces and opportunity for measurement possible.

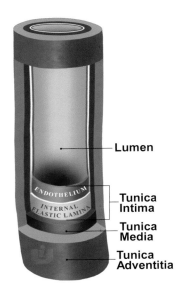

Arterial wall anatomy

Etiology (of carotid atherosclerosis)

- Endothelial dysfunction
- Hemodynamic forces

Risk Factors (to predict cardiovascular risk)

- Genetic predisposition
- Gender (Males >Females)
- Race
- Obesity
- Smoking
- Diabetes
- Radiation therapy

Indications for Exam

- History of early cardiovascular disease in an immediate family member (men <55 years and women <65 years of age).[1,2]
- Patients younger than 60 years of age who are not candidates for drug therapy but have severe abnormalities involving a single risk factor. [1]
- Women, younger than 60 years of age with >2 CVD risk factors. [1]

Contraindications/Limitations

- Suboptimal visualization by B-mode image (including, but not limited to the lack of visible "double line" along the far arterial wall, motion artifact from the jugular vein or deep vessels).
- Tortuous carotid arteries
- Intraobserver variability of CIMT measurements range between 3.7 - 7.8% according to published data.[2]

Location (of arteries for testing)

- Distal common carotid artery (most common)
- Carotid bifurcation
- Proximal internal carotid artery

Patient History

- CVD
- Risk factors for CVD [3]
  - Hypertension
  - Hyperlipidemia
  - Diabetes
  - Obesity
  - Sedentary lifestyle
  - Smoking
  - Stress
  - Poor diet

Physical Examination

- Carotid bruit (abnormal sound heard through auscultation caused by vibration of tissue from turbulent flow).

Carotid Intima Media Thickness (CIMT) Protocol

> *CIMT measurements should be performed using the far wall of the carotid artery. Near-wall CIMT is less accurate since the US beam has to travel from a more echogenic to a less echogenic interface.*

- The patient is examined in the supine position with the head elevated.
- Some patients may require the use of a range of transducers for superficial vessels including high frequency, linear-array (5-7 MHz) (8-15 MHz) transducers.
- The typical depth used for scanning is 4 cm, although increased depths may be necessary in patients with deeper arteries or larger necks.
- Evaluate the common carotid artery (CCA), carotid bifurcation and internal carotid artery (ICA) for any carotid plaque with grayscale and color imaging in both the transverse (short-axis) and longitudinal (sagittal) planes. Adjust the color scale to accurately fill the arterial lumen around any observed plaque without resulting in color-bleeding.

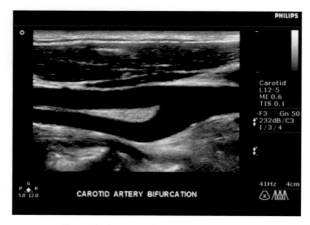

B-mode image of carotid bifurcation
Images courtesy of Philips Healthcare

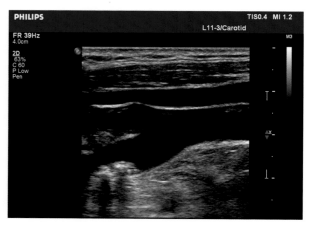

Plaque noted by B-mode imaging
Images courtesy of Philips Healthcare

- Document and report the location of carotid plaque (e.g., near/far wall, proximal/mid or distal CCA segment). Report the presence of any calcific arterial shadowing which may result in technically suboptimal images.

- Measure and record the peak systolic velocity (PSV) of the CCA and ICA in longitudinal view using pulsed wave Doppler (60° Doppler angle or less, with the angle cursor parallel to the vessel walls in the center of the flow stream).

- Identify a straight segment of the distal CCA in the longitudinal plane, approximately 1 cm from the flow divider. Using the heel-toe probe method, align the CCA so that the artery is perfectly horizontal on the ultrasound screen. Optimize the B-mode image to see the characteristic "double line" representing the lumen-intima-and media-adventitia interfaces.

> *(ASE consensus) Histologic studies have confirmed that the two echogenic lines produced by B-mode imaging correspond to the lumina-intima and media-adventitia interfaces.*

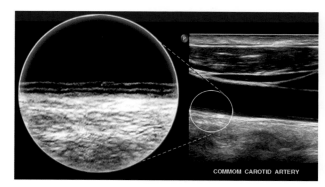

Characteristic "double line" between the lumen-intima and media-adventitia interfaces
Image courtesy of Philips Healthcare

- Record loops or still frames of this distal CCA segment using each of the carotid scan windows: anterior, anterio-lateral and posterior-lateral. Loops should consist of 3-5 cardiac cycles.

- Capture an image of the arterial wall when systolic-diastolic differences are at a minimum (during end-diastole). Capture multiple images of the distal CCA, concentrating on image optimization of the far-wall.

- Repeat the protocol for the contralateral carotid arteries.

- Use a manual or semiautomated border detection measuring technique to determine the CIMT value. It may be necessary to edit suboptimal borders generated by the automated programs.

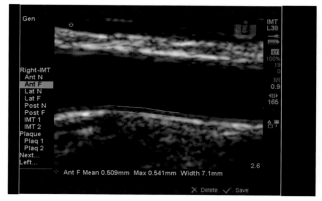

Manual CIMT trace method

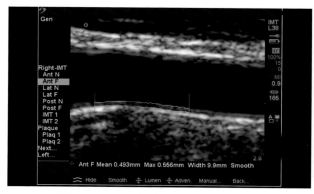

Auto CIMT trace method *Image courtesy of SonoSite FUJIFILM*

- Using the best images recorded, trace the intima and media adventitia interfaces of the far-wall. Using 1 cm length segments, repeat these measurements multiple times to ensure accuracy.
- Report the CIMT as an average of all of the recorded values. Mean CIMT values should also be reported using both right and left carotid data.

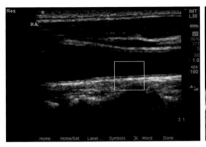 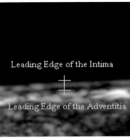

"Double-line" noted on the far wall of the carotid artery by B-mode imaging

Image courtesy of SonoSite FUJIFILM

TABLE 15: Carotid Intima Media Thickness Protocol at a Glance

1. Evaluate the CCA, bifurcation and ICA for disease in the transverse and longitudinal planes using B-mode and color imaging. Record representative images.
   - Record B-mode and color images. Document and describe the location of any carotid plaque.
   - Record representative PW Doppler waveforms of the CCA and ICA.
2. Identify a relatively straight segment of the distal CCA in the longitudinal plane, approximately 1 cm proximal to the flow divider and optimize visualization of the "double lined" far-arterial wall.
3. Record loops/stills of the distal CCA segment from three scan windows; anterior, anteriolateral and posteriolateral.
4. Repeat the protocol for the contralateral carotid artery.
5. Measure CIMT using manual or semiautomated detection software.
6. Report the average CIMT values for each side.

Interpretation

- Research shows that CIMT increases linearly with age from a mean value of 0.48 at age 40 to 1.02 by age 100.[4]

$$(0.009 \times age) + 0.116 = mean\ CIMT$$

CIMT measurements have not been proven to be particularly precise and are best reported as a range in order to account for technical differences (e.g., instrumentation and techniques) since the US beam has to travel from a more echogenic to a less echogenic interface. American Society of Echocardiography (ASE)

- CIMT values less than or equal to the 25th percentile are considered at low-risk for cardiovascular disease (CVD).[1,5]
- CIMT values in the 25th-75th percentile are considered average and suggest no change in CVD risk.[1,5]
- CIMT values >the 75th percentile are considered elevated and suggest increased risk of CVD.[1,5]

Repeat measurements should be within 0.05 mm of each other.

Interpretation at a Glance

TABLE 16: CIMT Diagnostic Criteria	
Description	**IMT**
Normal	<0.8
Abnormal	>0.8
Age, gender and race should be documented for risk assessment.	

Source: Stein JH, Fraizer MC, et al. (2004). Vascular age: Integrating carotid intima-media thickness measurements with global coronary risk assessment. *Clin Cardiol.* (388-392) 27.

Risk for CVD Based on CIMT Values	
Risk of CVD	**CIMT value (in percentile)**
Low	≤25th
Average	25-75th
High	>75th

Source: Stein JH MD FASE, Korcarz CE DVM RDCS FASE, Hurst RT MD, Lonn E MD MSc FASE, Kendall CB BS RDCS, Mohler ER MD, Najjar SS MD, Rembold CM MD, Post WS MD MS. (2008). Use of carotid ultrasound to identify subclinical vascular disease and evaluate cardiovascular risk: A consensus statement from the American society of echocardiography carotid intima-media thickness task force endorsed by the society for vascular medicine. *Journal of the American Society of Echocardiography* Feb; 21(2):93-106.

Correlation

- CT scan to measure coronary artery calcification score. (ARIC)
- Transesophageal echocardiography (TEE)
- Intravascular ultrasound (IVUS) during arteriography
- MRI

Medical Treatment and Prevention

- Statin therapy
- Modify risk factors (e.g., reduce cholesterol/HTN, manage DM, smoking cessation)
- Exercise regimen
- Antihypertensive medication

Points to Remember

- Carotid intima media thickness (CIMT) has been shown to be associated with increased risk of myocardial infarction (MI), stroke and/or death from heart disease.[1,5,6] There is a link between greater CIMT and more extensive/severe cases of coronary heart disease.
- CIMT testing is used to predict major critical CVD events in symptomatic and asymptomatic patients, with and without prevalent CVD.[1,7]

- CIMT is used by some clinicians to predict the likelihood and efficiency of treatment used to prevent atherosclerosis before it becomes symptomatic. [2]

- CIMT increases nearly 3 fold between the ages of 20 and 90 years of age. [1]

- CIMT evaluation using B-mode imaging is preferred over M-mode imaging since B-mode provides better perpendicular images and is capable of providing thickness values for longer segments of the artery, rather than just a single point. [1]

- A carotid plaque has been defined as CIMT $\geq$1.5 mm or <50% of the surrounding IMT by the Manheim Intima Media Thickness Consensus Panel. Some physicians consider CIMT >1.0 mm as a significant plaque. [6]

- An ultrasound phantom is suggested to ensure accurate resolution of the transducer. [1]

- To prevent image degradation, digital images (e.g., DICOM) are preferred for analysis over digitized video capture. [1]

- Imaging should not be performed in patients with known significant atherosclerotic disease or if results would not alter patient management. [1].

- Semiautomated border detection software is thought to improve reproducibility and shorten reading time. Some critics of automated programs believe CIMT are thicker than those measured manually with or without electronic calipers. [1]

- CIMT testing is a cardiovascular risk assessment tool and should not be used as a substitute for a clinically indicated carotid ultrasound duplex exam. [1]

- Increased CIMT has been associated with higher risks for peripheral vascular disease and stroke. [2]

- In cases where the wall interfaces are suboptimal, you can trace a segment <1 cm in length. Do not trace any interfaces that are not clearly visualized.

References

1. Stein JH MD FASE, Korcarz CE DVM RDCS FASE, Hurst RT MD, Lonn E MD MSc FASE, Kendall CB BS RDCS, Mohler ER MD, Najjar SS MD, Rembold CM MD, Post WS MD MS. (2008). Use of carotid ultrasound to identify subclinical vascular disease and evaluate cardiovascular risk: A consensus statement from the American society of echocardiography carotid intima-media thickness task force endorsed by the society for vascular medicine. *Journal of the American Society of Echocardiography.* Feb; 21(2):93-106.

2. Leon Jr, LR, Brewster LP, Labropoulos N. (2005). Non-invasive screening and utility of carotid intima-media thickness. In Mansour MA, Labropoulos N. (Eds.), *Vascular Diagnosis.* (157-173). Philadelphia: Elsevier Saunders.

3. National Heart Lung and Blood Institute. (12/3/2011 10:58 PM). Retrieved from http://www.nhlbi.nih.gov/.

4. Zwiebel, WJ. Pellerito JS. (2005). Ultrasound assessment of carotid plaque. In Zwiebel WJ, Pellerito JS (Eds.), In Introduction to Vascular Ultrasonography 5th ed, (155-169). Philadelphia: Elsevier Saunders.

5. Nambi J MD, Chambless L PhD, Folsom AR MD, He M, Hu Y, Mosley T PhD, Volcik V PhD, Boerwinkle E PhD, Ballantyne CM MD. Carotid intima-media thickness and presence or absence of plaque improves prediction of coronary heart disease risk in the Atherosclerosis Risk in Communities (ARIC) study. (2010). J Am Coll Cardiol. 2010 April 13; 55(15): 1600–1607.

6. Cobble M, Bale B (2010). Carotid intima-media thickness: knowledge and application to everyday practice. *Postgrad Med.* Jan; 122 (1): 10-8.

7. Tabor A RVT, Size GP RVT RVS RPhS FSVU (2007). What is IMT? Sonosite. PowerPoint slides].

8. Carotid intima-media thickness and presence or absence of plaque improves prediction of coronary heart disease risk in the Atherosclerosis Risk in Communities (ARIC) study. Nambi V, Chambless L, Folsom AR, He M, Hu Y, Mosley T, Volcik K, Boerwinkle E, and Ballantyne CM, Am Coll Cardiol. 2010 April 13; 55(15): 1600–1607. doi:10.1016/j.jacc.2009.11.075.

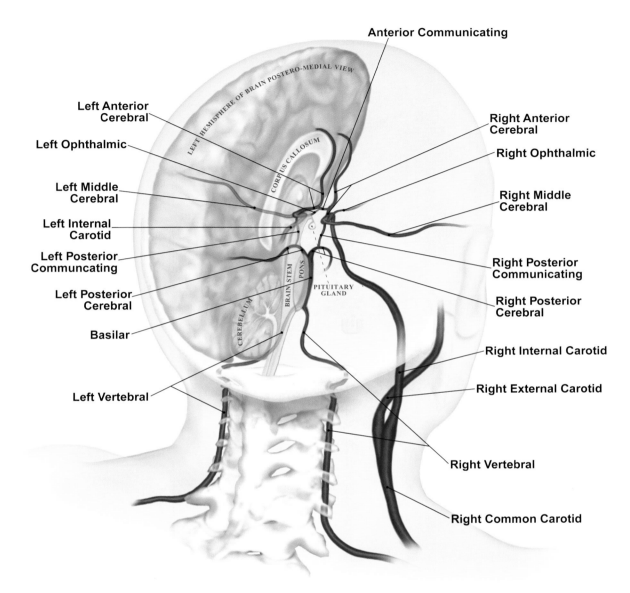

Anterior Communicating

Left Anterior Cerebral

Left Ophthalmic

Left Middle Cerebral

Left Internal Carotid

Left Posterior Communcating

Left Posterior Cerebral

Basilar

Left Vertebral

LEFT HEMISPHERE OF BRAIN POSTERO-MEDIAL VIEW

CORPUS CALLOSUM

CEREBELLUM

BRAIN STEM

PONS

PITUITARY GLAND

Right Anterior Cerebral

Right Ophthalmic

Right Middle Cerebral

Right Posterior Communicating

Right Posterior Cerebral

Right Internal Carotid

Right External Carotid

Right Vertebral

Right Common Carotid

Circle of Willis Posterior View

Definition

Intracranial cerebrovascular testing is performed to assess arterial patency and measure flow velocities within the Circle of Willis using transcranial Doppler (TCD) or transcranial imaging (TCI). The hemodynamic effects of stenosis or occlusion can be studied in real-time.

TCD and TCI are able to determine the extent and patterns of collateral circulation in patients with known cerebrovascular disease and can be used to monitor patients with vasospasm after subarachnoid hemorrhage and detect embolic events (e.g., during surgery).

Rationale

TCD uses range-gated pulsed wave (PW) Doppler to penetrate "windows" or openings through the cranium and assess intracranial cerebrovascular blood flow. TCI adds imaging and utilizes color flow as a guide during the examination.

Etiology of Intracranial Disease

- Atherosclerosis, resulting in stenosis or occlusion
- Embolus
- Thrombosis
- Vasculitis
- Carotid aneurysm
- Carotid dissection (spontaneous or post-traumatic)
- Arteriovenous malformations (AVM)
- Non-atherosclerotic causes; e.g., carotid coiling or kinking
- Fibromuscular dysplasia (FMD

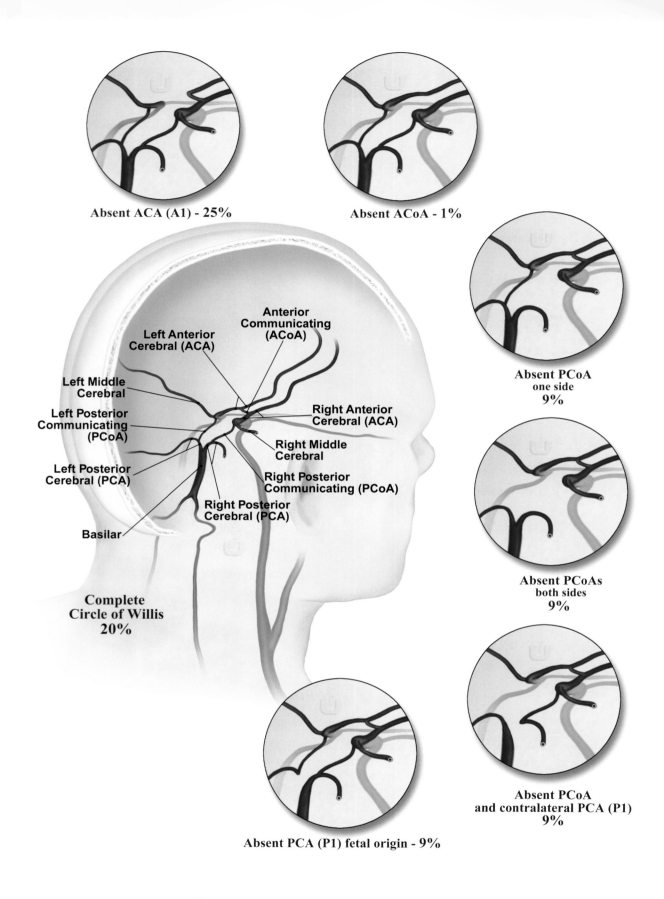

Absent ACA (A1) - 25%

Absent ACoA - 1%

Absent PCoA
one side
9%

Absent PCoAs
both sides
9%

Absent PCoA
and contralateral PCA (P1)
9%

Anterior
Communicating
(ACoA)

Left Anterior
Cerebral (ACA)

Left Middle
Cerebral

Left Posterior
Communicating
(PCoA)

Left Posterior
Cerebral (PCA)

Basilar

Right Anterior
Cerebral (ACA)

Right Middle
Cerebral

Right Posterior
Communicating (PCoA)

Right Posterior
Cerebral (PCA)

**Complete
Circle of Willis
20%**

Absent PCA (P1) fetal origin - 9%

Most Common Variations of the Circle of Willis

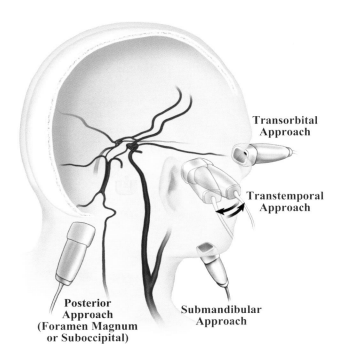

Acoustical windows used in transcranial testing

Risk Factors

- Hypertension
- Hypercholesteremia
- Diabetes
- Smoking
- Age
- Gender (Male >Female)
- History of peripheral vascular disease (PVD)
- History of coronary artery disease (CAD) or atrial fibrillation (A-fib)
- History of cerebrovascular disease (CVA, TIA, subarachnoid hemorrhage or intracranial aneurysm)
- Vasculitis
- Family history
- Trauma, especially to the cranium

Indications for Exam

- Detect hemodynamically significant stenosis (>65%) of the intracranial cerebral arteries
- Assess collateral circulation in patients with regions of known severe disease
- Determine the affects of hemodynamically significant stenosis/occlusion of the extracranial arteries on intracranial circulation
- Evaluate patients with cerebral vasospasm (e.g., subarachnoid hemorrhage patients)
- Detect AVM and determine flow patterns and supplying arterial flow
- Suspected intracranial aneurysm
- Embolism detection during operative procedures. Middle cerebral arterial (MCA) flow is monitored during carotid endarterectomy (CEA) and other revascularization procedures, such as cardiac surgery.
- Detection of cerebral ischemia during surgery (e.g., when cross-clamping)

- Detection and management of post-operative hyperemia
- Suspected carotid dissection, post-angiography
- Evaluation of pediatric patients with various blood vessel disease such as sickle cell disease, Moyamoya disease, etc. to assess the risk of stroke (CVA)
- Evaluate vasomotor reserve (VMR) with the use of CO_2 challenge testing
- Detection of right to left cardiac or pulmonary shunts using bubble studies (e.g., patent foramen ovale (PFO))
- Evaluate intracranial flow, post-cranial injury
- Evaluate patients for suspected brain death

Contraindications/Limitations

- Inadequate cranial windows preventing insonation of the Circle of Willis
  - Older patients, especially women have thicker bones (*hyperostosis*) which may inhibit visualization through the transtemporal window.
- Uncooperative or agitated patients (e.g., post-operative, patients with cranial injury or some pediatric patients, etc.)
- Exams can be time consuming.
- Exams can be limited due to severity of the patient's condition or poor patient positioning.
- Since the Circle of Willis anatomy can vary and TCD does not involve direct imaging, incorrect identification of vessels is possible.
- TCI imaging is dependent on color flow and vessel walls are not well visualized.
- PW Doppler can produce aliasing in very high intracranial stenoses.
- Collaterals or vasospasms can be misinterpreted as a stenosis.
- Transcranial testing is not sensitive for smaller intracranial aneurysms.
- Recent eye surgery

Circle of Willis

The Circle of Willis refers to the intracranial arteries. The polygonal shape of this "circle" allows blood to flow between the right and left hemispheres of the brain. There is an anterior (carotid) and posterior (vertebrobasilar) supply to the Circle of Willis.

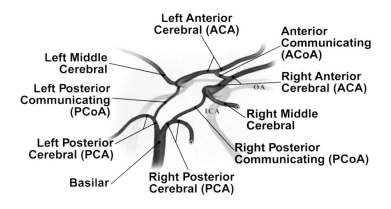

Location of the cranial windows (and their accessible arteries)

There are several acoustical windows used to access the intracranial vessels. These are thinner areas or openings (*foramina*) of the cranium that transcranial testing uses to visualize the following arteries:

- Transorbital
  - OA
  - Carotid siphon
- Transtemporal
  - MCA
  - ACA
  - MCA-ACA bifurcation
  - PCA
  - Terminal ICA
  - ACoA and/or PCoA (when functioning as collateral pathways)
- Submandibular (retromandibular)
  - Distal cervical portion of the ICA
- Transforamenal (suboccipital)
  - Vertebral arteries (VA)
  - Basilar artery (BA)

> *Staples, bandaging, scar tissue, etc. may limit scan windows.*

Mechanism of disease

Atheroscerotic cerebrovascular events are defined as brain tissue damage due to disruption of blood flow from a stenosis or occlusion. Types of cerebrovascular events include:

- Transient ischemic attack (TIA: neurological deficit (motor, sensory, speech deficit, etc.) lasting less than 24 hours.
- CVA: deficits lasting longer than 24 hours are considered a completed stroke.
- Types of stroke include:[5,6]
  - **Ischemic stroke**: (most common, approximately 85% of all strokes) due to a decrease in blood flow to the brain caused by an arterial narrowing or blockage. The five widely accepted sub classifications of ischemic stroke are:
  - **Cardioembolic (embolic)**: an embolus from a cardiac or pericardiac source causes a territorial infarction. Most common cause is atrial fibrillation, where there is pooling of the blood in the heart which can lead to the formation of blood clots. Plaque or fragments of an organized thrombus loosen and flow upstream. Emboli become lodged in a distant blood vessel, causing arterial occlusion and reduction of flow.
  - **Large vessel atherosclerosis**: (atherothrombotic), Occlusion or stenosis greater than 50% of the major intra- and extracranial arteries (internal carotid, common carotid, vertebral, basilar, middle cerebral, anterior cerebral or posterior cerebral) supplying the vascular territory of the stroke. Decrease in lumenal area due to atherosclerosis and/or thrombosis.

- **Lacunar**: (Small vessel disease) account for approximately 25% of all acute ischemic strokes.[6,7] Lacunar infarcts are small infarcts (3-20 mm in diameter) in the deeper noncortical parts of the cerebrum and brainstem. They result from occlusion or stenosis of penetrating branches of the large cerebral arteries.
  - **Stroke of other determined etiology**: these rare cases normally occur in the young who have no stroke risk factors. They include coagulopathies, vasculopathies, genetic disorders and metabolic disorders.
  - **Stroke of undetermined etiology**: In a significant number of cases (≤40%), no clear explanation can be found for an ischemic stroke despite an extensive diagnostic evaluation.
- **Hemorrhagic stroke**: (approximately 15% of all strokes) due to artery rupture or venous malformation in the brain. Blood accumulates and compresses the surrounding brain tissue. In addition there is no or little blood flow distal to the rupture site. Hemorrhagic strokes are classified as either subarachnoid hemorrhage or intracerebral hemorrhage.
- **Subarachnoid hemorrhage (SAH)**: most commonly due to trauma but also occur due to rupture of a cerebral aneurysm. In 10-20% of spontaneous, nontraumatic cases no cause is found.
- **Intracerebral hemorrhage**: (parenchymatous) Rupture of a blood vessel within the parenchyma often the result of chronic hypertension or an intrinsic vessel problem such as amyloid angiopathy or other vascular malformation. May also be caused by a brain tumor.
- **Vasospasm**: decreased perfusion caused by a gradual constriction of cerebral arterial flow in the subarachnoid space following subarachnoid hemorrhage. Normal arterial wall vasodilatation/vasoconstriction is disrupted due to the changes in metabolism and arterial wall structure A higher risk of cerebral infarction exists due to the constricted arterial flow caused by the surrounding blood clot.[8]
- **Vasculitis**: hyperactivity of the immune system causing inflammation of the vessel walls. Inflammation can lead to arterial narrowing and a subsequent decrease in cerebral perfusion.
- **Intracerebral aneurysm**: Aneurysmal disease results from weakening of the structural proteins (elastin and collagen) within the medial layer of the arterial wall. Large aneurysms can constrict surrounding arterial flow and also carry the risk of rupture, subsequent SAH and cerebral infarct. The basilar artery bifurcation, vertebral artery junction and ACoA are areas prone to aneurysmal formation because of the high wall sheer stress, hydrostatic and translumenal pressures through these segments. Also, individuals with an incomplete Circle of Willis may also have a higher risk for aneurysmal formation since there is greater flow resistance through their arterial pathways.[9]
- **Carotid dissection**: tears in the intimal layer of the arterial wall allowing blood flow to access the media. Trauma can cause a dissection, though it also occurs due to aging or connective tissue disorders when the breakdown of collagen and elastin fibers, render the arterial wall weak and at risk for tears.[10,13] Blood flows through the tear in the intimal layer and sometimes clots. Pulsatile flow and high blood pressure cause propagation of the dissection.[10] Dissection between the medial and adventitial layers may result in a false lumen, which can narrow the true carotid lumen.[10]

- **Arteriovenous malformations**: abnormal connection between an artery and vein where blood flows directly from the artery into the venous system without passing through the tissues and capillary bed. The exact cause of AVM is unknown. AVM can be a congenital condition, with the onset of symptoms occurring at any age.
- **Carotid coiling/kinking**: coils and kinks are thought to normally be present during the embryonic stage of development. The arteries typically straighten once the fetal heart and larger vessels descend into the thoracic cavity. In some patients, these coils/kinks linger.[11] Intralumenal folds involving all three arterial layers have been observed on histological study along with increased fibrous tissue, and a loss of elastic tissue and smooth muscle cell within the medial layer. Some believe that atherosclerotic occlusive disease must be present before patients with coils/kinks become symptomatic.[12]
- **Fibromuscular dysplasia**: non-atherosclerotic arterial disease which affects medium and large sized vessels, including the internal carotid artery (ICA). A significant decrease in blood flow through the ICA can result in decreased cerebral pefusion.

Location of Disease

- For stenosis: MCA, carotid siphon and terminal ICA
- For aneurysm: ACoA, MCA, PCA

Patient History

- Aphasia-difficulty expressing or understanding language
- Dysphagia- difficulty swallowing
- Dysarthria-language issues (ranging from slurred speech to mumbling)
- Visual disturbances
- Numbness/tingling
- Paresthesia (hemiparesis or monoparesis)
- Syncope
- Ataxia- gait disturbance

Physical Examination

- Assess responsiveness (ranging from awake and responsive to unresponsive)
- Ability to follow commands (grip objects, open and close eyes, etc.)
- Facial paralysis
- Ability to move arms/legs independently
- Sensory loss
- Language difficulties (e.g., aphasia, dysarthria)
- Visual loss (monocular or binocular)

Intracranial Testing Protocols

- Obtain a patient history to include symptoms and risk factors whenever possible.

Equipment and supplies

- A non-imaging TCD system or color duplex ultrasound for TCI exams with PW Doppler and bidirectional spectral analysis capabilities.
  - Real-time spectral Doppler waveforms will produce a bidirectional signal which will display flow toward the transducer, above the baseline and flow away from the transducer, below the baseline.

> Flow direction is relative to the transducer; toward, away from or in both directions (bidirectional) from the probe.

- Both non-imaging and imaging systems should allow for adjustment of sample gate, audiovisual output, permanent recording and measurement of velocities using manual calipers.
- A low frequency (1.0 to 2.0 MHz) PW Doppler transducer should be used for TCD imaging. A low frequency transducer (1.8 to 2.5 MHz) is used for TCI examinations.
- A small amount of ultrasound gel is needed to start. Additional gel may be necessary to maintain contact with the skin when having to tilt the probe in order to obtain the best angle.

Patient positioning

- The patient is examined in the supine position with the head supported and neck straight for evaluations through the transtemporal, transorbital and submandibular windows.

> The transforamenal window may also be studied in the prone position.

- Have the patient lie on their side or ask the patient to sit and lower their head towards their chest in order to access the transforamenal window.
- The technologist should try to be seated at the head of the bed whenever possible with their arms supported.
- When imaging through the transorbital window, ask the patient to gently close their eyelids during the examination and focus their eye to the opposite side that is being studied.

> Limit the amount of time spent imaging through the transorbital window and use the lowest output power possible in order to obtain the spectral tracing (10% or 17 mW/cm²).

TABLE 17: Windows for visualization of the intracranial arteries

Window	Arteries Visualized
Transtemporal	MCA
	ACA
	ACoA
	PCA
	PCoA
	Terminal ICA
Transorbital	OA
	Carotid siphon
Transforamenal	VA
	Basilar
Submandibular	ICA

Transcranial Doppler and Imaging Techniques

- Move over the various acoustical windows (transtemporal, transorbital, transforamenal and submandibular) while adjusting the depth, angle and location of the probe searching for the highest pitched signal (strongest signal: highest velocity and amplitude). Usually small maneuvers and minimal probe pressure are all that is necessary.

> *If no audible signal is located, try changing windows.*

- Use a large sample volume between 10-15 mm. When studying a child, a smaller sample volume (6 mm) may be used.
- Adjust the Doppler gain as needed throughout the examination to fill the peak velocity outline of the spectral waveform found on many types of transcranial equipment.
- Increase the output power while searching for intracranial signals if necessary. Once the signal has been located, consider lowering the output power to a level where signals can still be assessed.
- Record the peak-systolic velocity (PSV), end-diastolic velocity (EDV) and mean velocity (MV) in each vessel.

> *MV is more accurate than PSV since MV is unaffected by systemic factors (e.g., heart rate).*

- Use a 0° (zero) Doppler angle for TCI examinations. The exact angle is unknown between the ultrasound beam and the intracranial vessel, especially in TCD.
- During an abnormal TCI exam, the PRF, filters, color scales should be adjusted appropriately (e.g., low PRF and increased color scale for low-flow). Using both color and power Doppler may be helpful.
- The examination should be performed bilaterally.

Transtemporal Window

- Place the probe superior to the zygomatic arch, over the temporal bone. Set the sample volume depth for 50-60 mm and the output power to 100%. Locate the best sample area within this window. Once the signal is located, decrease the output power as much as possible without losing the arterial signal.

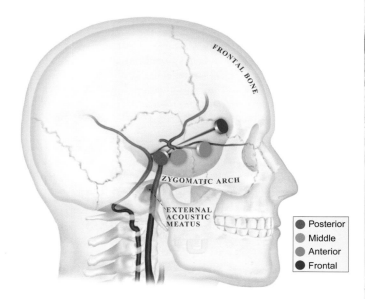

Transtemporal Probe Positioning

- There are three main areas of the transtemporal window: anterior, middle and posterior A fourth area known as the frontal is also considered by some technologists. Explore these areas, rotating the angle of the transducer and search for the best signal.

TABLE 18: Collateral Pathways of Intracranial Flow

Collateral path	Flow (Direction and Mean Velocity)			
	MCA	ACA	PCA	BA
ACA				
(Normal side)	Toward, normal	Away, elevated	P1: Toward, normal P2: Away, normal	Away, normal
(Diseased side)	Toward, normal/increased	Toward, turbulent	P1: Toward, normal P2: Away, normal	Away, normal
PCoA				
(Normal side)	Toward, normal	Away, elevated	P1: Toward, normal P2: Away, normal	Away, elevated-also expected elevated VA(s)
(Diseased side)	Toward, normal/increased	Toward, turbulent	P1: Toward, elevated P2: Away, normal	Away, normal
OA				
(Normal side)	Toward, normal	Away, normal	P1: Toward, normal P2: Away, normal	Away, normal
(Diseased side) *OA flow will be away, increased*	Toward, velocity dependent on capability of OA flow	Toward, velocity dependent on capability of OA flow	P1: Toward, normal P2: Away, normal	Away, normal

– Anterior: move the transducer 1.5 cm in front of the middle window, slightly superior to the zygomatic arch and angle posteriorly.

– Middle: move the transducer forward from the upper edge of the zygomatic arch, about 1.5 cm in front of the posterior window.

– Posterior: point the transducer anteriorly and superiorly, above the zygomatic arch and in front of the external auditory meatus. This area often provides the best access of the three.[4]

– Frontal: place the transducer over the frontal bone, superior and in front of the anterior window, angling posteriorly.

> Increase the sample volume depth to 60-70 mm if no signals are obtained at 50-60 mm in order to rule out MCA occlusion.

- **MCA**: Analyze the entire length of the MCA using a depth between 30-60 mm. Angle anteriorly and superiorly. Flow direction should be toward the transducer. Starting at the shallowest depth, adjust the sample volume deeper using small increments (2-5 mm) and small angle changes. Obtain and record the highest velocities in the proximal, mid and distal segments.

> The M2 segment can usually be found between 30-40 mm.

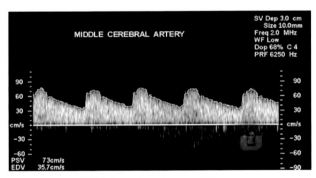

MCA Doppler signal at 30 mm

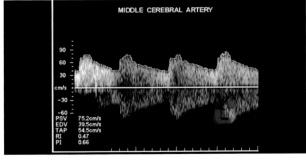

MCA signal at branch point

> You may need to angle differently for each artery if the MCA and ACA are not directly in line with each other.

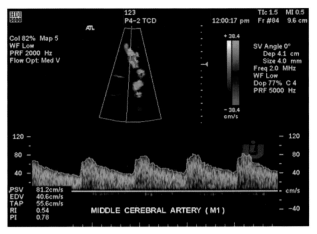

MCA using TCI

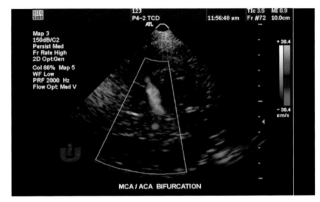

MCA/ACA bifurcation with TCI

- **Terminal ICA (tICA)**: Identify the terminal ICA (bifurcating segment into the MCA and ACA) for use as a reference point at a depth between 55-65 mm. Angle anteriorly and superiorly. Start at the MCA and increase the depth until bidirectional flow is noted. Blood flow toward and away from the probe represents simultaneous MCA and ACA flow. Obtain and record the highest velocity.

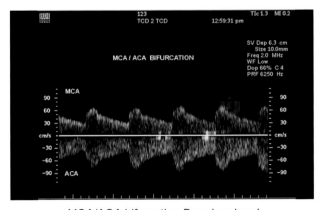

MCA/ACA bifurcation Doppler signal

- **ACA**: Increase the depth to about 60-80 mm from the terminal ICA to access the ACA. Angle anteriorly and superiorly. The A1 segment typically can be sampled between 70-80 mm depths. Flow direction should be away from the transducer. Obtain and record the highest velocity.

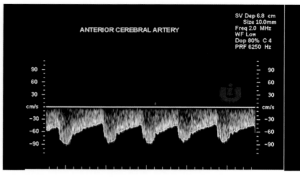

ACA Doppler signal

- **PCA**: Returning to the reference bifurcation, rotate the probe posteriorly and inferiorly using a depth between 60-70 mm. Flow direction should be toward the transducer. Adjust the sample volume using small increments and small angle changes. Obtain and record the highest velocities.
  - Flow should be toward the transducer in the P1 segment of the PCA.
  - The PCA signal should drop out at a depth of 55-60 mm.
  - Increase the depth to 70-80 mm in order to access the contralateral P1 segment of the PCA. Flow should be away from the transducer.
  - The ipsilateral P2 segment of the PCA can be analyzed by returning to a depth of 60-70 mm and angling more posteriorly. Flow should be away from the transducer.

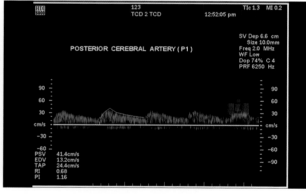

P1 segment Doppler signal

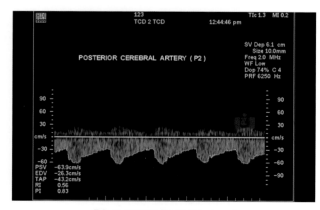

P2 segment Doppler signal

Artery	Mean Diameter	Mean Length of Artery
TABLE 19: Intracranial Artery Diameter and Length		
TICA	3.6-4.6 mm	–
PCoA	–	1.5 cm
MCA	2.5-3.8 mm	16.2 mm
ACA	1.8-3.0 mm	
PCA		
P1 segment	–	6.3 mm
P2 segment	1.96 mm	6.3 mm
BA	4.1 mm	–
	(distally)	

Source: Modified from Byrd-Raynor SA, Smith WB. (2010). Transcranial duplex imaging. In Zierler RE (Ed.), Strandess's duplex scanning disorders in vascular diagnosis 4th ed. (101-113).Philadelphia Wolters Kluwer Lippincott Williams & Wilkins

Collateral Vessels

- **ACoA**: When patent, the ACoA signal can be identified at a depth between 70-80 mm. Flow is usually toward the hemisphere being supported by this collateral. The ACoA also becomes active when one A1 segment of the ACA is congenitally absent.
- **PCoA**: When patent, the PCoA may be identified by angling the transducer posteriorly and slightly inferior from the terminal ICA. Expect turbulence and increased velocities.

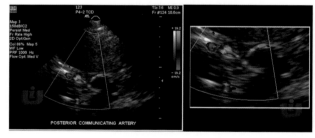

PCoA imaged using TCI

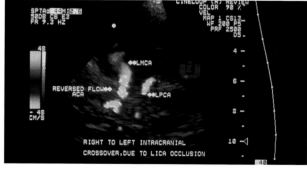

Collateralization observed using TCI

Transorbital Window

- **OA**: Place the probe on the orbital window, position laterally and point the probe medially. Adjust the depth to 40-60 mm and make small movements of the probe to access the OA. Flow should be toward the transducer. Obtain and record the highest velocity.

- **Carotid siphon**: Increase the depth to 60-80 mm in order to insonate the carotid siphon. Flow direction may vary due to tortuosity of this vessel in many individuals. Obtain and record the highest velocity.

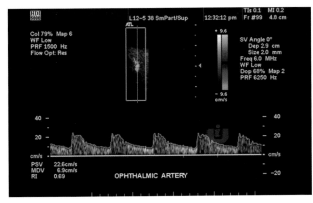

OA signal using TCI

Transforamenal Window

- **VA**: Place the probe at the midline of the nape of the neck. Make sure there is enough gel to ensure probe contact and aim the probe towards the patient's nose. Using a depth between 40-85 mm, move the probe slightly to either side of the midline. Flow direction should be away from the transducer.
- **BA**: Increase the depth from the vertebral arteries greater than 80 mm (90-100 mm in some cases) to insonate the basilar segment. Flow direction should be away from the transducer.

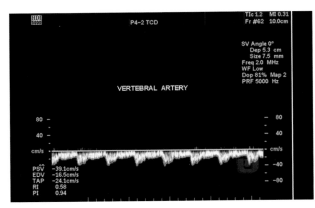

VA Doppler signal

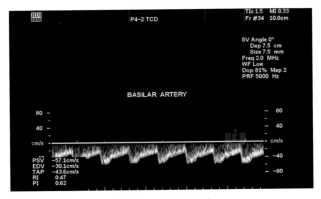

BA Doppler signal

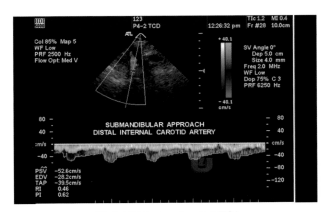

Distal ICA signal using TCI

Submandibular Window

- **Distal ICA** (proximal intracranial portion): Place the probe at the angle of the mandible and aim both slightly medial and toward the head. The ICA is usually found at a depth between 35-70 mm. Flow direction should be away from the transducer. Expect a low-resistant signal. *Note: You may be listening to the ECA if the signal obtained with this approach demonstrates high-resistance.*

Intraoperative Monitoring for Embolism (e.g., during CEA)

- Assess baseline intracranial velocities. Mark the transtemporal window on the skin for easier access peri-operatively.
- A head frame (or modified version of one) may be used to keep the transcranial equipment in place during the continuous MCA monitoring necessary during the procedure.
- Monitor the main trunk of the MCA with a 2 MHz probe at a depth of 45-55 mm. Adjust the sample volume to exclude any ACA or tICA flow signals.
- Determine an ischemic index by comparing the velocity at clamp time to the velocity pre-clamping. Other protocols suggest monitoring 10 minutes before CEA, as well as 10-15 minutes after CEA.[14]
- Document any signs of emboli (e.g., visible straight, bright lines through the spectral tracing) or changes in perfusion (e.g., mean velocities) during administration of anesthesia or during cross clamping procedures.
- Monitor for any of these changes during the different parts of the procedure (e.g., when the line is passed through the plaque to deploy the filter, balloon angioplasty, stent deployment, etc).

Arteriovenous Malformation (AVM) Evaluations

- Attempt to identify the artery feeding the AVM. Record flow velocities in the arterial branch.
- Record flow in the venous drainage vessel.
- Measure the diameter of the AVM when possible.

Evaluations for Subclavian Steal

- Evaluate the vertebral and basilar arteries, looking for reversed flow direction.
- If vertebrobasilar flow appears normal (no flow reversal or flow oscillates), there may be a "latent steal." The arm can be stressed if suspicion for steal is high:
  - Apply a blood pressure cuff to the ipsilateral arm with the suspected obstruction.
  - Monitor the ipsilateral VA flow. Inflate the cuff >20 mmHg above the systolic pressure for approximately 3 minutes. Rapidly release the pressure in the cuff.
  - Record any changes in the vertebral Doppler signal or flow direction throughout the process.
  - Repeat on the contralateral side.

Evaluations for Vasospasm

- Multiple exams are typically performed daily or every other day depending on the patient's symptoms and the level of clinical suspicion.
- Record the highest mean velocity from each artery.
- Record a cervical ICA velocity at a depth of 45-55 mm without adjusting the angle in order to calculate a hemispheric ratio.

Evaluations during tPA Infusion

- Perform a baseline transcranial evaluation. Document any occlusion or other abnormality.
- A head frame may be used to keep the transcranial equipment in place during the continuous intracranial monitoring necessary during the infusion of tPA.
- Note the time and record any changes to the Doppler signal (e.g., reappearance of the signal, increase in velocity, change in waveform shape or evidence of embolization).
- Adjust sample volume depth according to the location of the obstruction. For example, use 55-60 mm when the M1 segment is occluded and 80-100 mm for the basilar artery.

Evaluation for Right-to-Left Cardiac Shunts (RLS)

- Examine the patient in the supine position with their head slightly elevated. Perform what is referred to as a "PFO bubble study" using agitated saline solution injected into a peripheral vein, while TCD is continuously being monitored during normal respiration and while "straining" (Valsalva maneuver, for example).
- Perform a baseline transcranial evaluation of the MCA using a low frequency probe at a depth between 50-60 mm. Document any occlusion or other abnormality.
- A multigated TCD system is best for observation since screening multiple vessels and depths at the same time is possible and makes detection of HITS (*hyperintense transient signal*) often resembling a "chirp" or a "click" more reliable. Although a transtemporal window is preferred, observation of the distal ICA through the submandibular window is acceptable.[15]

- A head frame (or modified version of one) may be used to keep the transcranial equipment in place during the continuous MCA monitoring necessary during the procedure. Monitoring should be performed bilaterally. The gain should be set low and sweep speed should be slow.
- Obtain and record the highest velocities. Make sure the TCD transducers will not move from this position.
- Qualified personnel insert an IV typically at the antecubital fossa. A three-way stopcock device is attached to the inserted needle, along with two syringes. One syringe will remain empty while the other syringe will contain a mixture of 9 mL saline and 1 mL air.[15,16] A small amount of blood (0.5 mL) may be introduced into one of the syringes to optimize the procedure.[15,17] Once the stopcock is locked so no fluid can enter the vein, the saline-air mixture is agitated between the two syringes about 10 times in order to create microbubbles.[15] The saline is then introduced into the vein.

> *The pulmonary artery (PA) may also be monitored to determine how long it takes (number of cardiac cycles) for the microbubbles to reach the heart. Using a low frequency continuous-wave Doppler probe, listen for an audible signal similar to a "washing machine".[15]*

> *Knowing the number of cardiac cycles that will occur before the microbubbles reach the heart can be helpful. If the patient performs Valsalva after the microbubbles have left the heart, there is a greater chance for false-positive or non-diagnostic results.[15]*

- Begin monitoring the intracranial vessels after injection of the agitated saline solution while the patient is "at rest".
- Observe for visual and audible "HITS." Count and document the number of HITS, bilaterally.
- Repeat the observation while the patient performs the Valsalva maneuver; asking the patient to inhale deeply and hold their breath. While holding this breath, the patient will need to contract the abdomen (or bear down). Instruct the patient to release the breath and relax the abdomen after 10 seconds.

> *A valsalvometer can be used to performed a "calibrated Valsalva" which standardizes the Valsalva strain. The patient releases their breath into a tube for 10 seconds, trying to achieve 40 mmHg of pressure on the valsalvometer gauge.[15]*

- Observe for visual and audible "HITS" once again. Count and document the number of HITS, bilaterally.
- A third observation for HITS may be performed, this time without a calibrated Valsalva.
- When only unilateral monitoring is possible, the number of HITS reported should be doubled.[15]

Evaluation for Brain Death

- Use multiple windows and obtain recordings from several intracranial arteries.
- Repeat examinations can prevent false positive results.

Common Carotid Artery Compressions/ Oscillation Maneuvers

- A drop in pressure results when the CCA is compressed low in the neck or vibrated with brisk finger compressions (similar to a "temporal tap"). An affect on flow velocities, direction of flow and pulsatility of the intracranial vessels may be observed.
- Compression maneuvers should not be performed when there is evidence of high-grade stenosis/occlusion, low carotid bifurcations, calcification or complicated lesions in the CCA.
  - Palpate the CCA in the lower neck using the thumb, or first and second digits, above the clavicle and between the trachea and sternocleidomastoid muscle.
  - While insonating the intracranial vessel, apply downward pressure away from the trachea. Compress for 2-4 cardiac cycles and release.
  - Observe for any changes to intracranial flow.

Interpretation

General Considerations

- Expect a low-resistant signal similar to the extracranial ICA with diastolic flow throughout systole, since the Circle of Willis feeds the brain, a low-resistance vascular bed.
- Doppler waveforms, spectral analysis and direction of flow are utilized to pinpoint location of lesions and resulting collateralization. Comparisons should be made regarding the anterior and posterior circulation, as well as right/left sides. [1,3]
- **Mean velocity (MV)**: time mean of the peak velocity "envelope" The envelope refers to a trace of the PSV as a function of time. MV or TAMV=

$$MV= \frac{PSV + (EDV \times 2)}{3}$$

or

$$MV= \frac{(PSV - EDV)}{3} + EDV$$

- **Pulsatility index (PI)**: distal vascular resistance is measured through waveform analysis. PI is calculated using the *Gosling equation*; the difference between the maximum and minimum velocities divided by the mean velocity:

$$PI = \frac{PSV - EDV}{MV}$$

  - Elevated PI suggests increased vascular resistance.
  - Decreased PI suggests lower vascular resistance. PI <0.5 is considered abnormal.
- Responses to CCA compression would include obliteration, diminished flow, alternating flow or change in flow direction.
- **Hemispheric index**: Normal hemispheric index ranges from 1-3.
  - MCA/ICA ratio or hemispheric index- indicates global high or low flow states.

$$\frac{\text{Highest MCA velocity}}{\text{ICA velocity}}$$

Doppler waveforms and flow velocities:

Normal [1,4]

- MCA flow should be toward the transducer with a time average mean velocity (TAMV) = 55 ± 12 cm/s.

- Bifurcation (MCA/ACA) flow should be bidirectional with a TAMV= 55 ± 12 cm/s.
- ACA flow should be away from the transducer with a TAMV= 50 ± 11 cm/s.

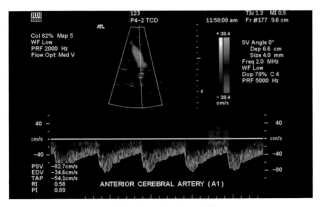

ACA signal using TCI

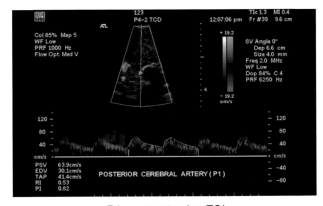

P1 segment using TCI

- PCA flow (P1 segment) should be toward the transducer with a TAMV= 39 ± 10 cm/s.
- P2 segment flow should be away from the transducer with a TAMV= 40 ± 10 cm/s.
- Terminal ICA flow should be toward the probe with TAMV= 39 ± 9 cm/s.
- OA flow should be toward the probe with TAMV= 21 ± 5 cm/s.

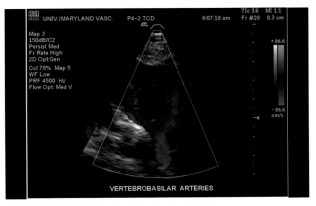

VA signal using TCI

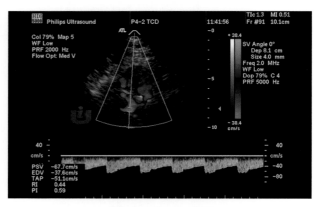

BA signal using TCI

- VA flow should be away from the probe, toward the head with a TAMV= 38 ± 10 cm/s.
- BA flow should be away from the probe, toward the head with a TAMV= 41 ± 10 cm/s.
- Since the carotid siphon is often tortuous, flow may be toward, bidirectional or away from the transducer with a TAMV= 47 ± 14 cm/s. The waveform is normally low-resistant.
- Distal ICA TAMV obtained from the submandibular approach are normally 37 ± 9 cm/s.

Abnormal

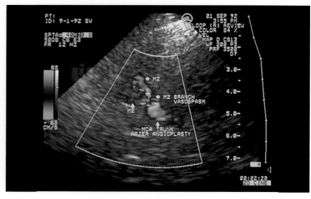

TCI image of vasospasm

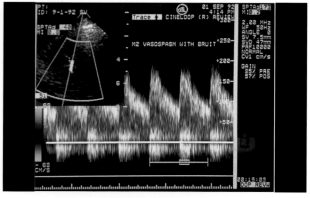

TCI signal representing vasospasm

- **Stenosis/Vasospasm:** A stenosis is characterized by a focal increase in velocity ≥30 cm/s at 1-2 sample depths, while a vasospasm is characterized by a long segment velocity increase over several sample depths.

  – A hemodynamically significant focal stenosis (≥50%) is characterized by a **minimum** two-fold increase in velocity compared to the proximal segment.[1]

  – Mean velocity criteria: A mean velocity of 80 cm/s suggests a significant stenosis in the MCA, ACA, PCA and terminal ICA.

    – When the mean velocity is 100 cm/s in the MCA, a ≥50 stenosis is highly suspected.[1]

    – A mean velocity of 70 cm/s is used to predict a stenosis in the VA.[1] Other studies suggest >80 cm/s as the threshold for VA vasospasm.[20]

> *The most common sites for stenoses are in the MCA, CS and the ICA bifurcation.[1]*

  – Hemispheric index:[1]

    – Mild stenosis/vasospasm is suggested by a hemispheric index between 3-5. The mean velocity in the MCA is usually 100-200 cm/s.[1]

    – Moderate stenosis/vasospasm is suggested by a hemispheric index between 5-7. The mean velocity in the MCA is usually 120-200 cm/s.

    – Severe stenosis/vasospasm is suggested by a hemispheric index >7. The mean velocity in the MCA is usually >200 cm/s.

> *Mean velocity increases >25 cm/s each day suggest a poor prognosis.*

- Additional findings that support intracranial stenosis include: turbulence, post-stenotic drop in velocity, bruit/musical murmurs and compensatory flow in branching vessels.[1]
- **Occlusion:** An MCA occlusion is suspected when there is absence of the MCA signal, but there is good window and recordable signals in the ipsilateral ACA, PCA and tICA. Increased ipsilateral ACA flow in such cases also supports MCA occlusion.[1]

> *The MCA can recanalize on serial TCD in cases of acute cerebral infarct.*

- **Collateralization:** Increased velocities are not uncommon in a vessel acting as a collateral. For example, a patent ACoA signal with turbulence and increased velocities is often a signal of ICA obstruction.

> *Multiple collateral paths can occur at the same time in individuals.*

- The most common collateral pathways include:[1,18]

  - **ACA (most common)**: carrying flow from hemisphere to hemisphere. Expect increased velocities in the contralateral ACA (above those recorded in the MCA) while flow in the ipsilateral ACA is reversed.

  - **PCoA**: carrying flow between the posterior and anterior circulation.

    - This collateral pathway can be activated when there is bilateral extracranial obstruction, or when either the ACA/ACoA is absent.[18]

    - The ipsilateral PCA will demonstrate increased velocities proximal to the PCoA origin, the PCA velocities will be decreased distally.

  - **OA**: Flow will be reversed in the OA in cases of severe ICA obstruction. The OA acts as a collateral from ECA branches and its waveform patterns will be low resistant, since the OA will now have to supply the brain.

- **Subclavian steal**: Flow will be reversed in the vertebral or basilar arteries (toward the probe, instead of away) in cases of subclavian steal. A vertebral to vertebral steal may also be observed.[1]

> *The BA is usually not affected unless the supplying VA is disease.*

- **Aneurysms**: When a larger intracranial aneurysm is present (>1 cm), decreased velocities, multiple systolic peaks, increased resistance, areas of turbulence and bruits may all be present.[1]

  - The neck of an aneurysm may project increased velocities.[1]

  - Compression by the aneurysm is reflected by focal increases in velocity in any adjacent arteries.[1]

  - **Arteriovenous malformations (AVM)**: In this condition, there is an abnormal tangle of blood vessels in the brain. The blood flows directly from an artery to a vein, without going through the capillaries. Surrounding tissue is at risk, since blood is automatically shunted away from the tissue into the vein.

    - Flow should be low resistant and the PI will be decreased.

    - The "feeder artery" that supplies the AVM is usually larger in diameter. Blood flow will typically demonstrate increased velocities and reduced pulsatility.

    - The veins involved will also be larger in diameter and flow will be pulsatile.

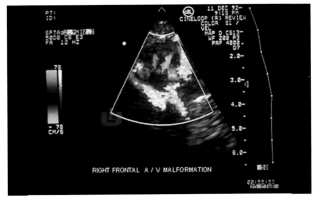

Image of an AVM using TCI

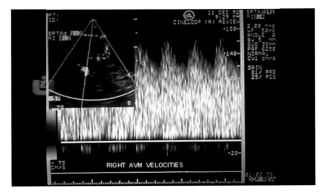

Doppler signal representing an AVM

- **Stroke prediction in sickle cell patients:**

  - MV is used for diagnosis rather than PSV in sickle cell cases to decrease the risk of false positive results. MV <170 cm/s are considered normal.[19]

  - MV between 171-199 cm/s are considered "conditional".[19] Some labs will repeat the exam within 3-6 months to monitor for disease progression.

  - Studies suggests that MCA velocities ≥200 cm/s on two separate exams indicate a higher stroke risk for the child.[1,20]

- **Intraoperative monitoring during CEA**: Microemboli are described as a change in signal which is unilateral, lasting <300 microseconds, with an amplitude that is at minimum 3 dB higher than the background flow signal. The audible signal or HITS often resembles a "chirp" or a "click."[1] HITS resemble straight, bright lines through the spectral tracing.

  - The degree of ischemia during cross-clamping is categorized as follows:[1]

    - Absent: >40%
    - Mild: 0-15%
    - Severe: 16-40%

  - A decrease in MV of >75-90% in the ipsilateral MCA is considered significant.[14]

- **Post-operative hyperperfusion**: Elevated MCA velocities >175% has been associated with hyperperfusion.[22]

- **RLS shunts (e.g., PFO)**: Observe for the appearance of microemboli after injection of the saline-contrast during the first 3-5 cardiac cycles. The criterion that exists in the literature predicts either the size of the opening or the amount of microemboli which may pass.

  - Contrast bubbles after 3-5 cardiac cycles often result from intrapulmonary AVM.

> *An initial decrease in velocities during the Valsalva maneuver indicates a good strain was performed.[15]*

- **Brain death**: Three different signals that are suggestive of brain death have been described:

  - The loss of EDV (to about 50% of the PSV) or loss of forward, antegrade flow through diastole.[1]

  - To and fro waveform, since blood flow oscillates within the blood column and does not perfuse the parenchyma of the brain. There will be an absence of net flow over time.[1,19]

  - Staccato signal- short systolic peak only.[1]

  - Net flow velocities in the MCA <10 cm/s also suggest brain death.[1]

TABLE 20: Quantification of RLS Shunts

Low-grade shunt	1-10 microbubbles
Mid-grade shunt	>10 microbubbles
High-grade shunt	numerous microbubbles which can no longer be identified separately ("curtain effect")

Source: Modified from Sarkar, S., S. Ghosh, et al. (2007). "Role of Transcranial Doppler ultrasonography in stroke." Postgrad Med J 83(985): 683-689.

TABLE 21: PFO Grading System[15,21]

Grade 0	No microemboli detected
Grade 1	1-10 embolic tracks
Grade 2	11-30 embolic tracks
Grade 3	31-100 embolic tracks
Grade 4	101-300 embolic tracks
Grade 5	>300 embolic tracks or "curtain effect"

Source: Modified from Sarkar, S., S. Ghosh, et al. (2007). "Role of Transcranial Doppler ultrasonography in stroke." Postgrad Med J 83(985): 683-689.

Differential Diagnosis

- Atherosclerosis
- Arterial dissection
- Vasculitis (giant cell arteritis, PAN, Wegener's, lupus, primary angiitis of CNS)
- Reversible cerebral vasoconstrictive syndrome
- Moyamoya disease
- CADASIL (cerebral autosomal dominant arteriopathy with subcortical infarcts and leukoencephalopathy)
- Syphilis
- Sarcoidosis
- Migranes
- Brain tumor
- Seizure
- Dementia, caused by Alzheimer's
- Stokes-Adams syndrome
- Bell's palsy
- Demyelinative diseases (multiple sclerosis, etc).

Correlation

- CT scan
- MRI/MRA
- Digital subtraction cerebral angiography
- **Spectamine scan**: nuclear medicine exam using radioisotope uptake to create images for assessment of cerebral blood flow.

TABLE 22: Protocol and Diagnostic Criteria Summary for Intracranial Cerebrovascular Techniques

Artery	Transducer Position	Depth of Sample Volume	Flow Direction	Spatial Relationship of ACA/MCA Bifurcation	Mean Velocity (cm/s)	Response of Ipsilateral Compression
MCA [M1]	Transtemporal	30-60	Toward	Same	55 ± 12	Obliteration Diminishment
ACA/MCA Bifurcation	Transtemporal	55-65	Bidirectional	–	–	Identical to ACA/MCA
ACA [A1]	Transtemporal	60-80	Away	Anterior and Superior	50 ± 11	Obliteration Diminishment Reversal
PCA [P1] *Fetal Origin	Transtemporal	60-70	Toward	Posterior and Inferior	39 ± 10	No Change Augmentation Diminishment* Obliteration*
PCA [P2] *Fetal Origin	Transtemporal	60-70	Away	Posterior and Inferior	40 + 10	No Change Diminishment* Obliteration*
TICA	Transtemporal	55-65	Toward	Inferior	39 ± 9	Obliteration Reversal
OA	Transorbital	40-60	Toward	–	21 ± 5	Obliteration
Carotid Siphon [Supraclinoid] [Genu] [Parasellar]	Transorbital	60-80	Away Bidirectional Toward	–	41 ± 11 – 47 + 14	Obliteration Reversal
VA	Transforamenal	60-90	Away	–	38 ± 10	–
BA	Transforamenal	80-120	Away	–	41 ± 10	–

Source– Fujioka KA, Douville CM. 1992. "Anatomy and Freehand Examination Techniques". Transcranial Doppler. Raven Press, Ltd. New York.

Medical Treatment

- Modify risk factors (e.g., reduce cholesterol, manage HTN and DM, smoking cessation)
- Anticoagulation (e.g., coumadin) or aspirin and statin therapy
- Heparin therapy, with monitoring for hemorrhage

Surgical Treatment

- EC-IC bypass (extracranial-intracranial bypass joining the superficial temporal to MCA)
- Aneurysm repair (e.g., clipping)
- Coil embolization

Endovascular Treatment

- Balloon angioplasty (vasospasm)
- Stenting

Points to Remember

- TCD is sometimes referred to as the "free-hand" method.[4]
- A quiet room is helpful when performing TCD examinations, otherwise headphones can also be used. Some technologists prefer using headphones to block out any background noise during transcranial exams.
- Visualization through the transtemporal window may be technically difficult in 10-15% of cases.[23]
- The size and location of the transtemporal window may vary from side to side on the same patient.
- Visualization may be difficult through the transforamenal window if the muscles are too tense from extending the patient's neck too far forward.[4]
- Expect higher velocities in the anterior versus the posterior circulation. MCA >ACA >PCA is often used to describe the normal velocity relationship between the three major intracranial arteries. When the PCA >MCA and ACA for example, this finding would suggest that the PCA is acting as a collateral pathway.[18]
- Some TCD machines use multigate or M-mode (power motion) Doppler to display multiple gates and depths of information (6.5 cm path). This enables capture of hemodynamic data from multiple depths simultaneously. This method may increase accuracy when detecting emboli.[1]
- The FDA in the United States does not condone using ultrasound through the transorbital window. Recommendations suggest lowering the overall power to 10% and minimizing scan time to 10 second intervals or 3 spectral tracings to avoid retinal damage.
- The PI should be higher in the OA since it supplies structures such as the ocular muscles and has anastomoses with ECA territories.[1]
- Improper gain adjustments can result in invalid automatic calculations by machines. Manual calculations for TAMV should be performed by placing the cursor at the point where the peak velocity area in systole and peak velocity area in diastole are equal. Manual calculation can also be performed for pulsatility index when necessary.[4]

- Significant extracranial disease can result in decreased ipsilateral intracranial artery velocities, a delay in systole, reduced PI and collateralization. In other cases of significant extracranial disease, there will be no affect on the Circle of Willis.[1]

- Intraoperative TCD monitoring can help surgeons decide between clamping or shunting. If there is a significant velocity decrease after clamping, shunting is suggested.

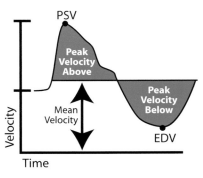

- During fetal development, there is normally an opening in the atrial septum known as the "*foramen ovale*". Through the foramen ovale, oxygenated blood can easily pass from the mother to the fetus without having to pass through the lung. This opening, which normally closes within a year after birth, remains open in approximately 20-25% of the population. The patent foramen ovale (PFO) is a flap-like opening within the heart which can grow and stretch as the individual ages. The high pressure of the left atrium usually keeps the flap closed, though certain straining actions like lifting, sneezing or coughing can result in a pressure gradient between the right and left atria. It is possible for an emboli to cross directly through this opening and travel to the brain, bypassing the lung filter. For this reason, patients with PFO are at risk for a cerebrovascular event. There is also the theory that maybe the PFO tunnel itself may develop thrombus and be a source of emboli.[15]

- Use of a valsalvometer provides a means of measurement during a RLS evaluation, ensuring adequate Valsalva strain. Adequate strain will likely increase the pressure gradient between the right and left atria and open the PFO.[15]

- Asking the patient to vigorously cough for 5 seconds is an alternative method used for a non-calibrated Valsalva technique.[17]

- The absence of "HITS" during a RLS bubble study does not definitively rule out PFO.[15]

- The ACoA is the most common site for an intracranial aneurysm, especially those associated with subarachnoid hemorrhage. The PCoA and MCA bifurcation are also common sites for aneurysm development.[1]

- An isolated stenosis of the PCA or ACA is rare.[1]

- The A2 segment is easier to access in patients that have a "burr hole" (hole in the skull, made in the frontal bone).

- A "false bifurcation" may be encountered near 50 mm depths in larger diameter ACA that course medially. Although the spectral trace will appear similar to the ACA/MCA, the "true" bifurcation will be deeper.[4]

- Hyperostosis causes increased density and thickness of the skull.[1] This condition is most often encountered in older, female and/or African American patients.[1,18]

- TCD monitoring has been used to support physicians during infusion of tPA (tissue plasminogen activator) in acute stroke cases.

- Examination of the proximal intracranial portion of the ICA through the submandibular window can be used for patients with subarachnoid hemorrhage (SAH).[1,4] Other uses for this window include detection of spontaneous ICA dissection and FMD which often occur above the level of the jaw. Flow velocity ratios between the extracranial ICA and MCA can help distinguish vasospasm versus hyperemia in trauma patients.[4]

- Patients with SAH and craniotomies will usually have bandaging covering their transtemporal windows which will need to be loosened in order to gain access for transcranial testing.

- Add approximately 2 cm/depth for vessel depth post-craniotomy when patients are experiencing swelling.[4]

> *SAH can last 12-16 days.*[19]

- The incidence of SAH in the United States is approximately 25,000 to 30,000 cases yearly. There is an 1.5-3 fold increased risk of death during the first 2 weeks after SAH. TCD has been shown to identify this condition 1-2 days before the patient becomes symptomatic, which can expedite treatment.[19,20]

- The onset of vasospasm is typically 3-5 days after the initial SAH and is usually at its worst between the 6-8th day.

- For sickle cell patients with mean velocities $\geq$200 cm/s, there is a estimated 40% stroke risk within 3 years.[19]

- The Stroke Prevention Trial in Sickle Cell Anemia (STOP) study revealed elevated MCA velocities by TCD followed by blood transfusion reduced the rate of the first stroke in children.

- Output power should be reduced when scanning patients with "burr holes" or removed and replaced pieces of the skull bone.

- Changes in heart rate, hematocrit levels, blood pressure, etc, can affect transcranial velocities and should be considered during the exam.

- Transcranial imaging can be used to study the affects of temporary vessel occlusion when treating patients with tumors, fistulas or aneurysms.

- The Glasgow coma scale is used for patients with brain injury to assess their level of consciousness. Eye movements and motor responses are considered. A normal score is 15. Noting changes in this score and correlating it to changes in serial transcranial exams may be a useful tool.

- Since there will be a lack of color flow, TCI is not an appropriate study to assess a thrombosed intracranial aneurysm. Plus vessel tortuosity and branching can be misdiagnosed as an aneurysm.[1]

- Transcranial testing can help surgeons detect hyperperfusion syndrome post-CEA; symptoms include headache, seizure and intracranial hemorrhage.[1,18] Preoperative screening (e.g., CO_2 challenge) and post-operative monitoring can be useful tools to identify patients at-risk.[22]

- The diameter of a child's head should be considered before TCD testing. Determining where the midline is on the child will assist in selection of proper depths to be used for analysis. Children have larger transtemporal windows than adults, so the overall power can be reduced before study. Note the child's demeanor during testing, since crying and sleeping for example can affect intracranial velocities.[1]

- It may be helpful to mark the transtemporal window for serial study on patients suspected of brain death.

- There should be little difference between the right and left sides in asymptomatic patients.

- Transcranial protocols may vary at different institutions.

References

1. Katz ML, Alexandrov AV. (2003). A Practical Guide to Transcranial Doppler Examinations. Littleton: Sumner Publishing.
2. McCartney JP, Lukes-Thomas KM, Gomez CR. (1997). Handbook of Transcranial Doppler. New York. Springer-Verlag
3. Naylor AR, Markose G. (2010) Cerebrovascular disease: diagnostic evaluation, In Cronenwett JL, Johnston KW. (Eds.) Rutherford's Vascular Surgery (7th ed). (Chapter 93). Philadelphia. Saunders Elsevier.
4. Fujioka KA, Douville CM. 1992. "Anatomy and Freehand Examination Techniques". Transcranial Doppler. Raven Press, Ltd. New York.
5. Easton JD, Saver JL, et al. (2009). "Definition and Evaluation of Transient Ischemic Attack." Stroke 40(6): 2276-2293.
6. Bamford J, Sandercock P., et al. (1987). "The natural history of lacunar infarction: the Oxfordshire Community Stroke Project." Stroke 18(3): 545-551.
7. Petty GW, Brown RD, et al. (2000). "Ischemic Stroke Subtypes: A Population-Based Study of Functional Outcome, Survival, and Recurrence." Stroke 31(5): 1062-1068.
8. Weir, B., R. L. Macdonald, et al. (1999). "Etiology of cerebral vasospasm." Acta Neurochir Suppl 72: 27-46.
9. Penn DL, Komotar RJ, et al. (2011). "Hemodynamic mechanisms underlying cerebral aneurysm pathogenesis." J Clin Neurosci 18(11): 1435-1438.
10. Rowe VL, Yellin AE, Weaver FA. (2005). Vascular injuries of the extremities. In Rutherford Vascular Surgery 6th edition. (1044-1058). Philadelphia. Elsevier Saunders.
11. Desai, B. and J. F. Toole (1975). "Kinks, coils, and carotids: a review." Stroke 6(6): 649-653.
12. Trackler, RT, Mikulicich AG. (1974). "Diminished cerebral perfusion resulting from kinking of the internal carotid artery." J Nucl Med 15(7): 634-635.
13. Bickerstaff LK, Pairolero PC, et al. (1982). "Thoracic aortic aneurysms: a population-based study." Surgery 92(6): 1103-1108.
14. Rowed, D. W., D. A. Houlden, et al. (2004). "Comparison of monitoring techniques for intraoperative cerebral ischemia." Can J Neurol Sci 31(3): 347-356.
15. Hughes JP, Dubin R, Harley M, Renz J. (2007). "Transcranial Doppler in the Detection of Patent Foramen Ovale. Vascular US Today 12(5):77-96.
16. Rubiera, M., L. Cava, et al. (2010). "Diagnostic criteria and yield of real-time transcranial Doppler monitoring of intra-arterial reperfusion procedures." Stroke 41(4): 695-699.
17. Sastry, S., A. MacNab, et al. (2009). "Transcranial Doppler detection of venous-to-arterial circulation shunts: criteria for patent foramen ovale." J Clin Ultrasound 37(5): 276-280.
18. Byrd-Raynor SA, Smith WB. (2010). Transcranial duplex imaging. In Zierler RE (Ed.), Strandess's duplex scanning disorders in vascular diagnosis 4th ed. (101-113).Philadelphia Wolters Kluwer Lippincott Williams & Wilkins.
19. Kassab, MY, Majid A, et al. (2007). "Transcranial Doppler: an introduction for primary care physicians." J Am Board Fam Med 20(1): 65-71.
20. Alexandrov, AV, Sloan MA, et al. (2010). "Practice Standards for Transcranial Doppler (TCD) Ultrasound. Part II. Clinical Indications and Expected Outcomes." J Neuroimaging. Epub ahead of print.
21. Spencer Vascular. (n.d.). Grading of Right-to-Left Shunt Conductance. Retrieved from http://spencervascular.com.
22. Nicholls SC. (2010). Transcranial Doppler monitoring for carotid interventions. In Zierler RE (Ed.), Strandess's duplex scanning disorders in vascular diagnosis 4th ed. (123-130).Philadelphia Wolters Kluwer Lippincott Williams & Wilkins
23. Nicholls SC. (2005). Transcranial Doppler: technique and application. In Mansour MA, Labropoulos N. (Eds.), Vascular Diagnosis, (113-129). Philadelphia: Elsevier Saunders

Definition

A non-invasive physiological test comparing the systolic pressure at the level of the ankle to the systolic pressure at the level of the brachial artery. Continuous-wave (CW) analog Doppler waveforms are recorded to support the pressure information.

Rationale

When narrowing of the arterial lumen reaches a critical level, distal arterial flow and pressure decrease significantly. Ankle brachial indices (ABI) define the resulting decrease in blood flow to the extremity at the ankle level.

Etiology

- Atherosclerosis
- Embolization
- Thrombus
- Intimal hyperplasia
- Trauma
- Traumatic occlusion
- Extrinsic compression
- Vasculitis
- AV fistula (abnormal connection between an artery and a vein)

Risk Factors

- Age (increased risk with age)
- Coronary artery disease
- Diabetes
- Family history
- Hyperlipidemia
- Hypertension
- Obesity
- Smoking
- Sedentary lifestyle
- Previous history of CVA or MI
- Elevated levels of homocysteine
- Excessive levels of C-reactive protein
- History of radiation

Indications for Exam

- Claudication (exercise-related limb pain)
- Follow-up of an abnormal ABI
- Limb pain at rest
- Absent peripheral pulses
- Extremity ulcer
- Gangrene
- Pre-operative assessment of healing potential
- Digital cyanosis
- Cold sensitivity
- Arterial aneurysm
- Trauma to an artery
- Follow-up after revascularization procedure

Contraindications/Limitations

- Calcified vessels which will falsely elevate pressure measurements (typically encountered in patients with diabetes or end-stage renal disease).
- Significant lesions with excellent collateral circulation, which may result in normal distal pressures and waveforms at rest.
- Patients with acute clot or venous thrombosis in the lower extremities should not have pressure cuffs inflated over their thrombus.
- Patients with extensive bandages or casts which are not removable.
- Any site of trauma, surgery, ulceration or graft placement which should not be compressed by the pressure cuff.

- Pressure measurements are typically prohibited on ipsilateral side of mastectomy or AVG/AVF.

Mechanism of disease

There are two major mechanisms that cause reduced arterial blood supply to the lower extremity: atherosclerotic plaque and embolism. Of these, atherosclerosis is more common.

- **Atherosclerosis** is the most common arterial disease. Atherosclerotic plaque forms in the artery to block flow by either narrowing it (arterial stenosis) or totally blocking the artery (arterial occlusion). The term "hemodynamically significant obstruction" refers to either a stenosis or an occlusion that results in a decrease in blood pressure or flow distal to the obstruction. Typically, a stenosis must narrow the diameter of the artery by at least 50% to decrease pressure and flow distally. An arterial occlusion is typically seen from one major branch to the next.
- **Emboli**: embolization of contents of a plaque and/ or fragments of an organized thrombus from the heart or proximal aneurysm which become lodged in a distant blood vessel.[2]
- **Extrinsic compression** from tumors, hematoma, etc., can result in stenosis or occlusion by placing enough pressure on arterial walls to compromise blood flow.[1]
- **Vasospasm** is a temporary constriction of the arteries (typically digital arteries) that may cause significant discomfort to the patient (uncommon). [3]
- **Aneurysmal** disease results from weakening of the structural proteins (elastin and collagen) within the medial layer of the arterial wall. Aneurysmal disease typically does not obstruct flow, but carries the risk of rupture and/or emboli.[4]

Location of Disease

- Arterial disease can be focal or diffuse and affect any level or multiple levels.
- The most common location of obstruction in the lower extremities is the superficial femoral artery at the adductor canal.
- Arterial bifurcations and the popliteal artery are other common locations of obstruction.

Patient History

- Claudication (exercise related)
- Rest pain
- Paralysis (weakness)
- Paresthesia ("pins and needles")
- Poikilothermia (ice-cold limbs)
- Previous ulceration/gangrene of feet/toes
- Previous therapeutic vascular procedure (e.g., bypass, stenting)

Physical Examination

- Pulselessness
- Pallor
- Cyanosis
- Dependent rubor
- Bruit (abnormal sound heard through auscultation caused by vibration of tissue from turbulent flow)
- Marked temperature difference between extremities
- Gangrene/necrosis (tissue death)
- Palpable thrill (vibration caused by turbulent blood flow as seen in AV fistulas)

Ankle-Brachial Indices Protocol

> *Pressure measurements should be taken in the supine position with the extremity at the same level as the heart. Pressures recorded while the patient is sitting will be falsely elevated due to the effects of hydrostatic pressure.* *For details see Points to Remember section.*

- Rest the patient for 5-10 minutes before beginning the exam in order for blood pressures to stabilize after "exercise" (walking into the exam room). You may use this time to obtain a patient history, including symptoms and risk factors and to place cuffs.
- Appropriately wrap blood pressure cuffs on the limbs. Cuffs should be placed "straight" rather than angled. All cuffs should fit snugly so that inflation of the bladder transmits the head of pressure into the tissue rather than into space between the bladder and the limb, producing falsely elevated readings.
  - Apply ankle cuffs with 10-12 cm bladder (in width) 2-3 cm above the medial malleolus, bilaterally.
  - Apply same sized cuffs on the arm to obtain brachial pressures.
- Locate the posterior tibial arterial (PTA) signal posterior to the medial malleolus using a high frequency (8 MHz) CW Doppler probe. (Use a lower frequency probe (e.g., 4 MHz) on obese patients or for deeper vessels when needed.)

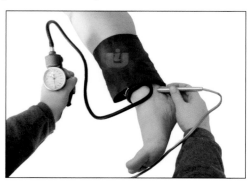

Pressure measurement at the PTA

- Angle between 45-60°, pointing the probe towards the heart.
- Place enough pressure on the probe to stay in place without compressing the artery.
- Manipulate the probe slightly to obtain the strongest arterial signal. Resting the hand on the foot is helpful in holding the probe in place during cuff inflation.
- Record several representative PTA waveforms. If no arterial signal is identified at the ankle, you can try for a signal more proximally along the medial calf. You may also have to reposition your pressure cuff higher on the leg. In such cases, document what level the pressure was taken.

The following instructions can be used when testing with an automatic cuff inflator or standard manometer:

- Inflate the air cuff 20-30 mmHg above the last audible arterial signal heard using the Doppler probe.

> *For patients with irregular heart beats decrease deflation speeds.*

- Deflate the cuff slowly (at a rate of 2-4 mmHg per second). The systolic pressure is recorded in mmHg as soon as the first audible arterial Doppler signal returns. The Doppler pulse must continue after hearing the first pulse to assure there is an actual pulse rather than motion artifact.

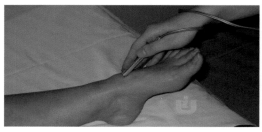

CW Doppler waveforms at the DPA

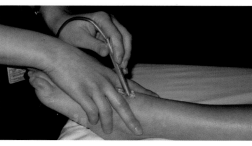

Place your fingers on the ankle bones to help locate the DPA

- Locate the dorsalis pedis arterial (DPA) signal and repeat the procedure using CW Doppler on the dorsum of the foot (about halfway between the toes and ankle). Record several representative waveforms. Avoid sampling too close to the toes, or you will likely be listening to the plantar arch or a digital vessel instead of the DPA (which may be receiving blood from the posterior tibial artery if the DPA or anterior tibial is occluded). If the signal is damped, retrograde or absent, move to the anterior ankle area and search for the anterior tibial (ATA) signal. If no arterial signal is identified, locate the peroneal artery (PerA) slightly anterior to the lateral malleolus.
- Obtain bilateral brachial artery (BrA) pressures.

> *If brachial pressures differ >20 mmHg or if brachial waveforms are different, examine the vertebral arteries to check flow direction. A retrograde vertebral on the side with the lower brachial pressure is indicative of subclavian steal syndrome.*

- Calculate the ankle-brachial index (ABI) by dividing the pedal pressure by the highest brachial pressure:

$$\frac{\text{pedal pressure}}{\text{highest brachial pressure}} = \text{ABI}$$

- Repeat on the contralateral leg when indicated.
- Determine severity of disease according to laboratory diagnostic criteria.

TABLE 23: **ABI Protocol Summary**

- Wrap pressure cuffs around limb
  - Arm
  - Leg-ankle level
- Using CW Doppler, record representative waveforms
  - DPA
  - PTA
  - BrA
- Inflate cuff 20-30 mmHg beyond the last audible arterial signal using a Doppler probe on the appropriate artery distal to the cuff.
- Deflation of the cuff should be at a rate of 2-4 mmHg per second. The pressure is recorded as soon as the first audible arterial Doppler signal returns.
- Calculate the ABI:

$$\frac{\text{pedal pressure}}{\text{highest brachial pressure}} = \text{ABI}$$

- Determine classification of disease according to laboratory diagnostic criteria.

Ankle-Brachial Pressure Worksheet

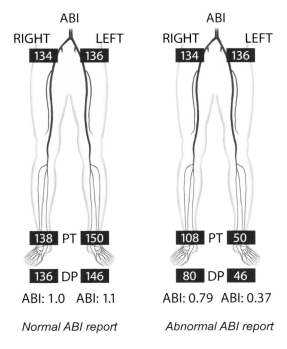

Normal ABI report   Abnormal ABI report

> The diagnostic criteria used to determine the severity of abnormal lower extremity ankle-brachial indices varies across institutions.

Interpretation

Normal Pressures

- Leg pressures are normally higher than the highest brachial pressure. According to research, the normal pressure difference between the arm and ankle is between 12 (±8) to 24 (±9) mmHg.[5]

- If the ABI is ≥1.0, the presence of a hemodynamically significant stenosis or occlusion is unlikely between the arm and ankle cuffs. The upper and lower limits of normal varies within the literature and is thought to depend on whether the patient is hypertensive or hypotensive.[6] An ABI >0.97 is often considered normal.[7] The ABI typically is no less than 0.92 in a normal limb.[5]

Normal Doppler Waveforms

- A normal triphasic signal is demonstrated by strong forward flow in late systole (sharp upstroke), followed by flow reversal in early diastole (below the baseline) plus a late diastolic component.[7] Many laboratories will accept a waveform with a reversed flow component as normal even if the third phase is missing.

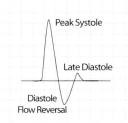

Normal, triphasic Doppler waveform

Abnormal Pressures

> The reason for decreased ankle pressures is almost always a hemodynamically significant proximal lesion.[5]

- An ABI of <1.0 suggests that functionally significant obstruction exists somewhere between the heart and the ankle cuff.[5]

- As the ABI lowers to 90% of the arm pressure, it is likely that a hemodynamically significant obstruction is present in the lower extremity above the level of the ankle.[8]

- The difference in ankle pressure between the dorsalis pedis and posterior tibial arteries in the same limb should be within 10mmHg.[5] A difference in ABI >15 mmHg suggests a proximal obstruction.[5,7,9]

- A change in the ABI of ≥0.15 from one study to the next is significant.[5,7,8]

- An ABI of >1.3 suggests calcific disease and is considered non-diagnostic. As an alternative means of estimating disease severity, use a toe/brachial index.[5,7] A diagnosis of disease severity (normal, mild, moderate, severe, critical) can also be made based solely on waveform analysis when calcific disease is present.[7]

Continuous Wave Arterial Doppler Signals

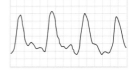

Moderately abnormal waveforms

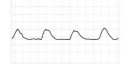

Severely abnormal waveforms

* Triphasic, biphasic, and monophasic waveforms have multiple definitions throughout the vascular ultrasound community. Although these waveforms may be labeled differently in different labs, most laboratories would identify the left waveform as moderately abnormal, and the right as severely abnormal. Some laboratories reserve the term biphasic only for waveforms with a reversed flow component but no third phase. It is likely that these would be considered normal due to the presence of the reversed component. Also, some labs may term any waveform without a reversed flow component as monophasic

Abnormal Doppler Waveforms

- There is controversy among vascular professionals regarding the terminology describing CW Doppler analog waveforms.

  - Essentially all vascular professionals agree that a waveform with a sharp, quick upstroke followed by reversed flow direction and a third forward phase is termed triphasic. This is considered a normal finding in the peripheral arteries.

  - A waveform with a reversed second phase that is missing the third forward phase may be described as "triphasic" or "biphasic" by laboratories. However, nearly all will interpret this as normal. Recently, some laboratories have adopted terminology that recognizes the reversed flow connection to normal by using an abbreviation NR for "normal-reversed" whether or not the third phase is present, and avoiding the confusing use of "triphasic" and "biphasic" terms.

  - Monophasic arterial Doppler waveforms are characterized by a slow upstroke, low amplitude, and broad peak with no evidence of the reversed flow component in late systole. The upstroke has a general direction of being tipped to the right. Continuous forward flow is typical in diastole, but diastolic flow may be absent if there is distal resistance from an additional high grade distal obstruction. For example, monophasic waveforms are typically present distal to an occlusion or a very high grade stenosis.

- An absent Doppler signal suggests arterial occlusive disease at the site of interrogation.[5] Absent Doppler signals in all pedal arteries of a limb suggest a critical decrease in perfusion to the lower extremity, particularly if the VPR or PPG waveforms at the toe are flat. Be aware that extensive calcification will obscure the Doppler signal, but the VPR and PPG waveforms are typically not affected.

TABLE 24: Diagnostic Criteria for ABI

ABI	Comment
≥1.0	Normal
0.90 to <1.0	Mild disease
0.50-0.90	Claudication
0.30-0.50	Severe occlusive disease
<0.30	Ischemia

Source: AbuRahma AF. (2000). Segmental Doppler pressures and Doppler waveform analysis in peripheral vascular disease of the lower extremities. In AbuRahma AF, Bergan JJ (Eds). *Non-invasive Vascular Diagnosis*. (213-229). London: Springer.

TABLE 25: University of Chicago Diagnostic ABI Criteria

ABI	Severity
≥1.0-0.95	Normal
0.80-0.94	Mild disease
0.50-0.79	Moderate disease
0.30-0.49	Severe disease
<0.29	Critical disease

Source: Internally validated at the University of Chicago Medical Center Vascular Laboratory.

TABLE 26: ABI Symptoms

ABI	Symptom
≥1.0	Normal
<0.80	Claudication
<0.40	Rest pain
<0.20	Impending gangrene

Source: Modified from Yao JST. (1970). Hemodynamic studies in peripheral arterial disease. Br J Surg. 57:761.

Differential Diagnosis

- Spinal stenosis
- Venous thrombosis
- Restless leg syndrome
- Compartment syndrome
- Nocturnal leg cramps
- Neuropathy
- Muscle/tendon strains
- Arthritis
- Abnormalities of adrenergic receptor/sympathetic nervous system
- Connective tissue disease (scleroderma)

Correlation

- Duplex ultrasound
- Spiral CT scan
- MRA
- Arteriography

Medical Treatment

- Modify risk factors (e.g., reduce cholesterol, manage HTN and DM, smoking cessation)
- Exercise regimen
- Antiplatelet medication (e.g., aspirin)
- Anticoagulation (warfarin)
- Thrombolysis (acute blockage)

Surgical Treatment

- Bypass grafting
- Atherectomy
- Endarterectomy
- Direct focal repair
- Resection (aneurysmal disease)
- Sympathectomy
- Amputation

Endovascular Treatment

- Angioplasty
- Stent
- Intra-arterial directed thrombolysis (acute blockage)

Points to Remember

- The ABI only evaluates the presence and severity of disease. The ABI should be combined with segmental pressures, volume pulse recording, Doppler waveforms or duplex imaging to determine location of disease.

- Pressure measurements should be taken in the supine position with the extremity at the same level as the heart. Pressures recorded while the patient is sitting will be falsely elevated due to the effects of hydrostatic pressure. For every 10 inches that the heart is elevated above the ankle level, pressure increases 18.67 mmHg. Since the heart level is 34 inches from the ankle on an average person while sitting, the blood pressure at the ankle will be affected about 63 mmHg (3.4 x 18.67 mmHg). If pressures can only be obtained while the patient is sitting, use the same method for follow-up exams for accurate comparison.

- Conversely, when the extremity is elevated above the heart level, misleadingly low pressure readings can result.

- If a pressure measurement needs to be repeated, the cuff should be fully deflated for approximately one minute prior to the repeat measurement. The systolic pressure is recorded as the pressure at which the first audible arterial Doppler signal returns. There should be a period of silence after inflation and prior to hearing the first pulse to be sure the cuff was inflated beyond the local arterial pressure. The Doppler pulse must continue after hearing the first pulse to assure there is an actual pulse rather than motion artifact.

- A foot ulcer is unlikely to heal if the ankle pressure is <80 mmHg in a diabetic patient.[13]

- The ABI examination may be combined with exercise stress testing to uncover obstructions unrecognizable at rest that become significant with exercise.

- A patient with claudication is likely to have an ABI <0.80.[12]

- A patient with rest pain is likely to have an ABI of <0.40.[7]

- An ABI <0.50 suggests multiple levels of disease.[5,7,8]

- Do not take a blood pressure over a bypass graft or dialysis access conduit or fistula without first consulting your medical director. Do not take a blood pressure on the arm of a patient with a history of mastectomy.

- Moderate to severely abnormal analog waveforms typically have a somewhat wider peak and a slightly slower upstroke. There may be a "multiphasic" downslope that stays above the baseline (no reversal of flow) but demonstrates what appears to be a "notch" or two in the downslope. This is the most difficult waveform to describe due to its very qualitative nature, but it is helpful to distinguish the moderately abnormal Doppler waveform from a severely abnormal one in practice, especially at the common femoral and pedal levels.

- Pulsed wave Doppler on a duplex scanner can also be used to obtain arterial waveforms when necessary. Be sure to keep the sample volume wide and the image in real time while measuring pressures to assure sample volume location during and after cuff inflation.

References

1. 1 Sumner DS, Zierler RE. (2005). Vascular physiology: essential hemodynamic principles. In *Rutherford Vascular Surgery 6th edition.* (75-123). Philadelphia. Elsevier Saunders.

2. 2 Fecteau SR, Darling III RC, Roddy SP. (2005). Arterial thromboembolism. In *Rutherford Vascular Surgery 6th edition.* (971-986). Philadelphia. Elsevier Saunders.

3. 3 Shepard RFJ. (2005). Raynaud's syndrome: vasospastic and occlusive arterial disease involving the distal upper extremity. In *Rutherford Vascular Surgery 6th edition.* (1319-1346). Philadelphia: Elsevier Saunders.

4. 4 Dawson DL, Lee ES, Lindholm K. (2010). Aortic and peripheral aneurysms. In Zierler RE (Ed.), *Strandess's duplex scanning disorders in vascular diagnosis 4th ed.* (157-168). Philadelphia: Wolters Kluwer Lippincott Williams & Wilkins.

5. 5 Zierler RE, Sumner DS. (2005). Physiologic assessment of peripheral arterial occlusive disease. . In *Rutherford Vascular Surgery 6th edition.* (197-222). Philadelphia. Elsevier Saunders.

6. 6 Nicolaides AN. (2003). Basic and practical aspects of peripheral arterial testing. In Bernstein EF (Ed.), *Vascular Diagnosis* (481-485). St. Louis: Mosby.

7. 7 Carter SA. (2003). Role of pressure measurements. In Bernstein EF (Ed.), *Vascular Diagnosis* (486-512). St. Louis: Mosby.

8. 8 Zierler, RE, (2005). Nonimaging Physiologic Tests for Assessment of Lower Extremity Arterial Occlusive Disease. In Zwiebel WJ, Pellerito JS (Eds.), *Introduction to Vascular Ultrasonography.* (275-295). Philadelphia: Elsevier Saunders.

9. 9 Nordness PJ, Money SR. (2005). In Mansour MA, Labropoulos N. (Eds.), *Vascular Diagnosis,* (207-214). Philadelphia: Elsevier Saunders.

10. 10 Needham T. (2005). In Mansour MA, Labropoulos N. (Eds.), *Vascular Diagnosis,* (215-222). Philadelphia: Elsevier Saunders.

11. 11 AbuRahma AF. (2000). Segmental Doppler pressures and Doppler waveform analysis in peripheral vascular disease of the lower extremities. In AbuRahma AF, Bergan JJ (Eds.) *Non-invasive Vascular Diagnosis.* (213-229). London: Springer.

12. 12 Yao JST. (1970). Hemodynamic studies in peripheral arterial disease. *Br J Surg. 57:761.*

13. 13 Raines JK, Darling RC, Both K et al. (1976). Vascular laboratory criteria for the management of peripheral vascular disease of the lower extremities. *Surgery 79:21-29,*

Definition

Systolic blood pressures and Doppler waveforms are compared at different segments of the lower extremities to identify the general location of a hemodynamically significant arterial obstruction. The term "obstruction" is used to describe either a stenosis or an occlusion of an artery. These techniques also define the resulting decrease in blood flow in terms of pressure and general perfusion of the lower extremity.

Rationale

When narrowing of the arterial lumen increases beyond the critical level, distal arterial flow and pressure decrease significantly. Segmental pressures define the level of disease by comparing the limb and brachial pressures from one level to the next. A pressure gradient (pressure difference) of 20-30 mmHg indicates a significant stenosis or occlusion between cuff levels. Higher gradients most likely represent an occlusion, rather than a stenosis. Doppler waveforms from the lower extremity arteries normally demonstrate a high resistance waveform pattern, whereas waveforms distal to a significant obstruction typically reflect a low resistance configuration. This lowered resistance is caused by the dilatation of the distal arterioles to encourage flow to the region.

Etiology

- Atherosclerosis
- Embolization
- Thrombus
- Intimal hyperplasia
- Trauma
- Traumatic occlusion
- Extrinsic compression
- Vasculitis
- AV fistula (abnormal connection between an artery and a vein)
- Radiation arteritis

Risk Factors

- Age (increased risk with age)
- Coronary artery disease
- Diabetes
- Family history
- Hyperlipidemia
- Hypertension
- Obesity
- Smoking
- Sedentary lifestyle
- Previous history of CVA or MI
- Elevated levels of homocysteine
- Excessive levels of C-reactive protein
- History of radiation

Indications for Exam

- Claudication (exercise-related limb pain)
- Follow-up of a previously abnormal segmental exam
- Limb pain at rest
- Absent peripheral pulses
- Extremity ulcer
- Gangrene
- Pre-operative assessment of healing potential
- Digital cyanosis
- Cold sensitivity
- Aneurysmal disease
- Dependent rubor
- Trauma to an artery
- Follow-up after revascularization procedure

Contraindications/Limitations

- Calcified vessels which will falsely elevate pressures (typically encountered in patients with diabetes or end-stage renal disease).
- Significant lesions with excellent collateral circulation, which may result in normal distal pressures and waveforms at rest.
- Pressure cuffs may not fit around very large thighs. When cuffs are too small they can elevate pressures considerably.
- Patients with acute clot or venous thrombosis in the lower extremities should not have pressure cuffs inflated over their clot.
- Patients with extensive bandages or casts which are not removable.
- Any site of trauma, surgery, ulceration or graft placement which should not be compressed by the pressure cuff.
- Pressure measurements typically prohibited on ipsilateral side of mastectomy or AVG/AVF.

Mechanism of disease

There are two major mechanisms that cause reduced arterial blood supply to the lower extremity; atherosclerotic plaque and embolism. Of these, atherosclerosis is more common.

- **Atherosclerosis** is the most common arterial disease. Atherosclerotic plaque forms in the artery to block flow by either narrowing it (arterial stenosis) or totally blocking the artery (arterial occlusion). The term "hemodynamically significant obstruction" refers to either a stenosis or an occlusion that results in a decrease in blood pressure or flow distal to the obstruction. Typically, a stenosis must narrow the diameter of the artery by at least 50% to decrease pressure and flow distally. An arterial occlusion is typically seen from one major branch to the next.
- **Emboli**: embolization of contents of a plaque and/ or fragments of an organized thrombus from the heart or proximal aneurysm which become lodged in a distant blood vessel.[2]
- **Extrinsic compression** from tumors, hematoma, etc., can result in stenosis or occlusion by placing enough pressure on arterial walls to compromise blood flow.[1]
- **Vasospasm**: is a temporary constriction of the arteries (typically digital arteries) that may cause significant discomfort to the patient (uncommon).[3]
- **Aneurysmal disease** results from weakening of the structural proteins (elastin and collagen) within the medial layer of the arterial wall. Aneurysmal disease typically does not obstruct flow, but carries the risk of rupture and/or emboli.[4]

Location of Obstructive Disease

- Arterial disease can be focal or diffuse and affect any level or multiple levels.
- The most common location of obstruction in the lower extremities is the distal superficial femoral artery at the adductor canal.
- Arterial bifurcations and the popliteal artery are other common locations of obstruction.

Patient History

- Claudication (exercise-related)
- Rest pain
- Paralysis (weakness)
- Paresthesia ("pins and needles")
- Poikilothermia (ice-cold limbs)
- Previous ulceration/gangrene of feet/toes
- Previous therapeutic vascular procedure (e.g., bypass, stenting)

Physical Examination

- Pulselessness
- Pallor
- Cyanosis
- Dependent rubor
- Bruit (abnormal sound heard through auscultation caused by vibration of tissue from turbulent flow)
- Marked temperature difference between extremities
- Gangrene/necrosis (tissue death)
- Palpable thrill (vibration caused by turbulent blood flow as seen in AV fistulas)

Lower Extremity Segmental Pressures and Doppler Waveforms Protocol

> *Pressure measurements should be taken in the supine position with the extremity at the same level as the heart. Pressures recorded while the patient is sitting will be falsely elevated due to the effects of hydrostatic pressure. For details see Points to Remember section.*

- Rest the patient before beginning the exam in order for blood pressures to stabilize after "exercise" (walking into the exam room). You may use this time to obtain a patient history, including symptoms and risk factors or wrap cuffs.
- Cuff positions may include:
  - Thigh, calf and ankle (a.k.a. "3-cuff method")
  - High thigh, low thigh, calf, and ankle (a.k.a. "4-cuff method")
- Choose appropriately sized pneumatic cuffs for each section of the limb:
  - 18-20 cm width on thigh (for 3-cuff method)
  - 12 cm width on upper/lower thigh (for 4-cuff method)
  - 12 cm width on arm, calf and ankle (Some labs prefer a 10 cm cuff at the arm and ankle. The cuff width should be at least 20% greater than the diameter of the limb).

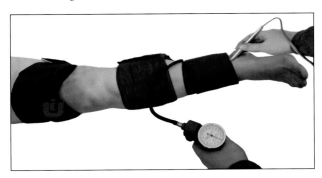

3-cuff method

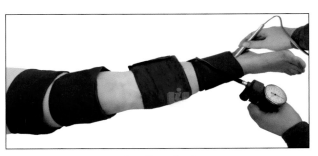

4-cuff method

- Appropriately wrap blood pressure cuffs on the limb. Cuffs should be placed "straight" rather than angled. All cuffs should fit snugly, particularly if they are to be used for the VPR technique following the pressures exam.
- Place the thigh cuff as high as possible on the thigh, the low thigh cuff above the knee, the calf cuff just below the knee and the ankle cuff just above the medial malleolus.
- Arterial physiologic exams are traditionally performed using a continuous wave (CW) Doppler. However, waveforms can be obtained at the same sites using a pulsed wave (PW) Doppler. The CW Doppler is recommended for segmental pressure measurement due to its capabilities for a larger sampling region. Use a high frequency (8 MHz) CW Doppler probe to locate arterial signals. Alternate transducers including a lower frequency probe (e.g., 4 MHz) may be needed for obese patients or for deeper vessels.

Segmental Doppler Waveforms

- Place the Doppler probe on the limb using a 45º-60º angle to the skin with enough pressure to keep contact, but not so much pressure that the artery is compressed by the probe:
- Document several representative Doppler waveforms at the following levels after moving or angling the probe appropriately to optimize the signal:
  - Dorsalis pedis artery*
  - Posterior tibial artery*
  - Popliteal artery

> *If the venous signal is interfering with the arterial waveform, try a slightly more proximal or distal location or manually compress the proximal limb to temporarily stop venous return.*

  - Superficial femoral (avoiding the deep femoral artery)
  - Common femoral artery

*If neither pedal artery is audible, try to obtain a waveform of the peroneal artery by placing the probe superior to the lateral malleolus, pointing inward.

Segmental Pressures

- Locate the best arterial signal at the ankle or use the popliteal signal for the thigh pressure(s) and the pedal arteries only for the calf and ankle pressures.

The following instructions can be used when testing with an automatic cuff inflator or standard manometer:

- Inflate cuffs 20-30 mmHg above the last audible arterial signal heard using the Doppler probe.

> *For patients with irregular heart beats, decrease deflation speeds.*

- Deflate the cuff slowly (at a rate of 2-4 mmHg per second). The systolic pressure is recorded as soon as the first audible arterial Doppler signal returns. The Doppler pulse must continue after hearing the first pulse to assure there is an actual pulse rather than motion artifact.

- The pressure is recorded in "mmHg" as soon as the first audible Doppler arterial signal returns at each level indicated; ankle, calf, low thigh and/or high thigh.

- Obtain bilateral brachial artery (BrA) pressures.

- Calculate ankle, calf, low-thigh, high-thigh brachial indices by dividing the systolic pressure at the particular level by the highest brachial pressure.

- Repeat for the contralateral leg when indicated.

Preliminary Analysis of Data

- Consider the segmental Doppler waveforms and pressures obtained. Determine severity of disease according to laboratory diagnostic criteria.

Interpretation

Normal Segmental Pressures

- Leg pressures are normally higher than the highest brachial pressure. The normal pressure difference between the arm and ankle is 12(±8) – 24 (±9)mmHg. [5]

- Segmental pressure ratios (leg pressure ÷ arm pressure) of the lower thigh, calf and ankle should be ≥1.0 at all levels. [5] There is normally no significant decrease in pressure (<20 mmHg) between the cuffs. [5-8]

- If using the 4-cuff method with a 12 cm thigh cuff, the upper thigh pressure is normally 30-40 mmHg higher than the arm pressure due to cuff artifact. [5-7] The high thigh ratio using a 12 cm cuff is normally ≥1.2-1.4. [5,7,9]

> *The third phase may be missing in older patients with less vessel compliance.*

TABLE 27: Lower Extremity Segmental Pressures Protocol Summary

- Apply appropriately sized pneumatic cuffs for each section of the limb:
    - For 3-cuff method: 18-20 cm width; thigh, 12 cm width; arm, calf and ankle*
    - For 4-cuff method: 12 cm width; arms, thigh, calf and ankle*

- Record representative Doppler waveforms for all lower extremity levels.

- Inflate each cuff 20-30 mmHg beyond the last audible arterial signal using a Doppler probe on the appropriate artery distal to the cuff.

- Deflation of the cuff should be at a rate of 2-4 mmHg per second.

- The pressure is recorded as soon as the first audible arterial Doppler signal returns.

- Obtain a pressure at each cuff consecutively and calculate the index at each level:

$$\frac{pedal,\ calf,\ thigh\ pressure}{highest\ brachial\ pressure}$$

- Determine classification of disease according to laboratory diagnostic criteria.

- Repeat for the contralateral side.

  * *(Some labs use a 10 cm cuff at the ankle)*

Segmental Pressure Worksheet

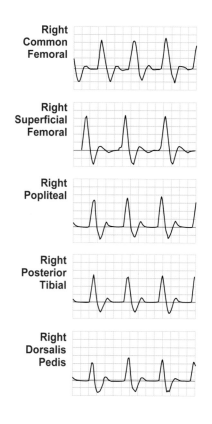

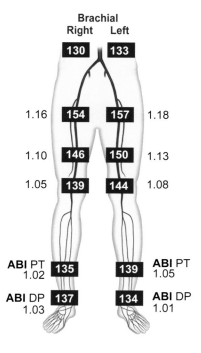

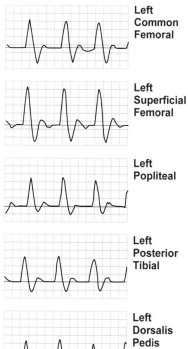

Normal Doppler Waveforms

- A normal triphasic Doppler waveform is demonstrated by strong forward flow with a sharp upstroke in systole followed by flow reversal in early diastole (below the baseline) and an additional short pulse of forward flow. Many laboratories will accept a waveform with a reversed flow component as normal even if the third phase is missing.[7,10]

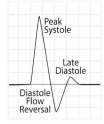

Normal, triphasic waveform

Abnormal Segmental Pressures

- A leg/brachial ratio <1.0 (or <1.2-1.4 at the upper thigh level) is abnormal and indicates a significant stenosis or occlusion at/ or proximal to the cuff.[5,9]

- If the ABI is <0.90-0.92 it is likely that a hemodynamically significant obstruction is present in the lower extremity above the level of the ankle.[5,7,9]

- A drop in pressure greater than 20-30 mmHg between adjacent cuffs (proximal to distal) indicates significant obstruction between these levels.[6-8,11]

- A change in the ABI of ≥0.15 from one study to the next is significant.[8,9]

> *If the ankle pressure is significantly higher than the calf, it is likely that calcification is causing a falsely high ankle pressure and should not be used for interpretation.*[7,10]

- An ABI of greater that 1.3 suggests calcific disease and is considered non-diagnostic.[6,10] As an alternative means of estimating disease severity, use a toe/brachial index.[6,10] A toe/brachial index <0.70 is abnormal.[10]

Abnormal Doppler Waveforms

- There is controversy among vascular professionals regarding the terminology describing CW Doppler analog waveforms.

  – Essentially all vascular professionals agree that a waveform with a sharp, quick upstroke followed by reversed flow direction and a third forward phase is termed triphasic and consider this a normal finding in the peripheral arteries.

  – A waveform with a reversed second phase that is missing the third forward phase may be described as "triphasic" or "biphasic" by laboratories. However, nearly all will interpret this as normal. Recently some laboratories have adopted terminology that recognizes the reversed flow connection to normal by using an abbreviation NR for "normal-reversed" whether or not the third phase is present, and avoiding the confusing use of "triphasic" and "biphasic" terms.

  – Monophasic arterial Doppler waveforms are characterized by a slow upstroke, low amplitude, and broad peak with no evidence of the reversed flow component in late systole. The upstroke has a general direction of being tipped to the right. Continuous forward flow is typical in diastole, but diastolic flow may be absent if there is distal resistance from an additional high grade distal obstruction, for example. Monophasic waveforms are typically present distal to an occlusion or a very high grade stenosis.

- Absent Doppler signals suggest arterial occlusion at the site of interrogation.[5] Absent Doppler signals in all pedal arteries of a limb suggest a critical decrease in perfusion to the lower extremity, particularly if the VPR or PPG waveforms at the toe are flat. Be aware that extensive calcification will obscure the Doppler signal, but the VPR and PPG waveforms are typically not affected.

Continuous Wave Arterial Doppler Signals

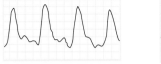

Moderately abnormal waveforms

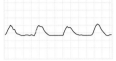

Severely abnormal waveforms

* Triphasic, biphasic, and monophasic waveforms have multiple definitions throughout the vascular ultrasound community. Although these waveforms may be labeled differently in different labs, most laboratories would identify the first waveform as normal, the second as moderately abnormal, and the third as severely abnormal. Some laboratories reserve the term biphasic only for waveforms with a reversed flow component but no third phase, but despite the term it is likely that these would be considered normal due to the presence of the reversed flow component.

TABLE 28: **Findings of the Lower Extremities and Level of Disease**	
Level of Disease	**Findings**
Aortoiliac	High thigh/brachial index <1.0 bilaterally
Iliac	High thigh/brachial index <1.0 unilaterally
Femoral (FA) disease	Gradient between high and low thigh cuffs
Distal FA/popliteal	Gradient between thigh and calf cuffs
Infrapopliteal	Gradient between calf and ankle cuffs

TABLE 29: **University of Chicago Diagnostic Criteria for ABI**	
ABI	**Severity**
≥1.0-0.95	Normal
0.80-0.94	Mild disease
0.50-0.79	Moderate disease
0.30-0.49	Severe disease
<0.29	Critical disease

Source: Internally validated at the University of Chicago Medical Center Vascular Laboratory.

TABLE 30: **Diagnostic Criteria for ABI Severity**	
ABI	**Severity**
≥1.0	Normal
0.90 to <1.0	Mild disease
0.50-0.90	Claudication
0.30-0.50	Severe occlusive disease
<0.30	Ischemia

Source: AbuRahma AF. (2000). Segmental Doppler pressures and Doppler waveform analysis in peripheral vascular disease of the lower extremities. In AbuRahma AF, Bergan JJ (Eds). *Non-invasive Vascular Diagnosis.* (213-229). London: Springer.

TABLE 31: Diagnostic Criteria for Occlusive Disease by Segmental Arterial Pressures Indices

One primary arterial occlusion

- Ankle brachial index is typically between 0.50-0.80 (Consider highest ABI)

Multilevel occlusive disease

- Ankle brachial index is typically <0.50 (Consider highest ABI)

Source: Zierler RE, Sumner DS. (2005). Physiologic assessment of peripheral arterial occlusive disease. In *Rutherford Vascular Surgery 6th edition*. (197-222). Philadelphia. Elsevier Saunders.

TABLE 32: ABI Symptoms

ABI	Symptom
≥1.0	Normal
<0.80	Claudication
<0.30	Rest pain
<0.20	Impending gangrene

Source: Kempczinski RF. (1982) Clinical application of non-invasive testing in extremity arterial insufficiency. In Kempczinski RF & Yao JST (Eds.), Practical Non-invasive Vascular Diagnosis (343-365). Chicago: Year Book Medical Publishers.

Differential Diagnosis

- Spinal stenosis
- Venous thrombosis
- Restless leg syndrome
- Compartment syndrome
- Nocturnal leg cramps
- Neuropathy
- Muscle/tendon strains
- Arthritis
- Abnormalities of adrenergic receptor/sympathetic nervous system
- Connective tissue disease (scleroderma)

Correlation

- Duplex ultrasound
- Spiral CT scan
- MRA
- Arteriography

Medical Treatment

- Modify risk factors (e.g., reduce cholesterol, manage HTN and DM, smoking cessation)
- Exercise regimen
- Antiplatelet medication (e.g., aspirin)
- Anticoagulation (warfarin)
- Thrombolysis (acute blockage)

Surgical Treatment

- Bypass grafting
- Atherectomy
- Endarterectomy
- Direct focal repair
- Resection (aneurysmal disease)
- Sympathectomy
- Amputation

Endovascular Treatment

- Angioplasty
- Stent
- Atherectomy
- Intra-arterial directed thrombolysis (acute blockage)

Points to Remember

- Pressure measurements should be taken in the supine position with the extremity at the same level as the heart. Pressures recorded while the patient is sitting will be falsely elevated due to the effects of hydrostatic pressure. For every 10 inches that the heart is elevated above the ankle level, pressure increases 18.67 mmHg. Since the heart level is 34 inches from the ankle on an average person while sitting, the blood pressure at the ankle will be affected about 63 mmHg (3.4 x 18.67 mmHg). If pressures can only be obtained while the patient is sitting, note the position and know that the actual pressure will be significantly lower than if the pressure was taken while supine. (If possible, try placing the foot on a chair to get it closer to the heart). Remember to use the same method for follow-up exams for accurate comparison.

- The 4-cuff method offers more information than the 3-cuff method; distinguishing inflow from femoral disease.

- A calf pressure ≥65-70 mmHg is typically needed to heal a below-knee amputation. [7,8]

- Significant collateral blood flow may result in a false negative pressure gradient of less than 20 mmHg between segments or a normal upper thigh brachial ratio.[8]

- Using too narrow a cuff for the width of the limb will result in higher pressures due to cuff artifact. [7,10,11]

- If a pressure measurement needs to be repeated, the cuff should be fully deflated for approximately one minute prior to the repeat measurement. Do not take a blood pressure over a bypass graft or dialysis access conduit or fistula without first consulting your medical director. Do not take a blood pressure on the arm of a patient with a history of mastectomy.

- Moderate to severely abnormal analog waveforms typically have a somewhat wider peak and a slightly slower upstroke. There may be a "multiphasic" downslope that stays above the baseline (no reversal of flow) but demonstrates what appears to be a "notch" or two in the downslope. This is the most difficult waveform to describe due to its very qualitative nature, but it is helpful to distinguish the moderately abnormal Doppler waveform from a severely abnormal one in practice, especially at the common femoral and pedal levels.

References

1. 1 Sumner DS, Zierler RE. (2005). Vascular physiology: essential hemodynamic principles. In *Rutherford Vascular Surgery 6th edition*. (75-123). Philadelphia. Elsevier Saunders.
2. 2 Fecteau SR, Darling III RC, Roddy SP. (2005). Arterial thromboembolism. In *Rutherford Vascular Surgery 6th edition*. (971-986). Philadelphia. Elsevier Saunders.
3. 3 Shepard RFJ. (2005). Raynaud's syndrome: vasospastic and occlusive arterial disease involving the distal upper extremity. In *Rutherford Vascular Surgery 6th edition*. (1319-1346). Philadelphia. Elsevier Saunders.
4. 4 Dawson DL, Lee ES, Lindholm K. (2010). Aortic and peripheral aneurysms. In Zierler RE (Ed.), *Strandess's duplex scanning disorders in vascular diagnosis 4th ed.* (157-168). Philadelphia Wolters Kluwer Lippincott Williams & Wilkins.
5. 5 Zierler RE, Sumner DS. (2005). Physiologic assessment of peripheral arterial occlusive disease. *In Rutherford Vascular Surgery 6th edition*. (197-222). Philadelphia. Elsevier Saunders.
6. 6 Carter SA. (2003). Role of pressure measurements. In Bernstein EF (Ed.), Vascular Diagnosis (486-512). St. Louis: Mosby.
7. 7 Zierler, RE, (2005). Nonimaging Physiologic Tests for Assessment of Lower Extremity Arterial Occlusive Disease. In Zwiebel WJ, Pellerito JS (Eds.), *Introduction to Vascular Ultrasonography*. (275-295). Philadelphia: Elsevier Saunders
8. 8 Hallett, JW, Brewster DC, Rasmussen TE, (2001) Non-invasive Vascular Testing, In *Handbook of Patient Care in Vascular Diseases*, (29-49). Philadelphia: Lippincott Williams & Wilkins.
9. 9 Moneta GL, Zacardi MJ, Olmsted KA. (2010). Lower extremity arterial occlusive disease. In Zierler RE (Ed.), Strandess's duplex scanning disorders in vascular diagnosis 4th ed. (133-147).Philadelphia Wolters Kluwer Lippincott Williams & Wilkins.
10. 10 Zwiebel, WJ. Pellerito JS. (2005). Basic concepts of Doppler frequency spectrum analysis and ultrasound blood flow imaging. In Zwiebel WJ, Pellerito JS (Eds.), *In Introduction to Vascular Ultrasonography 5th ed*, (61-89). Philadelphia: Elsevier Saunders.
11. 11 Needham T. (2005). In Mansour MA, Labropoulos N. (Eds.). *Vascular Diagnosis*, (215-222). Philadelphia: Elsevier Saunders.

Definition

Volume pulse recording (VPR) uses air plethysmography to detect volume changes related to blood flow. VPR determines whether peripheral arterial disease is present, its effects on arterial perfusion to the extremity, and the segmental location of the obstruction.

Rationale

Each arterial pulse creates a change in volume under a pressure cuff. These limb volume changes result in proportional changes in the air pressure in the cuffs. The air pressure changes are monitored by a pressure transducer in the VPR instrument and recorded as a waveform.

Etiology of Disease

- Atherosclerosis
- Embolization
- Thrombus
- Extrinsic compression
- Intimal hyperplasia
- Trauma
- Traumatic occlusion

Risk Factors

- Age (increased risk with age)
- Coronary artery disease or MI
- Diabetes
- Family history
- Hyperlipidemia
- Hypertension
- Obesity
- Smoking
- Sedentary lifestyle
- Previous history of CVA
- Elevated levels of homocysteine
- Excessive levels of C-reactive protein
- History of radiation
- Occupational exposure to toxic substances

Indications for Exam

- Claudication (exercise-related limb pain)
- Abnormal ABI (VPR used to confirm decrease in perfusion and identify general location of obstruction)
- Limb pain at rest
- Absent peripheral pulses
- Extremity ulcer
- Gangrene
- Aneurysmal disease
- Trauma to an artery
- Follow-up after revascularization procedure
- Popliteal artery entrapment

Contraindications/Limitations

- Patients with acute venous thrombosis (there is a slight risk of embolization by the pressure cuff).
- VPR cannot be performed over extensive bandages or casts which are not removable.
- Any site of trauma, recent surgery, ulceration or graft placement which should not be compressed by the pressure cuff.
- Good collaterals around a short occlusion may normalize the VPR waveform.

Mechanism of disease

- **Atherosclerosis** [1] is the most common arterial disease. Atherosclerotic plaque forms in the artery to block flow by either narrowing it (arterial stenosis) or totally blocking the artery (arterial occlusion). The term "hemodynamically significant obstruction" refers to either a stenosis or an occlusion that results in a decrease in blood pressure or flow distal to the obstruction. Typically, a stenosis must narrow the diameter of the artery by at least 50% to decrease pressure and flow distally. An arterial occlusion is typically seen from one major branch to the next.
- **Emboli** may occur as contents of a plaque or fragments of an organized thrombus from the heart or aneurysm loosen and flow downstream. Emboli become lodged in a distant blood vessel, causing arterial occlusion and reduction of flow. [1]
- **Vasospasm** is a temporary constriction of the arteries (typically digital arteries) that may cause significant discomfort to the patient or be a sign of a more serious underlying disease.[2]
- **Extrinsic compression** from tumors, hematoma, etc., can result in stenosis or occlusion by placing enough pressure on arterial walls to compromise blood flow. [1]

Location of Disease

- Location of disease can be focal or diffuse and affect any level or multiple levels
- The most common location of obstruction in the lower extremities is the superficial femoral artery at the adductor canal.
- The popliteal artery is another common location.
- Arterial bifurcations
- Subclavian artery, palmar arch and/or digital arteries

Patient History

- Claudication (exercise related)
- Rest pain
- Acute occlusion
  - Pain
  - Paralysis (weakness)
  - Paresthesia ("pins and needles")
  - Poikilothermia (ice-cold limb)
  - Pulselessness
  - Pallor
- Previous ulceration/gangrene of feet/toes or hands/digits
- Previous therapeutic vascular procedure (e.g., bypass, stenting)

Physical Examination

- Pulselessness
- Pallor
- Gangrene/necrosis (tissue death)
- Cyanosis
- Dependent rubor
- Bruit (abnormal sound heard through auscultation caused by vibration of tissue from turbulent flow)
- Marked temperature difference between extremities, especially if one is ice cold
- Palpable thrill (vibration caused by turbulent blood flow as seen in AV fistula)

Volume Pulse Recording Protocol

- Rest the patient for 5 minutes before beginning the exam in order for blood pressures to stabilize after "exercise" (walking into the exam room). You may use this time to obtain a patient history, including symptoms and risk factors, explain the procedure, and wrap the cuffs.

- Patient is examined in the supine position. Elevating the foot onto a pillow or towel momentarily may make it easier to wrap cuffs around the leg for a lower extremity exam, but be careful not to hyperextend the knee during testing and risk possibly compressing the popliteal artery.

- Cuffs should be placed "straight" rather than angled. Choose appropriately sized pneumatic cuffs for each section of the limb:

  - 12 cm width; arm, thigh, calf and ankle

  Place the cuffs with equal snugness on the limb; this will affect the height of the VPR waveform.

  - Most labs use two 12 cm cuffs on the thigh, but some may choose to use one 18 cm cuff on the thigh instead. Also, some labs prefer a 10 cm cuff at the arm and ankle. Whichever you chose, the suggestion is to use the same size cuff on both the arm and ankle.

  - 7 cm width; hand/foot

  - 1.9-2.5 cm width; digital*

  *A 2.5 cm cuff is highly preferred if the cuff will also be used for digital pressures.

  Ask the patient to lay as still as possible to eliminate motion artifact on the tracings.

- Place the cuffs with equal snugness on the limb; the volume of air needed to obtain the appropriate pressure will affect the height of the VPR waveform. If one cuff is very loosely applied, it will take more air to fill the cuff, affecting the wave height. Ask the patient if the cuffs feel equally snug and adjust as necessary.

- An obese thigh will create a VPR waveform with a lower amplitude than normal, but may still demonstrate a normal contour. Note this for the interpreting physician and make an interpretation based on a change in the waveform shape rather than a change in amplitude from one level to the next.

- During the exam, cuffs will be inflated at each level according to the pressure indicated by the manufacturer of the VPR unit. See tables 33-34 for sample manufacturer settings. This will ensure appropriate contact is made with the limb to transfer the volume pulse from the limb to the cuff. A volume pulse tracing is then recorded using the indicated gain settings for the extremity.

- Record VPR waveforms at each level using the appropriate gain settings. Consider the factory settings of the VPR equipment being used.

- The size of the VPR tracing in the lower extremities may need to be adjusted during testing to account for the decrease in distal tissue volumes. The calf tracing typically augments 25% in normal limbs and may bound off the chart. (If the size was decreased for the calf, remember to return back to initial settings for the ankle.)

- When adjustments are made, you must be consistent with these settings on the contralateral leg at the same level.

- When assessing for popliteal artery entrapment syndrome, place the patient's heel up on a firm pillow or roll of towels to create a hyperabduction of the knee. Have the patient slowly plantar and dorsiflex their foot. A resting plantarflexion and dorsiflexion VPR waveform should be documented.

- The VPR trace setting for "size" in the upper extremity is usually consistent for each level (see recommended factory settings of the VPR equipment being used). If you need to change the size of the tracing (i.e., the amplitude of the trace bounds off the chart at any level), remember to be consistent and use the same size for the rest of the levels.

- Determine severity of disease according to shape and relative amplitude of the tracings. Use comparisons between "typical" normal, the tracing of proximal segments and to the contralateral limb. [3]

TABLE 33: VPR Settings for Upper Extremities

Cuff Level	Cuff Size	Pressure	Gain
Arm	10-12 cm	65 mmHg	2.5
Forearm	10-12 cm	65 mmHg	2.5
Hand	7 cm	65 mmHg	6.0
Finger	2.5 cm	40 mmHg	10.0

TABLE 34: VPR Settings for Lower Extremities

Cuff Level	Cuff Size	Pressure	Gain	Size
*High Thigh	12 cm	65 mmHg	2.5	3
*Low Thigh	12 cm	65 mmHg	2.5	3
Calf	10 cm	65 mmHg	2.5	3
Ankle	10 cm	65 mmHg	2.5	3
Foot	7 cm	65 mmHg	2.5	6

* Both a high-thigh and low-thigh cuff are used for the "four cuff method". Only one 18 cm wide thigh cuff is used for the "three-cuff method".

Interpretation

- The volume pulse waveform is primarily interpreted by its contour (shape) and amplitude (height) relative to the amplitude of the adjacent proximal cuff.

- The tracings are described as being normal, mildly abnormal, moderately abnormal or severely abnormal:

TABLE 35: Volume Pulse Recording Protocol Summary

- Wrap appropriately sized pneumatic cuffs for each section of the limb:
  - 12 cm width; arm, thigh, calf and ankle*
  - 7 cm width; hand/foot
  - 1.9-2.5 cm width; digital **
- Inflate cuffs at each level according to the pressure and gain settings indicated by the manufacturer of the VPR unit. Refer to tables 33-34 for sample manufacturer settings. Record representative VPR waveforms.
- Determine classification of disease according to laboratory diagnostic criteria.

  * *Most labs use two 12 cm cuffs on the thigh, but some may choose to use one 18 cm cuff on the thigh instead. Also, some labs prefer a 10 cm cuff at the arm and ankle. Whichever you chose, the suggestion is to use the same size cuff on both the arm and ankle.*

  ** *A 2.5 cm cuff is highly preferred if the cuff will also be used for digital pressures.*

Normal VPR Waveform Interpretation

- Waveform has a quick upstroke, sharp peak and a dicrotic notch on its downslope or bows toward the baseline when the dicrotic notch is absent. [4,5]
- The presence of the dicrotic notch eliminates the possibility of significant arterial occlusive disease. [5]
- The calf tracing should be approximately 25% larger than the thigh tracing. [5,6]
- The thigh tracing should generally be the same amplitude as the ankle tracing. [4,5]

TABLE 36: Normal Amplitudes for Lower Extremity VPR

Level	Amplitude
Thigh	>15 mm
Calf	>20 mm
Ankle	>15 mm

Source: Sumner DS, Zierler RE. (2005). Physiologic assessment of peripheral arterial occlusive disease. In Rutherford Vascular Surgery 6th edition. (197-222). Philadelphia. Elsevier Saunders.

VPR Waveforms [4-6]

Normal

- Sharp upstroke
- Sharp systolic peak
- Gradual downslope bowing towards baseline
- Dicrotic notch, however some patients may have inward bowing on the downslope

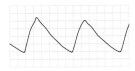

Mildly Abnormal

- Sharp upstroke
- Rounded systolic peak
- Loss of dicrotic notch
- Downslope bends slightly away from the baseline

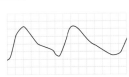

Moderately Abnormal

- Prolonged upstroke
- Rounded systolic peak
- Loss of dicrotic notch
- Relatively low amplitude compared to normal and proximal tracings
- Upslope and downslope time nearly equal

Severely Abnormal

- Very prolonged upstroke
- Rounded systolic peak
- No dicrotic notch
- Upslope, downslope time nearly equal
- Very low amplitude or flat, non-pulsatile tracing

TABLE 37: Lower Extremity VPR Changes Based on Location of Disease

Level of disease	PVR Amplitude		
	Thigh	Calf	Ankle
Aoil stenosis*	Abnormal	Abnormal	Abnormal
Aoil occlusion *	Abnormal	Abnormal	Abnormal
Low SFA occlusion	Normal	Abnormal	Abnormal
High SFA occlusion w/o AI disease	Abnormal	Abnormal	Abnormal
Aoil + SFA disease	Abnormal	Abnormal	Abnormal
Tibial disease	Normal	Normal	Abnormal
Small vessel disease	Normal	Normal	Normal

* open distal system

Source: Modified from Raines JK. (1993). The pulse volume recording in peripheral arterial disease. In Bernstein EF (Ed). Vascular Diagnosis 4th ed. (p. 538). St Louis: Mosby.

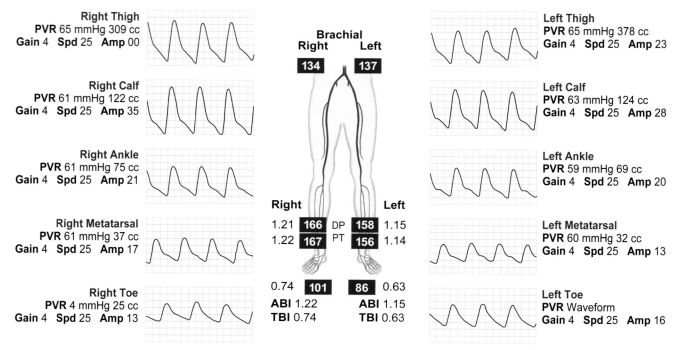

Right Thigh
PVR 65 mmHg 309 cc
Gain 4 **Spd** 25 **Amp** 00

Right Calf
PVR 61 mmHg 122 cc
Gain 4 **Spd** 25 **Amp** 35

Right Ankle
PVR 61 mmHg 75 cc
Gain 4 **Spd** 25 **Amp** 21

Right Metatarsal
PVR 61 mmHg 37 cc
Gain 4 **Spd** 25 **Amp** 17

Right Toe
PVR 4 mmHg 25 cc
Gain 4 **Spd** 25 **Amp** 13

Brachial
Right   Left
134   137

Right   Left
1.21 166 DP 158 1.15
1.22 167 PT 156 1.14

0.74 101   86 0.63
ABI 1.22   **ABI** 1.15
TBI 0.74   **TBI** 0.63

Left Thigh
PVR 65 mmHg 378 cc
Gain 4 **Spd** 25 **Amp** 23

Left Calf
PVR 63 mmHg 124 cc
Gain 4 **Spd** 25 **Amp** 28

Left Ankle
PVR 59 mmHg 69 cc
Gain 4 **Spd** 25 **Amp** 20

Left Metatarsal
PVR 60 mmHg 32 cc
Gain 4 **Spd** 25 **Amp** 13

Left Toe
PVR Waveform
Gain 4 **Spd** 25 **Amp** 16

Normal VPR Examination of the Lower Extremity

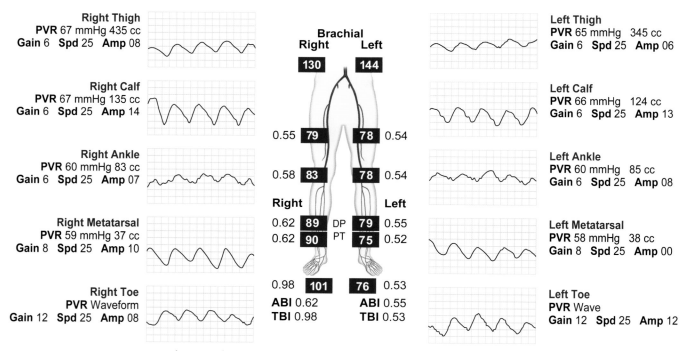

Right Thigh
PVR 67 mmHg 435 cc
Gain 6 **Spd** 25 **Amp** 08

Right Calf
PVR 67 mmHg 135 cc
Gain 6 **Spd** 25 **Amp** 14

Right Ankle
PVR 60 mmHg 83 cc
Gain 6 **Spd** 25 **Amp** 07

Right Metatarsal
PVR 59 mmHg 37 cc
Gain 8 **Spd** 25 **Amp** 10

Right Toe
PVR Waveform
Gain 12 **Spd** 25 **Amp** 08

Brachial
Right   Left
130   144

0.55 79   78 0.54

0.58 83   78 0.54
Right   Left
0.62 89 DP 79 0.55
0.62 90 PT 75 0.52

0.98 101   76 0.53
ABI 0.62   **ABI** 0.55
TBI 0.98   **TBI** 0.53

Left Thigh
PVR 65 mmHg 345 cc
Gain 6 **Spd** 25 **Amp** 06

Left Calf
PVR 66 mmHg 124 cc
Gain 6 **Spd** 25 **Amp** 13

Left Ankle
PVR 60 mmHg 85 cc
Gain 6 **Spd** 25 **Amp** 08

Left Metatarsal
PVR 58 mmHg 38 cc
Gain 8 **Spd** 25 **Amp** 00

Left Toe
PVR Wave
Gain 12 **Spd** 25 **Amp** 12

Abnormal VPR Examination of the Bilateral Lower Extremities

Abnormal VPR Tracing: *Note the decrease in amplitude of the thigh tracings. Abnormally rounded systolic peaks and loss of dicrotic notch are noted on both sides. The left ankle is abnormal; note having the same amplitude as the L-thigh.*

Abnormal VPR Waveform Interpretation

- Abnormal VPR waveforms occur distal to the obstructed arterial segment.[4,6]

- The abnormal VPR has a slower upstroke, rounded peak and a downslope that bows away from the baseline.[4]

- The dicrotic notch disappears.[5]

- As disease progresses, the VPR waveform becomes more rounded and loses amplitude.[3,5,6]

- An aortoiliac obstruction produces abnormal VPR waveforms at all levels, though the calf amplitude can be greater than at the thigh.[4,5]

- A low amplitude, abnormally shaped thigh VPR may indicate aortoiliac or proximal SFA obstruction.[4]

- A calf VPR amplitude that is equal to or lower than the ipsilateral thigh VPR amplitude with the same settings is the most indicative finding of superficial femoral artery (SFA) disease.[4,5]

- Tibial artery obstruction will result in normal calf augmentation but demonstrate an abnormal ankle VPR waveform.[6]

- Significant decrease or obliteration of the VPR waveform will occur during provocative maneuvers if a patient has popliteal artery entrapment.[7]

Differential Diagnosis

- Spinal stenosis
- Venous thrombosis causing pain
- Restless leg syndrome
- Compartment syndrome
- Nocturnal leg cramps
- Neuropathy
- Muscle/tendon strains
- Arthritis
- Abnormalities of adrenergic receptor/sympathetic nervous system
- Connective tissue disease (scleroderma)

Correlation

- Duplex ultrasound
- Spiral CT scan
- MRA
- Arteriography

Medical Treatment

- Modify risk factors (e.g., cessation of tobacco usage, avoidance of cold)
- Antiplatelet medication (e.g., aspirin)
- Anticoagulation (warfarin)

Surgical Treatment

- Bypass grafting
- Atherectomy
- Endarterectomy
- Direct focal repair
- Resection (aneurysmal disease)
- Sympathectomy
- Amputation

Endovascular Treatment

- Angioplasty
- Stent
- Intra-arterial directed thrombolysis (acute blockage)

Points to Remember

- Good collateralization can normalize the VPR waveform in a short occlusion.[5]

- The VPR amplitude is influenced by a number of physiologic variables including cardiac stroke volume, blood pressure, blood volume, vasoconstriction, motor tone, loose cuff application and size of limb.[5]

- VPR may be helpful in assessing a patient for popliteal entrapment syndrome; the ankle VPR tracing will be normal at rest and flatten with plantarflexion or dorsiflexion with knee hyperextension as the gastrocnemius contracts and compresses the popliteal artery.[7]

- Tremors can cause waveform artifact.[4]

- VPR waveforms are not affected by calcified vessels.[5,6]

- When the VPR waveform exhibits a dicrotic notch, the presence of occlusive disease can be excluded. The absence of a dicrotic notch is less important since it may not be present even in normal patients when resistance is lowered, such as after exercise.[4]

References

1. 1 Sumner DS, Zierler RE. (2005). Vascular physiology: essential hemodynamic principles. In Rutherford Vascular Surgery 6th edition. (75-123). Philadelphia. Elsevier Saunders

2. 2 Shepard RFJ. (2005). Raynaud's syndrome: vasospastic and occlusive arterial disease involving the distal upper extremity. In Rutherford Vascular Surgery 6th edition. (1319-1346). Philadelphia. Elsevier Saunders

3. 3 Talbot, SR, Zwiebel WJ. (2005). Assessment of Upper Extremity Arterial Occlusive Disease. In Zwiebel WJ. Pellerito JS (Eds.), Introduction to Vascular Ultrasonography 5th ed. (297-323). Philadelphia: Elsevier Saunders

4. 4 Kempczinski RF. (1982). Segmental volume plethysmography: The pulse volume recorder. In: Kempczinski RF and Yao SJS. Practical Noninvasive Vascular Diagnosis. (105--117). Chicago: Yearbook Medical.

5. 5 Sumner DS, Zierler RE. (2005). Physiologic assessment of peripheral arterial occlusive disease. In Rutherford Vascular Surgery 6th edition. (197-222). Philadelphia. Elsevier Saunders.

6. 6 Raines JK. (1993). The pulse volume recording in peripheral arterial disease. In Bernstein EF (Ed). Vascular Diagnosis 4th ed. (534-553). St Louis: Mosby

7. 7 Hallett JW, Brewster DC, Rasmussen TE. (2001). Noninvasive vascular testing. In: Handbook of Patient Care in Vascular Diseases. (29-49), Philadelphia Lippincott Williams & Wilkins.

Defintion

Noninvasive physiological tests which compare the systolic pressure at the level of the brachial artery to the systolic pressure of the toes in the foot (TBI) and detect arterial pulsations in the terminal portions of the digits (PPG).

Rationale

The sensors of a photoplethysmography (PPG) transducer consist of an infrared light-emitting diode and a phototransistor. Infrared light is transmitted into the superficial tissue and a reflection is received by the phototransistor. The signal received relates to the quantity of red blood cells in the cutaneous circulation. Each arterial pulse creates a change in blood volume under the sensor. These cutaneous volume changes result in a proportional change in the reflection of the infrared light from the tissue. The changes in reflection are monitored in the instrument and recorded as a pulse waveform when the instrument is set in arterial or AC mode. If set in the venous or DC mode, the PPG can be used to monitor slower volume changes related to venous reflux, as opposed to quick changes seen during the arterial pulse cycle.

Etiology

- Atherosclerosis
- Trauma
- Embolization
- Thrombus
- Aneurysm
- Pseudoaneurysm
- Intimal hyperplasia
- Traumatic occlusion
- Extrinsic compression
- AV fistula (abnormal connection between an artery and a vein)
- Buerger's disease
- Vasculitis
- Radiation arteritis
- Vasospasm

Risk Factors

- Age (increased risk with age)
- Coronary artery disease
- Diabetes
- Family history
- Hyperlipidemia
- Hypertension
- Smoking
- Obesity
- Aneurysm
- History of radiation
- Fibromuscular dysplasia
- Occupational exposure to toxic substances

Indications for Exam

- Exercise-related pain (claudication symptoms)
- Limb or digital pain at rest
- Extremity ulcer/gangrene
- Digital cyanosis
- Cold sensitivity
- Absent peripheral pulses
- Arterial trauma and aneurysms
- Bruit
- Raynaud's syndrome/ phenomenon

Contraindications/Limitations

- Calcified vessels which will falsely elevate ankle pressures (typically encountered in patients with diabetes or end-stage renal disease). Calcification rarely affects digital arteries.
- Significant lesions with excellent collateral circulation, which may result in normal distal pressures and waveforms.
- Pressure cuffs may not fit well around very large or very small digits.
- Any site of trauma, surgery or ulceration which should not be compressed by the pressure cuff.
- Patients with extensive bandages or casts.

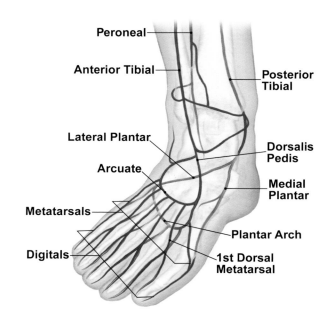

Lower Extremity: Distal Limb and Digital Arteries

Mechanism of Disease

There are two major mechanisms that cause reduced arterial blood supply to the lower extremity; obstruction from atherosclerotic plaque and embolism. Of these, atherosclerosis is more common.

- **Atherosclerosis** is the most common arterial disease. Atherosclerotic plaque forms in the artery to block flow by either narrowing it (arterial stenosis) or totally blocking the artery (arterial occlusion). The term "hemodynamically significant obstruction" refers to either a stenosis or an occlusion that results in a decrease in blood pressure or flow distal to the obstruction. Typically, a stenosis must narrow the diameter of the artery by at least 50% to decrease pressure and flow distally. An arterial occlusion is typically seen from one major branch to the next.

- **Emboli**: embolization of contents of a plaque and/or fragments of an organized thrombus from the heart or proximal aneurysm which become lodged in a distant blood vessel. [2]
- **Vasospasm** is a temporary constriction, typically of the digital arteries, that may cause significant discomfort to the patient.
- **Extrinsic compression** from tumors, hematoma, etc., can result in stenosis or occlusion by placing enough pressure on arterial walls to compromise blood flow. [1]

Patient History

- Claudication (exercise related)
- Pain
- Paralysis (weakness)
- Paresthesia ("pins and needles")
- Poikilothermia (ice cold limbs)
- Previous ulceration/gangrene of feet/toes
- Previous therapeutic vascular procedure (e.g., bypass, stent)

Physical Examination

- Pulselessness
- Cyanosis
- Gangrene/necrosis (tissue death)
- Pallor
- Dependent rubor
- Marked temperature difference between digits and/or extremities
- Bruit (abnormal sound heard through auscultation caused by turbulent flow)
- Palpable thrill (vibration caused by turbulent blood flow as seen with an AV fistula)

Lower Extremity Digital Evaluation Protocol

- Obtain a patient history to include symptoms and risk factors.
- Patient is examined in a warm room in the supine position to eliminate the effects of hydrostatic pressure.
- Apply a 2-2.5 cm cuff around the digit to be studied while avoiding cuff placement over the bony joint. Smaller cuffs will result in falsely elevated pressures due to the narrow cuff width. Follow up studies should use same width cuff for comparison.
- Attach the PPG photocell to the pad of the digit using double-stick tape placed between the photocell and the skin. Avoid taping the entire digit like a cuff since a tightly placed PPG could obliterate a low pressure pulse.
- Run the PPG recording at high speed (25 mm/sec) to record the shape of the digital waveform at rest, ensuring that the PPG tracing is centered. Ideally the baseline is horizontal between pulses.

> *Use a towel to cover the foot to eliminate any room light which may cause an artifact in the PPG tracing.*

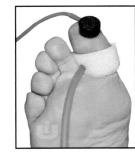

Lower Extremity TBI and PPG Evaluation Placement of the Digital Cuff and PPG Sensor

> *The size control on the PPG device is kept at "10" for standardization of tracings. If the waveform "goes off" the strip chart recording paper, the size is reduced to "5" and the change is documented.*

- Reduce PPG recording speed to 5 mm/sec and inflate the pressure cuff on the digit until the PPG waveforms are no longer visible.
- Slowly deflate the cuff (at rate of 2-4 mmHg/sec) until the PPG waveforms return. Note the pressure when the first pulse returns, but be sure that the pulse is continuous. If the pulse does not continue, consider that this was not a true pulse, but rather a motion artifact.
- If data is abnormal at rest, consider warming the affected toes for several minutes and repeating the measurements. False positive results may occur if the digits are cold during testing.
- Repeat procedure on other digits as necessary.
- Repeat on the contralateral leg.
- Apply pressure cuffs with 10-12 cm bladder (in width) on the mid upper arms.
- Locate the brachial artery (BrA) near the antecubital fossa using a Doppler probe.
- Inflate the cuff on the mid arm 20-30 mmHg beyond the last audible arterial Doppler signal.
- Deflate the cuff slowly (at a rate of 2-4 mmHg per second). The systolic pressure is recorded as soon as the first audible Doppler arterial signal returns.
- Calculate the toe-brachial index (TBI) by dividing the digital pressures by the highest brachial artery pressure (toe pressure ÷ highest brachial pressure = TBI).
- Determine severity of disease according to laboratory diagnostic criteria.

TABLE 38: Lower Extremity Digital Protocol Summary

- Wrap pressure cuffs around toes.
- Tape PPG sensor to the pad of the digit with double stick tape.
- Record representative tracing of PPG waveforms.
- Inflate digital cuff 20-30 mmHg beyond the last visualized PPG tracing. Be sure that a couple seconds pass before the first pulse.
- Deflate cuff at a rate of 2-4 mmHg per second. The pressure is recorded as soon as the PPG waveforms return. Check for subsequent pulses to confirm it was a "first pulse" rather than motion artifact.
- Wrap pressure cuff around the mid upper arms for a brachial pressure.
- Inflate cuff 20-30 mmHg beyond the last audible Doppler arterial signal.
- Calculate toe-brachial indices using the highest brachial pressure.
- Determine severity of disease according to laboratory diagnostic criteria.

TABLE 39: **Lower Extremity TBI Symptoms**	
TBI Range	**Symptoms**
0.80-0.90	Normal
0.35 + 15	Claudication
0.11 + 10	Rest pain/ulceration

Source: Zierler, RE, (2005). Nonimaging physiologic tests for assessment of lower extremity arterial occlusive disease. In Zwiebel WJ, Pellerito JS (Eds.), *Introduction to Vascular Ultrasonography 5th ed..* (275-295). Philadelphia: Elsevier Saunders.

PPG Digital Waveforms

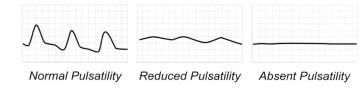

Normal Pulsatility   *Reduced Pulsatility*   *Absent Pulsatility*

Interpretation

Normal

- If the TBI is >0.70, the presence of a hemodynamically significant stenosis or occlusion is unlikely from the heart to the digits in the lower extremities. [3]
- Normal PPG waveforms exclude the presence of significant disease. Normal PPG waveform characteristics include: [4]
  - Short onset to peak (subjective)
  - Downslope that bows toward the baseline
  - A dicrotic notch in the downslope

Abnormal

- A difference in systolic pressures between the ankle and toe indicates pedal or digital artery obstruction. An abnormal difference is >44 mmHg in younger patients and >64 mmHg in older patients. [4]
- A TBI of <0.60 in the toes indicates a significant obstruction at or proximal to the digits and indicates a decrease in perfusion at the digital level. [5]
- An absolute toe pressure of <20 mmHg is associated with toe ischemia. [4,6]
- Abnormal ("reduced") PPG waveform characteristics (secondary to obstruction) include: [4]
  - Prolonged onset to peak (subjective)
  - Rounded peak
  - Downslope that bows away from the baseline
- An "absent" or non-pulsatile digital waveform is reported when the PPG tracing reflects a flat-line.

> *Digits with pressures of less than 20 mmHg may not produce a waveform.*

TABLE 40: **Diagnostic Criteria for Lower Extremity Digital Testing**

Normal: no hemodynamically significant disease
- TBI ≥0.70
- Normal waveform characteristics include:
  - Short onset to peak (subjective)
  - Downslope that bows toward the baseline or
  - A dicrotic notch in the downslope

Abnormal: hemodynamically significant disease
- TBI <0.60
- Pressure difference between the ankle and toes (>44 mmHg in younger patients and >64 mmHg in older patients)
- Abnormal waveform characteristics include:
- Prolonged onset to peak (subjective)
  - Rounded peak
  - Downslope that bows away from the baseline
  - Absence of tracing
- Absolute pressure <20 mmHg (toe ischemia)

TABLE 41: **University of Chicago Lower Extremity TBI Diagnostic Criteria**	
Severity	**Toe Brachial Index (TBI)**
Normal	>0.70
Mild	0.60-0.69
Moderate	0.59-0.40
Severe	<0.39

Source: Internally validated at the University of Chicago Medical Center Vascular Laboratory

Differential Diagnosis

- Buerger's disease
- Scleroderma
- Connective tissue disorders
- Abnormalities of adrenergic receptor/sympathetic nervous system
- Neuropathy
- Muscle/tendon strains
- Arthritis

Correlation

- Duplex ultrasound
- Spiral CT scan
- MR Angiography
- Arteriography

Medical Treatment

- Risk factor management (e.g., smoking cessation)
- Cold temperature avoidance
- Antiplatelet medication (e.g., aspirin)
- Anticoagulation (warfarin)
- Thermal biofeedback
- Thrombolysis (acute blockage)

Surgical Treatment

- Sympathectomy
- Endarterectomy
- Bypass grafting
- Direct focal repair
- Resection (aneurysmal disease)
- Amputation

Points to Remember

- Skin integrity of the digit must be intact to properly assess digital circulation.
- Digital analysis should be routinely performed on all diabetics, symptomatic toes and in patients with calcified ankle pressures.
- Digits should be room temperature for accurate data collection. Use hot packs or warming devices with care to achieve if necessary.
- Calcified digital artery pressures are rarely a problem.
- Exposure to cold conditions or stressful situations can exacerbate digital symptoms.
- A patient presenting with an embolic event such as "blue toe syndrome" should be worked up for an abdominal aortic aneurysm. Embolization is associated with abdominal aortic aneurysm, but is relatively uncommon.
- A toe pressure >30 mmHg is associated with healing. With a toe pressure <30 mmHg, healing is doubtful. [7,8]

References

1. Sumner DS, Zierler RE. (2005). Vascular physiology: essential hemodynamic principles. In *Rutherford Vascular Surgery 6th edition.* (75-123). Philadelphia. Elsevier Saunders.

2. Fecteau SR, Darling III RC, Roddy SP. (2005). Arterial thromboembolism. In *Rutherford Vascular Surgery 6th edition.* (971-986). Philadelphia. Elsevier Saunders.

3. Needham T. (2005). Peripheral atherosclerotic occlusive disease. In Mansour MA, Labropoulos N. (Eds.), *Vascular Diagnosis,* (215-222). Philadelphia: Elsevier Saunders.

4. Zierler RE, Sumner DS. (2005). Physiologic assessment of peripheral arterial occlusive disease. In *Rutherford Vascular Surgery 6th edition.* (197-222). Philadelphia. Elsevier Saunders.

5. Bridges RA, Barnes RW. (1982). Segmental limb pressures. In: Kempczinski RF and Yao SJS. *Practical Noninvasive Vascular Diagnosis.* (79-93). Chicago: Yearbook Medical.

6. Carter SA, Lezack JD. (1971). Digital systolic pressures in the lower limb in arterial disease. *Circulation.* 43: 905-913.

7. Hallett JW, Brewster DC, Rasmussen TE. (2001). Noninvasive vascular testing. In: *Handbook of Patient Care in Vascular Diseases.* (29-49), Philadelphia Lippincott Williams & Wilkins..

8. Ramsey DE, Manke DA, Sumner DS. (1983). Toe blood pressure. A valuable adjunct to ankle pressure measurement for assessing peripheral arterial disease. *J Card Surg.* Jan-Feb;24(1):43-8.

9. Zierler, RE, (2005). Nonimaging physiologic tests for assessment of lower extremity arterial occlusive disease. In Zwiebel WJ, Pellerito JS (Eds.), *Introduction to Vascular Ultrasonography 5th ed..* (275-295). Philadelphia: Elsevier Saunders.

Definitions

Treadmill testing evaluates the arterial hemodynamics of the lower extremities and determines the functional significance of disease by evaluating walking distance limitations and whether walking induced pain is secondary to nonvascular conditions, such as musculoskeletal or cardiopulmonary disease that may affect exercise performance.

Post-occlusive reactive hyperemia (PORH) is a form of stress testing used on patients with contraindications to other forms of stress testing (e.g., patients with amputation, physical disability, etc.). In this method, exercise is simulated by inflating an arterial cuff (usually placed on the thigh) above the suprasystolic pressure for 3-5 minutes to create a brief period of distal limb ischemia.

Rationale

Exercise increases blood flow which will exaggerate a pressure gradient that may not be appreciated at rest according to Poiseuille's Law (Q = Δ P / R). Upon exercise, an individual's distal vascular bed vasodilates, decreasing resistance and increasing blood flow in response to the demand. If a patient cannot exercise, the reactive hyperemia technique is an alternative means of increasing blood flow in order to elicit a pressure gradient that is not present at rest. The ankle pressure will decrease in the presence of increased flow and a significant arterial obstruction.

Indications for Exam

- Claudication (exercise-related limb pain) in the presence of normal ABI's at rest
  - PORH is useful when a patient cannot exercise via treadmill or toe raises.

Contraindications/Limitations

- Calcified vessels which will falsely elevate pressures (typically encountered in patients with diabetes or end-stage renal disease)
- Avoid reducing flow further by doing treadmill testing or PORH on patients with rest pain, gangrene, or ulceration.
- Patients with acute venous thrombosis
- Any site of trauma, surgery, ulceration or graft placement which should not be compressed by the pressure cuff
- Patients with extensive bandages or casts which are not removable
- Pressures typically prohibited on ipsilateral side of mastectomy or AVG/AVF

Specific treadmill limitations

- Patients with lower extremity amputation
- Inability of the patient to walk (e.g., arthritis, joint disease, stroke, obesity)
- History or suggestion of angina, myocardial infarction (MI) or need to carry nitroglycerin on order of a personal physician
- Significant shortness of breath at rest

Mechanism of Reduction in Peripheral Vascular Resistance

- Muscular vessels dilate and divert blood away from the cutaneous tissue in response to exercise, reducing oxygen levels in the tissues. Unless arterial inflow is compromised, this reduction will not be measurable. [1]
- An oxygen shortage (hypoxia) is created during cuff occlusion with a build-up of vasodilator metabolites, such as adenosine. [2]
- Dilatation of arterioles results, decreasing vascular resistance. [2]
- Once cuff occlusion is released, flow increases creating a hyperemic state. [2]
- When flow is increased, a significant decrease in pressure may occur distal to an arterial obstruction in diseased limbs during the hyperemic period. [2]
- Once tissues reoxygenate, vasodilator metabolites are excreted from the tissue resulting in baseline resistance. [2]

Location of Disease

- Location of disease can be focal or diffuse and affect any level or multiple levels.

Patient History

- Claudication (exercise-related)
- Rest pain

Physical Examination

- Pulselessness
- Pallor
- Gangrene/ulceration
- Dependent rubor
- Bruit

Treadmill Testing Protocol

- Rest the patient for 5-10 minutes before beginning the exam in order for blood pressures to stabilize after "exercise" (walking into the exam room). You may use this time to obtain a patient history, including symptoms and risk factors and to place cuffs. It also helps to fully explain the procedure to the patient and possibly demonstrate how they will walk on the treadmill and then move quickly back to the bed.
- Before starting the exercise portion of the examination, baseline pressures are taken while the patient is in the supine position.
- Appropriately wrap blood pressure cuffs on the limbs (arm and ankle). All cuffs should be placed "straight" rather than angled with the bladder of the cuff over the artery. Apply the ankle cuff with 10-12 cm bladder (in width) 2-3 cm above the medial malleolus.
- Obtain resting ankle-brachial indices (ABI) for comparison to post-exercise values.

The following instructions can be used when testing with an automatic cuff inflator or standard manometer:

- Inflate cuffs 20-30 mmHg above the last audible arterial Doppler signal using a Doppler probe.

- Deflation of the cuff should be at a rate of 2-4 mmHg per second. The pressure is recorded as soon as the first audible Doppler arterial signal returns.

- The ankle cuffs and the cuff on the arm with the higher brachial pressure remain on the patient (tape cuff ends if necessary). Prepare continuous-wave Doppler and recording equipment for immediate use after completion of the exercise.

> *Marking the location of the arteries with an indelible marker helps to locate the arterial signals quicker after exercise.*

> *Treadmill settings may be altered to accommodate the needs of the patient. Any changes should be documented in the exam report.*

- A treadmill with speed variability and a changeable grade or elevation is required. A stopwatch, watch or clock with second hand is also needed.

- The treadmill grade is initially set at 10%, at a speed of 2 miles/hour.

- Record the exercise start time. As the patient walks on the treadmill, ask if symptoms have improved, worsened or remained unchanged. Record what interval of time has passed when any symptoms begin (*initial claudication*). Also record the time at which the patient can no longer continue walking (*absolute claudication*). Note other pertinent observations (e.g., complaints of shortness of breath). Record the time exercise ends. The patient will not need to walk longer than 5 minutes.

- Stop the treadmill. The patient returns promptly to the supine position on the bed or stretcher after exercise. Obtain ABI measurements within the first minute post-exercise.

> *Take the pressures in the symptomatic extremity or the extremity with the lower ABI at rest first.*

- Retake the ankle and brachial pressures every 2 minutes until returning to within 10 mmHg of the baseline pressure or for approximately 5-10 minutes. If the ABI immediately after exercise are equal to or greater than the resting pressures, no additional pressures are taken.

TABLE 42: Treadmill Testing Protocol Summary

- Apply pneumatic cuffs on the arm and ankle.
- Measure pre-exercise ankle-brachial indices (ABI).
- Have the patient walk on the treadmill at a 10% grade and speed of 2 mph for 5 minutes or until claudication or other restrictions occur.
- Quickly re-measure ABI within the first minute post-exercise.
- Retake the ABI every 2 minutes until ankle pressures return to within 10 mmHg of the baseline pressure or for 5-10 minutes (whichever comes first).
- Determine classification of disease according to laboratory diagnostic criteria.

Reactive Hyperemia Testing Protocol

- *NOTE: This procedure places uncomfortable pressure on the limb, resulting in numbness and pain in the extremity for 3-5 minutes. This should be thoroughly explained to the patient before the exam begins.*

- Obtain a patient history to include symptoms and risk factors.

- Patient is examined in the supine position.

> *Try making small talk with the patient during the procedure in order to take their mind off the discomfort.*

- Since the response to reactive hyperemia typically has a very short duration after release of the cuff occlusion, it is important to take the first ankle pressure within the first minute after deflation. Perform this procedure on only one limb at a time.

- Appropriately wrap blood pressure cuffs on the limbs (arm, thigh and ankle). All cuffs should be placed "straight" rather than angled with the bladder of the cuff over the artery. Apply the thigh cuff as high as possible on the thigh. Apply the ankle cuff with 10-12 cm bladder (in width) 2-3 cm above the medial malleolus.

- Obtain baseline ankle-brachial indices (ABI).

The following instructions can be used when testing with an automatic cuff inflator or standard manometer:

- Inflate cuffs 20-30 mmHg above the last audible arterial Doppler signal using a Doppler probe.

- Rapid deflation of the cuff should be at a rate of 2-4 mmHg per second. The pressure is recorded as soon as the first audible Doppler arterial signal returns.

- Inflate the thigh cuff 40-50 mmHg above the highest brachial systolic pressure for approximately 3-5 minutes.

- Be sure to monitor the pressure in the cuff during the occlusion period to make sure that the suprasystolic pressure is maintained for the full 3-5 minute period.

- Rapid deflate the thigh cuff and quickly re-measure the ABI.

- Retake the ankle and brachial pressures every 30 seconds until the ankle pressure returns to within 10 mmHg of the baseline pressure or for approximately 5 minutes since the recovery time is faster than treadmill testing.

- Determine classification of disease according to laboratory diagnostic criteria.

- If necessary, repeat on the contralateral side.

> *For patients with irregular heart beats, decrease deflation speeds.*

TABLE 43: Post-Occlusive Reactive Hyperemia Protocol Summary

- Apply pneumatic cuffs on the arm, thigh and ankle.
- Measure baseline ankle-brachial indices (ABI).
- Inflate thigh cuff 40-50 mmHg above the highest brachial systolic pressure for 3-5 minutes.
- Rapid deflate thigh cuff and quickly re-measure ABI.
- Retake ABI every 30 seconds until ankle pressure returns to within 10 mmHg of the baseline pressure or for 5 minutes (whichever comes first).
- Determine classification of disease according to laboratory diagnostic criteria.

Interpretation

Treadmill Testing

Normal

- There should be little to no drop in ankle pressure after 5 minutes of exercise.[1,3] The ABI may even increase. [1] The drop in post-exercise systolic ankle pressure should be <20% of the resting pressure and should return to baseline within 3 minutes after exercise. [4]
- Brachial pressures should increase post-exercise. [1]

Abnormal

- An immediate drop in ankle pressure post-exercise indicates significant arterial obstruction involving the arteries which supply the gastrocnemius and soleal muscles. The distance a patient can walk and the absolute pressure drop relates to the severity of disease. [1,3] For example, patients with multilevel disease will walk for a shorter distance and there will be a greater pressure decrease. [1]

  > *Post-exercise ankle pressure may be unobtainable in cases of severe disease for ≥15 minutes.[1,5]*

- A difference in brachial-ankle pressure ≥20 mmHg indicates significant arterial disease. [1]
- The drop in post-exercise systolic ankle pressure should be >20% of the resting pressure and takes >3 minutes to return to baseline after exercise. [4]
- A recovery time between 2-6 minutes suggests single level disease. Multilevel disease typically requires 6-12 minutes before pressures return to baseline levels. [5,6]

TABLE 44: Diagnostic Criteria for Post-Reactive Hyperemia Ankle-Brachial Index

% Pressure Decrease	Classification
17-34%	Normal
35-50%	Single-level disease
>50%	Multi-level disease

Source: Strandess DE, Zierler RE. (1993). Exercise ankle pressure measurements in arterial disease. In Bernstein EF (Ed.), Vascular Diagnosis (547-553). St. Louis: Mosby

---

TABLE 45: Diagnostic Criteria for Post-Treadmill Exercise Ankle-Brachial Indices and Recovery Times

Recovery Time	Classification
<3 minutes *	Normal
2-6 minutes **	Single-level disease
6-12 minutes **	Multi-level disease
>15 minutes **	Severe occlusive disease

* The post-exercise systolic ankle pressure drops <20% compared to the resting systolic pressure.

** The post-exercise systolic ankle pressure drops >20% compared to the resting systolic pressure.

Source: Modified from Strandess DE, Zierler RE. (1993). Exercise ankle pressure measurements in arterial disease. In Bernstein EF (Ed.), Vascular Diagnosis (54 553). St. Louis: Mosby.

Reactive Hyperemia

Normal

- The initial drop in pressure is the most important measurement post-occlusion. [5,7]
- A 17-34% drop in ankle pressure is normal after release of the cuff occlusion. [5,7]
- Pressures should return to 90% of their baseline value within the first 60 seconds after release of the cuff occlusion. [1,7]

  > *Following cuff occlusion, "no change" in pressure after or a slight decrease is a normal result.*

Abnormal

- Pressure drops >35% of the baseline pressure immediately after occlusion are abnormal. [8]
- Ankle pressures do not return to baseline within 1 minute after cuff deflation. [1,7]
- Single-level arterial disease usually results in a <50% drop in ankle pressure. [5,7]
- Multi-level arterial disease usually results in a >50% drop in ankle pressure. [5,7]

Differential Diagnosis

- Spinal stenosis
- Venous thrombosis
- Restless leg syndrome
- Compartment syndrome
- Nocturnal leg cramps
- Neuropathy
- Muscle/tendon strains
- Arthritis

Correlation

- Duplex ultrasound
- Spiral CT scan
- MRA
- Arteriography

Medical Treatment

- Modify risk factors (e.g., reduce cholesterol, manage HTN and DM, smoking cessation)
- Exercise regimen
- Antiplatelet medication (e.g., aspirin)
- Anticoagulation (warfarin)

Surgical Treatment

- Bypass grafting
- Endarterectomy
- Direct focal repair
- Amputation

Endovascular Treatment

- Angioplasty
- Stent
- Atherectomy
- Intra-arterial directed thrombolysis (acute blockage)

Points to Remember

- If a treadmill cannot be utilized, exercise may consist of walking a predetermined distance down the hallway.

- Arterial obstructions involving the tibial arteries may not result in claudication or a decrease in post-exercise pressures. [1]

- The changes in ABI during PORH testing are similar to those observed during treadmill testing in patients with arterial disease, though recovery is typically much faster. [1,9]

- PORH protocol may be difficult or impossible to perform on some patients due to marked numbness and discomfort that the patient experiences from temporary ischemia or from the cuff pressure itself. The technique is not typically used when resting measurements are enough to evaluate the patient, but is only used in selected patients when stress testing with walking cannot be done and is necessary to fully assess the patient's condition.

- PORH has also been used to diagnose subclavian steal syndrome when the vertebral artery demonstrates pendulum (to and fro) flow direction or has questionable reversed flow direction present. Inflate a pressure cuff over the brachial artery (30 mmHg above the highest brachial pressure) for 5 minutes to cause temporary ischemia in the arm. After cuff deflation, investigate the flow direction of the ipsilateral vertebral artery using the duplex scanner as you would during a carotid exam. If the flow direction of the vertebral artery is retrograde, this finding suggests a subclavian steal on that side. [10]

- "Toe-up" exercises are an alternative stress testing method when treadmill testing or PORH is not possible. Although this method is not as quantifiable as the other methods, it is a form of exercise and stress, especially at the calf levels. A fairly normal achievement is 100 toe-ups; however, this is variable. To perform:
  - The patient stands facing the side of the bed, balancing their hand on the examination table for support.
  - At a moderate speed, the patient rises onto the toes as much as possible, then drops down to a flat-footed position. Performing this maneuver along with the patient can help the patient maintain a moderate speed.
  - Record post-exercise ABI measurements as described.

- If a pressure measurement needs to be repeated, the cuff should be fully deflated for approximately one minute prior to the repeat measurement.

- The systolic pressure is recorded as the pressure at which the first audible arterial Doppler signal returns. There should be a period of silence after inflation and prior to hearing the first pulse to be sure the cuff was inflated beyond the local arterial pressure. The Doppler pulse must continue after hearing the first pulse to assure an actual pulse rather than motion artifact.

References

1. Zierler RE, Sumner DS. (2005). Physiologic assessment of peripheral arterial occlusive disease. In Rutherford Vascular Surgery 6th edition. (197-222). Philadelphia. Elsevier Saunders.

2. Sumner DS, Zierler RE. (2005). Vascular physiology: essential hemodynamic principles. In *Rutherford Vascular Surgery 6th edition.* (75-123). Philadelphia. Elsevier Saunders.

3. Baker JD. (2005). The role of noninvasive procedures in the management of extremity arterial disease. In Zwiebel WJ. Pellerito JS (Eds.), Introduction to Vascular Ultrasonography 5th ed. (254-260). Philadelphia: Elsevier Saunders.

4. Zaccardi MJ, Olmsted KA. (2002) Peripheral arterial evaluation, In Strandess DE. (Ed.). *Duplex Scanning Disorders 3rd edition.* (253-266). Philadelphia: Lippincott Williams & Wilkins.

5. Strandess DE, Zierler RE, (1993) Exercise ankle pressure measurements in arterial disease. In Bernstein EF (Ed.), *Vascular Diagnosis* (547-553). St. Louis: Mosby.

6. Leon, Labropoulos, N, Mansour MA. (2005). Hemodynamic principles as applied to diagnostic testing. In Mansour MA, Labropoulos N. (Eds.), Vascular Diagnosis, (7-21). Philadelphia: Elsevier Saunders.

7. Zierler, RE. (2005). Nonimaging physiologic tests for assessment of lower extremity arterial occlusive disease: In Zwiebel WJ, Pellerito JS (Eds.). *Introduction to Vascular Ultrasonography 5th ed.* (275-295). Philadelphia: Elsevier Saunders.

8. Baker DJ, (1982) Stress Testing. In Kempczinski RF & Yao JST (Eds.), *Practical Noninvasive Vascular Diagnosis.* (93-103). Chicago: Year Book Medical Publishers.

9. Gerlock A, Giyanani VL, Krebs C (1988): Noninvasive assessment of the lower extremity arteries. In Gerlock A, Giyanani VL, Krebs C (Eds.) Applications of Noninvasive Vascular Techniques. (310). Philadelphia: WB Saunders.

10. Longo MG, Pearce WH, Sumner DS. (2005). Evaluation of upper extremity ischemia. In Rutherford Vascular Surgery 6th edition. (1274-1293). Philadelphia. Elsevier Saunders.

TABLE 46: Lower Arterial Exam with Exercise Report

Ankle/Toe Pressures

Location		Press	BI	Waveforms
Right	Brachial	116		
	Dor. Pedis	90	0.71	Triphasic
	Post. Tibial	94	0.75	Triphasic
	Great Toe			
Left	Brachial	126		
	Dor. Pedis	82	0.65	Triphasic
	Post. Tibial	90	0.71	Triphasic
	Great Toe			

Post-Exercise Pressures

	Right			Left		
	Brachial	Ankle	ABI	Brachial	Ankle	ABI
0 min	152	58	0.38		42	0.28
2 min	128	58	0.45		42	0.33
5 min	120	58	0.48		42	0.35
10 min	110	64	0.58		56	0.51
Rec. Time	>10 min			>10 min		
% DROP	49%			61%		

Onset of Symptoms
45 sec.

Symptoms
Lt. buttock pain after 45 sec. on treadmill.
Rt calf pain after 1.5 min. on treadmill.
Lt. calf pain after 2.5 min. of walking

Walking Duration
4 min.

This abnormal treadmill exam reports a significant pressure drop in both legs, post-exercise.
The recovery time was >10 minutes suggesting the presence of multilevel disease.

Definition

The combination of real time B-mode imaging with pulsed wave and color flow Doppler (duplex scan) to evaluate the lower extremity arteries.

Etiology

- Atherosclerosis
- Embolization
- Thrombus
- Pseudoaneurysm
- Aneurysm
- Intimal hyperplasia
- Trauma
- Traumatic occlusion
- Extrinsic compression
- External radiation
- AV fistula (abnormal connection between an artery and a vein)
- Popliteal entrapment (extrinsic compression of the popliteal artery)

Risk Factors

- Age (increased risk with age)
- Coronary artery disease
- Diabetes
- Family history
- Hyperlipidemia
- Hypertension
- Obesity
- Smoking
- Sedentary lifestyle
- Previous history of CVA or MI
- Elevated levels of homocysteine
- Excessive levels of C-reactive protein
- Post-op cardiac catheterization

Indications for Exam

- Claudication (exercise-related leg pain)
- Limb pain at rest
- Extremity ulcer
- Gangrene
- Absent peripheral pulses
- Digital cyanosis
- Arterial trauma
- Abnormal ABI
- Aneurysmal disease
- Dependent rubor
- Evaluation prior to dialysis access
- A decrease in ankle brachial index (ABI) >0.15 compared to the previous exam

Contraindications/Limitations

- Patients with extensive bandages or casts.
- Poor visualization due to vessel depth secondary to obesity/severe leg edema.
- Diffuse arterial wall calcification (such as in diabetics and end-stage renal failure patients) may interfere with acquisition of duplex information.
- Patients who cannot be adequately positioned.

Mechanism of disease

- **Atherosclerosis** is the most common arterial disease. Atherosclerotic plaque forms in the artery blocking flow by either narrowing it (arterial stenosis) or totally blocking the artery (arterial occlusion). The term "hemodynamically significant obstruction" refers to either a stenosis or an occlusion that results in a decrease in blood pressure or flow distal to the obstruction. Typically, a stenosis must narrow the diameter of the artery by at least 50% to decrease pressure and flow distally. [1] An arterial occlusion is typically seen from one major branch to the next.
- **Emboli** may occur as contents of a plaque or fragments of an organized thrombus from the heart or aneurysm loosen and flow downstream. Emboli become lodged in a distant blood vessel, causing arterial occlusion and reduction of flow. [1]
- **Vasospasm** is a temporary constriction of the arteries (typically digital arteries) that may cause significant discomfort to the patient or be a sign of a more serious underlying disease. [2]
- **Extrinsic compression** from tumors, musculoskeletal configuration, hematoma, etc. can result in stenosis or occlusion by placing enough pressure on arterial walls to compromise blood flow. [1]
- **Entrapment syndrome** occurs in certain leg positions, when the gastrocnemius muscle compresses the popliteal artery resulting in loss of distal pulses. [3]
- **Aneurysmal disease** results from weakening of the structural proteins (elastin and collagen) within the medial layer of the arterial wall. [4]
- A **pseudoaneurysm** (PA) or "false aneurysm" forms due to trauma to all three layers of the arterial wall. The "false aneurysm" is actually a hematoma, receiving its blood supply via communication with an artery through a patent "neck." [5]
- An **arteriovenous fistula** or abnormal connection between artery and vein can result from trauma or complications during invasive procedures (e.g., cardiac catheterization). In such cases, blood flows directly from the artery into the venous system without passing through the tissues and capillary bed. [6]
- **Arterial dissections** are caused by tears in the intimal layer of the arterial wall and allow blood flow to access the media. Dissection between the medial and adventitial layers may result in true and false lumens. The false lumen can progressively dilate into a pseudoaneurysm. [7]

Location of Disease

- Location of disease can be focal or diffuse and affect any level or multiple levels.
- The most common location of atherosclerotic obstruction in the lower extremities is the distal superficial femoral artery.
- Arterial bifurcations
- Popliteal artery (entrapment syndrome)

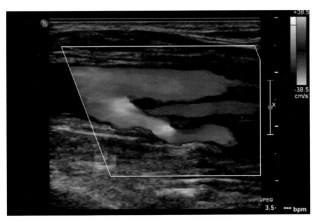

Bifurcation of the common femoral artery into the superficial femoral and deep femoral arteries

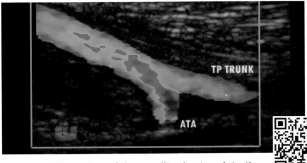

Bifurcation of the popliteal artery into the anterior tibial artery and tibioperoneal trunk

Patient History

- Claudication (exercise-related limb pain)
- Limb pain at rest
- Paralysis (weakness)
- Paresthesia ("pins and needles")
- Poikilothermia (ice-cold limb)
- Previous ulceration/gangrene of feet/toes
- Previous therapeutic vascular procedure (e.g., bypass, stent)

Physical Examination

- Pulselessness
- Cyanosis
- Pallor
- Dependent rubor
- Bruit (abnormal sound heard through auscultation caused by turbulent flow)
- Pulsatile mass
- Marked temperature difference between extremities
- Gangrene/necrosis (tissue death)
- Palpable thrill (vibration caused by turbulent blood flow as seen in an AV fistula)

Lower Extremity Arterial Duplex Protocol

- Obtain a patient history to include symptoms, risk factors, past vascular interventions and general dates.
- Obtain bilateral ankle-brachial indices (ABI's) using posterior tibial and dorsalis pedis artery waveforms with continuous-wave (CW) or pulsed-wave (PW)Doppler (Refer to section on "ABI").

- The patient is examined in the supine position with the leg externally rotated.
- Some patients may require the use of a range of transducers, including high-frequency (5-7 MHz) (8-15 MHz) transducers and a lower frequency (1-4 MHz) transducer to assist in the Hunter's canal.
- Locate the common femoral artery and vein at the groin in the transverse (short axis) plane. Rotate your probe onto the common femoral artery in the longitudinal (sagittal) plane. As you move the probe distally down the leg, obtain and record grayscale images in longitudinal view of the following:
    - Common femoral artery (CFA)
    - Deep femoral artery (DFA)
    - Superficial femoral artery (SFA)
    - Popliteal artery (POPA)
- Position the probe in the abdomen to record additional grayscale images from the abdominal aorta, common iliac (CIA) and external iliac (EIA) arteries when indicated. Color flow Doppler will be a useful guide to help identify these arteries. Locate the artery and vein in the transverse plane and rotate the probe longitudinally onto the artery for documentation.
- Position the probe behind the knee and scan distally (or begin from the ankle and scan proximally) to record additional grayscale images from the tibial arteries when indicated. Color flow Doppler will be a useful guide to help identify these arteries. Locate the artery and veins in the transverse plane and rotate the probe longitudinally onto the artery for documentation.
- Measure and record the peak systolic velocity (PSV) in longitudinal view of the following using pulsed wave Doppler (60° Doppler angle or less, with the angle cursor parallel to the vessel walls in the center of the flow stream):
    - Common femoral artery (CFA)
    - Proximal deep femoral artery (DFA)
    - Proximal, mid and distal superficial femoral artery (SFA)
    - Popliteal artery (POPA)
    - Dorsalis pedis (DPA) and posterior tibial (PTA) arteries
    - Highest obtainable velocity through any area(s) of stenosis
    - Proximal and distal to any stenosis
    - Abdominal aorta, common iliac (CIA), external iliac (EIA), anterior tibial and peroneal arteries (when indicated)
- Document grayscale and color images in areas of suspected stenosis. Measure lumenal reduction, especially caused by a hemodynamically significant lesion to provide backup information for the velocity data.

> *Color flow can obscure the true lumenal reduction if the color gain is set too high. Measure lumenal reduction in grayscale whenever possible.*

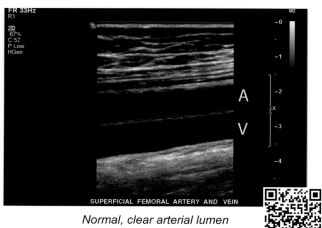

Normal, clear arterial lumen
Image courtesy of Philips Healthcare

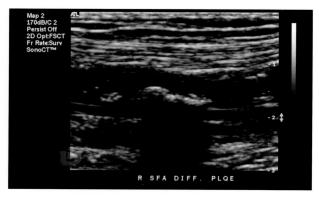

Abnormal artery: lumenal reduction and calcific plaque

- Determine classification of stenosis according to laboratory diagnostic criteria *(see criteria tables)*.
- Document any additional abnormal findings with grayscale and color imaging (e.g., aneurysmal formation, plaque, thrombus, wall irregularity, aneurysm, AV fistula, etc.). Retrograde arterial flow direction is another possible abnormal finding that requires additional documentation.

> *Decrease color and velocity scales to detect low velocity flow and confirm occlusion.*

- When arterial occlusion is suspected, document the lack of flow with PW Doppler and any visualized collateral branches by color and PW Doppler. Also note the anatomic level of flow reconstitution when visualized.
- Repeat protocol for the contralateral extremity.

Duplex Evaluation for Popliteal Entrapment Syndrome

- Ask the patient to lie on his/her side for best access to the popliteal during the positional maneuvers required for this exam.
- Measure and record the PSV in longitudinal view of the distal popliteal artery at the level of the gastrocnemius muscle heads using pulsed wave Doppler (60º Doppler angle or less, with the angle cursor parallel to the vessel walls in the center of the flow stream).
- Document grayscale images of the popliteal artery at rest and measure anterior-posterior (AP) and transverse diameter measurements.

- Instruct the patient to hyperextend the knee and point the foot downward (plantarflexion).
- Re-measure AP and transverse diameter measurements on images of the popliteal artery taken while the foot was pointed downward.
- Repeat the PW Doppler measurements while the patient hyperextends the knee and points their toes upward (dorsiflexion).

Plaque and Lesion Descriptions/Characteristics

- **Diffuse plaque**: long segment of the artery lined with plaque, but <50% diameter reduction at any point.
- **Stenotic**: lumen is narrowed and velocity increases. Hemodynamically significant stenosis typically occurs when narrowing results in a >50% diameter reduction (75% area reduction). A stenosis can be focal or involve a long segment.
- **Calcific**: highly reflective plaque(s) with acoustic shadowing
- **Occluded**: complete occlusion of the vessel
- "**Moving**"/"**Mobile**": debris within the lumen is poorly adhered to the vessel wall, e.g., moving thrombus.

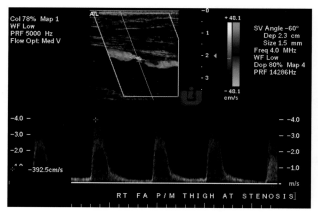

Abnormal, stenotic arterial waveform

TABLE 47: **Lower Extremity Arterial Duplex Summary**

Scan longitudinal (sagittal) view with grayscale, color and PW Doppler

1. CFA	• Measure and record the peak systolic velocity (PSV) for all segments.
2. Proximal DFA	
3. Proximal SFA	• When an area of stenosis is identified, "walk" the sample gate through the area of stenosis and obtain representative waveforms at the narrowest point of stenosis, as well as proximal and distal to the stenosis.
4. Mid SFA	
5. Distal SFA	
6. POPA	
7. PTA *	
8. DPA *	
9. EIA (optional)	• Determine classification of stenosis according to laboratory diagnostic criteria.
10. ATA (optional)	
11. Per A (optional)	* *Waveforms may be taken with either CW or PW Doppler.*

Interpretation

- Determine:
  - Plaque location and plaque characteristics
  - Peak systolic velocity (PSV) and flow direction
  - V_2/V_1 peak systolic velocity ratio (Vr); where V_2 represents the maximum PSV of a stenosis and V_1 is the PSV of the proximal normal segment
  - Any change in spectral waveform analysis (e.g., triphasic to biphasic to monophasic)

Normal (absence of a hemodynamically significant stenosis, <50%)

- **Doppler waveforms and flow velocities:**
  - Normal lower extremity arterial waveforms are triphasic. A triphasic signal is demonstrated by strong forward flow in arterial systole (sharp upstroke), followed by flow reversal in late systole or early diastole (below the baseline), plus a late diastolic forward component. [8-14]
  - PSV and Vr are relatively uniform throughout the sampled arterial segment. [8]
- **General grayscale and color characteristics:** The artery is free of intraluminal echoes. When utilized, color Doppler fills the entire arterial lumen. [9]

TABLE 48: **Normal PSV of Lower Extremity Arteries**	
Artery	**PSV cm/s (angle-corrected)**
EIA	119 ± 22
CFA	114 ± 25
SFA (proximal)	91 ± 14
SFA (distal)	94 ± 14
PopA	69 ± 14

Source: Modified from Jager KA, Ricketts HJ, Strandess DE Jr. (1985). Duplex scanning for the evaluation of lower limb arterial disease. In Bernstein EF (Ed.), Noninvasive diagnostic techniques in vascular disease. St. Louis: Mosby

Abnormal

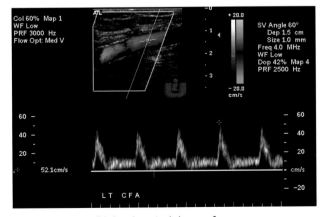

Biphasic arterial waveform

Note: Triphasic, biphasic, and monophasic waveforms have multiple definitions throughout the vascular ultrasound community. Some laboratories reserve the term biphasic only for waveforms with a reversed flow component but no third phase. Other labs describe a biphasic waveform as one with a sharp peak but continuous forward flow throughout the waveform. Some labs describe any waveform without a reversed flow component as monophasic whether or not it has a sharp peak.

- **Doppler waveforms and flow velocities:**
  - Biphasic arterial signals are characterized by strong forward flow in arterial systole (sharp upstroke) with a loss of flow reversal in early diastole (no flow below the baseline) and either forward flow or no flow in the late diastolic component. [14]
  - Monophasic arterial signals are characterized by reduced pulsatility or forward flow in late systole (blunted upstroke). A diastolic flow component may or may not be apparent. **Parvus tardus** is an alternative term for "monophasic" used by some laboratories to describe a waveform with continuous forward flow and a slow, blunted systolic component. [15] Monophasic waveforms are common distal to a hemodynamically significant stenosis or occlusion. [9-11,14]

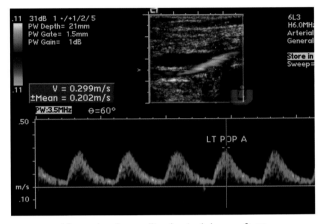

Monophasic popliteal arterial waveform

  - A hemodynamically significant lesion (>50%) will result in a focal velocity increase (at least double the velocity in the proximal arterial segment), change in spectral waveform (from triphasic to biphasic or biphasic to monophasic), post-stenotic turbulence and a possible color bruit. [8,10,11,13,16]
  - A hemodynamically significant lesion (>70%) will result in a focal velocity increase at least triple the velocity in the proximal arterial segment. [13]

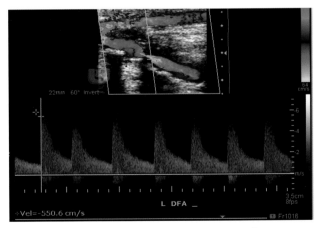

Hemodynamically significant stenosis of the deep femoral artery

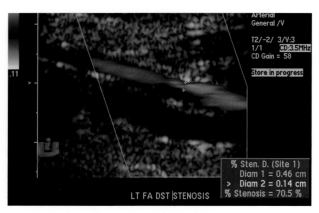

Lumenal reduction of the superficial femoral artery

- Use indirect signs to evaluate hemodynamically significant lesions in regions where a proximal velocity is technically difficult to obtain or a ratio cannot be calculated (e.g., distal to calcified plaque), such as:
  - Increased velocities (with lumenal reduction) followed by a waveform change
  - Change in spectral waveform from one segment to the next
  - Comparison of arterial waveform in the contralateral extremity at the same site

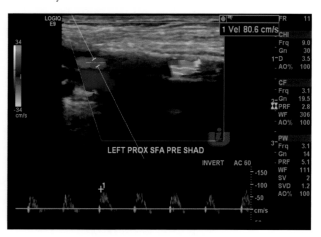

PW Doppler-pre-shadowing

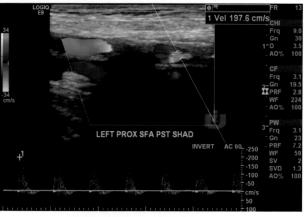

PW Doppler post-shadowing

> The criterion for abnormal lower extremity arterial duplex varies across institutions.

- **General grayscale and color characteristics:** Intralumenal echoes are visualized within the artery resulting in a measurable lumenal reduction. When utilized, color Doppler does not fill the entire arterial lumen.
  - A color jet can be visualized through the narrowed lumen. [12]
  - A mosaic color pattern can be observed due to turbulent flow in the post-stenotic region. [9,10]

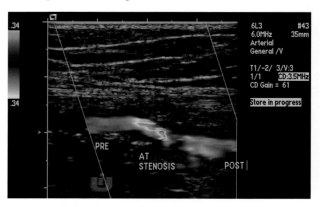

Color changes through a stenotic area

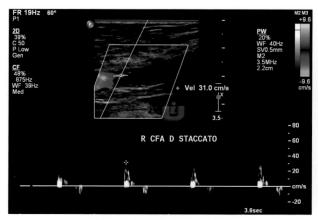

Staccato arterial waveform (pre-occlusive)

Occlusion:

- A "staccato" waveform often indicates that there is downstream occlusion. [8,12]

> Use flow in the adjacent vein as a guide to identify an occluded artery. Always confirm flow by placing the Doppler sample volume in the vessel lumen.

- An occlusion of the artery is present when no flow is detected by color or spectral Doppler. Determine the extent of the occlusion. [8,9,12]

- Often a large collateral can be identified at the proximal and distal ends of the occlusion. These collaterals often exit and enter the artery at 90° angles.

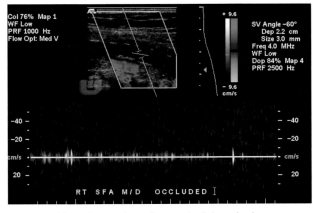

Absent waveform from arterial occlusion

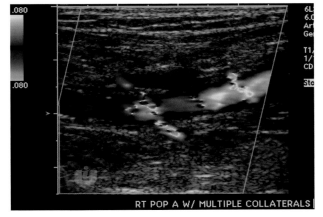

Collaterals at the distal end of an occlusion

– Blood flow may reverse in arteries supplying collateral flow, especially near arterial bifurcations when the proximal artery is occluded (e.g., retrograde arterial flow from the DFA will supply the SFA in cases of CFA occlusion). [17]

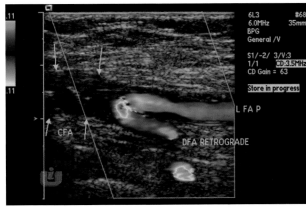

Retrograde deep femoral arterial flow by color Doppler feeding the SFA in cases of CFA occlusion

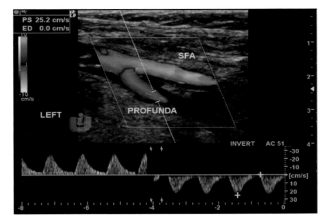

Doppler waveforms documenting forward flow direction in the SFA and reversed flow direction of the DFA

Other Pathology

- **Arteriovenous fistula (AVF):** An arteriovenous fistula between any artery and an adjacent vein is characterized by color bruit on duplex image along with high velocity, low-resistance spectral waveforms at the same site by pulsed-wave Doppler. [7]

- The arterial segment proximal to the AVF typically demonstrates a low resistance configuration as the arterial flow feeds the low resistance vein. The venous segment immediately proximal to the AVF will demonstrate a pulsatile, turbulent waveform.

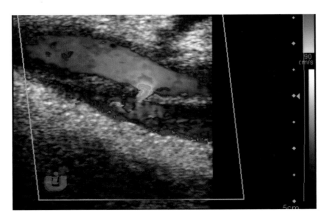

Arteriovenous fistula by color duplex

- **Pseudoaneurysm (PA):** A pulsatile mass observed communicating with a native artery is indicative of a pseudoaneurysm. A to-and-fro Doppler flow pattern will be apparent within the "neck" of the PA. The size of a pseudoaneurysm varies in diameter, but is typically between 1-5 cm. [18]

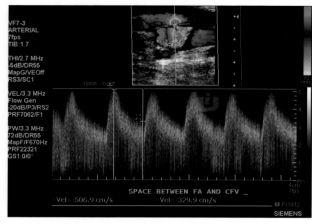

*Doppler waveforms at the site of
an arteriovenous fistula*

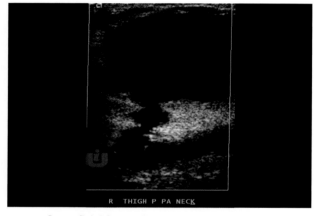

Superficial femoral artery pseudoaneurysm

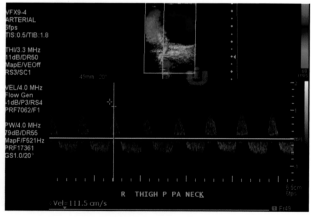

Pseudoaneurysm: characteristic "to-and-fro" waveform

- **Aneurysm:** An aneurysm is defined as a focal enlargement of an artery at least twice the diameter of the proximal segment. Intralumenal thrombus may be observed and is a possible source of distal emboli. [12] PSV are typically reduced with abnormal flow patterns within an aneurysm. [10]

  - **Arteriomegaly:** The term used to describe a uniform arterial dilation throughout an artery. [19]

- An artery can also be described as "**ectatic**" (dilatation of a circular tube) when diameters are somewhat larger through a segment, though not yet aneurysmal. The dilated areas of the artery may or may not be uniform.

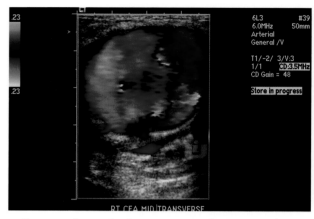

Common femoral artery aneurysm: transverse plane

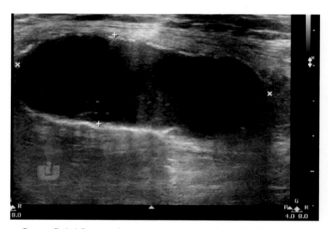

Superficial femoral artery aneurysm: longitudinal plane

- **Arterial dissection:** A dissection of the arterial lumen is recognized by two distinct flow channels by B-mode and/or color Doppler separated by the dissected intima seen as a white line within the lumen. One lumen is known as the "true lumen" while the other is referred to as the "false lumen." Each lumen has a distinctly different flow pattern or one lumen may be occluded. [7]

- **Popliteal entrapment syndrome:** A reduction in arterial diameter while the patient points their foot downward with resulting stenosis or loss of arterial pulse may indicate popliteal entrapment syndrome. [10,20]

> *The use of duplex testing to diagnose popliteal entrapment syndrome is controversial. Some believe the reduction in arterial diameter is a normal response when pointing the foot downward.*

- **Adventitial cystic disease (ACD):** Duplex findings of ACD include focal stenosis or occlusion of the popliteal artery and observance of compression on the arterial lumen by the cyst. [20,21]

TABLE 49: University of Washington Arterial Duplex Diagnostic Criteria

% Stenosis	Waveform	Spectral Broadening	Velocity/ Ratio	Distal Waveform
Normal	Triphasic	None	None	Normal
1-19%	Triphasic	Minimal spectral broadening	<30% increase in PSV from proximal segment	Waveforms remain normal proximally and distally
20-49%	Tri/biphasic	Prominent spectral broadening	30-100% increase in PSV from proximal segment	Waveforms remain normal proximally and distally
50-99%	Monophasic	Extensive spectral broadening	>100% increase in PSV from proximal segment	Waveform becomes monophasic distally
Occlusion	No flow (pre-occlusive thump may be heard proximal to occluded segment)	None	None	Collateral waveforms are monophasic with reduced PSV

Source: Moneta GL, Zacardi MJ, Olmsted KA. (2010). Lower extremity arterial occlusive disease. In Zierler RE (Ed.), *Strandess's duplex scanning disorders in Vascular Diagnosis 4th ed.* (133-147).Philadelphia:Wolters Kluwer Lippincott Williams & Wilkins.

TABLE 50: University of Chicago Arterial Duplex Diagnostic Criteria

% Stenosis	Waveform	Velocity Ratio	Spectral Broadening	Distal Waveform
Normal	Triphasic	0-2.0	None	Normal, triphasic
1-49%	Triphasic	0-2.0	Minimal	Normal, triphasic
50-99%	Bi/ monophasic	>2.1	Pronounced, significant spectral broadening	Bi/monophasic
Occluded	Absent	None	None	Collateral flow (monophasic) or absent flow

Source: Modified from Vandenberghe,NJ. (1994). Duplex scan assessment of arterial occlusive disease. Journal of Vascular Technology. 18:287-293.

TABLE 51: Duplex Imaging Diagnostic Criteria

% Stenosis	Peak Velocity	Velocity Ratio
Normal	<150 cm/s	<1.5: 1
30-49%	150-200 cm/s	1.5:1-2:1
50-74%	200-400 cm/s	2:1-4:1
>75-99%	>400 cm/s	>4:1
Occlusion	No color saturation	NA

Source: Cossman DV, Ellison JE, et al (1989). Comparison of contrast arteriography to arterial mapping with color flow duplex imaging in the lower extremity *The Journal of Vascular Surgery*, Nov; 10(5):522-8; discussion 528-9.

Differential Diagnosis

- Spinal stenosis
- Venous thrombosis
- Restless leg syndrome
- Compartment syndrome
- Nocturnal leg cramps
- Neuropathy
- Muscle/tendon strains
- Arthritis
- Cystic disease (such as popliteal)

Correlation

- Spiral CT scan
- MRA
- Arteriography

Medical Treatment

- Modify risk factors (e.g., reduce cholesterol/HTN, manage DM, smoking cessation)
- Exercise regimen
- Antiplatelet medication (e.g., aspirin)
- Anticoagulation (warfarin)

Surgical Treatment

- Bypass grafting
- Endarterectomy
- Direct focal repair
- Amputation

Endovascular Treatment

- Angioplasty
- Stent
- Atherectomy
- Intra-arterial directed thrombolysis

Points to Remember

- Arterial duplex ultrasound can identify the presence, exact location, extent and severity of disease. The course of the arteries, collaterals and disease can be visualized using B-mode and color while the measurement of Doppler velocity and waveform changes can estimate the severity of obstructions and flow direction.

- Color Doppler can underestimate plaque and diameter reductions due to bleeding of the color flow over the plaque seen in B-mode. For increased accuracy when assessing disease, measure in B-mode whenever possible and consider reductions together with Doppler velocity ratios.

- Besides atherosclerosis, narrowing of an arterial lumen can result from intimal hyperplasia or cellular damage after radiation therapy. [23,24]

- Surgical repair is suggested for peripheral aneurysms measuring 2.5-3 cm or more in diameter. [25]

- Monophasic CFA waveforms combined with a PSV <45 cm/s is highly indicative of ipsilateral iliac artery occlusion. [26]

- An acceleration time >144 cm/s in the EIA suggests iliac disease. [27]

- Calcific shadowing can prohibit Doppler and color flow analysis of a specific arterial segment. Comparing the Doppler waveform proximal and distal to the calcified segment can point to a hemodynamically significant obstruction under the calcific shadowing (e.g., if severe post-stenotic turbulence is present distal to the shadowing, there could be a stenosis in the calcified segment, or conversely, if there is essentially no change in the waveform pattern, it is unlikely that a significant obstruction exists under the calcific area).

- An important complication of popliteal artery aneurysms is emboli from intramural thrombus, not rupture. [25]

- Popliteal aneurysms usually occur bilaterally. [25]

- The most common peripheral artery aneurysm is in the popliteal artery. Approximately 64% of male patients with a popliteal artery aneurysm will have an abdominal aortic aneurysm. [19]

- 3% of patients with a femoral artery aneurysm also have a popliteal artery aneurysm. [25]

- Arteriovenous fistulas can be congenital or result from penetrating, blunt or iatrogenic trauma. [28]

References

1. Sumner DS, Zierler RE. (2005). Vascular physiology: essential hemodynamic principles. In *Rutherford Vascular Surgery 6th edition*. (75-123). Philadelphia. Elsevier Saunders.

2. Shepard RFJ. (2005). Raynaud's syndrome: vasospastic and occlusive arterial disease involving the distal upper extremity. In *Rutherford Vascular Surgery 6th edition*. (1319-1346). Philadelphia. Elsevier Saunders

3. Levien LJ. (2005). Nonatheromatous causes of popliteal artery disease. In *Rutherford Vascular Surgery 6th edition*. (1236-1255). Philadelphia. Elsevier Saunders.

4. Schermerhorn ML, Cronenwett JL. (2005). Abdominal aortic and iliac aneurysms. In *Rutherford Vascular Surgery 6th edition*. (1408-1452). Philadelphia. Elsevier Saunders.

5. Casey, PJ, LaMuraglia GM. (2005). Anastomotic aneurysms. In *Rutherford Vascular Surgery 6th edition*. (894-902). Philadelphia. Elsevier Saunders

6. Rutherford RB. (2005). Diagnostic evaluation of arteriovenous fistulas and vascular anomalies. In *Rutherford Vascular Surgery 6th edition*. (1602-1612). Philadelphia. Elsevier Saunders.

7. Baker JD. (2005). The role of noninvasive procedures in the management of extremity arterial disease. In Zwiebel WJ. Pellerito JS (Eds.), Introduction to Vascular Ultrasonography 5th ed. (254-260). Philadelphia: Elsevier Saunders.

8. Moneta GL, Zacardi MJ, Olmsted KA. (2010). Lower extremity arterial occlusive disease. In Zierler RE (Ed.), *Strandess's duplex scanning disorders in Vascular Diagnosis 4th ed*. (133-147).Philadelphia Wolters Kluwer Lippincott Williams & Wilkins.

9. Zierler RE. (2005). Ultrasound assessment of lower extremity arteries. In Zwiebel WJ, Pellerito JS (Eds.), *Introduction to Vascular Ultrasonography 5th ed*, (341-356). Philadelphia: Elsevier Saunders.

10. Thrush A, Hartshorne, T. (2005). "Duplex assessment of lower limb arterial disease" In *Peripheral Vascular Ultrasound, How Why and When, 2nd ed*. (111-131). Edinburgh: Elsevier Churchill Livingstone.

11. Kohler TR. (1993). Duplex scanning for the evaluation of lower limb arterial disease. In Bernstein EF (Ed.). *Vascular Diagnosis 4th ed*. (520-526). St. Louis: Mosby.

12. Kerr TM, Bandyk DF. (1993). Color duplex imaging of peripheral arterial disease before angioplasty or surgical intervention. In Bernstein EF (Ed.). *Vascular Diagnosis 4th ed*. (527-533). St. Louis: Mosby.

13. Ascher E, Salles-Cunha SX, Hingorani A, Markevich N. (2005). Duplex ultrasound and arterial mapping before infrainguinal revascularization. In *Mansour MA, Labropoulos N. (Eds.), Vascular Diagnosis*. (237-246). Philadelphia: Elsevier Saunders.

14. 14 Zierler RE, Sumner DS. (2005). Physiologic assessment of peripheral arterial occlusive disease. In *Rutherford Vascular Surgery 6th edition*. (197-222). Philadelphia. Elsevier Saunders

15. Armstrong PA, Bandyk DF. (2010). Vascular laboratory: arterial duplex scanning . In *Rutherford Vascular Surgery 7th edition*. (Chapter 15). Philadelphia. Elsevier Saunders.

16. Rzucidlo EM, Zwolak RM. (2005). Arterial duplex scanning. In *Rutherford Vascular Surgery 6th edition*. (233-253). Philadelphia: Elsevier Saunders.

17. Kalman PG. (2005). Profundaplasty: isolated and adjunctive applications. In *Rutherford Vascular Surgery 6th edition*. (1174-1180). Philadelphia: Elsevier Saunders.

18. Burke BJ, Friedman SG. (2005). Ultrasound in the diagnosis and management of arterial emergencies. In Zwiebel WJ. Pellerito JS (Eds.), *Introduction to Vascular Ultrasonography 5th ed*. (254-260). Philadelphia: Elsevier Saunders.

19. Cronenwett JL. (2005). Abdominal aortic and iliac aneurysms. In *Rutherford Vascular Surgery 6th edition*. (1408-1452). Philadelphia. El Sevier Saunders.

20. Levien LJ. (2005). Nonatheromatous causes of popliteal artery disease. In *Rutherford Vascular Surgery 6th edition*. (1236-1255). Philadelphia. Elsevier Saunders.

21. Flanigan DP, Burnham SJ, Goodreau JJ, Bergan JJ. *Summary of cases of adventitial cystic disease of the popliteal artery*. Ann Surgery 1979 Feb: 189 (2): 165-75.

22. Cossman DV, Ellison JE, et al (1989). Comparison of contrast arteriography to arterial mapping with color flow duplex imaging in the lower extremity *The Journal of Vascular Surgery*, Nov; 10(5):522-8; discussion 528-9.

23. Davies MG. (2005). Intimal hyperplasia: basic response to arterial and vein graft injury and reconstruction. In *Rutherford Vascular Surgery 6th edition*. (149-172). Philadelphia. El Sevier Saunders

24. Shepard RJ, Rooke T. (2005). Uncommon arteriopathies. In *Rutherford Vascular Surgery 6th edition*. (453-474). Philadelphia. Elsevier Saunders.

25. Van Bockel JH, Hamming JF. (2005). Lower extremity aneurysms. In *Rutherford Vascular Surgery 6th edition*. (1534-1551). Philadelphia. El Sevier Saunders

26. Shaalan WE; French-Sherry, E; Castilla MS; Lozanski L; Bassiouny Hisham S. (2003). Reliability of common femoral artery hemodynamics in assessing the severity of aortoiliac inflow disease *The Journal of Vascular Surgery*, May; 37(5):960-9.

27. Burnham SJ, Jaques P, Burnham CB. (1992). Noninvasive detection of iliac artery stenosis in the presence of superficial femoral artery obstruction. J Vasc Surg. Sep;16(3):445-51; discussion 452.

28. Brawley JG, Modrall JG. (2005). Traumatic arteriovenous fistulas. In *Rutherford Vascular Surgery 6th edition*. (1619-1626). Philadelphia. El Sevier Saunders.

Arterial Testing (Lower Extremity)
Arterial Bypass and Stent Surveillance Duplex Ultrasound

Definition
The use of a combination of real time B-mode imaging with pulsed wave and color flow Doppler (duplex scan) to evaluate the patency of bypass grafts or stents in the upper or lower extremities.

Etiology
- Intimal hyperplasia
- Atherosclerosis
- Thrombosis
- Aneurysm
- Pseudoaneurysm
- Embolization
- Trauma
- Traumatic occlusion
- Extrinsic compression
- AV fistula (abnormal connection between an artery and a vein)

Risk Factors
- Age (increased risk with age)
- Coronary artery disease
- Diabetes
- Family history
- Hyperlipidemia
- Hypertension
- Obesity
- Smoking
- Sedentary lifestyle
- Previous history of CVA or MI
- Elevated levels of homocysteine
- Excessive levels of C-reactive protein

Indications for Exam
- Post-operative follow-up exams
- New symptoms of claudication, pain, ulcer/ gangrene post-intervention
- A decrease in ankle brachial index (ABI) >0.15 compared to the previous exam
- Absent peripheral pulses
- Pulsatile mass near an anastomotic or intervention site
- Digital cyanosis
- Dependent rubor

Contraindications/Limitations
- Patients with extensive bandages or casts
- Obesity/severe edema may cause poor visualization due to vessel depth
- Diffuse arterial wall calcification (often seen in diabetics and end-stage renal failure patients) may interfere with acquisition of duplex information
- Patients who cannot be adequately positioned

Graft Location
Bypass grafts can be located between any two vessels and are named for the two arteries they connect. Examples of typical arterial grafts encountered for surveillance include:

- Aorto-Iliac (abdominal aorta to unilateral or bilateral iliac)
- Aorto-Fem (abdominal aorta to unilateral or bilateral femoral)
- Ax-Fem (axillary to common femoral, axillary to superficial femoral or axillary to deep femoral)
- Fem-Fem (right common femoral artery to left common femoral artery or vice versa)
- Fem-Pop (common or superficial femoral artery to proximal or distal popliteal artery)
- Fem-Tib (common or superficial femoral artery to any one of the tibial arteries)

Graft Types (Graft Conduits)
- Dacron and PTFE grafts are easily differentiated from each other by their unique ultrasound pattern, PTFE has a bright double line and Dacron a single line with a "saw tooth" or wavy appearance.

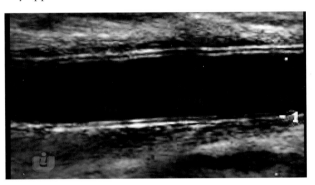

PTFE (non-ringed)

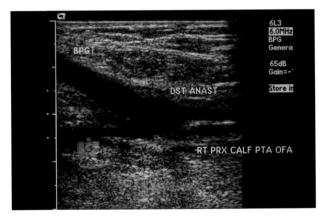

Vein

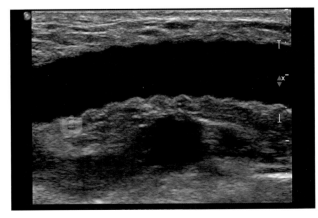

Dacron

Types of Lower Extremity Bypass Graft Material

Synthetic

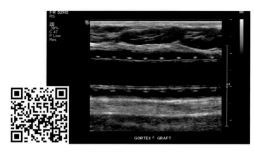

PTFE (ringed)
Image courtesy of Philips Healthcare

- PTFE (Polytetrafluoroethylene)
- Dacron

Autogenous (a.k.a. autologous)
Vein bypasses using any of the following:

- In-situ vein (vein left in original anatomic location with valves cut and branches ligated)
- Reversed vein (vein is ligated, reversed and attached to arteries)
- Autogenous veins commonly used:
  - Great saphenous vein
  - Small saphenous vein
  - Basilic vein
  - Cephalic vein
- Modified biologic grafts
  - Human umbilical vein
  - Cryopreserved saphenous vein
  - Bovine

Composite

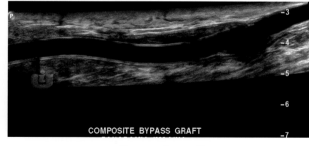

Composite graft

- Synthetic graft connected to an autogenous vein

Bypass Anastomoses

- End-to-end
- End-to-side
- Side-to-side

Types of Bypass Graft Anastomoses

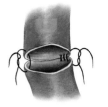 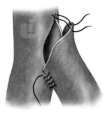 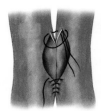

End to end *End to side* *Side to side*

Types of Stents *(include but are not limited to):*

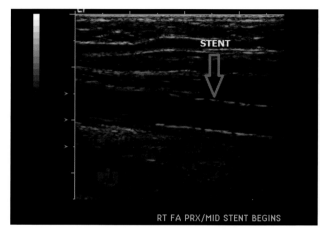

Stent in superficial femoral artery

- Drug-eluting stents (coated with a drug that should decrease the chance of intimal hyperplasia)
- Self expanding Nitinol stents
- Balloon expanding stents
- Covered stents (graft material covers the stent to exclude the severely diseased native arterial lumen)

Mechanism of Graft Failure

- Early graft failure (<30 days) is most likely due to technical errors in construction of the bypass (e.g., poor choice of inflow or outflow vessels, retained valves, clamp injury etc.). [1,2,3]
- Hemodynamically significant graft stenoses resulting from intimal hyperplasia often occurs between one month and 2 years of graft placement .[1,2,4]
- Hemodynamically significant graft stenoses resulting from atherosclerotic progression in the inflow/outflow beds often occurs in grafts older than 2 years. [1,2,4]
- Patient has undiagnosed hypercoagulable disorder. [3,4]
- Graft infection is possible though rare, occurring in 0.2-5% of operations. [4,5]
- Aneurysmal degeneration can occur in mature vein grafts. [2]
- Trauma to the graft can result in thrombosis.[4]
- Thromboembolism [1-4]
- Early graft failure can occur even without an identifiable mechanical defect or cause. [2,3]

Mechanism of Stent Failure

- Stenting is increasingly being used to treat more complicated lesions and technical failures may occur acutely (<30 days post-op). Technical failure is more common after percutaneous transluminal angioplasty for an occlusion than for stenosis. [1,6]
- Recurrent arterial re-stenosis is believed to be the cause for failures occurring >30 days post-operatively. [6]

Location of Disease

- Location of disease can be focal or diffuse and affect any level or multiple levels.
- Common locations of graft obstruction:
  - Valve sites (vein grafts)
  - Graft anastomoses
  - Inflow arterial tract
  - Outflow arterial tract
  - Graft kink
- Common locations for stent placement:
  - Iliac arteries
  - Femoral-popliteal arteries
  - Tibial arteries (less often)

Patient History

- Claudication (exercise-related)
- Rest pain
- Paralysis
- Paresthesia
- Poikilothermia
- Current and previous ulceration of feet/toes
- All vascular therapeutic procedures (e.g., bypass, stenting)

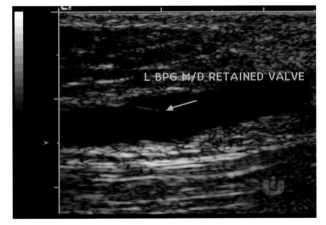

Vein graft at valve site

Physical Examination

- Pulselessness
- Cyanosis
- Pallor
- Dependent rubor
- Bruit (abnormal sound heard through auscultation caused by turbulent flow)
- Significant temperature difference between extremities
- Palpable thrill (vibration caused by turbulent blood flow as seen in AV fistula)
- Ulceration
- Gangrene/necrosis (tissue death)
- Pulsatile mass

Arterial Bypass Graft/Stent Surveillance Protocol

- Obtain a patient history to include symptoms, risk factors and past vascular interventions and general dates. This will assist in locating the graft, particularly when multiple grafts are present.
- Obtain past surgical reports/records, including type of bypass graft or stent placed and general date of surgery if available.
- Patient is typically examined in the supine position for grafts and stents. A prone position may be useful to study a stent or graft at or below the knee.
- Obtain bilateral ABI's (never put a blood pressure cuff over a bypass graft or stent without first consulting the medical director of the lab or according to lab protocol).
- Some patients may require the use of a range of transducers, including high-frequency (5-7 MHz) (8-15 MHz) transducers and a lower frequency (1-4 MHz) transducer with deeper structures, for example the distal anastomosis.
- Evaluate for graft or stent abnormalities while scanning (e.g., thrombosis, stenosis, valves, aneurysm, kinks, intimal hyperplasia, perigraft fluid, etc.).

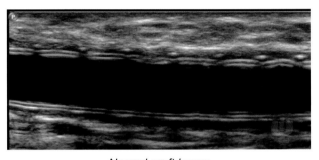

Normal graft lumen

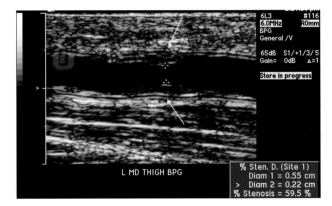

Lumenal reduction within graft by B-mode image

Transverse Scan and Images

- Scanning the limb in the transverse (short-axis) plane assists in locating the anastomotic sites, gives information about the length of the graft or stent and locates any previously occluded grafts.
- Once the location of the graft/stent is determined, record transverse images with and without color flow Doppler of the:
  - Inflow/proximal native artery
  - Proximal anastomosis
  - Proximal graft or stent
  - Mid graft or stent
  - Distal graft or stent
  - Distal anastomosis
  - Outflow/distal native artery

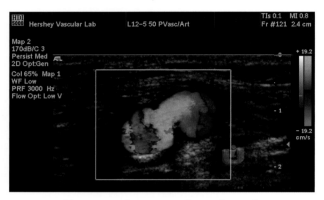

Transverse bypass graft anastomosis

Longitudinal Scan and Images

- Record images in a longitudinal (sagittal) view with and without color flow of the:
  - Inflow/proximal native artery
  - Proximal anastomosis
  - Proximal graft or stent
  - Mid graft or stent
  - Distal graft or stent
  - Distal anastomosis
  - Outflow/distal native artery

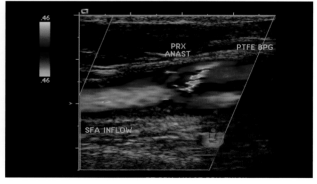

Proximal anastomosis

Doppler Scan and Images

> *Early post-operative flow patterns (within the first 2 months) may not be triphasic due to reactive hyperemia. The waveform will demonstrate a low resistance pattern with forward flow throughout diastole in initial scans that eventually changes to triphasic in follow up scan.*

- Scroll or "walk" the Doppler sample volume through the bypass graft/stent checking for focal changes in velocity and waveform configuration.
- Record and measure the peak systolic velocity (PSV) in longitudinal view using pulsed wave Doppler (≤60° Doppler angle with the angle cursor parallel to the vessel walls and sample volume within the center of the flow stream) at the following levels:
  - Inflow/proximal native artery, at least 2 cm proximal to the anastomosis
  - Proximal anastomosis
  - Proximal graft or stent
  - Mid graft or stent
  - Distal graft or stent
  - Distal anastomosis
  - Outflow/distal native artery
- When an area of stenosis is identified, "walk" the sample gate through the area of stenosis and obtain representative waveforms within 2 cm proximal to the stenosis, at the highest point of velocity within the stenosis and distal to the stenosis. Post-stenotic turbulence and color bruit should be documented when present. Measure any lumenal reductions in the longitudinal and sagittal planes when possible to support the Doppler data.
- **Note that longer bypass grafts need B-mode and Doppler data recorded at additional locations.** Consider that a thorough femoral-distal tibial bypass graft, for example, requires documentation including:
  - Inflow/proximal native artery
  - Proximal anastomosis
  - Proximal thigh graft
  - Mid thigh graft
  - Distal thigh graft
  - Graft at knee level
  - Proximal calf graft
  - Mid calf graft
  - Distal calf graft
  - Distal anastomosis
  - Outflow/distal native artery
- Repeat protocol for other grafts/stents if necessary.

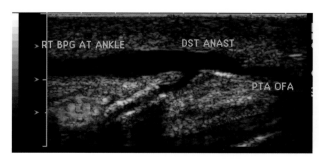

Longitudinal view of distal anastomosis near the ankle plane

Preliminary Analysis of Data

- Determine classification of stenosis according to laboratory diagnostic criteria.

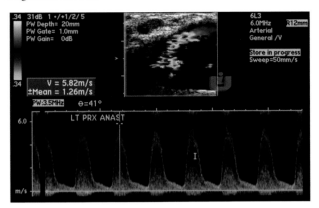

Abnormal spectral waveforms of bypass graft (anastomotic stenosis)

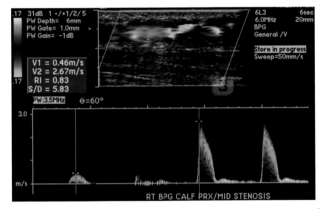

"Pre" and "at" stenosis spectral waveforms in a bypass graft

Interpretation

> *The severity of a stenosis within a graft depends on the type of graft material.*

- Analyze all of the following data from the duplex exam:
  - Ankle-brachial indices (ABI) or wrist-brachial indices (WBI)
  - Peak systolic velocity (PSV) and flow direction
  - Velocity ratios (Vr), where highest peak systolic velocity at stenosis (V_2) is divided by the PSV of the proximal normal segment (V_1)
  - Waveform configurations and changes through the extremity, including flow direction. Determine if post-stenotic turbulence is present.
  - Image information (e.g., presence of intralumenal echoes, diameter of vessel, color Doppler, unusual pathology)
  - Reasons image and velocity data may not agree

Normal
(absence of a hemodynamically significant stenosis, <50%)

- **General grayscale and color characteristics**:
  Normally, there is no echogenic material within the native arterial, graft or stent lumen.[7] Color fills the lumen wall-to-wall in transverse and longitudinal views with appropriate settings.

  - Synthetic grafts have a characteristic "double-line" appearance on B-mode image.
  - Stent walls can typically be seen within the lumen of clearly visualized arteries, though deeper stents may be difficult to identify with certainty.

TABLE 52: **Arterial Bypass Graft or Stent Surveillance Protocol Summary**

Scan transverse (short-axis) view with grayscale and color flow	**Scan longitudinal (sagittal) view with grayscale, color flow and PW Doppler**
• Inflow/proximal native artery	• Inflow/proximal native artery*
• Proximal anastomosis	• Proximal anastomosis*
• Proximal graft or stent	• Proximal graft or stent*
• Mid graft or stent	• Mid graft or stent*
• Distal graft or stent	• Distal graft or stent*
• Distal anastomosis	• Distal anastomosis*
• Outflow/distal native artery	• Outflow/distal native artery*
	• Proximal, at and distal to any stenosis*

- Record and measure the peak systolic velocity (PSV). Include additional locations for longer grafts as described in the protocol section.

- Evaluate for graft or stent abnormalities.

- Determine classification of stenosis according to laboratory diagnostic criteria.

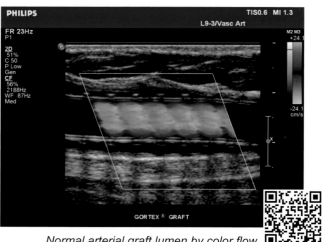

Normal arterial graft lumen by color flow

Image courtesy of Philips Healthcare

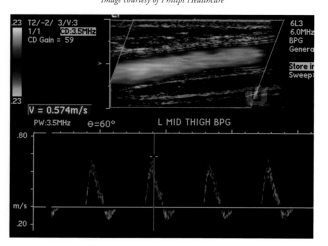

Normal arterial graft by Doppler waveforms

- **Inflow artery**: Normal inflow artery waveform configuration is triphasic. Velocity ratios are less than 2.0 in the inflow or outflow tracts. [8]

- **Proximal anastomosis**: Normal velocity ratios (Vr) are less than 2.0.[4] Waveforms may demonstrate the typical disturbed flow patterns seen at bifurcations/branches or areas of angulation.[7] These changes are focal at the anastomosis and normalize distally. A large inflow artery feeding a small diameter graft may result in a higher velocity ratio due to the size change. The image should be scrutinized for the presence of intralumenal echoes.

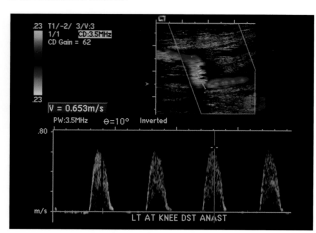

Normal bypass graft spectral waveforms at an anastomosis

- **Body of graft/stent**:
  - PSV are <180 cm/s and Vr <2.0 throughout the graft body. [4,9] PSV are at least >40-45 cm/s in vein grafts ≤4 mm in diameter. Larger conduits (e.g., PTFE conduits or veins >4 mm) may demonstrate lower velocities[7]; approximately 35 cm/s in a normal setting. [9]
  - PSV <190 cm/s and Vr <1.5 are normally expected in a superficial femoral artery stent. [10]
  - Waveform configurations remain essentially the same as in the inflow artery throughout a non-obstructed conduit, unless the bypass graft was placed very recently and hyperemic flow is present throughout the graft. [7]

- **Distal anastomosis:** In a bypass graft, there is often a size change between the wider bypass graft and smaller diameter native artery which results in a velocity increase. A normal distal anastomosis demonstrates a velocity ratio <3.0. The image should be scrutinized for the presence of intralumenal echoes. Waveform configuration may be disturbed due to vessel angulation and size change. [7]

- **Outflow artery:** Velocities remain fairly constant with Vr <2.0. Waveforms are similar from the graft/stent body to the outflow artery.[8] Flow direction may normally be retrograde in the native artery proximal to the distal anastomosis. [7]

Abnormal

General findings that indicate an abnormality in any arterial intervention include:

- A significant decrease in ABI >0.15 on serial exam is indicative of significant disease progression in the inflow, graft, stent or outflow arteries. [1,9]

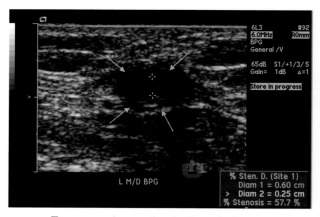

Transverse lumenal reduction of a bypass

- **General grayscale and color characteristics**:
  - Echogenic material within the native arterial, graft or stent lumen suggest lumenal reduction (intimal hyperplasia, for example). [7]
  - Color does not fill the lumen wall to wall in transverse and longitudinal views with appropriate settings. Color flow aliasing will be noted in stenotic segments. [7]
  - Moving, residual valve cusps can also be identified by B-mode imaging. [7]
  - Aneurysmal dilatations and intralumenal thrombus may be observed as a graft ages. [7]

> *The criterion for abnormal arterial duplex of a peripheral stent varies across institutions.*

- **Inflow artery:**
  - Velocity ratios >2.0 within the inflow artery associated with post-stenotic turbulence and waveform changes (from triphasic to biphasic to monophasic) indicate a hemodynamically significant stenosis (≥50%). [8]
  - Low resistance waveform patterns (at least 2 cm proximal to the anastomosis) indicate a significant inflow artery obstruction. [8]

- **Proximal anastomosis:**
  - Velocity ratios >2.0 (or >3.0 if the graft has a much smaller diameter than the inflow vessel) with elevated velocities, stenotic waveform patterns, spectral broadening and post-stenotic turbulence indicate a hemodynamically significant stenosis (≥50%). [7]
  - Duplex images may demonstrate echogenic material at the point of highest velocity.

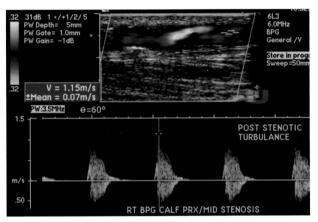

Post-stenotic turbulence in a bypass graft by color flow and PW Doppler

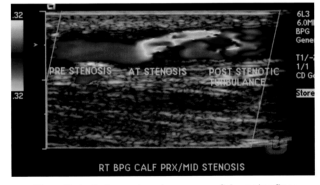

Stenotic turbulence in a bypass graft by color flow

- **Body of graft/stent:**
  - PSV >180 cm/s in a graft that result in a Vr >2.0 indicates a moderately significant (≥50%) stenosis.[9] PSV >300 cm/s and a Vr >3.5 indicates a high grade stenosis (>70%) in any graft body. [1,9,11,12]
  - PSV >190 cm/s in a superficial femoral artery stent that result in a Vr >1.5 indicates a >50% stenosis. PSV >275 cm/s and a Vr ≥3.5 indicates an >80% stenosis in the stent.[10]
  - Generally, PSV <40-45 cm/s *throughout* a normally sized vein graft (<4 mm in diameter) are associated with impending graft failure. [1,7,11]

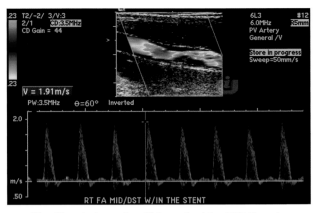

Significant stenosis within a stent by PW Doppler

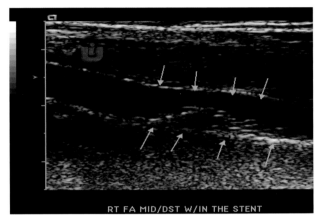

Lumenal reduction by B-mode within the stent

  - Monophasic waveforms in the graft (blunted, slow upstroke with or without diastolic flow) indicate an obstruction in the inflow tract.
  - Graft waveforms that demonstrate high-resistance, with no end diastolic velocity or a "staccato" pattern, indicate a distal anastomotic or outflow tract obstruction. [9]

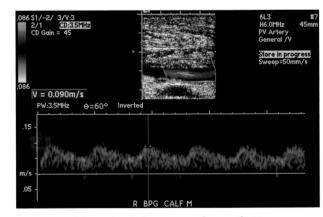

Monophasic bypass graft waveform

Arterial Bypass and Stent Surveillance Duplex Ultrasound

Arterial Testing (Lower Extremity)

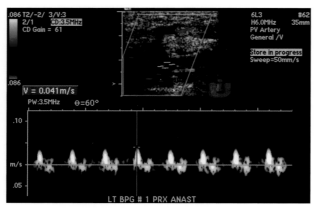

Staccato bypass graft waveform

- **Distal anastomosis**:
  – A velocity ratio >3.0 is indicative of a hemodynamically significant stenosis (≥50%), particularly if post-stenotic turbulence is present and the waveform pattern changes distally compared to the pre-anastomotic waveform pattern.[7]

> *It is important to look at the images for intralumenal defects at the anastomosis or marked diameter changes that may account for velocity increases.[7]*

- In the absence of intralumenal echoes at the distal anastomotic site, a velocity increase due to size mismatch between the bypass and outflow artery should be considered.

Graft/Stent Occlusion

> *An occlusion should never be based on color flow alone. Always confirm occlusions with PW Doppler.*

An occlusion of the graft or stent is present when no flow is detected by spectral Doppler or color in transverse and longitudinal views. [7] Intralumenal echoes may be observed.

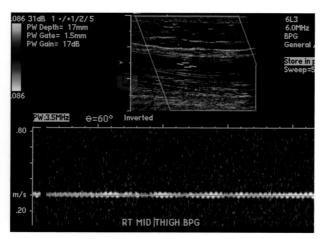

Bypass graft occlusion by PW Doppler

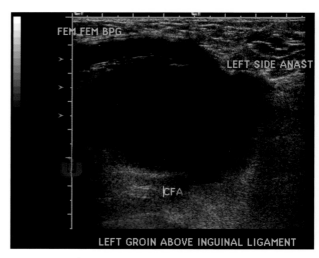

Aneurysm at an anastomotic site

Other Pathology

- **Pseudoaneurysm**: A pseudoaneurysm is diagnosed when a pulsatile mass is identified by color and Doppler flow (often near an anastomotic site) which is observed communicating with the bypass or native artery through a patent "neck".[7] The neck must demonstrate to and fro (pendulum) Doppler flow patterns to indicate a pseudoaneurysm.

- **Aneurysmal dilatation**: Arterial diameters that show a focal enlargement twice the proximal arterial segment indicate significant aneurysmal dilatation. Intramural thrombus may be observed within the aneurysm. [7]

- **Entrapment of a graft** can occur at the knee. Normal flow is recorded with the leg slightly bent (flexion). However, when the knee is straightened, no flow will be detected in the graft by Doppler or color flow. [7]

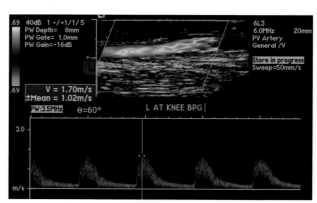

Bypass waveforms with the leg extended

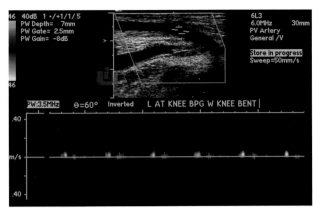

Graft occludes with flexion of the knee

– Perigraft fluid is suspected when anechoic, fluid-filled structures appear to surround the bypass conduit. Ultrasound cannot determine the exact fluid substance which may be related to infection, hematoma, etc.

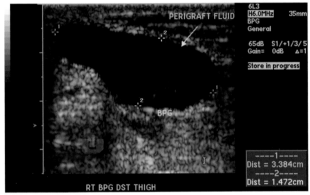

Transverse image of perigraft fluid surrounding the graft

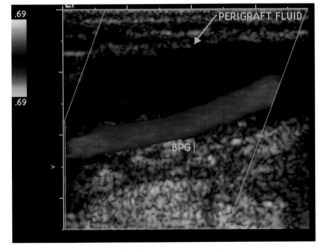

Longitudinal image of a graft with evidence of perigraft fluid

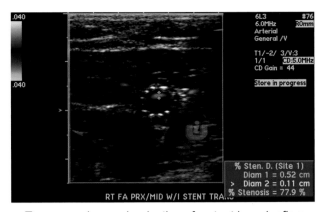

Transverse lumenal reduction of a stent by color flow

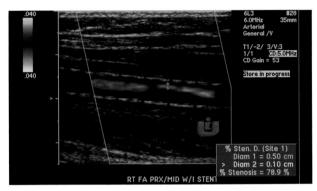

Longitudinal lumenal reduction of a stent by color flow

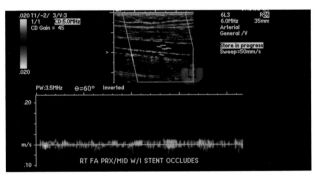

Absent flow through the stent by PW Doppler

TABLE 53: Duplex Diagnostic Criteria for In-Stent Restenosis of the Superficial Femoral Artery

	PSV	Vr
≥50% stenosis	≥190 cm/s	>1.5
≥80% stenosis	≥275 cm/s	≥3.5

• Significant decrease in ABI >0.15 was also useful to predict restenosis

Source: Baril DT, et al, Duplex criteria for determination of in-stent restenosis after angioplasty and stenting of the superficial femoral artery. *J Vasc Surg.* 2009, Jan:49(1): 133-8

TABLE 54: Diagnostic Criteria for Prosthetic Graft Surveillance

	Peak Systolic Velocity (PSV)	Velocity Ratio (Vr)
Normal	<180 cm/s	<2.0
Moderate stenosis	180-300 cm/s	>2.0
High grade stenosis*	PSV >300 cm/s	>3.5
Impending graft failure*	PSV <45 cm/s	NA
Occlusion	No flow signal or color saturation identifiable	

* A decrease in ABI >0.15 supports the presence of significant disease progression.

Source: Modified from Bandyk DF, Armstrong PA. (2010). Surveillance of infrainguinal bypass grafts. In Zierler RE (Ed.), *Strandess's Duplex Scanning Disorders in Vascular Diagnosis 4th ed.* (341-349). Philadelphia Wolters Kluwer Lippincott Williams & Wilkins.

TABLE 55: Diagnostic Criteria for Vein Graft Surveillance

	PSV	Vr
Normal	>45 cm/s	<2.0
Moderate stenosis	250-300 cm/s	>3.0
High grade stenosis*	>350 cm/s	>3.5
Occlusion	No flow signal or color saturation identifiable	

* A decrease in ABI >0.15 supports the presence of significant disease progression.

Source: Modified from Mofidi R, Kelman J, Bennett BS, Murie JA, Dawson ARW. (2007). Significance of the early post-operative duplex result in infrainguinal vein bypass surveillance. Eur J Vasc Endovasc Surg. Sep: 34, 327-332.

TABLE 56: Diagnostic Criteria for Femoropopliteal Arterial Duplex After Endovascular Intervention

	PSV	Vr
<50% stenosis	<180 cm/s	<2.5
>50% stenosis	>180 cm/s	>2.5
>70% stenosis	>300 cm/s	

• For patients suffering from rest pain or non-healing ulceration; a lower PSV >240 cm/s is the threshold for consideration of re-intervention.

• Significant decrease in ABI >0.15 was also useful to predict restenosis.

Source: Shames ML. (2007). Duplex surveillance of lower extremity endovascular interventions. *Perspectives in Vascular Surgery and Endovascular Therapy.* Dec. 19(4), 370-374.

Differential Diagnosis

- Spinal stenosis
- Venous thrombosis
- Restless leg syndrome
- Compartment syndrome
- Nocturnal leg cramps
- Neuropathy
- Muscle/tendon strains
- Arthritis

Correlation

- Spiral CT scan
- MRA
- Arteriography

Medical Treatment

- Modify risk factors (e.g., smoking cessation, etc.)
- Antiplatelet medication (e.g., aspirin)
- Anticoagulation (warfarin)

Surgical Treatment

- Balloon catheter thromboembolectomy
- Open surgical endarterectomy
- Graft revision (e.g., "jump graft" where another bypass is created to flow around a troubled area of the original bypass)
- Direct focal repair
- Amputation

Interventional Treatment

- Angioplasty, with or without stenting
- Intra-arterial directed thrombolysis
- Mechanical clot-removing endoluminal devices (i.e., Angiojet)
- Aspiration thromboembolectomy

Points to Remember

- The majority of infrainguinal bypass grafts use autogenous vein as conduit.[1] Look for incisional scars on the extremity to give you a hint what type of graft there is or where the graft anastomosis might be if a report of the operation is unavailable. Do not confuse incisions from vein harvesting with bypass graft incision sites.

- It may be contraindicated to place a blood pressure cuff over a graft due to the high risk of occluding the graft. Check the laboratory protocol or with the medical director for guidance.

- Immediate post-operative duplex scanning of a prosthetic bypass graft (e.g., PTFE, Dacron) can be technically difficult due to air within the walls of the graft, which ultrasound cannot penetrate.[3] This limitation is temporary.

- Duplex scanning has been shown to be more reliable than ABI's alone for predicting graft failure, but recent studies have shown how important the ABI remains in graft surveillance exams.

- Graft flow velocity (GFV) is an average of peak systolic velocities measured from 3-4 non-stenotic graft segments. Normal GFV ranges from 40-45 cm/s, though larger diameter grafts may average less (30-50 cm/s). [13]

- Color Doppler can overestimate diameter reductions due to bleeding of the color flow over plaque or vessel walls. For increased accuracy, measure in B-mode whenever possible or carefully set color to avoid bleeding over B-mode echoes.

- Disturbed flow may occur at anastomotic sites, areas of valve cusps and vessel diameter changes.

- In-situ vein grafts have more problems than reverse saphenous vein grafts due to size mismatch and valve site trauma.[11]

- Intraoperative duplex scans can identify technical defects resulting in hemodynamically significant lesions in bypass grafts. Immediate correction of these defects can occur in the operating room to prevent a graft thrombosis which might have occurred.[3,9]

- Iliac angioplasty has a longer patency rate than femoral-popliteal arterial angioplasty.[6]

- Below the iliacs, angioplasty is more successful in patients experiencing claudication when the lesion is short (<2 cm in length) and there is good distal arterial flow. Angioplasty is less successful for longer lesion and occlusions.[2] Studies suggest that stenting often does not improve long-term patency of lesions.[10]

References

1. Mills JL. (2005). Infrainguinal bypass. In *Rutherford Vascular Surgery 6th edition.* (1154-1174). Philadelphia. Elsevier Saunders.

2. Veith FJ, Lipsitz EC, Gargiulo NJ, Ascher E. (2005). Secondary arterial reconstruction in the lower extremity. In *Rutherford Vascular Surgery 6th edition.* (1181-1191). Philadelphia. Elsevier Saunders.

3. Walsh D. (2005). Post-operative graft thrombosis: prevention and management. In *Rutherford Vascular Surgery 6th edition.* (938-957). Philadelphia. Elsevier Saunders.

4. Pomposelli FB, LoGerfo FW. (2005). The autogenous vein. In *Rutherford Vascular Surgery 6th edition.* (695-715). Philadelphia. Elsevier Saunders.

5. 5 Bandyk DF, Back MR. (2005). Infection in prosthetic vascular grafts. In *Rutherford Vascular Surgery 6th edition.* (875-894). Philadelphia. Elsevier Saunders.

6. Schneider PA. (2005). Endovascular surgery in the management of chronic lower extremity ischemia. In *Rutherford Vascular Surgery 6th edition.* (1192-1222). Philadelphia. Elsevier Saunders.

7. Thrush A, Hartshorne T. (2005). Graft surveillance and preoperative vein mapping for bypass surgery. In *Peripheral Vascular Ultrasound, How Why and When, 2nd ed.* (207-224). London: Elsevier Chruchill Livingstone.

8. Zwiebel, WJ (2005). Ultrasound assessment of lower extremity arteries. In Zwiebel WJ, Pellerito JS (Eds.), *Introduction to Vascular Ultrasonography 5th ed,* (341-356). Philadelphia. Elsevier Saunders.

9. Bandyk, DF, (2005). Ultrasound assessment during and after peripheral intervention. In Zwiebel WJ, Pellerito JS (Eds.), *Introduction to Vascular Ultrasonography 5th ed,* (357-379). Philadelphia: Elsevier Saunders.

10. Baril, DT, Rhee RY, Kim J, Mararoun MS, Caer RA, Marone LK (2009). Duplex criteria for in-stent restenosis after angioplasty and stenting of the superficial femoral artery. J Vasc Surg. Jan: 49(1) 133-8.

11. Patel, ST, Mills Sr, JL. (2005). The preoperative, intraoperative and post-operative noninvasive evaluation of infrainguinal vein bypass grafts. In Mansour MA, Labropoulos N. (Eds.), *Vascular Diagnosis,* (277-292). Philadelphia: Elsevier Saunders.

12. Mofidi R, Kelman J, Bennett BS, Murie JA, Dawson ARW. (2007). Significance of the early post-operative duplex result in infrainguinal vein bypass surveillance. Eur J Vasc Endovasc Surg. Sep: 34, 327-332.

13. Tinder CN, Bandyk DF. (2009). Detection of imminent vein graft occlusion: what is the optimal surveillance program. *Seminars in Vasc Surgery,* Dec. 22(4) (252-260).

Description

A non-invasive physiological test comparing the systolic pressure at the level of the brachial artery to the systolic pressure at the level of the forearm/wrist. Doppler-derived pressure measurements can identify the location of a significant obstruction in an arterial segment and define the resulting decrease in terms of pressure. The term "obstruction" is used to describe either a stenosis or an occlusion of an artery.

Rationale

When narrowing of the arterial lumen increases beyond the critical level, distal arterial flow and pressure decrease significantly. Segmental pressures define the level of disease using a comparison of the brachial pressure to the forearm/wrist pressures, known as wrist-brachial index (WBI). A *pressure gradient* (pressure difference) of 20-30 mmHg indicates a significant stenosis or occlusion between cuff levels.

Etiology

- Atherosclerosis
- Embolization
- Thrombus
- Intimal hyperplasia
- Trauma
- Traumatic occlusion
- Extrinsic compression
- Vasculitis
- AV fistula (abnormal connection between an artery and a vein)
- External radiation
- Radiation arteritis

Risk Factors

- Age (increased risk with age)
- Coronary artery disease
- Diabetes
- Family history
- Hyperlipidemia
- Hypertension
- Obesity
- Smoking
- Sedentary lifestyle
- Previous history of CVA or MI
- Elevated homocysteine
- Excessive levels of C-reactive protein
- Post-op cardiac catheterization through the brachial artery
- History of radiation
- Occupational exposure to toxic substances

Indications for Exam

- Claudication
- Follow-up of a previously abnormal pressure index
- Limb pain at rest
- Absent peripheral pulses
- Extremity ulcer
- Gangrene
- Pre-operative assessment of healing potential
- Pre-operative assessment prior to creation of dialysis access
- Pre-operative assessment prior to radial artery harvest for CABG
- Abnormal vertebral artery waveforms
- Bruit
- Digital cyanosis
- Cold sensitivity
- Aneurysmal disease
- Trauma to an artery
- Raynaud's syndrome/phenomenon
- Thoracic outlet symptoms
- Abnormal arterial arm pressures, including BP differential of >20 mmHg between arms

Contraindications/Limitations

- Calcified vessels which will falsely elevate pressures (typically encountered in patients with diabetes or end-stage renal disease).
- Significant lesions with excellent collateral circulation, which may result in normal distal pressures and waveforms.
- Patients with acute clot or venous thrombosis in the upper extremities should not have pressure cuffs inflated over their clot.
- Any site of trauma, surgery, ulceration or graft placement which should not be compressed by the pressure cuff.
- Patients with extensive bandages or casts which are not removable.
- Pressures typically prohibited on ipsilateral side of a mastectomy or dialysis AVG/AVF.

Mechanism of disease

- **Atherosclerosis** is the most common arterial disease. Atherosclerotic plaque forms in the artery to block flow by either narrowing it (arterial stenosis) or totally blocking the artery (arterial occlusion). The term "hemodynamically significant obstruction" refers to either a stenosis or an occlusion that results in a decrease in blood pressure or flow distal to the obstruction. Typically, a stenosis must narrow the diameter of the artery by at least 50% to decrease pressure and flow distally. [1] An arterial occlusion is typically seen from one major branch to the next.

- **Emboli** may occur as contents of a plaque or fragments of an organized thrombus from the heart or aneurysm loosen and flow downstream. Emboli become lodged in a distant blood vessel, causing arterial occlusion and reduction of flow. [1]

- **Vasospasm** is a temporary constriction of the arteries (typically digital arteries) that may cause significant discomfort to the patient or be a sign of a more serious underlying disease. [2]

- **Extrinsic compression** from tumors, musculoskeletal configuration, hematoma, etc. can result in stenosis or occlusion by placing enough pressure on arterial walls to compromise blood flow. [1]

- **Mechanical compression** of arterial vessels in the thoracic outlet. Anatomical defects, such as a congenital abnormality of the first rib or fracture of the clavicle, are examples of possible sources of this compression. [3]

- A **pseudoaneurysm** (PA) or "false aneurysm" forms due to trauma to all three layers of the arterial wall. The "false aneurysm" is actually a hematoma, receiving its blood supply via communication with an artery through a patent "neck". [4]

- An **arteriovenous fistula** or abnormal connection between artery and vein can result from trauma or complications during invasive procedures (e.g., cardiac catheterization). In such cases, blood flows directly from the artery into the venous system without passing through the tissues and capillary bed. [5]

Location of Disease

- Location of disease can be focal or diffuse and affect any level or multiple levels
- Subclavian artery, palmar arch and/or digital arteries
- Axillary artery
- Arterial bifurcations

Patient History

- Claudication (exercise-related)
- Rest pain
- Acute occlusion
  - Pain
  - Paralysis (weakness)
  - Paresthesia ("pins and needles")
  - Poikilothermia (ice-cold limb)
  - Pulselessness
  - Pallor
- Previous ulceration/gangrene of hands/digits
- Previous therapeutic vascular procedure (e.g., bypass, stenting)

Physical Examination

- Pulselessness
- Cyanosis
- Pallor
- Dependent rubor
- Bruit (abnormal sound heard through auscultation caused by turbulent flow vibration)
- Marked temperature difference between hand/fingers, especially if one is ice cold.
- Gangrene/necrosis (tissue death)
- Palpable thrill (vibration caused by turbulent blood flow as seen in AV fistula)

Upper Extremity Segmental Pressures and Doppler Waveforms Protocol

- Obtain a patient history to include symptoms, risk factors and general dates of past vascular interventions. Obtain past surgical reports/records, including type of bypass graft or stent placed and general date of surgery if available.

- Patient is examined in the supine position. The patient can also sit in a chair with their arm extended on a pillow if unable to lie down for the exam.

- Appropriately wrap blood pressure cuffs on the limb. Apply cuffs with 10-12 cm bladders (in width) on the mid-arm and forearm. All cuffs should be placed "straight" rather than angled. All cuffs should fit snugly.

- Arterial physiologic exams are traditionally performed using a continuous wave (CW) Doppler. However, waveforms can be obtained at the same sites using a pulsed wave (PW) Doppler. The CW Doppler is recommended for segmental pressure measurement due to its capabilities for a larger sampling region.

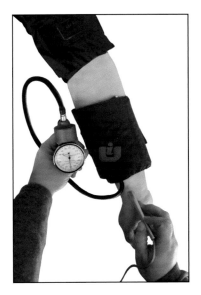

- Use a high frequency (8 MHz) CW Doppler probe to locate arterial signals. Alternate transducers, including a lower frequency probe (e.g. 4 MHz), may be needed for obese patients or for deeper vessels.

- Place the Doppler probe on the limb using a 45-60° angle to the skin, with enough pressure to keep contact but not so much pressure that the artery is compressed by the probe.

- Locate the brachial artery (BrA) near the antecubital fossa. Record several representative Doppler waveforms. If the signal is damped, retrograde or absent at this level, move proximally and search for a better signal to be used for the brachial pressure.

- The following instructions can be used when testing with an automatic cuff inflator or standard manometer:
  - Inflate the cuff on the mid-arm 20-30 mmHg above the last audible arterial signal using a Doppler probe.
  - Deflate the cuff slowly (at a rate of 2-4 mmHg per second). The brachial systolic pressure is recorded as soon as the first audible arterial Doppler signal returns. The Doppler pulse must continue after hearing the first pulse to assure there is an actual pulse rather than motion artifact.
  - Locate the radial artery (RA) along the lateral (thumb) side of the arm using the Doppler probe. Record several representative Doppler waveforms. If the signal is damped, retrograde or absent at this level, move proximally and search for a better signal.
  - Inflate the cuff on the forearm 20-30 mmHg beyond the last audible arterial signal using a Doppler probe. Deflate the cuff slowly. The systolic pressure is recorded as soon as the first audible arterial Doppler signal returns.
  - Repeat procedure using the ulnar arterial (UA) signal found along the medial (pinky) side of the arm.
  - Repeat on the contralateral arm when indicated.

- Record additional representative waveforms proximally in the subclavian and axillary arteries when indicated.

> For patients with irregular heart beats, decrease deflation speeds.

Preliminary Analysis of Data

- Consider the segmental Doppler waveforms and pressures obtained. Determine classification of disease according to laboratory diagnostic criteria.

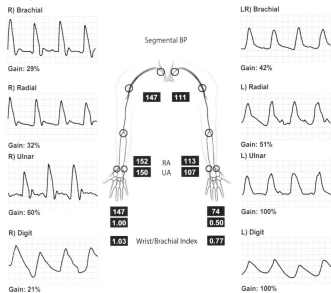

Abnormal WBI and DBI Physiologic Report

TABLE 57: Upper Extremity Segmental Pressures and Doppler Waveforms Protocol Summary

- Wrap pressure cuffs around limb:
  - Arm
  - Forearm
- Record representative Doppler waveforms at the following levels:
  - SA
  - AxA
  - BrA
  - RA
  - UA
- Inflate each cuff 20-30 mmHg beyond the last audible arterial signal using a Doppler probe on the appropriate artery distal to the cuff.
- Deflation of the cuff should be at a rate of 2-4 mmHg per second.
- The pressure is recorded as soon as the first audible arterial Doppler signal returns.
- Calculate the pressure index at each level:

$$\frac{\text{brachial, wrist pressure}}{\text{highest brachial pressure}}$$

- Repeat for the contralateral side.
- Determine classification of disease according to laboratory diagnostic criteria.

Continuous Wave Arterial Doppler Signals

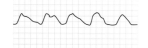

Moderately Abnormal Waveforms

Severely Abnormal Waveforms

Triphasic, biphasic, and monophasic waveforms have multiple definitions throughout the vascular ultrasound community. Although these waveforms may be labeled differently in different labs, most laboratories would identify the first waveform as normal, the second as moderately abnormal, and the third as severely abnormal. Some laboratories reserve the term biphasic only for waveforms with a reversed flow component but no third phase, though despite the term it is likely that these would be considered normal due to the presence of the reversed component.

Interpretation

- It is very helpful to compare the right and left sides when evaluating pressure and waveform changes in the upper extremities.

Normal Segmental Pressures

- There should be no greater than 20 mmHg difference between the right and left brachial pressures. [6,7]
- If the WBI is ≥1.0, the presence of a hemodynamically significant stenosis or occlusion is unlikely between the arm and forearm cuffs. [6,8]
- There is normally no decrease in pressure between the arm and forearm cuffs. [6]

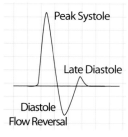

Peak Systole

Late Diastole

Diastole Flow Reversal

Normal, triphasic Doppler waveform

Normal Doppler Waveforms

- A normal triphasic signal is demonstrated by strong forward flow in late diastole (sharp upstroke), followed by flow reversal in early diastole (below baseline) plus a late diastolic component. [6,7]
- Biphasic arterial signals can be a normal finding for some patients, such as the elderly. If arterial pressures are normal, consider the possibility that the biphasic signal may also be normal. [6]

Abnormal Segmental Pressures

- An absolute pressure difference between the right and left brachial cuffs greater than 20 mmHg indicates a hemodynamically significant obstruction on the side with the lower pressure. [6,9,10]
- A WBI of <1.0 indicates that disease exists somewhere between the arm cuffs and the wrist. [8]
- The pressure difference between the brachial/forearm and forearm/digital levels should not exceed 15 mmHg. [6,8]
- A difference of 10-30 mmHg between radial and ulnar artery pressures suggests obstruction in the vessel with the lower pressure. A difference >30 mmHg confirms obstruction in the vessel with the lower pressure. [10]
- A change in the WBI of ≥0.15 from one study to the next is significant.
- A WBI ≥1.3 suggests calcific disease and is considered non-diagnostic. As an alternative means of estimating disease severity, use the digital/brachial index.

Abnormal Doppler Waveforms

- *If arterial pressures are abnormal, consider the possibility that the biphasic signal may also be abnormal.*
- There is controversy among vascular professionals regarding the terminology describing CW Doppler analog waveforms.
  - Essentially all vascular professionals agree that a waveform with a sharp, quick upstroke followed by reversed flow direction and a third forward phase is termed triphasic and consider this a normal finding in the peripheral arteries.
  - A waveform with a reversed second phase that is missing the third forward phase may be described as "triphasic" or "biphasic" by laboratories. However, nearly all will interpret this as normal. Recently some laboratories have adopted terminology that recognizes the reversed flow connection to normal by using an abbreviation NR for "normal-reversed" whether or not the third phase is present, and avoiding the confusing use of "triphasic" and "biphasic" terms.
  - Monophasic arterial Doppler waveforms are characterized by a slow upstroke, low amplitude, and broad peak with no evidence of the reversed flow component in late systole. The upstroke has a general direction of being tipped to the right. Continuous forward flow is typical in diastole, but diastolic flow may be absent if there is distal resistance from an additional high grade distal obstruction. For example, monophasic waveforms are typically present distal to an occlusion or a very high grade stenosis.
- Absent Doppler signals suggests arterial occlusive disease at the site of interrogation. [6]

Subclavian Steal Syndrome

- A significant difference in brachial artery pressures >20 mmHg, along with bi/monophasic arterial waveforms and retrograde vertebral artery flow is indicative of subclavian steal in the arm with the lower pressure. If the lower extremities are free of disease, the ankle pressures may be compared to the upper extremity for an arterial ratio.[6]

Differential Diagnosis

- Spinal stenosis
- Venous thrombosis
- Thoracic outlet syndrome
- Neuropathy
- Muscle/tendon strains
- Cervical arthritis
- Abnormalities of adrenergic receptor/sympathetic nervous system
- Connective tissue disease (scleroderma)

Correlation

- Duplex ultrasound
- Spiral CT scan
- MRA
- Arteriography

Medical Treatment

- Modify risk factors (e.g., reduce cholesterol, manage HTN and DM, smoking cessation)
- Antiplatelet medication (e.g., aspirin)
- Anticoagulation (warfarin)
- Cold temperature avoidance

Surgical Treatment

- Bypass grafting
- Endarterectomy
- Direct focal repair
- Amputation

Endovascular Treatment

- Angioplasty
- Stent
- Atherectomy
- Intra-arterial directed thrombolysis (acute blockage)

Points to Remember

- Arterial disease in the upper extremity is uncommon, accounting for less than 5% of patients presenting with extremity ischemia. [8] When disease is present, it is more likely to be small vessel disease (e.g., digital) rather than large vessel disease. [9]

- The combination of upper extremity and digital arterial examinations will differentiate between large and small vessel disease.

- The WBI only answers presence and severity of obstructive disease. The WBI should be combined with segmental pressures, volume pulse recording (VPR), Doppler waveforms or duplex imaging to determine location of disease.

- A specific WBI criterion is not well established. Many labs use the same criteria to classify WBI as ABI values.

- Two primary limitations to the WBI test are: calcified vessels (e.g., diabetics, end-stage renal disease and general atherosclerosis) and functionally significant lesions with good collateral circulation. Doppler waveforms should be obtained to ensure accuracy of WBI in calcified vessels.

- The source of embolic disease to the upper extremities' arteries can be from a cardiac source, the subclavian artery or a proximal aneurysm.

- If a pressure measurement needs to be repeated, the cuff should be fully deflated for approximately one minute prior to the repeat measurement. The systolic pressure is recorded as the pressure at which the first audible Doppler arterial signal returns. There should be a period of silence after inflation and prior to hearing the first pulse to be sure the cuff was inflated beyond the local arterial pressure. The Doppler pulse must continue after hearing the first pulse to assure there is an actual pulse rather than motion artifact.

- Additional contraindications to testing include:
  - Patient intolerance of cuff pressures.
  - Exposure to cold conditions or stressful situations can exacerbate digital symptoms.

- Pulsed wave Doppler on a duplex scanner can be used to obtain arterial waveforms when necessary. Be sure to keep the sample volume wide and the image in real time while measuring pressures to assure sample volume location.

- The bladder of the cuff must compress soft tissue, not bony structures. Failure to adhere to these guidelines will produce falsely elevated pressure readings.

- Arterial pressures obtained in the supine position will be falsely elevated due to the effects of hydrostatic pressure. If pressures can only be obtained while the patient is sitting, use the same method for follow-up exams for accurate comparison.

References

1. Sumner DS, Zierler RE. (2005). Vascular physiology: essential hemodynamic principles. *In Rutherford Vascular Surgery 6th edition.* (75-123). Philadelphia. Elsevier Saunders

2. Shepard RFJ. (2005). Raynaud's syndrome: vasospastic and occlusive arterial disease involving the distal upper extremity. In *Rutherford Vascular Surgery 6th edition.* (1319-1346). Philadelphia. Elsevier Saunders

3. Kreienberg PB, Shah, DM, Darling III, RC, Change BB, Paty SK, Roddy SP, Ozsvath KJ, Manish,, (2005). Thoracic Outlet Syndrome. In *Mansour MA, Labropoulos N. (Eds.),* Vascular Diagnosis, (517-522). Philadelphia,: Elsevier Saunders.

4. Casey, PJ, LaMuraglia GM. (2005). Anastomotic aneurysms. *In Rutherford Vascular Surgery 6th edition.* (894-902). Philadelphia. Elsevier Saunders

5. Rutherford RB. (2005). Diagnostic evaluation of arteriovenous fistulas and vascular anomalies. *In Rutherford Vascular Surgery 6th edition.* (1602-1612). Philadelphia. Elsevier Saunders

6. Longo MG, Pearce WH, Sumner DS. (2005). Evaluation of upper extremity ischemia. In *Rutherford Vascular Surgery 6th edition.* (1274-1293). Philadelphia. Elsevier Saunders.

7. Talbot, SR, Zwiebel WJ. (2005). Assessment of upper extremity arterial occlusive disease. In Zwiebel WJ. Pellerito JS (Eds.), *Introduction to Vascular Ultrasonography 5th ed.* (297-323). Philadelphia: Elsevier Saunders.

8. Moneta GL, Partsafas A, Zacardi M. (2010). Noninvasive diagnosis of upper extremity arterial disease. In Zierler RE (Ed.), *Strandess's duplex scanning disorders in vascular diagnosis 4th ed.* (149-156). Philadelphia Wolters Kluwer Lippincott Williams & Wilkins.

9. Talbot, SR, Zwiebel WJ. (2005). Assessment of upper extremity arterial occlusive disease. In *Introduction to Vascular Ultrasonography 5th ed.* (297-323). Philadelphia: Elsevier Saunders.

10. Myers K, Clogh A, (2004). Disease of vessels to the upper limbs. In *Making Sense of Vascular Ultrasound.* (227-254). London: Hodder Arnold.

Definition

Non-invasive physiological tests which compare the systolic pressure at the level of the brachial artery to the systolic pressure at the level of the digits in the hand (DBI) and detect arterial pulsations in the terminal portions of the digits (PPG).

Rationale

The sensors of a photoplethysmograph (PPG) consist of an infrared-light-emitting diode and a phototransistor. Infrared light is transmitted into the superficial tissue and a reflection is received by the phototransistor. The signal received relates to the quantity of red blood cells in the cutaneous circulation. Each arterial pulse creates a change in blood volume under the sensor. These cutaneous volume changes result in proportional changes in the reflection of the infrared light from the tissue. The changes in reflection are monitored in the instrument and recorded as a pulse waveform when the instrument is set in arterial or AC mode. If set in the venous or DC mode, the PPG can be used to monitor slower volume changes related to venous reflux, as opposed to quick changes seen during the arterial pulse cycle.

Etiology

- Atherosclerosis
- Buerger's disease
- Embolization
- Vasculitis
- Vasospasm (e.g., Raynaud's phenomenon)
- Trauma
- Connective tissue disease (e.g., scleroderma)
- Traumatic-occupational occlusion (e.g., hypothenar hammer syndrome)
- Vascular steal related to dialysis arteriovenous fistula/graft
- Radiation arteritis
- Thrombus

Risk Factors

- Age (increased risk with age)
- Coronary artery disease
- Diabetes
- Family history
- Smoking
- Hypertension
- Hyperlipidemia
- Post-op cardiac catheterization through the brachial artery
- History of radiation
- Fibromuscular dysplasia
- Occupational exposure to toxic substances
- Arteriovenous fistula or graft for kidney dialysis

Indications for Exam

- Exercise-related pain (claudication symptoms)
- Limb or digital pain at rest
- Extremity ulcer/gangrene
- Digital cyanosis
- Cold sensitivity
- Absent peripheral pulses
- Arterial trauma and aneurysms
- Bruit
- Raynaud's syndrome/ phenomenon
- Abnormal vertebral artery waveforms (UE exam)
- Thoracic outlet symptoms (UE exam)
- Abnormal arterial arm pressures, including BP differential of >20 mmHg between arms (UE exam)
- Steal syndrome (dialysis patients)

Contraindications/Limitations

- Calcified vessels which will falsely elevate pressures (typically encountered in arteries proximal to the digits in patients with diabetes or end-stage renal disease).
- Significant lesions with excellent collateral circulation, which may result in normal distal pressures and waveforms
- Any site of trauma, surgery, ulceration or graft placement which should not be compressed by the pressure cuff
- Patients with extensive bandages or casts

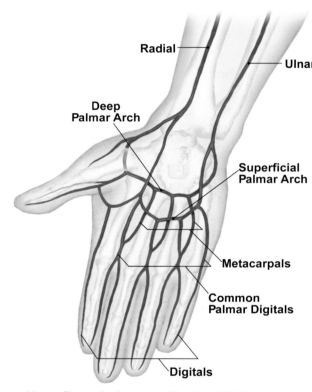

Upper Extremity Anatomy: Hand and Digital Arteries

Mechanism of Disease

There are two major mechanisms that cause reduced arterial blood supply to the upper extremity; atherosclerotic plaque and embolism. Of these, atherosclerosis is more common.

- **Atherosclerosis** is the most common arterial disease. Atherosclerotic plaque forms in the artery to block flow by either narrowing it (arterial stenosis) or totally blocking the artery (arterial occlusion). The term "hemodynamically significant obstruction" refers to either a stenosis or an occlusion that results in a decrease in blood pressure or flow distal to the obstruction. Typically, a stenosis must narrow the diameter of the artery by at least 50% to decrease pressure and flow distally. An arterial occlusion is typically seen from one major branch to the next.
- **Emboli**: embolization of contents of a plaque and/or fragments of an organized thrombus from the heart or proximal aneurysm which become lodged in a distant blood vessel. [2]

- **Mechanical compression** in the thoracic outlet region. [3]
- **External compression** is a much less common cause of obstruction in the upper extremity arteries. Extrinsic compression from tumors, hematomas, etc. can result in stenosis and/or occlusion by placing enough pressure on arterial walls to compress blood flow. [1]
- **Vasospasm** causes obstruction to digital flow and is typically intermittent and associated with Raynaud's phenomenon. Secondary Raynaud's may result in more serious obstruction from the underlying diseases. [3]
  - Digital smooth muscle cells constrict in an abnormal response to cold or stress stimuli.

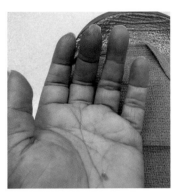

Upper extremity digital ischemia
Image courtesy of Heather Hall MD

Patient History

- Claudication (exercise related)
- Pain
- Paralysis (weakness)
- Paresthesia ("pins and needles")
- Poikilothermia (ice cold limbs)
- Previous ulceration/gangrene of hands/fingers

Physical Examination

- Pulselessness
- Cyanosis
- Pallor
- Gangrene/necrosis (tissue death)
- Marked temperature difference between hand/ fingers
- Rubor
- Bruit (abnormal sound heard through auscultation caused by turbulent flow)
- Palpable thrill (vibration caused by turbulent blood flow as seen in AV fistula)

Upper Extremity Digital Evaluation Protocol

> *Use a towel to cover the hand to eliminate any room light which may cause an artifact in the PPG tracing.*

- Obtain a patient history to include symptoms and risk factors.
- Patient is examined in the supine position, in a warm room.

> *The size control on the PPG device is kept at "10" for standardization of tracings. If the waveform "goes off" the strip chart recording paper, the size is reduced to "5" and the change is documented.*

Upper Extremity DBI and PPG Evaluation

- Apply a 2-2.5 cm cuff around the mid phalanx of the digit to be studied while avoiding cuff placement over the bony joint. Smaller cuffs will result in falsely elevated pressures due to the narrow width of the cuff. Follow up studies should use same width cuff for comparison.

Digital cuff and PPG sensor placement on the finger

- Attach the PPG photocell to the pad of the digit using double-stick tape placed between the photocell and the skin. Avoid taping the entire digit like a cuff since a tightly placed PPG could obliterate a low pressure pulse.
- Run the PPG recording at high speed (25 mm/sec) to record the shape of the digital waveform at rest, ensuring that the PPG tracing is centered. Ideally the baseline of a series of pulses is horizontal.
- Deduce PPG recorder speed to 5 mm/sec and inflate the pressure cuff on the digit until the PPG waveforms are no longer visible.
- Slowly deflate the cuff (at rate of 2-4 mmHg/sec) until the PPG waveforms return. Note the pressure in mmHg when the first pulse returns, but be sure that the pulse continues. If the pulse does not continue, consider that this was not a true pulse, but rather a motion artifact.
- If data is abnormal at rest, consider warming the affected fingers for several minutes and repeating the measurements. False positive results will occur if the digits are cold during testing.
- Repeat procedure on other digits as necessary.
- Repeat on the contralateral arm.
- Apply pressure cuffs with 10-12 cm bladder (in width) on the mid-arms.
- Locate the brachial artery (BrA) near the antecubital fossa using a Doppler probe.
- Inflate the cuff on the mid-arm 20-30 mmHg beyond the last audible arterial Doppler signal.
- Deflate the cuff slowly (at a rate of 2-4 mmHg per second). The systolic pressure is recorded as soon as the first audible Doppler arterial signal returns.
- Calculate the digital-brachial index (DBI) by dividing the digital pressures by the highest brachial artery pressure (digital pressure ÷ highest brachial pressure= DBI).
- Determine severity of disease according to laboratory diagnostic criteria.

Upper Extremity Palmar Arch Evaluation

- Evaluate the palmar arch of the hand using the PPG probe on either the thumb or index finger and the fifth digit. (CW Doppler of the digital pulse with an analog waveform may also be used if unavailable).

> *The superficial palmar arch is incomplete in 1 of 5 patients.*

- Run the PPG recording at low speed (5 mm/sec).

- With your hand, compress the radial artery (RA) and ulnar artery (UA) simultaneously, resulting in a flat-line PPG tracing, to verify that the compressions are being performed properly (cessation of flow). This is best achieved by placing your hand under the wrist and compressing the RA and UA with your index finger and thumb.
- Release compression of the RA and observe for return of the PPG pulse waveform.
- Compress the RA again to be sure that flow stops. Compress the UA. Release compression of the UA and observe for return of the waveform.

TABLE 58: Upper Extremity Digital Protocol Summary

- Wrap pressure cuffs around digits of hand.
- Tape PPG sensor to digit with double stick tape.
- Record representative tracing of PPG waveforms.
- Inflate digital cuff 20-30 mmHg beyond the last visualized PPG tracing.
- Deflate cuff at a rate of 2-4 mmHg per second. The pressure is recorded as soon as the PPG waveforms return. Be sure that a couple seconds pass before the first pulse and check for subsequent pulses to confirm it was a "first pulse" rather than motion artifact.
- Wrap pressure cuff around the mid arm for a brachial pressure.
- Inflate cuff 20-30 mmHg beyond the last audible Doppler arterial signal.
- Calculate digital-brachial indices using the highest brachial pressure.
- Determine severity of disease according to laboratory diagnostic criteria.

TABLE 59: PPG Digital Waveforms

Normal Pulsatility   Reduced Pulsatility   Absent Pulsatility

Interpretation

Normal Digital Pressures

- An absolute pressure ≥70 mmHg is normal for a digit. [4]
- If the DBI is ≥0.80, the presence of a hemodynamically significant stenosis or occlusion is unlikely between the arm and digital pressure cuffs in the upper extremities. [5,6]
- Normal digital artery pressures are within 20-30 mmHg of the brachial pressures in the arms. [5-7]

Normal Digital Waveforms

- Normal waveforms exclude the presence of significant disease. [8] Normal PPG waveform characteristics include: [4,6,7,9]
  - Short onset to peak (subjective)
  - Downslope that bows toward the baseline
  - A dicrotic notch in the downslope
- During palmar arch evaluation, if the PPG trace remains while the UA is compressed and RA is not and vice versa, the palmar arch is complete. [4,10] One artery may suggest being more dominant than the other should the amplitude of the PPG tracing increase with compression.

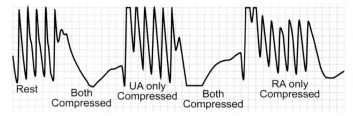

CW Doppler analysis recorded at 5 cm/s demonstrating a complete palmar arch

Abnormal Digital Pressures

- Decreased digital pressures in the presence of otherwise normal arm pressures indicates palmar or digital obstruction. [4]
- An absolute pressure <70 mmHg is abnormal for a digit. [4]
- A DBI <0.80 indicates a significant obstruction at or proximal to the digits and indicates a decrease in perfusion at the digital level. [5,6] Equally decreased finger pressures in a hand indicate disease in the distal radial and ulnar arteries or the palmar arch. [4]
- A pressure difference >15 mmHg is abnormal between fingers. [4]
- When pressures are decreased on only one side of the hand, palmar arch disease is present. [4]

Abnormal Digital Waveforms

- Abnormal ("reduced") PPG waveform characteristics (secondary to obstruction) include: [4,6,9]
  - Prolonged onset to peak (subjective)
  - Rounded peak
  - Downslope that bows away from the baseline

> Digits with pressures of less than 20 mmHg may not produce a pulsatile waveform.

- An "absent" or non-pulsatile digital waveform is reported when the PPG tracing reflects a flat-line. An obstruction is suspected. [4]
- A PPG waveform with a "double peak" (or early anacrotic notch with high dicrotic notch) is often seen in patients with Raynaud's disease. [4,7-9]

Abnormal "Double Peak" PPG Waveform

- During palmar arch evaluation, if the PPG tracing remains flat-lined or the waveform amplitude significantly decreases after release of UA or RA compressions, the palmar arch is incomplete. [4,10] Specifically:
  - A flat PPG tracing with radial artery (RA) compression (while the UA is not compressed) suggests the RA alone is feeding the palmar arch. [4]
  - A flat PPG tracing with ulnar artery (UA) compression (while the RA is not compressed) suggests the UA alone is feeding the palmar arch. [4]

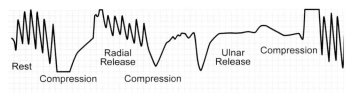

CW Doppler analysis recorded at 5 cm/s demonstrating an incomplete palmar arch fed by the radial artery

Differential Diagnosis

- Buerger's disease
- Scleroderma
- Connective tissue disorders
- Abnormalities of adrenergic receptor/sympathetic nervous system
- Neuropathy
- Muscle/tendon strains
- Arthritis

Correlation

- Duplex ultrasound
- Spiral CT scan
- MR Angiography
- Arteriography

Medical Treatment

- Risk factor management (e.g., smoking cessation)
- Cold temperature avoidance
- Antiplatelet medication (e.g., aspirin)
- Anticoagulation (warfarin)
- Thermal biofeedback
- Thrombolysis (acute blockage)

Surgical Treatment

- Sympathectomy
- Endarterectomy
- Bypass grafting
- Direct focal repair
- Resection (aneurysmal disease)
- Amputation

Points to Remember

- Skin integrity of the digit must be intact to properly assess digital circulation.

- Digits should be room temperature for accurate data collection. Use hot packs or warming devices with care to achieve if necessary. [4,6]

- Calcified digital artery pressures are rarely a problem.

- The combination of upper extremity arterial and digital artery examinations will differentiate between large and small vessel disease. Exposure to cold conditions or stressful situations can exacerbate digital symptoms. [7]

- Flow in the hand is tremendously variable because of the large number of arteriovenous shunts in the skin of the fingertips. [6]

- Digital disease can affect a single digit or multiple digits at a time.

TABLE 60: Diagnostic Criteria for Upper Extremity Digital Testing

Normal: no hemodynamically significant disease

- Absolute pressure ≥70 mmHg
- DBI ≥0.80
- Digital artery and brachial pressures are within 20-30 mmHg of each other.
- Normal waveform characteristics include:
    - Short onset to peak (subjective)
    - Downslope that bows toward the baseline or a dicrotic notch in the downslope
    - Complete palmar arch (PPG pulse wave remains or increases with compression)

Abnormal: hemodynamically significant disease

- Absolute pressure <70 mmHg
- DBI <0.80
- Pressure difference >15 mmHg between fingers
- Abnormal waveform characteristics include:
    - Prolonged onset to peak (subjective)
    - Rounded peak
    - Downslope that bows away from the baseline
    - Absence of tracing (obstruction)
    - Double-peaked tracing (Raynaud's disease)
- Incomplete palmar arch (PPG pulse wave remains flat-lined or decreases with compression)

References

1. Sumner DS, Zierler RE. (2005). Vascular physiology: essential hemodynamic principles. In *Rutherford Vascular Surgery 6th edition.* (75-123). Philadelphia. Elsevier Saunders.

2. Fecteau SR, Darling III RC, Roddy SP. (2005). Arterial thromboembolism. In *Rutherford Vascular Surgery 6th edition.* (971-986). Philadelphia. Elsevier Saunders.

3. Eskandari MK, Yao JST. (10-30-2009). Upper extremity occlusive disease: workup. *eMedicine.* Retrieved from: http://emedicine.medscape.com/article/462289-overview. (12-10-2010).

4. Longo MG, Pearce WH, Sumner DS. (2005). Evaluation of upper extremity ischemia. In Rutherford Vascular Surgery 6th edition. (1274-1293). Philadelphia. Elsevier Saunders.

5. Karkoski JK, Johnson B, Dalman RL. (2005). Upper extremity ischemia: diagnosis techniques and clinical applications. In Mansour MA, Labropoulos N. (Eds.), Vascular Diagnosis, (325-330). Philadelphia. Elsevier Saunders.

6. Moneta GL, Partsafas A, Zacardi M. (2010). Non-invasive diagnosis of upper extremity arterial disease. In Zierler RE (Ed.), *Strandess's duplex scanning disorders in vascular diagnosis 4th ed.* (149-156). Philadelphia Wolters Kluwer Lippincott Williams & Wilkins.

7. Edwards JM, Porter JM. (1998). Upper extremity arterial disease: Etiologic considerations and differential diagnosis. (60-68). Seminars in Vascular Surgery. Vol 11(2).

8. Edwards JM, Porter JM. (1993). Evaluation of upper extremity ischemia. In Bernstein EF (ed). *Vascular Diagnosis 4th ed.* (630-640). St. Louis: Mosby.

9. Sumner DS, Zierler RE. (2005). Physiologic assessment of peripheral arterial occlusive disease. In Rutherford *Vascular Surgery 6th edition.* (197-222). Philadelphia. Elsevier Saunders.

10. Zaccardi MJ, Mokadam NA. (2005). Radial artery evaluation before coronary artery bypass grafts. In Zierler RE (Ed.), *Strandess's duplex scanning disorders in vascular diagnosis 4th ed.* (385-398).Philadelphia Wolters Kluwer Lippincott Williams & Wilkins.

Definition

The use of a combination of real time B-mode ultrasonography with pulsed wave and color flow Doppler (duplex scan) to evaluate the upper extremity arteries

Etiology

- Atherosclerosis
- Embolization
- Thrombus
- Intimal hyperplasia
- Pseudoaneurysm
- Aneurysm
- Trauma
- Traumatic occlusion
- Extrinsic compression
- Vasculitis
- AV fistula (abnormal connection between an artery and a vein)
- External radiation
- Radiation arteritis

Risk Factors

- Age (increased risk with age)
- Coronary artery disease
- Diabetes
- Family history
- Hyperlipidemia
- Hypertension
- Smoking
- Obesity
- Post-op cardiac catheterization through the brachial artery
- History of radiation
- Fibromuscular dysplasia
- Occupational exposure to toxic substances
- Previous history of CVA or MI
- Elevated homocysteine
- Excessive levels of C-reactive protein

Indications for Exam

- Absent peripheral pulses
- Abnormal arterial arm pressures, including BP differential of >20 mmHg between arms
- Thoracic outlet symptoms
- Cold sensitivity
- Digital cyanosis
- Raynaud's syndrome/ phenomenon abnormal vertebral artery waveforms
- Bruit (abnormal sound heard through auscultation caused by vibration of tissue from turbulent flow)
- Claudication (exercise-related arm pain)
- Rest pain
- Extremity ulcer
- Gangrene
- Trauma to an artery
- Arterial aneurysm

Contraindications/Limitations

- Patients with extensive bandages or casts
- Subclavian or peripheral IV line placements may make it difficult to image an area.
- Poor visualization due to vessel depth (e.g., near clavicular area)
- Diffuse arterial wall calcification (such as in diabetics and end-stage renal failure patients) may interfere with acquisition of duplex information.

Upper Extremity Arterial Anatomy

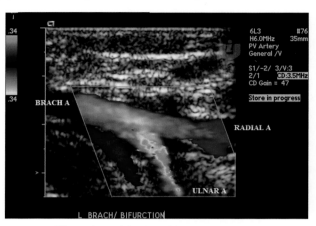

Bifurcation of the brachial artery into the radial artery and ulnar artery

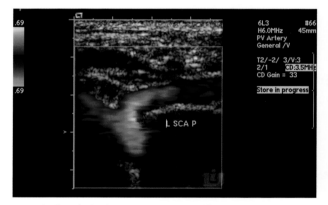

Left subclavian artery comes off the aortic arch

Mechanism of disease

- **Atherosclerosis** is the most common arterial disease. Atherosclerotic plaque forms in the artery to block flow by either narrowing it (arterial stenosis) or totally blocking the artery (arterial occlusion). The term "hemodynamically significant obstruction" refers to either a stenosis or an occlusion that results in a decrease in blood pressure or flow distal to the obstruction. Typically, a stenosis must narrow the diameter of the artery by at least 50% to decrease pressure and flow distally.[1] An arterial occlusion is typically seen from one major branch to the next.

- **Emboli** may occur as contents of a plaque or fragments of an organized thrombus from the heart or aneurysm loosen and flow downstream. Emboli become lodged in a distant blood vessel, causing arterial occlusion and reduction of flow.[1]

- **Vasospasm** is a temporary constriction of the arteries (typically digital arteries) that may cause significant discomfort to the patient or be a sign of a more serious underlying disease.[2]

- **Extrinsic compression** from tumors, musculoskeletal configuration, hematoma, etc. can result in stenosis or occlusion by placing enough pressure on arterial walls to compromise blood flow.[1]

- **Mechanical compression** of arterial vessels in the thoracic outlet can compromise flow. Anatomical defects, such as a congenital abnormality of the first rib or fracture of the clavicle, are examples of possible sources of this compression.[3]
- **Aneurysmal disease** results from weakening of the structural proteins (elastin and collagen) within the medial layer of the arterial wall. [4]
- A **pseudoaneurysm** (PA) or "false aneurysm" forms due to trauma to all three layers of the arterial wall. The "false aneurysm" is actually a hematoma, receiving its blood supply via communication with an artery through a patent "neck". [5]
- An **arteriovenous fistula** or abnormal connection between artery and vein can result from trauma or complications during invasive procedures (e.g., cardiac catheterization). In such cases, blood flows directly from the artery into the venous system without passing through the tissues and capillary bed. [6]
- **Arterial dissections** are caused by tears in the intimal layer of the arterial wall that allows blood flow to access the media. Dissection between the medial and adventitial layers may result in true and false lumens. The false lumen can progressively dilate into a pseudoaneurysm. [7]

Location of Disease

- Location of disease can be focal or diffuse and affect any level or multiple levels.
- At the origin of the great vessels
- Subclavian or axillary artery
- Palmar arch and/or digital arteries

Patient History

- Claudication (exercise related limb pain)
- Limb pain at rest
- Paralysis
- Paresthesia
- Poikilothermia
- Previous therapeutic vascular procedure (e.g., bypass, stenting)

Physical Examination

- Pulselessness
- Cyanosis
- Pallor
- Rubor
- Bruit (abnormal sound heard through auscultation caused by turbulent flow vibration)
- Marked temperature difference between hand/fingers
- Palpable thrill (vibration caused by turbulent blood flow as seen in an AV fistula)
- Gangrene/necrosis (tissue death)
- Pulsatile mass

Upper Extremity Arterial Duplex Protocol

- Obtain a patient history to include symptoms, risk factors and past vascular interventions and general dates.
- Patient is examined in the supine position with the arm angled approximately 45-90° and externally rotated away from the body for probe placement. The patient may be examined from the head of the bed to achieve ergonomically correct and excellent access from the central arteries to the antecubital fossa. The forearm vessels can often also be accessed in this position.
- Some patients may require the use of a range of transducers; including high-frequency (5-7 MHz) (8-15 MHz) transducers and a lower frequency (1-4 MHz) transducer for the area around the clavicle.
- Locate the subclavian artery (SCA) and vein in the supraclavicular fossa in the transverse (short axis) plane. Rotate your probe in the longitudinal (sagittal) plane to follow the artery proximal to its origin. Record grayscale and color images in a longitudinal view of the proximal SCA.
- As you move the probe distally down the arm, record grayscale and color images in a longitudinal view of the:
  - Distal SCA (below the clavicle)
  - Axillary artery (AXA)
  - Brachial artery (BrA)
  - Right distal innominate artery (optional)
- Record the peak systolic velocity (PSV) in longitudinal view using pulsed wave Doppler (60° Doppler angle or less, with the angle cursor (angle correct) parallel to the vessel walls in the center of the flow stream) in the following:
  - Subclavian artery (SCA)
  - Axillary artery (AXA)
  - Brachial artery (BrA)
  - Radial (RA) artery
  - Ulnar (UA) artery
  - Right distal innominate artery (optional)

> *The left SCA should be evaluated above the clavicle as proximally as possible.*

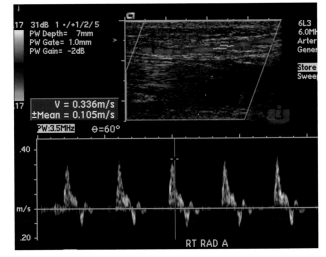

Normal radial artery waveforms

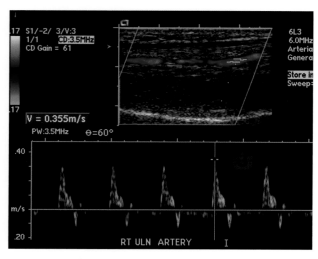

Normal ulnar artery waveforms

- Document additional grayscale and color images at areas of suspected stenosis.
  - When an area of stenosis is identified, "walk" the sample gate through the area of stenosis and obtain representative waveforms within 2 cm proximal to the stenosis, at the highest point of velocity within the stenosis and distal to the stenosis.
  - Post-stenotic turbulence and color bruit should be documented when present.
  - Measure diameter reduction in longitudinal and/or transverse planes, especially if this is a hemodynamically significant plaque.
- Determine classification of stenosis according to laboratory diagnostic criteria.
- Document any additional abnormal findings with grayscale and color imaging (e.g., aneurysmal formation, plaque, thrombus, wall irregularity, aneurysm, AV fistula, etc.).
- Repeat for the left side (omitting innominate artery visualization).

Subclavian Steal Syndrome Examination

- Arterial duplex can be used to diagnose subclavian steal syndrome. Patients present with abnormal arterial arm pressures, including a BP differential of >20 mmHg between arms. [8]
  - Using the duplex scanner, record a waveform in the vertebral artery ipsilateral to the arm with the lower blood pressure. Note the direction of flow.
  - Additional interrogation may be performed:
    - Use PW Doppler to insonate the ipsilateral subclavian artery to identify a significant velocity increase or occlusion proximal to the origin of the vertebral artery.
    - Identify any lumenal reduction by B-mode or color flow in the SCA. (Always use in combination with PSV documentation).
    - Compare bilateral axillary waveforms using PW Doppler.
    - Post occlusive reactive hyperemia (PORH) has also been used to diagnose subclavian steal syndrome when the vertebral artery demonstrates pendulum (to and fro) flow direction or has questionable reversed flow direction present. [8]

- Inflate a pressure cuff over the brachial artery (30 mmHg above the highest brachial pressure) for 5 minutes to cause temporary ischemia in the arm.
- After cuff deflation, investigate the flow direction of the ipsilateral vertebral artery using the duplex scanner as you would during a carotid exam.

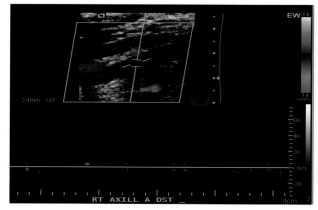

Occlusion of the AXA by spectral Doppler

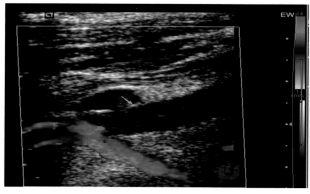

Arterial occlusion by color flow. Note patent collateral

Plaque and Lesion Descriptions/Characteristics

- **Diffuse:** long segment of artery lined with plaque, but less than 50% at any point.
- **Stenotic:** lumen is narrowed and velocity increases. Hemodynamically significant stenosis typically occurs when narrowing results in a >50% diameter reduction (75% area reduction). A stenosis can be focal or for a long segment.
- **Calcific:** highly reflective plaque(s) with acoustic shadowing.
- **Occluded:** complete occlusion of the vessel.
- **"Moving"/"Mobile":** debris within the lumen appears to be in motion (e.g., moving thrombus).

TABLE 61: Upper Extremity Arterial Protocol Summary

Scan longitudinal (sagittal) view with grayscale, color and PW Doppler

1. SCA
2. AXA
3. BrA
4. Right distal innominate artery (optional)
5. RA
6. UA

- Record the peak systolic velocity (PSV) for any segment interrogated.
- When an area of stenosis is identified, "walk" the sample gate through the area of stenosis and obtain representative waveforms at the tightest point of stenosis (highest velocity), as well as proximal and distal to the stenosis.
- Determine classification of stenosis according to laboratory diagnostic criteria.

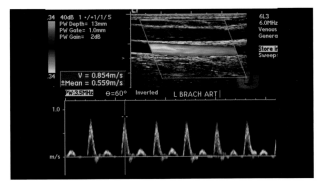

Normal, triphasic arterial waveforms

TABLE 62: Normal PSV of Upper Extremity Arteries[7]

Artery PSV (angle-corrected)
SCA and AXA 70-120 cm/s
BrA 50-120 cm/s
RA and UA 40-90 cm/s
Palmar arch and digits Lower

Source: Baker JD. (2005). The role of non-invasive procedures in the management of extremity arterial disease. In Zwiebel WJ. Pellerito JS (Eds.), Introduction to Vascular Ultrasonography 5th ed. (254-260). Philadelphia: Elsevier Saunders

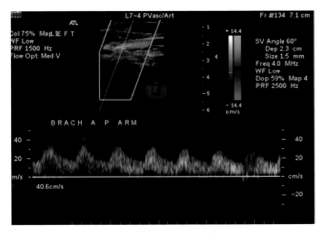

Abnormal, monophasic arterial waveforms

> *Triphasic, biphasic, and monophasic waveforms have multiple definitions throughout the vascular ultrasound community. Some laboratories reserve the term biphasic only for waveforms with a reversed flow component but no third phase. Some labs may term any waveform without a reversed flow component as monophasic.*

Interpretation

- Determine:
  - Plaque location, plaque characteristics
  - Peak systolic velocity (PSV)
  - V_2/V_1, peak systolic velocity ratio where V_2 represents the maximum peak systolic velocity of a stenosis; V_1 is the peak systolic velocity of the proximal normal segment. Generally, the same criterion for the legs is used to grade upper extremity disease.[9]
  - Any change in spectral waveform analysis (e.g., triphasic to biphasic to monophasic).

Normal (absence of a hemodynamically significant stenosis, <50%)

- **General grayscale and color characteristics:**
  - No intralumenal echoes are visualized within the artery and color Doppler will fill the entire arterial lumen wall-to-wall.
- **Doppler waveforms and flow velocities:**
  - Normal upper extremity arterial waveforms are triphasic. A triphasic signal is demonstrated by strong forward flow in late systole (sharp upstroke), followed by flow reversal in early diastole (below the baseline), plus a late diastolic component. [8-12]
  - Normal, biphasic upper extremity waveforms are not uncommon [8] (especially in older individuals).

Definitive criterion for upper extremity arterial stenosis has not been widely addressed in the literature so it varies across institutions. Some labs use the same criterion for the upper and lower extremities.

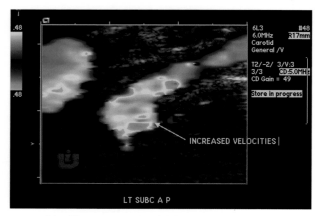

Significant stenosis of SCA by color Doppler

- **General grayscale and color characteristics:**
  - Intralumenal echoes are visualized within the artery, resulting in a measurable lumenal reduction.
  - When utilized, color Doppler does not fill the entire arterial lumen. Instead, a color jet can be visualized through the narrowed lumen. [9,11]
  - A mosaic color pattern can be observed due to turbulent flow in the post-stenotic region. [9]
- **Doppler waveforms and flow velocities:**
  - Biphasic arterial signals are characterized by strong forward flow in late systole (sharp upstroke) with a loss of flow reversal in early diastole (no flow below the baseline) and a reduction of the late diastolic component. [8]
  - Monophasic arterial signals are characterized by reduced pulsatility and no reversed flow in late systole. A diastolic flow component may or may not be apparent. [9,12]
  - **Stenosis:** A hemodynamically significant lesion (>50%) will result in a focal velocity increase (at least double the velocity in the proximal arterial segment), changes in spectral waveform (from triphasic to biphasic or monophasic), post-stenotic turbulence, color aliasing with proper settings and possible color bruit. [8-11]

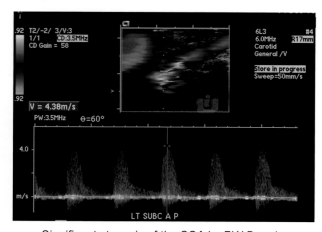

Significant stenosis of the SCA by PW Doppler

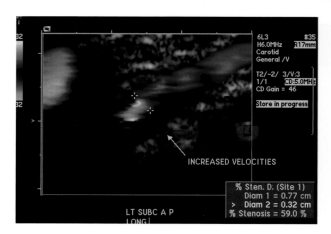

Lumenal reduction of the SCA by color flow

TABLE 63: Diagnostic Criteria for Arterial Stenosis[8,9,11]

- PSV* ratio >2 indicates significant stenosis
- Changes in velocity measurements or waveform shape on serial examinations warrant close interval follow-up
- PSV ratio= PSV (V_2) distal ÷ PSV (V_1) proximal

*PSV = Peak systolic velocity

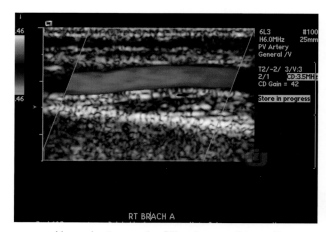

Normal artery; color filling from wall to wall

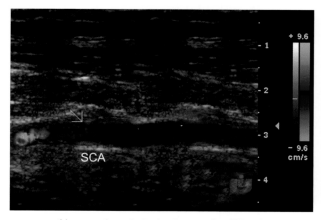

Abnormal occluded artery; color filling is absent with a collateral visualized

– Occlusion:

- A "staccato" waveform often indicates that there is a distal occlusion.
- An occlusion of the artery is present when no flow is detected by color and spectral Doppler. [8-11] The extent of the occlusion can often be determined by identifying a large collateral

> *Use flow in the adjacent vein as a guide to identify an occluded artery. But always confirm lack of flow by placing the Doppler sample volume in the artery.*

at the proximal and distal end of the occlusion. [9] These collaterals often exit or enter the artery at a 90° angle to the vessel.
- Blood flow may reverse direction, especially near arterial bifurcations, when the proximal artery is occluded and the vessel is supplying collateral flow.

- Use indirect signs to evaluate hemodynamically significant lesions in regions where a proximal velocity is technically difficult to obtain and a ratio cannot be calculated [10] (e.g., distal to a calcified plaque) such as:
    - Increased velocities (with lumenal reduction) with post-stenotic turbulence. [8,11]
    - Change in spectral waveform from one segment to the next (e.g., triphasic to monophasic). [10,11]
    - Comparison of arterial waveform in the contralateral extremity at the same site.

Other Pathology

- **Thoracic outlet syndrome**
- **Arteriovenous fistula (AVF):** An AVF between any artery and an adjacent vein is characterized by color bruit on duplex image along with high velocity, low-resistance spectral waveforms at the same site by pulsed wave Doppler.[11] The turbulent, pulsatile waveform typically continues for a short distance in the vein proximal to the AVF and slowly loses its pulsatility more proximally. The Doppler signal proximal to the AVF is clearly different than the venous signal distal to the AVF.

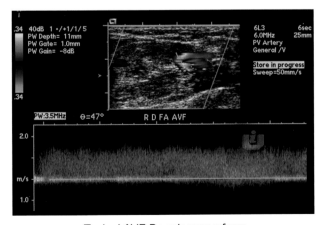

Typical AVF Doppler waveform

- **Pseudoaneurysm:** A pulsatile mass observed communicating with a native artery is indicative of a pseudoaneurysm. To-and-fro Doppler flow patterns will be apparent within the "neck" of the PA.[5]

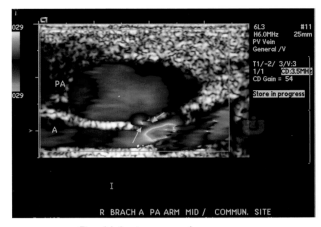

Brachial artery pseudoaneurysm

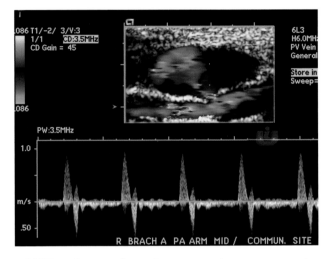

PW Doppler waveforms from a pseudoaneurysm neck

- **Aneurysm:** Arterial diameters that show a focal enlargement which is at least 1.5-2 times the size of the proximal arterial segment indicate significant aneurysmal dilatation.[9] Intralumenal thrombus may be present and is a possible source of distal emboli. [10]

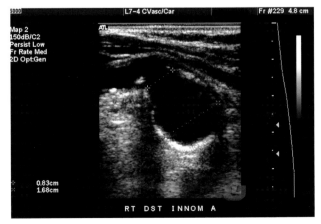

Innominate artery aneurysm

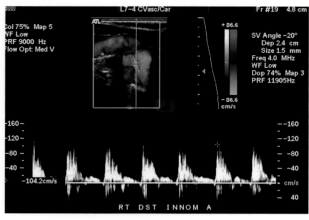

PW Doppler waveforms within the aneurysm

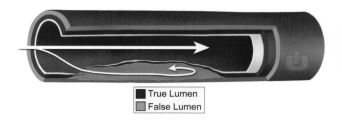

□ True Lumen
□ False Lumen

Artery with True and False Lumen

- **Subclavian steal syndrome:** A significant difference in brachial artery pressures >20 mmHg warrants additional interrogation of the arm with the lower blood pressure. Arterial flow in the ipsilateral vertebral, subclavian and axillary arteries is considered during interpretation. Reversed flow direction in the vertebral artery, combined with a significant difference in arm pressures, is indicative of a subclavian steal.

  - **By duplex:**
    - A focal velocity increase in the ipsilateral subclavian artery proximal to the origin of the vertebral artery that is at least double the velocity in the proximal arterial segment indicates a hemodynamically significant stenosis (>50%). Additional duplex findings including; changes in spectral waveform (from triphasic to biphasic or monophasic), post-stenotic turbulence and color bruit all support this finding. [8,9]
    - No flow detected by color or spectral Doppler (occlusion) in the SCA proximal to the origin of the vertebral artery is another possible abnormal finding. [9,10]
  - **By PORH:** [8]
    - Suspicion of subclavian steal, despite a non-significant difference in brachial pressures or a to-and-fro flow in the vertebral artery at rest, PORH followed by interrogation of the ipsilateral vertebral artery may be used for diagnosis.
    - If the flow direction of the vertebral artery becomes retrograde after the PORH technique, this finding suggests a subclavian steal on that side.

- **Arterial dissection:** A dissection of the arterial lumen is recognized by two distinct flow channels by B-mode and/or color Doppler separated by an intimal echo. One lumen is known as the "true lumen" while the other is referred to as the "false lumen". One of the lumens may be occluded or demonstrate reversed or unusual flow direction. [7,11]

> *The SCA is the most likely artery of the upper extremity to demonstrate a dissection, though it can occur elsewhere.*

Differential Diagnosis

- Spinal stenosis
- Venous thrombosis
- Thoracic outlet syndrome
- Neuropathy
- Muscle/tendon strains
- Cervical arthritis
- Abnormalities of adrenergic receptor/sympathetic nervous system
- Connective tissue disease (scleroderma)

Correlation

- Spiral CT scan
- MRA
- Arteriography

Medical Treatment

- Modify risk factors, (e.g., smoking cessation, especially for Raynaud's symptoms, reduce cholesterol/HTN, manage DM)
- Antiplatelet medication (e.g., aspirin)
- Anticoagulation (warfarin)
- Steroids
- Cold temperature avoidance

Surgical Treatment

- Bypass grafting
- Embolectomy
- Direct focal repair
- Resection (aneurysmal disease)
- Amputation

Endovascular Treatment

- Angioplasty
- Stent
- Atherectomy
- Intra-arterial directed thrombolysis (acute blockage)

Points to Remember

- Arterial duplex ultrasound can identify the presence, exact location, extent, and severity of disease. The course of the arteries, collaterals and disease can be visualized using B-mode and color, while the measurement of Doppler velocity and waveform changes can estimate the severity of obstructions and flow direction.
- Color Doppler can underestimate plaque and diameter reductions due to bleeding of the color flow over the plaque seen in B-mode. For increased accuracy, measure in B-mode whenever possible in two planes at the point of tightest stenosis.

- Besides atherosclerosis, narrowing of an arterial lumen can result from intimal hyperplasia or cellular damage after radiation therapy.
- Since the left subclavian artery originates directly from the aortic arch, its origin is often not seen in a routine examination. [9,11]
- The rate of subclavian steal involving the left arm is 85%. [9]
- The most common locations for upper extremity atherosclerotic plaques and aneurysms involve the SCA and AXA. [9,11] Obstruction of the RA and UA is less common, though can result from low-flow states or embolization. [9]
- The typical shape of an aneurysm in the upper extremity is fusiform. [9]
- A proximal branch of the SCA, the internal thoracic (internal mammary) artery, is frequently used as conduit for cardiac surgery and surgically grafted to the heart. [11] The artery can often be visualized coming off the SCA at a 90º angle to the vessel. Typical Doppler waveforms for the internal thoracic artery exhibit high diastolic flow when used to perfuse the heart. [11]
- The thoracic outlet is comprised of the clavicle, the first rib and the scalene muscle. Compression of the subclavian vessels is a common issue. Complete or partial compression of the vessels is possible, which over time may lead to damage of the arterial wall or formation of thrombus. Oftentimes symptoms are experienced with certain positional changes. [12]
- Calcific shadowing can prohibit Doppler and color flow analysis of a specific arterial segment(s). Comparing the Doppler waveform proximal and distal to the calcified segment may indicate a hemodynamically significant obstruction under the calcific shadowing (i.e., if severe post-stenotic turbulence is present distal to the shadowing, there could be a stenosis in the calcified segment, or if there is essentially no change in the waveform pattern it is unlikely that a significant obstruction exists under the calcific area).

References

1. Sumner DS, Zierler RE. (2005). Vascular physiology: essential hemodynamic principles. In Rutherford Vascular Surgery 6th edition. (75-123). Philadelphia. Elsevier Saunders

2. Shepard RFJ. (2005). Raynaud's syndrome: vasospastic and occlusive arterial disease involving the distal upper extremity. In Rutherford Vascular Surgery 6th edition. (1319-1346). Philadelphia. Elsevier Saunders

3. Kreienberg PB, Shah, DM, Darling III, RC, Change BB, Paty SK, Roddy SP, Ozsvath KJ, Manish,, (2005). Thoracic Outlet Syndrome. In Mansour MA, Labropoulos N. (Eds.), *Vascular Diagnosis*, (517-522). Philadelphia,: Elsevier Saunders.

4. Schermerhorn ML, Cronenwett JL. (2005). Abdominal aortic and iliac aneurysms. In *Rutherford Vascular Surgery 6th edition*. (1408-1452). Philadelphia. Elsevier Saunders.

5. Casey, PJ, LaMuraglia GM. (2005). Anastomotic aneurysms. In Rutherford Vascular Surgery 6th edition. (894-902). Philadelphia. Elsevier Saunders

6. Rutherford RB. (2005). Diagnostic evaluation of arteriovenous fistulas and vascular anomalies. In Rutherford Vascular Surgery 6th edition. (1602-1612). Philadelphia. Elsevier Saunders.

7. Baker JD. (2005). The role of non-invasive procedures in the management of extremity arterial disease. In Zwiebel WJ. Pellerito JS (Eds.), Introduction to Vascular Ultrasonography 5th ed. (254-260). Philadelphia: Elsevier Saunders.

8. Longo MG, Pearce WH, Sumner DS. (2005). Evaluation of upper extremity ischemia. In Rutherford Vascular Surgery 6th edition. (1274-1293). Philadelphia. Elsevier Saunders.

9. Talbot SR, Zwiebel WJ. (2005). Assessment of upper extremity arterial occlusive disease. In Zwiebel WJ. Pellerito JS (Eds.), Introduction to Vascular Ultrasonography 5th ed. (297-323). Philadelphia: Elsevier Saunders

10. Moneta GL, Partsafas A, Zacardi M. (2010). Non-invasive diagnosis of upper extremity arterial disease. In Zierler RE (Ed.), Strandess's duplex scanning disorders in vascular diagnosis 4th ed. (149-156). Philadelphia Wolters Kluwer Lippincott Williams & Wilkins.

11. Thrush, A, Hartshorne, T. (2005). Duplex assessment of upper extremity arterial disease. In Peripheral Vascular Ultrasound (2nd ed). (133-144). Philadelphia: Elsevier

12. Myers K, Clough A. (2004). Diseases of vessels to the upper limb. In Making sense of vascular ultrasound: A hands on guide. (227-254). London: Hodder Arnold.

Definition

A non-invasive physiological test or duplex evaluation comparing upper extremity waveform patterns at rest and during provocative postural maneuvers.

Rationale

The thoracic outlet is comprised of the clavicle, first rib and the scalene muscle. Either the subclavian vessels or nerve network, known as the brachial plexus, can be compressed by these structures at the thoracic outlet as they leave the chest (TOS-thoracic outlet syndrome).

Arterial compression can cause flow disturbance in certain arm or shoulder positions, disruption of the intimal layer, aneurysm, thrombosis or embolism. This compression can be reflected in the arterial waveform as a marked reduction or cessation of the arterial flow signal.

The nerve and/or vein may also be compressed at the thoracic outlet but this chapter refers to non-invasive arterial, and to a lesser extent, venous testing from compression of the thoracic outlet.

Etiology (of symptoms from TOS)

- Extrinsic compression of artery, vein and/or nerve at the thoracic outlet
- Thrombus in the SCV
- Atherosclerosis
- Trauma to the vessel
- Embolization from the subclavian/axillary arteries
- Aneurysm

Risk Factors

- Anatomical variations of the cervical ribs
- Head or neck trauma
- Large pectoral muscles
- Hyperlipidemia
- Excessive breast tissue
- Obesity
- History of radiation
- Klipple-Fiel Syndrome

Indications for Exam

- Thoracic outlet symptoms (numbness, tingling, arm pain in certain positions)
- Claudication (exercise-related arm pain)
- Bruit (abnormal sound heard through ausculation caused by turbulent flow vibration)
- Limb pain at rest
- Digital cyanosis
- Arterial aneurysm
- Upper extremity swelling indicates venous testing

Contraindications/Limitations

- Upper extremity venous thrombosis is a contraindication to arterial testing.
- Patient's inability to perform functional maneuvers
- Direct imaging of the subclavian vessels is limited by the clavicle.
- Patients with extensive bandages or casts which cannot be removed limit direct insonation at the bandage and movement.
- Obesity or severe edema (depth of vessels)
- Open wounds can limit access of the imaging probe.

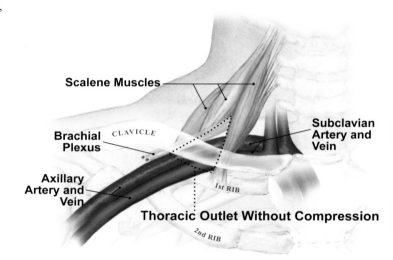

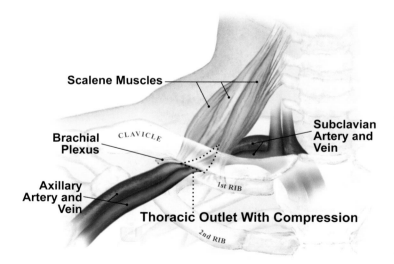

Upper Extremity Arterial and Venous Anatomy:
Thoracic Outlet Region

Mechanism of syndrome

Mechanical compression of the subclavian vein or artery can occur in the thoracic outlet region. Anatomical defects, such as a congenital abnormality of the first rib or fracture of the clavicle, are examples of possible sources of this compression. There are three types of thoracic outlet syndrome: neurogenic, venous and arterial.

Types of thoracic outlet syndrome[1]

- **Neurogenic** (most common): compression of the brachial plexus from the cervical ribs, first rib, anterior scalene muscles, congenital myofascial bands and ligaments

- **Venous**: also known as **effort thrombosis** or **Paget-Schroetter syndrome** results from repetitive trauma to the subclavian vein (SCV).[5] Arm abduction causes the SCV to be compressed against the first rib and scalenus anticus muscle, causing the trauma. Venous thrombosis can result.

- **Arterial** (least common): The head of the humerus can cause arterial compression when the arm is abducted and externally rotated, extrinsic compression of the SCA, post-stenotic dilatation or aneurysmal develops. The typical pathogenesis then is focal compression, dilation, ulceration, and thrombus formation. [1]

- Venous or arterial compression results in:
  - **Stenosis**: Significant narrowing of the artery or vein, decreasing the vessel lumen and possibly resulting in decreased blood flow.
  - **Occlusion**: Plaque, thrombus, or external compression of the artery completely blocking blood flow in that arterial segment.
  - **Embolization**: Contents of a plaque and/or fragments of an organized thrombus become lodged in a distant blood vessel.
  - **Swelling**: Significant compression of the subclavian vein causes limb swelling.

Location of Disease

- Subclavian vein
- Subclavian artery
- Distal obstruction caused by emboli from a thoracic outlet artery

Patient History

- Cold/painful/numb extremity during certain limb positions
- Claudication
- Limb pain at rest
- Acute arterial occlusive symptoms
- Previously fractured clavicle
- History of upper extremity venous thrombosis
- Swelling
- Regular exercise of upper extremity (e.g., weight lifting)

Physical Examination

- Most of these patients will present with thromboembolic symptoms.
- Patients also present with ischemic complications secondary to repeated episodes of embolization.
- Bruit (abnormal sound heard through auscultation caused by turbulent flow vibration)
- Cyanosis
- Marked temperature difference between hand/fingers
- Pallor
- Pulselessness
- Rubor
- Palpable thrill (vibration caused by turbulent blood flow)
- Swelling

Thoracic Outlet Testing Protocol

- Obtain a patient history to include symptoms and risk factors.

- Patient is examined in a sitting position with the hands palm up on the patient's lap and resting on a pillow.

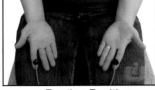

Resting Position

NOTE: A baseline upper extremity arterial physiologic exam at rest is recommended prior to performing provocative maneuvers to check for arterial TOS.

- Perform a baseline exam at rest of either the digits using photoplethysmography (PPG), or of the arms using volume pulse recording (VPR). Duplex imaging of the subclavian vessels may also be used as an additional baseline study.

PPG

- Attach the PPG photocell to the pad of the digit using double-stick tape. Typically the index finger is used. However, any symptomatic digit may also be tested.

- The PPG device with strip chart recorder or computer monitor is set to "arterial" or AC setting.

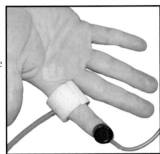

PPG Placement on Digit

- Run the PPG recording at a slow speed (5 mm/sec) to record the amplitude of the waveform. Center the PPG tracings on the paper or monitor.

- Continue recording while performing the functional maneuvers listed at the end of this section. Observe for significant waveform changes.

VPR

- Apply cuffs with 10-12 cm bladder (in width) on the upper arm and forearm bilaterally.

- Inflate the cuff to 65 mmHg. Set the gain settings appropriately to create a waveform that is moderate in amplitude. Settings should not be changed while the positional maneuvers are being performed.

> *Particular VPR gain settings are not necessary for TOS testing, as long as waveforms are moderately sized.*

- Record baseline VPR waveforms at each level.

- Record VPR waveforms while performing the functional maneuvers listed at the end of this section. Observe for any waveform changes.

Duplex Imaging

Venous Duplex

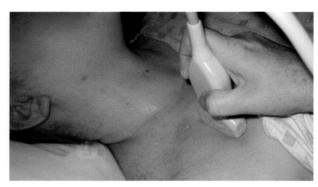

Probe position for visualization of the distal subclavian-proximal axillary arteries and veins

– Locate the subclavian vein (SCV) and axillary vein (AXV). Observe for venous thrombosis.

– Record baseline waveforms and peak systolic velocities (PSV) in the proximal and distal SCV and AXV.

– Have the patient perform the functional maneuvers listed at the end of this section slowly while re-recording the distal SCV and AXV waveforms. Observe for any waveform changes.

– Record additional PSV and waveforms proximal, at and distal to any venous stenosis.

– Note any symptoms the patient experiences during these maneuvers. Patients may test positively without any symptoms so this is also very important to note.

Arterial Duplex

– Locate the subclavian artery (SCA) above the clavicle and the proximal axillary artery (AXA) below the clavicle and record baseline waveforms and PSV.

– Ask the patient to slowly perform the functional maneuvers listed at the end of this section while re-recording the SCA and AXA waveforms and measuring the PSV. Observe for any waveform and velocity changes.

– Record additional waveforms proximal, at and distal to any stenosis.

Thoracic Outlet Functional Maneuvers [2,3]

Note: Some labs choose to constantly move the arm through any and all positions while recording tracings, describing what positions cause a change and symptoms. Other labs prefer to document responses to certain standard positions.

> *The most important positions are with the shoulder back and the arm back at 180 degrees and any position the patient reports causing symptoms.*

These positions can be performed one arm at a time, or simultaneously if equipment allows monitoring of both arms at once.

– **Adson's maneuver:** Instruct the patient to take a deep breath in, hold it, and look over the right shoulder, then over the left shoulder while recording the waveforms.

– **Costoclavicular maneuver:** The shoulders are in exaggerated "**military**" position (back and down). Instruct the patient to look over the right and left shoulders while recording the waveforms.

– **Hyperabduction:** The arms are extended straight out to the side (90°) with the shoulders back and while the patient looks to their right and left. Next the arms are positioned straight over-head (180°) while the shoulders are back and the patient looks to their right and left sides. Record waveforms during each maneuver.

– **Alternative positions:** Question the patient whether there is a special position they know to cause symptoms. Record waveforms during these maneuvers. Determine if there is signal loss at the same time the patient experiences symptoms.

Typical Patient Positioning for TOS using PPG

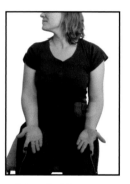

Adson's Maneuver with Head Turned

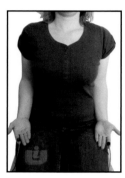

Costoclavicular maneuver:

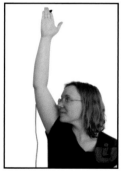

Arm Abducted 180° with Head Turned

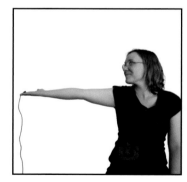

Arm Abducted 90° with Head Turned

Functional positions for TOS testing.

TABLE 64: **Thoracic Outlet Examination Protocol Summary**

- Using PPG, VPR or duplex scanning, obtain baseline arterial waveforms in the upper extremity with the patient in a neutral position (e.g., sitting). Duplex scanning is the method used to obtain baseline venous waveforms.
- Instruct the patient to perform functional maneuvers while re-recording vessel waveforms.
- Typical maneuvers include:
  - Adson's
  - Costoclavicular
  - Hyperabduction
  - Any alternative position the patient can describe which evokes symptoms
- Compare baseline waveforms to those performed during exercise.
- Ask the patient if the symptoms develop during the maneuvers and observe for the presence or absence of pulses/color flow at that time.

PPG Waveforms: TOS Testing

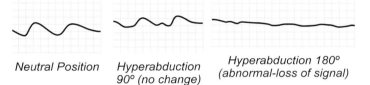

Neutral Position   Hyperabduction 90° (no change)   Hyperabduction 180° (abnormal-loss of signal)

Interpretation- Arterial Waveforms

Normal

- The amplitude of any waveform tracing during maneuvers should remain unchanged or increase compared to baseline. A slight decrease (without patient complaint of symptoms) is not suggestive of significant TOS. [4-6]

Abnormal

- **Thoracic outlet compression** is suggested when the arterial signal demonstrates a highly significant, persistent decrease in waveform amplitude or the waveform completely disappears during functional maneuvers and the patient experiences symptoms during the loss of pulse. [4,6]
- **Arterial stenosis**: A subclavian artery (SCA) stenosis is identified by duplex scan during functional maneuvers. A significant stenosis is at least a two-fold increase from the baseline velocity followed by post-stenotic turbulence. [5]

> It is very important to ensure the Doppler sample volume remains within the artery and has not moved off during positional changes.

Interpretation- Venous Waveforms

Normal

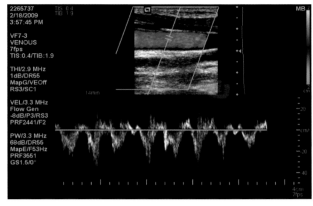

Normal venous Doppler waveform during TOS testing

- The phasic respirations expected of any venous tracing should remain unchanged or increase compared to baseline waveforms during maneuvers. A slight decrease (without patient complaint of symptoms) is not suggestive of significant TOS. [4,5]

Abnormal

- **Thoracic outlet compression** is suggested when the venous signal significantly loses phasic respiration or the signal completely disappears during functional maneuvers [7] and the patient experiences symptoms during loss of the signal.
- **Venous thrombosis:** Partial or totally occlusive venous thrombosis in the subclavian vein segment visualized by B-mode or color flow. [5]

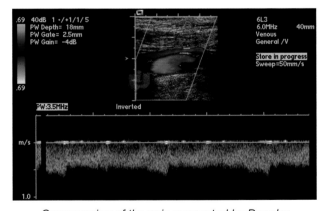

Compression of the vein suspected by Doppler waveform during TOS maneuvers

- **Venous stenosis** A hemodynamically significant venous stenosis is diagnosed when there is a velocity ratio of at least 2.5 in comparison to the adjacent venous segment. [8] An increased velocity may be demonstrated as the vein is compressed, followed by cessation of venous flow if the vein becomes totally occluded by the compression. The increased flow velocity may only be demonstrated if insonation is at or very near the point of compression.

TABLE 65: Diagnostic Criteria for TOS Disease

Normal

- Amplitude of the arterial waveform remains unchanged or increases compared to baseline.
- Phasic respirations of venous tracings remain unchanged or increase compared to baseline.

Abnormal

- Amplitude of the arterial waveform decreases compared to baseline during functional maneuvers AND the patient experiences symptoms during loss of pulse.
- Phasic respirations of venous tracings decreases compared to baseline or is completely lost during functional maneuvers AND the patient experiences symptoms during loss of signal.

Differential Diagnosis (for arterial or venous TOC)

- Nerve compression or nerve diseases
- Vascular compression by tumors
- Musculoskeletal problems
- Venous thrombosis, without venous compressions at the thoracic outlet
- Arterial obstruction or emboli proximal or distal to the thoracic outlet

Correlation

- Duplex ultrasound
- Spiral CT scan
- MRA
- Arteriography

Medical Treatment

- Modify risk factors (e.g., reduce cholesterol, manage HTN and DM, smoking cessation)
- Anti-inflammatory meds
- Muscle relaxants
- Physical therapy
- Anticoagulation (warfarin)

Surgical Treatment

- Removal of the first rib or cervical rib
- Dividing scalene muscle attachments and fibromuscular bands
- Cervical sympathectomy
- Resection (aneurysmal disease)
- Embolectomy
- Breast reduction

Endovascular Treatment

- Angioplasty
- Stent
- Intra-arterial directed thrombolysis

Points to Remember

- The cause of thoracic outlet syndrome (TOS) is neurogenic in 93% of cases. A venous cause is present in 5%, while an arterial cause is present in only 1% of cases. [9] A combination of these causes is also possible.[1]
- A flat PPG tracing or obliteration of the CW Doppler signal may occur even in normal patients when raising the arm overhead. [3] In such cases, question whether the patient is experiencing symptoms at the time. If not, such findings are suggestive of asymptomatic TOS.
- Approximately 25% of the population have asymptomatic compression. [6]
- Continuous wave Doppler is not recommended for TOS testing since one can easily slip off the vessel and misinterpret an occlusion.

References

1. Kreienberg PB, Shah, DM, Darling III, RC, Change BB, Paty SK, Roddy SP, Ozsvath KJ, Manish,, (2005). Thoracic Outlet Syndrome. In Mansour MA, Labropoulos N. (Eds.), *Vascular Diagnosis*, (517-522). Philadelphia,: Elsevier Saunders.
2. Daigle, R. (2002). Arterial evaluation of the upper extremities. In Daigle, R. (Ed.) *Techniques in non-invasive vascular diagnosis*. (187-196). Littleton: Summer Publishing..
3. Myers K, Clogh A, (2004). Disease of vessels to the upper limbs: In *Making Sense of Vascular Ultrasound*, (227-254). London: Hodder Arnold.
4. Talbot, SR, and Zwiebel, WJ. (2005). Assessment of upper extremity arterial occlusive disease. In Zwiebel, WJ (Ed.) *Introduction to Vascular Ultrasonography (5th ed)* (297-323). Philadelphia: Elsevier.
5. Longo MG, Pearce WH, Sumner DS. (2005). Evaluation of upper extremity ischemia. In *Rutherford Vascular Surgery 6th edition*. (1274-1293). Philadelphia. Elsevier Saunders
6. Raines JK. (1993). The pulse volume recording in peripheral arterial disease. In Bernstein EF (Ed). Vascular Diagnosis 4th ed. (534-553). St Louis: Mosby
7. Green RM. (2005). Subclavian-axillary vein thrombosis. In *Rutherford Vascular Surgery 6th edition*. (1371-1384). Philadelphia. Elsevier Saunders.
8. Leon, LR, Labropoulos, N, Mansour MA. (2005). Hemodynamic principles as applied to diagnostic testing. In Mansour MA, Labropoulos N. (Eds.), Vascular Diagnosis, (7-21). Philadelphia: Elsevier Saunders.
9. Thompson RW, Bartoli MA. (2005). Neurogenic thoracic outlet syndrome. In *Rutherford Vascular Surgery 6th edition*. (1347-1365). Philadelphia. Elsevier Saunders.

Defintion

Non-invasive physiological testing used to detect cold-induced vasospasm by comparing digital pressures, waveforms and temperatures (optional) at rest to those obtained after immersion in an ice bath.

Rationale

In the presence of Raynaud's disease, digits take longer to increase their blood flow after exposure to cold due to prolonged arterial vasospasm and there is a greater recovery time for fingers to rewarm back to baseline temperatures compared with normal subjects.

The sensors of a photoelectric plethysmography (PPG) consist of an infrared light-emitting diode and phototransistor receiver. Infrared light is transmitted into the superficial tissue and a reflection from the tissue is received by the phototransistor. The signal received relates to the quantity of red blood cells in the cutaneous circulation. Each arterial pulse creates a change in the volume of red blood cells reflecting the light. These changes are monitored by the PPG instrument and recorded as a pulse waveform when the instrument is set in arterial or AC mode.

Etiology

- Atherosclerosis
- Buerger's disease
- Vasculitis
- Trauma
- Embolization
- Thrombus
- Aneurysm
- Pseudoaneurysm
- Intimal hyperplasia
- Traumatic occlusion
- Extrinsic compression
- AV fistula (abnormal connection between an artery and a vein)
- Radiation arteritis

Risk Factors (increased risk for Raynaud's)

- Atherosclerosis
- Age (increased risk with age)
- Female
- Family history
- Smoking
- Inhabitants of colder climates
- Occupational exposure to toxic substances
- Occupational stress (those who use vibrating tools, for example)
- Immunology and connective tissue disorders
- Obstructive arterial disease
- Drug-induced Raynaud's

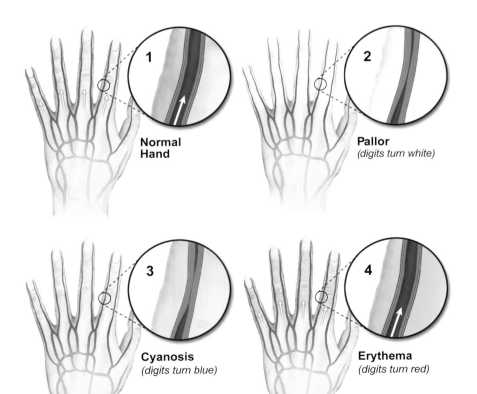

Normal Hand

Pallor
(digits turn white)

Cyanosis
(digits turn blue)

Erythema
(digits turn red)

Raynaud's Phenomenon

Example of Digital Color Changes due to Stress: White to Blue to Red

Indications for Exam

- Intermittent digital pallor, cyanosis and/or rubor
- Cold sensitivity
- Raynaud's disease
- Thoracic outlet symptoms

Contraindications/Limitations

- Digital ulceration or gangrene
- Severe rest pain
- Intolerance to ice bath used during examination
- Severely abnormal pressure values at rest, indicating a fixed obstruction

Mechanism of disease

- Current theory suggests the amount of receptors responsible for controlling body temperature on smooth muscle cells affect cold sensitivity. Refer to Raynaud's in Vascular Disease.
- Cold sensitivity due to Raynaud's phenomenon is caused by vasospasm in addition to an underlying fixed vessel obstruction. [1]
- Raynaud's phenomenon is characterized as primary or secondary.
  - *Primary* Raynaud's phenomenon is intermittently vasospastic in nature and has no underlying disease. [1]
  - *Secondary* Raynaud's phenomenon is associated with an underlying disease such as scleroderma and also involves a fixed obstruction. [1]

Location of Vasospastic Disease

- Location of disease can be focal and/or diffuse and affect any arterial level(s).
- Palmar arch arteries
- Digital vasospasm

Patient History

- Pain
- During stress, digits change colors; from white to blue to red

Physical Examination (all may be intermittent)

- Cyanosis
- Rubor
- Pallor
- Significant temperature difference between digits/extremities
- Pulselessness possible with proximal obstruction

Cold Immersion Testing Protocol

- Obtain a patient history to include symptoms and risk factors.
- Patient is examined in the supine or sitting position.
- Apply a 2.0-2.5 cm digital cuff around the mid-phalanx of the digit to be studied while avoiding cuff placement over the bony joint. Smaller cuffs will result in falsely elevated pressures due to the narrow width of the cuff.
- Attach the PPG photocell to the pad of the first digit to be examined using double-stick tape placed between the photocell and the skin. Avoid taping the entire digit like a cuff since a tightly placed PPG could obliterate a low pressure pulse.
- Apply pressure cuff with 10-12 cm bladder (in width) on the mid-arm.
- Locate the brachial artery (BrA) near the antecubital fossa with the Doppler probe.

- Inflate the pressure cuff on the mid-arm 20-30 mmHg beyond the last audible arterial signal using a Doppler probe. Deflate the cuff slowly and record the brachial systolic pressure as soon as the first audible Doppler arterial signal returns.
- Obtain the brachial pressure on the contralateral arm using the same technique.
- Use the highest brachial artery pressure to calculate the pre-submersion digital-brachial index (DBI).

> *Use a towel to cover the hand to eliminate any light artifact which may disrupt the PPG tracing.*

- Initiate the PPG (AC coupled) device with strip chart recorder or computer monitor.
- Run the PPG recording at high speed (25 mm/sec) to record the shape of the waveform, ensuring that the PPG tracing is centered. Ideally, the baseline is horizontal between pulses.
- Reduce the recorder speed to 5 mm/sec.
- Inflate the pressure cuff around the finger until the PPG waveforms are flat (no longer visible) and then inflate another 20-30 mmHg.
- Slowly deflate the pressure cuff (at rate of 2-4 mmHg/sec) until the PPG waveforms return. Note the pressure when the first pulse returns. Be sure that the pulse continues and if not, consider that this was not a true pulse, but rather a motion artifact.
- When using a computerized system, move the cursor back to the first pulse.
- Repeat this procedure on remaining digits.
- Repeat this procedure on contralateral digits for comparison, especially on any symptomatic contralateral digits.

- In addition, thermometry can be used to measure baseline digital temperatures with the use of a temperature probe sensitive for temperatures ranging from 0-55° C, placed on the tip of the finger.
- Immerse digits in an ice bath (approximately 1° C) for 1-3 minutes if able. Record the amount of time tolerated by the patient.

You can place the hand in a plastic bag to keep the hand dry.

- Remove the hand promptly. Quickly pat the fingers dry or remove the plastic covering. Do not attempt to warm the fingers with the towel.
- Promptly determine post-submersion digital waveforms, digital pressures and/or digital temperatures.
- Repeat digital pressure, waveforms and/or digital temperature measurements every 2-3 minutes until baseline values return, or for 10 minutes. Record the length of post-submersion study time.

Cold Immersion: PPG Waveforms

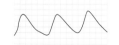

Pre-immersion tracing 2nd digit; 110 mmHg

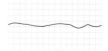

Immediate post-immersion tracing 2nd digit 104 mmHg

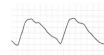

5 minutes post-immersion tracing 2nd digit 108 mmHg

Normal Recovery and Response Time

Interpretation

Normal

> *Normal waveforms are typically lower in amplitude following immersion, but it is most important to check that the waveforms pressures and temperatures return to baseline values within 10 minutes of cold immersion.*

- Baseline finger pressures, waveforms and temperatures return within 10 minutes. [1-3]
- Absolute digital artery pressure only decreases 16 mmHg ±3% at a skin temperature of 10° C. [4]

TABLE 66: Cold Immersion Protocol Summary

- Wrap pressure cuffs around:
  - Brachial artery
  - Digits
- Tape PPG sensor to digit with double stick tape.
- Record representative digital PPG waveforms from tips of fingers.
- Determine pre-submersion digital-brachial indices (DBI)
  - Inflate cuffs 20-30 mmHg beyond the last audible Doppler brachial artery signal and visualized PPG waveform(s).
  - Slowly deflate cuff (rate of 2-4 mmHg per second). Record the systolic pressure as soon as the PPG waveform or brachial artery Doppler signal returns.
- Obtain baseline temperatures (optional).
- Immerse digits in an ice bath for 1-3 minutes.
- Record post-submersion digital waveforms and pressures (temperature-optional).
- Repeat post-submersion digital waveforms and pressures every 2-3 minutes for 10 minutes or until baseline values return (temperature optional).
- Determine classification of disease according to lab diagnostic criteria.

- Normal baseline PPG waveforms characteristics include: [4-7]
  - Short onset to sharp peak (subjective)
  - Downslope that bows toward the baseline
  - A dicrotic notch in the downslope

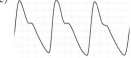

Normal PPG

Abnormal

- Baseline finger pressures, waveforms and temperatures return in >10 minutes. [1,4]
- Abnormal ("reduced") baseline PPG waveform characteristics (secondary to obstruction, not vasospasm) include: [4,5,7]
  - Prolonged onset to peak (subjective)
  - Rounded peak
  - Downslope that bows away from the baseline

> *Digits with pressures of <20 mmHg may not produce a pulsatile waveform.*

- An "absent" digital waveform is reported when the PPG tracing reflects a flat-line after stress testing. This is considered a positive study for Raynaud's phenomenon. (If the flat-line tracing was pre-immersion, a fixed obstruction would be suspected.) [4]

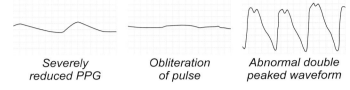

| Severely reduced PPG | Obliteration of pulse | Abnormal double peaked waveform |

- A digital pressure drop of greater than 17% from baseline indicates a significant digital artery vasospasm. [8]
- A PPG waveform with a "double peak" (or early anacrotic notch with high dicrotic notch) are often seen in patients with Raynaud's phenomenon. [4,7]

TABLE 67: Cold Immersion Thermometry Worksheet

Cold Tolerance Thermometry

	Base	1 min	5 min	10 min	15 min	20 min
R 1st	73.8	67.5	65.9	66.2	67.3	67.5
R 2nd	74.4	68.3	67.0	68.0	68.4	69.1
R 3rd	74.4	74.4	67.0	68.6	67.3	67.4
R 4th	74.0	66.9	67.5	67.1	68.4	67.5
R 5th	74.4	65.0	69.1	67.2	68.9	67.9
L 1st	74.7	67.3	67.9	67.4	71.5	68.2
L 2nd	74.6	66.7	68.5	67.5	69.0	69.3
L 3rd	74.2	66.1	67.1	67.5	67.8	68.7
L 4th	74.2	64.2	67.2	66.4	67.8	68.7
L 5th	74.4	65.0	65.7	66.5	68.9	68.4

Interpretation of Worksheet

This abnormal cold stress exam reports a recovery time >10 minutes for finger pressures to return to baseline values bilaterally.

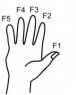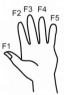

Differential Diagnosis

- Buerger's disease
- Scleroderma
- Connective tissue disorder
- Abnormalities of adrenergic receptor/sympathetic nervous system
- Neuropathy
- Muscle/tendon strains
- Arthritis
- Emboli
- Thoracic outlet syndrome

Correlation

- Duplex ultrasound
- MRA
- Contrast angiography
- Nailfold capillary microscopy

Medical Treatment

- Cold temperature avoidance
- Risk factor management (cessation of tobacco usage, avoidance of cold)
- Calcium channel blocker
- Alpha adrenergic antagonist
- Angiotensin antagonist
- Serotonin uptake inhibitor
- Prostaglandins
- Thermal biofeedback

Surgical Treatment

- Bypass grafting
- Thoracoscopic sympathectomy
- Amputation

Points to Remember

- Digital symptoms that involve pain and/or color changes may be due to obstructive arterial disease and/or vasospastic disease. Arterial obstruction should be ruled out first by completing an upper extremity exam at rest including digital brachial pressures and digital waveform analysis (*see chapter on Upper Extremity Digital Evaluations*). If digital brachial pressure indices (DBI) and PPG waveforms are abnormal at rest, obstructive arterial disease is probably the cause and the cold immersion test is unnecessary.
- In Raynaud's syndrome, digits display episodes of cyanosis or pallor due to vasoconstriction of the small, digital arteries or arterioles during times of cold or emotional stress.
- Cold immersion testing can also be referred to as cold stress testing.
- Skin integrity of the digit must be intact to properly assess digital circulation.
- Make sure the exam room is warm and comfortable.
- Recovery time for baseline digital pressures, waveforms and temperatures may be 30 minutes or more in some Raynaud's patients.[1,4]

- Patients can suffer from either Raynaud's disease or Raynaud's phenomenon.
  - Raynaud's disease is a primary vasospastic disorder without an identifiable underlying cause.
  - In Raynaud's phenomenon, vasospasm is secondary to some underlying condition and includes arterial obstruction. It is unlikely that cold immersion testing is needed for a patient with Raynaud's symptoms where fixed arterial obstructions are evident at rest.
- Cold stress evaluations cannot differentiate between the two types of Raynaud's syndrome.[1]
- Cold immersion testing can also be performed on toes.
- The most frequent cause of upper extremity ischemia is small artery occlusive disease of the palmar and digital arteries.
- DO NOT conduct a cold-immersion test on a patient with ulcerations or other signs of severe Raynaud's phenomenon (unless followed up with sympathectomy), since it may be difficult to reverse the resulting vasospasm. [2]
- A sympathectomy may be performed in conjunction with a cold stress evaluation. A local anesthetic is injected into a nerve to inactivate its tone. PPG waveforms are repeated and if normal, this suggests vasodilator therapy may be helpful. [2]

Cold Immersion with Injection of Local Anesthetic: PPG Waveforms

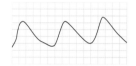

Pre-immersion tracing

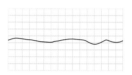

Post-immersion and xylocaine injection (The abnormal, flat PPG tracing suggests vasodilator therapy would not be helpful for this patient)

References

1. 1 Shepherd RFJ. (2005). Raynaud's syndrome: vasospastic and occlusive arterial disease involving the distal upper extremity. In Rutherford Vascular Surgery 6th edition. (1319-1346). Philadelphia. Elsevier Saunders.

2. 2 Talbot, SR, Zwiebel WJ. (2005). Assessment of upper extremity arterial occlusive disease. In Zwiebel WJ, Pellerito JS (Eds.), Introduction to Vascular Ultrasonography. (297-323). Philadelphia: Elsevier Saunders.

3. 3 Hallett, JW, Brewster DC, Rasmussen TE (2001). Upper extremity arterial disease and vasospastic disorder. In Handbook of Patient Care in Vascular Diseases, 4th ed. (238-247). Philadelphia. Lippincott Williams and Wilkins.

4. 4 Longo GM, Pearce WH, Sumner DS. (2005). Evaluation of upper extremity ischemia. In Rutherford Vascular Surgery 6th edition. (1274-1293). Philadelphia. Elsevier Saunders.

5. 5 Moneta GL, Partsafas A, Zacardi M. (2010). Non-invasive diagnosis of upper extremity arterial disease. In Zierler RE (Ed.), Strandess's duplex scanning disorders in vascular diagnosis 4th ed. (149-156).Philadelphia Wolters Kluwer Lippincott Williams & Wilkins.

6. 6 Edwards JM, Porter JM. (1998). Upper extremity arterial disease: Etiologic considerations and differential diagnosis. (60-68). Seminars in Vascular Surgery. Vol 11(2).

7. 7 Sumner DS, Zierler RE. (2005). Physiologic assessment of peripheral arterial occlusive disease. In

8. Rutherford Vascular Surgery 6th edition. (197-222). Philadelphia. Elsevier Saunders.

9. 8 Segall JA, Moneta GL. (2006). Non-invasive diagnosis of upper extremity vascular disease. In AbuRahma AF, Bergan JJ (Eds.), Non-invasive Vascular Diagnosis: A Practical Guide to Therapy. 2nd edition. (317-323). London. Springer-Verlag.

10. 9. http://www.nytimes.com "Getting to the Root of Raynaud's". New York Times. 4/29/10 by Winnie Yu interviewing Dr. Frederick Wigley .

Defintion

The use of a combination of real time B-mode imaging with pulsed wave and color flow Doppler to evaluate peripheral arterial vessels, dialysis conduits or arterial grafts for pseudoaneurysm.

A pseudoaneurysm (PA) or "false aneurysm" forms due to trauma to all three layers of the arterial wall. The "false aneurysm" is actually a pulsating hematoma, receiving its blood supply via communication with an artery through a patent "neck". These "necks" vary in size and length.

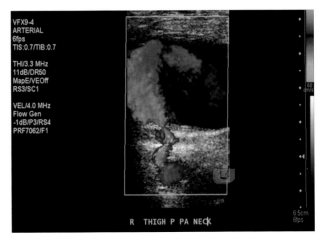

Pseudoaneurysm of the superficial femoral artery-transverse image

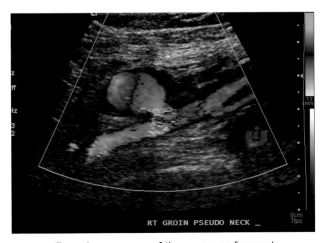

Pseudoaneurysm of the common femoral artery-longitudinal image

Etiology (of pseudoaneurysm development)

- Iatrogenic arterial puncture
- Trauma

Risk Factors

- Post-cardiac catheterization
- Post-angiography
- Post-endarterectomy
- Patients on renal dialysis (It is common to develop PA in synthetic grafts)

Indications for Exam

- Presence of pulsatile mass at anastomotic, catheterization or puncture sites
- Bruit (abnormal sound heard through auscultation caused by vibration of tissue from turbulent flow)

Contraindications/Limitations

- Allergy to thrombin or bovine products prohibits PA injection as a repair option
- Patients on medication for anticoagulation make thrombosis of PA technically difficult.
- Size and width of PA neck can influence treatment options.
- Ischemia of the distal limb being treated
- Skin infection at PA site

Mechanism of disease

- A pseudoaneurysm (PA) or "false aneurysm" forms due to trauma to all three layers of the arterial wall. The "false aneurysm" is actually a hematoma, receiving its blood supply via communication with an artery through a patent "neck."
- Insertion of a needle for diagnostic or therapeutic purposes is still a trauma to the arterial wall.
- Repeated puncture of hemodialysis grafts lead to formation of subcutaneous hematomas and pseudoaneurysms.

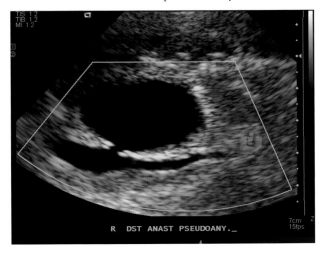

Pseudoaneurysm of a bypass graft at the distal anastomosis

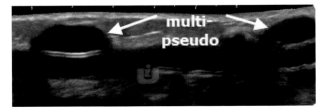

Multiple pseudoaneurysms of a dialysis access

- Reasons for pseudoaneurysm at an anastomotic site include, infection, tension at the anastomosis, thin-walled arteries, suture deterioration or improper suture technique.
- A reduction in tensile strength, post-endarterectomy may weaken arterial walls, increasing the risk of pseudoaneurysm.

Location of Disease

- Common femoral artery
- Superficial femoral artery
- External iliac artery
- Deep femoral artery
- Brachial artery
- Axillary artery
- Radial artery
- Carotid artery
- Anastomotic sites
- Hemodialysis grafts or AV fistulas

Patient History

- Recent percutaneous arterial catheterization/puncture
- History of arteriovenous graft (AVG)
- Recent surgery
- Trauma

Physical Examination

- Tenderness/swelling at puncture site
- Pain in vicinity of puncture
- Pulsatile mass
- Bruit near puncture site
- Palpable thrill (vibration caused by turbulent blood flow)

Duplex Examination for Suspected Pseudoaneurysm

- Obtain a patient history to include approximate location where catheter/needles were injected. If catheterization of the artery was recent, an entry point can usually be identified by physical exam on the skin. A pseudoaneurysm is likely to be located at or proximal to the entry point.
- Patient is examined in the supine position.
- Some patients may require the use of a range of transducers, including high-frequency (5-7 MHz) (8-15 MHz) transducers and lower frequency (1-4 MHz) transducers.

Transverse Scan and Images

- Document grayscale and color images in areas of suspected pseudoaneurysm (PA). Begin imaging in the transverse plane so more than one vessel can be visualized at one time.
- Moving the probe through the suspected area in every direction- cephalad, caudad, lateral and medial- observe the regional arteries and veins.

> There is often a pulsatile mass on physical exam which can guide your probe placement to locate the PA.

- Survey for evidence of tissue mass, hematoma or fluid collection.
  - If a mass is detected, color Doppler is useful to distinguish between a pulsatile and non-pulsatile mass. Areas of flow disturbance or flow absence prompt close observation by color Doppler. Adjust the color scale sensitivity (low-sensitivity versus high-sensitivity) depending on the flow states encountered.

- Obtain a color flow image of the mass. A pseudoaneurysm typically displays a half red-half blue appearance in at least one view, denoting flow into the mass and circling around it. An occluded pseudoaneurysm will show echogenic material and little to no color flow or may be a mass with another etiology.
- Measure the anterior-posterior and transverse diameters of any mass noted.

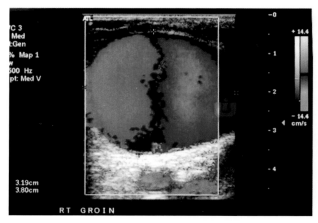

Typical color flow within a pseudoaneurysm

- Determine the communication point between any pulsatile mass (pseudoaneurysm) and a native artery by locating the "neck" using color Doppler. Place the sample volume in the neck and obtain a Doppler spectral display. A to-and-fro Doppler flow pattern is characteristic of a pseudoaneurysm whereby pulsatile flow escapes the native artery or graft, enters the mass, circles around the mass, and then returns to the artery.

> Use dual screen to measure a larger PA.

- Document the presence of any intramural thrombus present by B-mode image within the pseudoaneurysm.

> The groin is a common location for pseudoaneurysm.

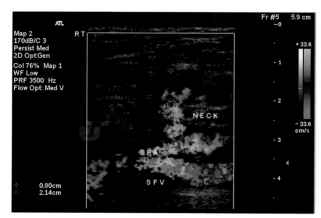

Color flow observed in a PA neck

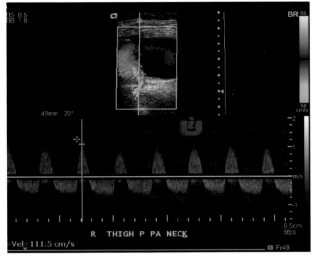

Characteristic "to and fro" flow pattern in a PA neck. Attempt to measure the length and diameter of the neck using equipment calipers

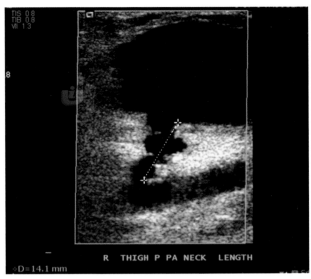

Pseudoaneurysm neck length

- Estimate the distance between top of the pseudoaneurysm cavity and skin to help choose an appropriate length needle for possible PA repair procedure.
- Document Doppler flow within the pseudoaneurysm. Use color flow imaging as a guide to place the sample volume for this recording. Measure peak systolic velocity (PSV) when directed.

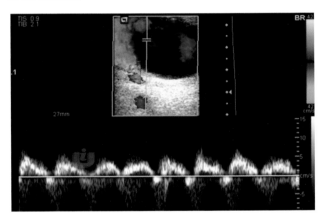

Flow within the pseudoaneurysm cavity

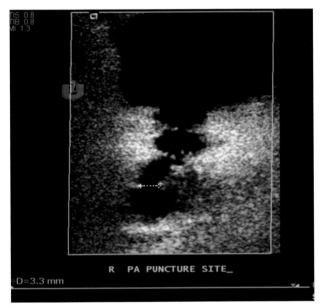

Pseudoaneurysm neck diameter

Longitudinal Scan and Images

- **Scan arteries:** Perform Doppler spectral waveform analysis in the adjacent arteries above and below the PA and its neck. Measure PSV.

    Example: *For a groin PA, assess common femoral, proximal superficial femoral and deep femoral arteries.*

- **Scan veins:** Perform Doppler spectral waveform analysis in the adjacent veins as well as above and below the PA and its neck. Assess for spontaneity, phasicity and augmentation of these venous signals.

    Example: *For a groin PA, assess common femoral, proximal great saphenous, femoral and deep femoral veins.*

- Occasionally, there may be multiple lobes or multiple pseudoaneurysms present. Evaluate all lobes or pseudoaneurysms in the same manner described above.

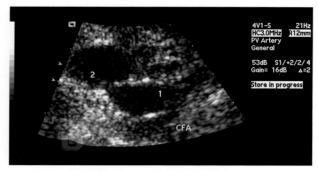

Bi-lobed pseudoaneurysm by B-mode image

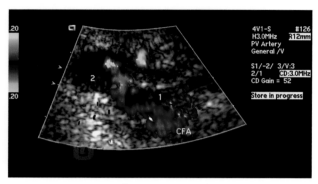

Bi-lobed pseudoaneurysm with color flow

Ultrasound-Guided Pseudoaneurysm Repair Using Thrombin Injection[1]

> Pre and post-procedural ABI measurements can detect embolic complications resulting from repair procedures.

- Document pre-injection pedal pulses and/or ABIs.
- Create a sterile field for the injection procedure. Probe covers and sterile gel may be used.
- Pain medication or local anesthetic is administered to the patient before injection at the physician's discretion.
- Place the transducer over the PA so it can be visualized by B-mode image, while leaving sufficient access for injection needles.
- The physician will typically insert a 21-22 gauge endoscopic needle with an echogenic tip containing thrombin at 1000 U/mL. A biopsy guide may be used.
- After confirming with duplex that the echogenic needle tip is within the PA cavity, turn on color Doppler.
- The physician will slowly inject the thrombin into the cavity. Observe for immediate thrombosis of the PA upon injection.

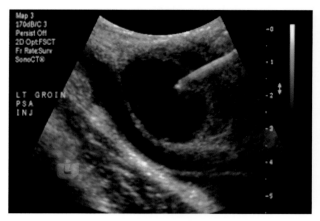

Confirm needle is within PA by B-mode

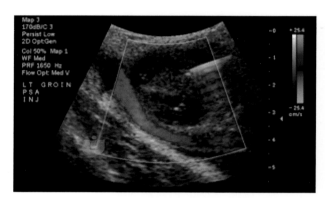

Once thrombin is injected into PA, thrombosis is noted

- Additional thrombin may need to be redirected to other areas within the PA cavity should partial color flow remain. However, avoid injecting too close to the exit site of the native artery as this may introduce thrombin into the native vessel.
- Reassess for flow within the PA cavity using color and PW Doppler.
- Document post-injection pedal pulses and/or ABIs.
- Re-image the PA and surrounding area 20 minutes post-injection to confirm total thrombosis.

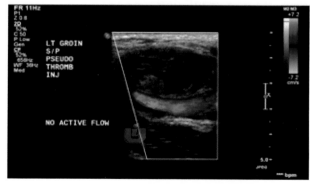

No color flow in pseudoaneurysm cavity post-injection

Interpretation

Pre-Intervention

- A pulsatile mass observed communicating with a native artery or arterial graft is indicative of a pseudoaneurysm. To-and-fro Doppler flow patterns will be apparent within the "neck" of the PA.
- Intramural thrombus may or may not be observed by duplex within the pseudoaneurysm.
- Changes in spectral waveform (from triphasic to biphasic or monophasic), post stenotic turbulence and color bruit may be observed in the arterial segments above and below the pseudoaneurysm, but are more likely to be unchanged except for the very localized area at the exit site.

Post-Thrombin Injection

> Pseudoaneurysms may thrombose spontaneously (without treatment), so all pseudoaneurysms do not require treatment.

- Expect thrombus to form immediately after thrombin injection and color flow to cease as a result while imaging.
- There should be no change between pre-injection and post-injection ABI/pedal pulses. A significant change in either is indicative of intra-arterial thrombus or embolization, post-injection.
- It is important to check the peri-mass native artery for thrombus formation following injection.

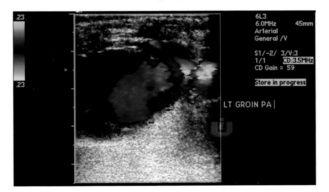

Pseudoaneurysm pre-injection by color flow

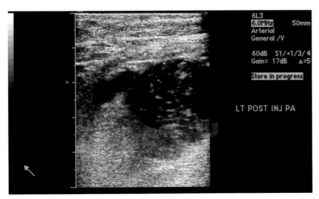

*Same pseudoaneurysm post-injection.
Note echoic thrombus in B-mode*

Note: There is a change in the echogenicity within the pseudoaneurysm cavity from pre-injection (echolucent) to post injection (echogenic).

TABLE 68: Pseudoaneurysm Duplex Protocol Summary

- Document suspected area of PA using grayscale and color Doppler.
- Measure AP and transverse diameters of any pulsatile or non-pulsatile masses noted.
- Document depth of PA from skin.
- Identify communication site (or neck) between arterial source and PA. Measure diameter and length of neck.
- Document Doppler waveforms within the neck of the PA.
- Document flow within the PA using color and PW Doppler.
- Document PSV and waveform patterns in the arterial and venous segments above and below the level of the PA.

TABLE 69: Ultrasound-Guided Pseudoaneurysm Injection Protocol Summary

- Document pre-injection pedal pulses and/or ABIs.
- Image PA using B-mode while physician inserts a needle into the PA cavity.
- Using color duplex, monitor flow within the PA cavity as physician injects thrombin.
- Confirm complete thrombosis of PA using color flow and PW Doppler.
- Document post-injection ABIs and arterial Doppler waveforms in peri-PA arteries.

Differential Diagnosis

- Hematoma without communication to an artery
- Hyperemic lymph nodes
- Arteriovenous fistula
- Vascular mass

Correlation

- CT angiography
- Angiography

Medical Treatment

- Follow-up observation of pseudoaneurysms <2 cm in diameter
- Thrombin injection under duplex ultrasound-guidance
- Duplex-guided compression repair

Surgical Treatment

- Open repair to evacuate the hematoma and repair the arterial wall
- In hemodialysis conduits: resection of the pseudoaneurysm site and surrounding graft
- Interposition graft placement or bypass around the affected section

Additional Arterial Testing

Pseudoaneurysm Duplex Ultrasound

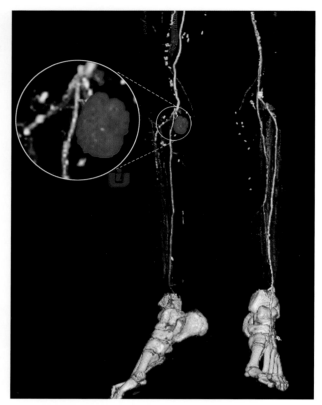

CT angiogram (in 3-D) of a pseudoaneurysm of a bypass graft

Endovascular Treatment

- Covered stent

Points to Remember

- The size of a pseudoaneurysm varies in diameter, but is typically between 1-5 cm.

- Pseudoaneurysms may spontaneously thrombose. [3]

- Pseudoaneurysm formation is less common in autogenous AV fistulas compared to prosthetic grafts. [4]

- In dialysis conduits, there are risks of graft thrombosis, infection and bleeding associated with pseudoaneurysms. [4]

- Contraindications for ultrasound guided pseudoaneurysm injection repair include:
  - Patients currently on anticoagulation (thrombus will not form in the PA)
  - The size and width of the PA neck (there may be less success when larger necks are present)
  - Known allergy to thrombin or bovine products

- Observe patients for complaints of local or distal symptoms (e.g., sudden lower extremity numbness or pain, toe discoloration) which may result from thrombosis of local arteries or micro thrombotic embolization during any repair.

Duplex Guided Compression Repair

- An alternative to thrombin injection for pseudoaneurysm treatment is **duplex guided compression repair**. Significant strength, stamina and time are often necessary to successfully thrombose a PA in this manner.
  - Using the ultrasound transducer, the technologist must apply enough pressure over the PA for 10-minute intervals to occlude the PA neck and cavity until the PA is thrombosed.
  - Approximately one hour of these 10-minute intervals may be necessary before noting any progress in thrombosis of the PA.
  - Pain medications are recommended for the patient prior to duplex-guided compression repair.

- Contraindications for ultrasound-guided pseudoaneurysm compression repair include: [2]
  - Anticoagulation medications (thrombus will not form or the PA can reoccur)
  - Obesity
  - Location and depth of PA
  - Patients with low pain threshold
  - Width and length of PA neck (easier to compress thin, long necks)
  - Skin ischemia
  - Infection at PA site
  - Limb threatening ischemia

Resources

1. 1 Kang, SS, (2005). Pseudoaneurysm: diagnosis and treatment. In Mansour MA, Labropoulos N. (Eds.), Vascular Diagnosis, (319-323). Philadelphia: Elsevier Saunders.
2. 2 Lenartova M, Tak T. (2003). Iatrogenic pseudoaneurysm of femoral artery: case report and literature review. *Clinical Medicine & Research*. 1(3): 243 -247
3. Burke BJ, Friedman SG. (2005). Ultrasound in the diagnosis and management of arterial emergencies. In Zwiebel WJ, Pellerito JS (Eds.), Introduction to Vascular Ultrasonography 5th ed, (381-399). Philadelphia: Elsevier Saunders
4. 3 Lumsden AB, Peden E, Bush RL, Lin PH. (2005). Complications of endovascular procedures. In Rutherford *Vascular Surgery 6th edition*. (809-820) Philadelphia. Elsevier Saunders.
5. 4 Adams ED, Sidway AN. (2005). Nonthrombotic complications of arteriovenous access for hemodialysis. In Rutherford *Vascular Surgery 6th edition*. (1692-1706) Philadelphia. Elsevier Saunders.

Additional Arterial Testing

Duplex of Arteriovenous Fistulas and Grafts for Hemodialysis Access

Defintion

The use of a combination of real time B-mode imaging with pulsed wave and color flow Doppler (duplex scan) to evaluate maturity of arteriovenous fistulas (AVF) prior to hemodialysis and to assess patency of dialysis fistulas or grafts (AVG) already in use.

Rationale

Hemodialysis requires high flow in a vessel that is easily accessible and can withstand multiple punctures with the dialysis catheters. To accomplish this, an arteriovenous fistula is often created surgically by connecting an artery and a vein together, so that a high flow situation is created as blood flows directly from a large high pressure artery to the vein. When an AVF is not an option, an AVG may be surgically inserted, which also connects an artery to a vein for hemodialysis access using a prosthetic graft or transposing a vein as conduit.

Etiology (for complications of hemodialysis access)

- Intimal hyperplasia
- Atherosclerosis
- Thrombosis
- Aneurysm
- Pseudoaneurysm
- Embolization
- Trauma (e.g., punctures)
- Extrinsic compression
- External radiation

Risk Factors (for renal disease)

- Age (increased risk with age)
- Hypertension
- Race (African Americans having the highest risk)
- Diabetes
- Kidney disease
- Family history of kidney disease
- Smoking
- Hyperlipidemia
- Obesity
- Coronary artery disease

Indications for Exam

- Abnormal measurements during a dialysis session including: elevated recirculation, elevated venous pressures or low urea reduction rates
- Onset of extremity symptoms post-intervention
- Decreased bruit or thrill in the access conduit
- Evaluation of AVF maturity
- Pulsatile mass

Contraindications/Limitations

- Obesity or severe edema/swelling may cause poor visualization due to vessel depth.
- Extensive bandaging or any open wounds limiting access by the ultrasound probe
- IV lines
- Severe hypotension affecting velocities/volume flow
- Extreme angles at anastomotic sites may limit visualization.

Types of Configurations for Hemodialysis Access

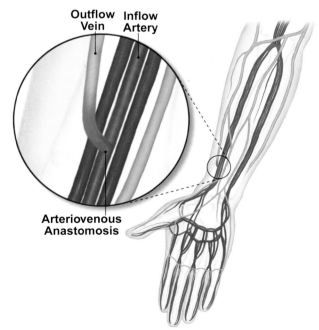

Arteriovenous Fistula (AVF) with an End-to-Side Anastomosis

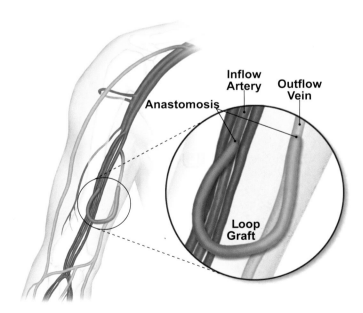

Arteriovenous Graft (AVG) Loop Graft Configuration

> *"Transposition" refers to removal and tunneling of a vein to a more superficial level.*

Common Connections of AVF/AVG

- Brescia-Cimino (radial artery-cephalic vein)
- "Snuffbox" fistula (thenar branch of the radial artery-cephalic vein)
- Radial artery-basilic vein forearm transposition
- Brachial artery-upper arm basilic vein transposition
- Brachial artery-cephalic vein (antecubital area)
- Brachial artery-cephalic vein (upper arm)
- Thigh graft connections involve:
  - Great saphenous, common femoral or femoral vein
  - Common femoral artery or superficial femoral artery
- Axillary artery-axillary vein
- Axillary artery-ipsilateral or contralateral jugular vein
- Subclavian artery-contralateral subclavian vein "necklace graft"

Graft Types- Configurations

- Straight graft in forearm or upper arm
- Loop graft in forearm or upper arm
- Thigh grafts (typically loop)

Graft Types-Materials Used

- Prosthetic
  - **Biological**: bovine heterografts, cryopreserved veins
  - **Synthetic**: Dacron or PTFE (Polytetrafluoroethylene)
- Autogenous
  - **In-situ vein**: using native veins as conduit
    - Basilic vein
    - Cephalic vein
    - Great saphenous vein
    - Femoral veins

Inflow Sites

- Radial artery at the wrist
- Brachial artery at the antecubital fossa
- Proximal brachial artery
- Axillary artery
- Common femoral artery
- Superficial femoral artery
- Subclavian artery

Outflow Sites

- Cephalic vein
- Median antecubital vein
- Basilic vein
- Great saphenous vein
- Femoral vein
- Subclavian vein
- Access anastomoses
  - End-to-side
  - End-to-end
  - Side-to-side

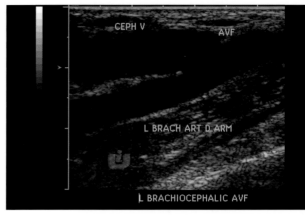

Brachiocephalic AVF: end-to-side anastomosis

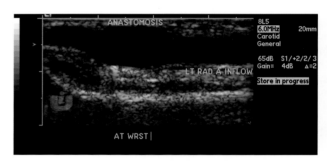

Radiocephalic AVF: end-to-end anastomosis

Mechanism of Access Complication/Failure

- A hemodynamically significant stenosis at the anastomosis or in the venous outflow track of an AVF can occur due to intimal hyperplasia and the inherent turbulent flow conditions of the access. [1-3] Hyperplasia typically occurs within 1 month to 2 years of access placement. Prosthetic dialysis grafts can also develop stenoses from intimal hyperplasia, typically at the venous anastomosis. [4]

- Hemodynamic abnormalities can arise in a vein after being arterialized. Besides venous intimal hyperplasia, abnormalities may be caused by valve position, venous wall thickening or a central venous stenosis.

- Thrombosis can occur early in the post-operative period due to technical errors in the construction of the access (e.g., poor choice of inflow/outflow, anastomotic configuration) undiagnosed hypercoaguable states or poor cardiac output (hypotension). [4]

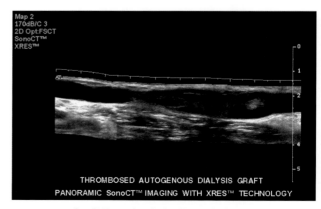

Graft thrombosis by B-mode image
Image courtesy of Philips Healthcare

- **AVF immaturity**: Venous branches which are significantly larger than the outflow vein of a fistula, can be the reason for AVF immaturity. When the branches are surgically ligated, oftentimes the AVF can mature. [2,3]

- **Steal syndrome**: Blood flow in the tissues distal to the AVF may be "stolen" by the fistula when the AVF offers lower resistance to flow than the distal arteries. In this case, the flow in the artery distal to the AVF is reversed, flowing proximally from the hand and "stealing" flow from the hand and digits. In the presence of a steal in the upper extremity, flow to the digits may be compromised, unless adequate collateral circulation is present. Note: AV grafts can also develop a steal. [2,4]

- **Pseudoaneurysm**: Insertion of a needle during a dialysis session creates "trauma" to the fistula or prosthetic graft. Over time, the access wall can weaken and a pseudoaneurysm or aneurysmal degeneration can develop in mature access conduits. [5,6]

- Early graft failure can occur even without an identifiable mechanical defect or cause. [6]

Patient History

- End-stage renal disease (ESRD)
- Previous dialysis access conduits
- Chronic arterial disease
- Extremity pain
- Claudication

> *The outflow tract may appear "lumpy" on physical exam due to the presence of multiple aneurysmal dilatation aneurysms.*

Physical Examination

- Steal phenomenon symptoms include hand coolness or pain and tingling of the digits, which may worsen during dialysis.
- Absent "thrill" within the fistula or graft
- Pulsatile mass
- Signs of infection, (e.g., fever of unknown origin)
- Presence of an indwelling catheter being used for dialysis, (e.g., in the jugular or subclavian veins)

Duplex Protocol of Arteriovenous Fistulas and Grafts for Hemodialysis

- Obtain a patient history to include any symptoms experienced during a dialysis session and past vascular interventions with general dates.

- Obtain past surgical reports/records if available, especially concerning creation of any dialysis access conduits. Dialysis patients can usually point out which access is currently being used when questioned.

- The patient is typically examined in the supine position with the arm resting at the side. The patient can also sit in a chair with the arm extended on a pillow if unable to lie down for the exam, as long as the graft/fistula can be adequately assessed.

- Some patients may require the use of a range of transducers; including high-frequency (5-7 MHz) (8-15 MHz) transducers and a lower frequency (1-4 MHz) transducer.

- Use your hand to feel for the "thrill" or pulsatility of the graft or fistula. This information can help with probe placement when trying to locate the fistula or graft.

- Identify any abnormalities during scanning (e.g., thrombosis, occlusion, stenosis, perigraft fluid, pseudoaneurysm, aneurysm).

Duplex protocols vary depending on the configuration and type of hemodialysis access in place. Protocols for three typical access types (prosthetic-loop graft, prosthetic-straight graft and arteriovenous fistula) are as follows:

Prosthetic Dialysis- Loop Graft Protocol

Transverse Scan and Images

- Follow the dialysis graft in transverse to determine its course. Locate the arterial and venous anastomoses in the transverse (short-axis) plane.

- Record transverse images of the: inflow artery, arterial anastomosis, arterial limb of the graft, venous limb of the graft, venous anastomosis and venous outflow using duplex, with color flow Doppler on and off.

Longitudinal Scan and Images

- Scan the entire inflow artery in long view in color, looking for any flow or lumenal abnormalities.

- Record longitudinal (sagittal) images of the inflow artery, arterial anastomosis, arterial limb of the graft, venous limb of the graft, venous anastomosis and venous outflow using duplex, with color flow on and off.

- Return the probe back to the arterial anastomosis and concentrate on the inflow. Rotate your probe onto the inflow artery above the anastomosis in the longitudinal plane. Record a longitudinal image with color flow Doppler on and off, using small probe manipulations to capture the inflow artery and arterial anastomosis in the same image. Observe for any lumenal reduction or other abnormality.

- When recording peak systolic velocities (PSV) in the longitudinal plane with pulsed-wave (PW) Doppler, use a ≤60° Doppler angle with the angle cursor parallel to the vessel walls and a sample volume that is in the center of the flow stream.

  - Record the PSV of the inflow (afferent) artery, at least 2 cm proximal to the arterial anastomosis.

  - Record the PSV of the inflow artery 2 cm distal to the arterial anastomosis. Determine flow direction to check for steal syndrome.

  - Record the highest PSV at the arterial anastomosis. Observe for any lumenal reduction or other abnormality.

  - Move the probe longitudinally through the arterial limb of the graft. Record the highest PSV in the arterial limb. Observe for any lumenal reduction or other abnormality.

  - As the graft curves around, the venous limb of the graft will be observed. Record the highest PSV in the venous limb. Observe for any lumenal reduction or other abnormality.

> *Since there is typically a high-flow state, set scales high to avoid aliasing color or waveforms.*

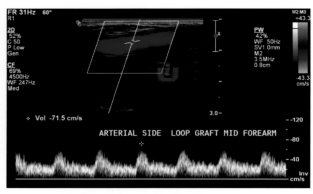

Spectral tracing-arterial limb of graft

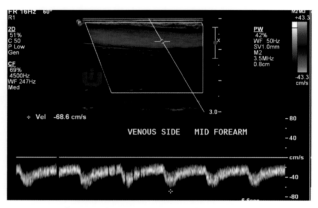

Spectral tracing-venous limb of graft

– Using small probe manipulations, insonate the venous limb of the graft as it connects to the venous anastomosis. Record the highest PSV at the venous anastomosis. Observe for any lumenal reduction or other abnormality.

• Record images with color flow on and off of the venous anastomosis. Use either a longitudinal or transverse approach depending on the angulation at the anastomosis. Observe for any lumenal reduction or other abnormality.

• Record the PSV of the venous outflow (efferent vein) in longitudinal using pulsed wave Doppler and a ≤60° Doppler angle with the angle cursor parallel to the vessel walls and a sample volume that is in the center of the flow stream.

– If the cephalic vein is the outflow, evaluate the cephalic-subclavian venous confluence. Record images of the confluence with color flow on and off. Record sample waveforms from this site and assess for spontaneity, phasicity and augmentation. Measure a PSV if possible.

– If the basilic is the outflow vein, record images and assess PW Doppler waveforms from the basilic-brachial vein confluence and the axillary vein.

– Record PW Doppler waveforms from the subclavian and internal jugular veins.

• Record additional velocities proximal, at and distal to any stenosis.

• Measure diameter of any aneurysmal dilatations or lumenal reductions at points of stenosis or thrombus.

• Determine classification of stenosis according to laboratory diagnostic criteria.

Prosthetic Dialysis- Straight Graft Protocol

> *Since there is typically a high-flow state, set scales high to avoid aliasing color or waveforms.*

Transverse Scan and Images

• Locate the arterial anastomosis in the transverse (short-axis) plane. Follow the dialysis graft in transverse to determine its course.

• Record transverse views of the inflow artery, arterial anastomosis, body of the graft, venous anastomosis and venous outflow using duplex, with and without color flow.

Longitudinal Scan and Images

• Record longitudinal (sagittal) views of the inflow artery, arterial anastomosis, body of the graft, venous anastomosis and venous outflow using duplex, with and without color flow Doppler.

• Return the probe back to the arterial anastomosis and concentrate on the inflow. Rotate your probe onto the inflow artery above the anastomosis in the longitudinal plane. Record a longitudinal image with color flow on and off, using small probe manipulations to capture the inflow artery and arterial anastomosis in the same image. Observe for any lumenal reduction or other abnormality.

• When recording peak systolic velocities (PSV) in the longitudinal plane with pulsed-wave (PW) Doppler, use a ≤60° Doppler angle with the angle cursor parallel to the vessel walls and a sample volume that is in the center of the flow stream.

– Record the PSV of the inflow (afferent) artery, at least 2 cm proximal to the arterial anastomosis.

– Record the PSV of the inflow artery, 2 cm distal to the arterial anastomosis. Determine flow direction to check for steal syndrome.

– Record the highest PSV at the arterial anastomosis.

– The access created should run in a straight line. Record several representative samples of flow within the body of the graft and measure the highest PSV.

– Using small probe manipulations, capture an image of the body of the graft as it connects to the venous anastomosis. Record the highest PSV at the venous anastomosis. Observe for any lumenal reduction or other abnormality.

• Record images with color flow on and off at the venous anastomosis. Use either a longitudinal or transverse approach depending on the angulation at the anastomosis. Observe for any lumenal reduction or other abnormality.

• Record the PSV of the venous outflow (efferent vein) in the longitudinal plane.

– If the cephalic vein is the outflow, evaluate the cephalic-subclavian venous confluence. Record images of the confluence with color flow on and off. Record sample waveforms from this site and assess for spontaneity, phasicity and augmentation. Measure a PSV if possible.

– If the basilic is the outflow vein, record images and assess PW Doppler waveforms from the basilic-brachial vein confluence and the axillary vein.

– Record PW Doppler waveforms from the subclavian and internal jugular veins.

– Record additional velocities proximal, at and distal to any stenosis.

- Measure diameter of any aneurysmal dilatations or lumenal reductions at points of stenosis, thrombus.
- Determine classification of stenosis according to laboratory diagnostic criteria.

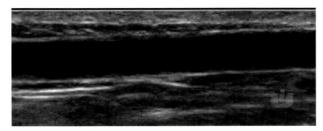

Normal graft with clear vessel lumen

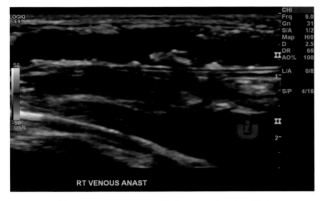

Abnormal access with lumenal reduction

Arteriovenous Fistula Protocol

Transverse Scan and Images

> There is a single connection between the arterial and venous system in these access types, the AVF anastomosis.

- Locate the anastomosis of the AVF in the transverse (short-axis) plane. Follow the fistula in transverse to determine its course.
- Record transverse views of the inflow artery, anastomosis and several representations of the outflow vein using duplex, with and without color flow.

Longitudinal Scan and Images

- Record longitudinal (sagittal) views of the: inflow artery, anastomosis and several representations of the outflow vein using duplex, with and without color flow Doppler.
- Return the probe back to the anastomosis and concentrate on the inflow. Rotate your probe onto the inflow artery above the anastomosis in the longitudinal plane. Record a longitudinal image with color flow Doppler on and off, using small probe manipulations to capture the inflow artery and arterial-venous anastomosis in the same image. Observe for any lumenal reduction or other abnormality.

> Be careful not to "create" a stenosis by putting too much compression on the outflow vein since these vessels are very superficial.

When recording peak systolic velocities (PSV) in the longitudinal plane with pulsed-wave (PW) Doppler, use a ≤60° Doppler angle with the angle cursor parallel to the vessel walls and a sample volume that is in the center of the flow stream.

- Record the PSV of the inflow (afferent) artery in the longitudinal plane, at least 2 cm proximal to the arterial anastomosis.
- Record the PSV of the inflow artery in the longitudinal plane, 2 cm distal to the arterial anastomosis. Determine flow direction to check for steal syndrome.
- Record the highest PSV at the arterial-venous anastomosis.

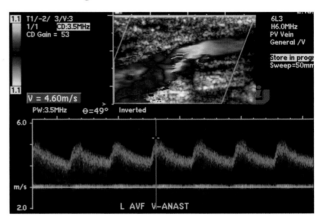

Spectral tracing at an AV fistula anastomosis

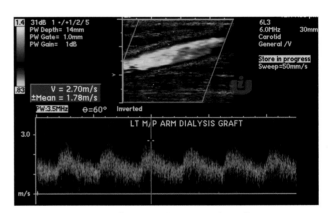

Normal efferent vein spectral tracings

- Record several representative samples of flow within the outflow (efferent) vein or body of the access and measure the highest PSV. Take several samples and annotate according to the anatomical level, i.e., "outflow-mid arm".
  - Assess for spontaneity, phasicity and augmentation. Measure a PSV if possible.
  - If the cephalic is the outflow vein, evaluate the cephalic-subclavian venous confluence.
  - If the basilic is the outflow vein, evaluate the basilic-brachial vein confluence and the axillary vein.
  - Subclavian and internal jugular veins
- Record additional velocities proximal, at and distal to a stenosis

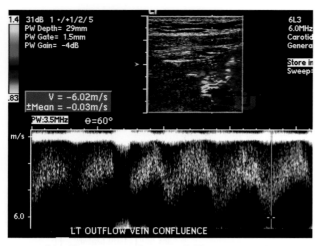

Significant stenosis at an AVF anastomosis

- Measure diameter of any lumenal reductions from stenosis or thrombus and any aneurysmal dilatations.
- Velocity increases can also occur in AVF conduits due to valve cusps. Determine if the velocity increase is significant by calculating the peak systolic velocity ratio (Vr) in the vicinity of the valve.

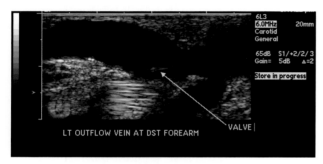

Valve cusp within an AVF

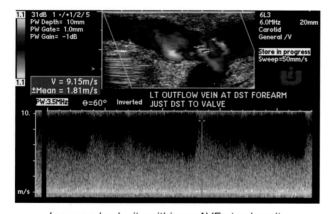

Increased velocity within an AVF at valve site

- Determine classification of stenosis according to laboratory diagnostic criteria.
- Measure several outflow vein diameters to assess for fistula maturity (e.g., distal, mid and proximal arm).
- Measure the distance from the skin to the anterior wall of the outflow vein. This can be reported to the dialysis center and may assist dialysis technicians when cannulating the conduit.

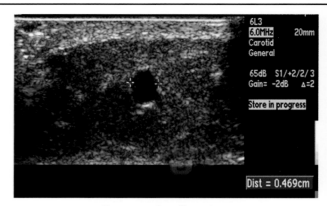

Pre-operative diameters

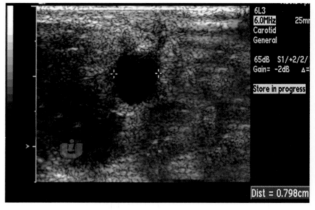

Post-operative diameters

*Transverse venous diameter measurements
before and after access creation*

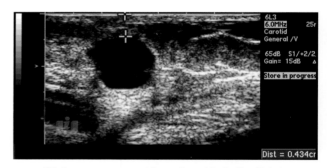

Distance measured from the skin to the fistula

Evaluation of Volume Flow

- Calculate volume flow using a straight, non-tapering segment of the access. Activate the "time average maximum" calculation or its equivalent on the duplex scanner.
  - Measure the diameter of the segment, placing the calipers perpendicular to the vessel wall.
  - At the same location, open the Doppler gate to include the entire width of the vessel. Measure at least one cycle (PSV to PSV or EDV to EDV) on the spectral tracing to obtain volume flow (mL/min). Use complete cycles if measuring more than one.
- Repeat these steps in one or two additional areas of the dialysis access. Use an average volume flow or choose the highest value if all flow calculations are similar.

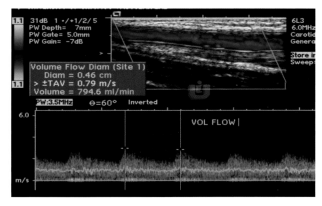

Volume flow calculation of an AV fistula

Evaluation for Steal Syndrome

- Obtain baseline photoplethysmography (PPG) waveforms and digital pressures in the affected digits. Additional evaluation of non-affected digits can be used for comparison. *For instructions, see chapter on PPG testing.*

- Repeat PPG waveforms and digital pressures while compressing the fistula or graft just beyond the anastomosis until you can no longer feel a "thrill" within the dialysis conduit.
- Compare pre-compression digital pressures and PPG waveforms to those taken during compression of the fistula or graft.
- Duplex imaging can also be used to illustrate steal syndrome.
  - Assess for retrograde flow in the inflow artery distal to the anastomosis.
  - Observe for large outflow venous branches. Measure PSV before the branch, in the branch, and after the branch to see how it affects flow in the fistula.

> *Be careful not to compress the inflow artery, only the graft or fistula just beyond the anastomosis.*

TABLE 70: Dialysis Arteriovenous Fistula Protocol Summary

Scan transverse (short-axis) with grayscale and color flow	Scan longitudinal (sagittal) with grayscale, color flow and PW Doppler
• Inflow/proximal to arterial anastomosis	• Inflow/proximal to arterial anastomosis*
• Inflow artery distal to arterial anastomosis	• Inflow artery distal to arterial anastomosis**
• Arterial-Venous anastomosis	• Arterial-Venous anastomosis*
• Body of the fistula	• Several points within the body of the fistula*
• Venous outflow	• Venous outflow*
• Cephalic (CV)-subclavian (SCV) confluence (if cephalic is outflow)	• Cephalic (CV)-subclavian (SCV) confluence (if cephalic is outflow)*
• Basilic (BSV)-brachial (BRV) confluence (if basilic is outflow)	• Basilic (BSV)-brachial (BRV) confluence (if basilic is outflow)*
• Subclavian and internal jugular vein	• Subclavian and internal jugular vein*
	• Proximal, at and distal to a stenosis*
	• Measure volume flow

* Record peak systolic velocity (PSV).

** Record peak systolic velocity (PSV) and check for flow direction.

Evaluate for dialysis access abnormalities. Measure diameter of any lumenal reductions and any aneurysmal dilatations.

Determine classification of stenosis according to laboratory diagnostic criteria.

TABLE 71: University of Chicago Diagnostic Criteria for ≥50% Stenosis in a Hemodialysis AVF

	PSV (V2) distal/ PSV (V1) proximal ratio*
Hemodynamically significant stenosis(arterial inflow or venous outflow)	>2.0
Hemodynamically significant stenosis at the anastomosis	>3.0

- **Occlusion:** Absent signal, No color saturation identifiable in an occlusion
- **Normal volume flow:** >500 mL/min

Source: Grogan J, Castilla M, Lozanski L, Griffin A, Loth F, Bassiouny, H. (2005). Frequency of critical stenosis in primary arteriovenous fistulae prior to hemodialysis access: should duplex ultrasound surveillance be the standard of care? *The Journal of Vascular Surgery*, June 41(6), 1000-1006

TABLE 72: Prosthetic Dialysis-Loop Graft Protocol Summary

Loop Configuration

Scan transverse (short-axis) with grayscale and color flow	Scan longitudinal (sagittal) with grayscale, color flow and PW Doppler
• Inflow/proximal to arterial anastomosis *	• Inflow/proximal to arterial anastomosis*
• Inflow artery distal to arterial anastomosis **	• Inflow artery. distal to arterial anastomosis**
• Arterial anastomosis *	• Arterial anastomosis*
• Mid arterial limb of graft *	• Mid arterial limb of graft*
• Mid venous limb of graft *	• Mid venous limb of graft*
• Venous anastomosis *	• Venous anastomosis*
• Venous outflow *	• Venous outflow*
• Cephalic-subclavian confluence (if cephalic is outflow) *	• Cephalic-subclavian confluence (if cephalic is outflow)*
• Basilic-brachial confluence (if basilic is outflow)	• Basilic-brachial confluence (if basilic is outflow)*
• Subclavian and internal jugular veins *	• Subclavian and internal jugular veins*
• Proximal, at and distal to a stenosis*	• Proximal, at and distal to a stenosis*

* Record peak systolic velocity (PSV)
** Record peak systolic velocity (PSV) and check for flow direction
Evaluate for graft abnormalities. Measure diameter of any lumenal reductions and any aneurysmal dilatations.
Determine classification of stenosis according to laboratory diagnostic criteria.

TABLE 73: Prosthetic Dialysis-Straight Graft Protocol Summary

Straight Configuration

Scan transverse (short-axis) with grayscale and color flow	Scan longitudinal (sagittal) with grayscale, color flow and PW Doppler
• Inflow/proximal to arterial anastomosis *	• Inflow/proximal to arterial anastomosis*
• Inflow artery distal to arterial anastomosis **	• Inflow artery distal to arterial anastomosis.**
• Arterial anastomosis *	• Arterial anastomosis*
• Body of graft *	• Body of graft *
• Venous anastomosis *	• Venous anastomosis*
• Venous outflow *	• Venous outflow*
• Cephalic-subclavian confluence (if cephalic is outflow) *	• Cephalic-subclavian confluence (if cephalic is outflow)*
• Basilic-brachial confluence (if basilic is outflow)	• Basilic-brachial confluence (if basilic is outflow)*
• Subclavian and internal jugular veins *	• Subclavian and internal jugular veins*
• Proximal, at and distal to a stenosis*	• Proximal, at and distal to a stenosis*

* Record peak systolic velocity (PSV).
** Record peak systolic velocity (PSV) and check for flow direction.
Evaluate for graft abnormalities. Measure diameter of any lumenal reductions and any aneurysmal dilatations.
Determine classification of stenosis according to laboratory diagnostic criteria.

TABLE 74: **Diagnostic Criteria for Prosthetic Hemodialysis Grafts**

	Peak Systolic Velocity (PSV)	PSV (V_2) distal/ PSV (V_1) proximal ratio	Diameter reduction
Within normal limits (0-49%)	NA	<50% increase	0-49%
Hemodynamically significant (50-74%)		>2.0	50-74%
Hemodynamically significant at venous anastomosis	>400 cm/s	1.9	
Hemodynamically ≥ 75%		>3.0	≥75%
Occlusion	absent signal		
• No color saturation identifiable in an occlusion			

Source: Mark E. Lockhart, M.D, Michelle L. Robbin, M.D. Hemodialysis Access Ultrasound
UltrasoundQuarterly Vol. 17, No. 3, pp. 157-167 © 2001 Lippincott Williams & Wilkins, Inc., Philadelphia

Interpretation

- Peak systolic velocity ratios (V_2/V_1) are used more than absolute velocities in most cases to determine the severity of stenosis.

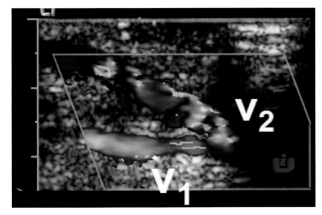

Example of velocity ratio points for V_r calculation

Normal

- **General grayscale and color characteristics**:
  - No lumenal reduction by B-mode image[7]
  - Color flow will fill the vessel lumen from wall-to-wall. [7]
- **Waveforms:** Normal hemodialysis conduit waveforms reflect high-flow states (a low resistance waveform with elevated peak systolic and end diastolic velocities).[7]
- **Depth:** A depth of less than 5 mm from the skin surface is needed for successful access of a fistula for hemodialysis.[2,8]
- **Peak systolic velocity and ratios:** PSV <400 cm/s is considered normal for both dialysis grafts and fistulas.
  - Dialysis grafts:
    - Normal PSV are 100-400 cm/s with EDV between 60-200 cm/s.[7]
    - A normal peak systolic velocity ratio (V_2/V_1) is <2.0.[9]
    - Normal PSV in the outflow vein is expected to be 30-100 cm/s.[7]
  - Dialysis fistulas: A normal peak systolic velocity ratio is <2.0. A ratio <3.0 is considered normal at the fistula anastomosis.[9,10]

- **Volume flow:** A volume flow greater than 800 mL/min is suggested for optimal dialysis graft performance.[11] A volume flow greater than 500 mL/min is suggested for optimal fistula performance.[12]

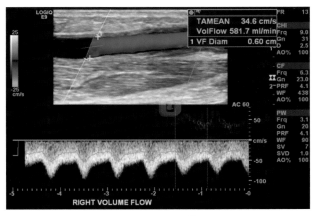

Normal volume flow

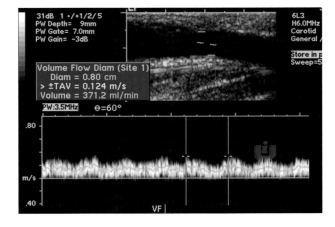

Abnormal volume flow

- **Arterial inflow:** waveforms should normally be low resistant above the anastomosis and high resistant below the anastomosis.[7]

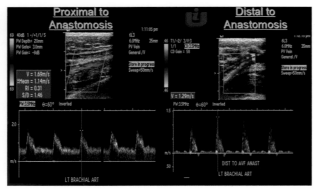

Typical waveform resistance proximal (low-resistance) and distal to the anastomosis (high-resistance)

Note: The patient's head is to the right in these images since the patient was reversed on the cart during scanning for ergonomic issues.

Abnormal

- **General grayscale and color characteristics**:
  - Lumenal reduction by B-mode image (e.g., intimal hyperplasia).[7]
  - High velocity color jet together with increased velocities and post-stenotic turbulence support the presence of a significant stenosis. Take care to note a diameter change in the vessel with lumenal debris that may explain an increased velocity in the smaller diameter section of the vessel.[7] Alternately, a dilated area will have lower velocities that increase as the sample volume is moved to a normal diameter segment of the vessel.

- **Waveforms:**
  - Decreased venous spontaneity and respirophasicity suggests the presence of obstruction (thrombus, stenosis, etc.) in the outflow vein.[7]
  - Evaluate the spontaneity, phasicity and pulsatility of the subclavian and internal jugular veins. Abnormal pulsatility, lack of spontaneity or decreased phasicity suggests central venous obstruction.[7]

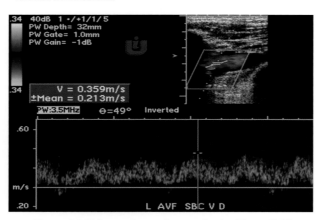

Normal SCV waveforms in a patient with an AVF

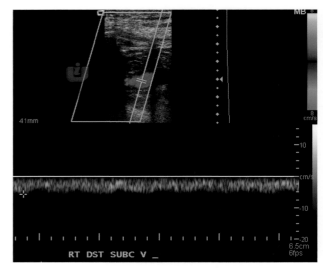

Abnormal SCV waveform with non-phasic, non-pulsatile flow in an AVF patient

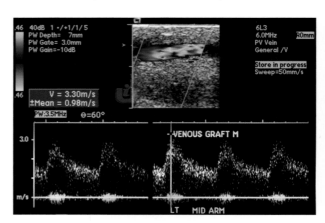

Stenosis in the venous limb of a graft

- **Peak systolic velocity:**
  - (PSV) >400 cm/s[9,13,14] **AND** a peak systolic velocity ratio (V_2/V_1) ≥1.9[9] indicates a hemodynamically significant stenosis (≥50%) at the venous anastomosis of a prosthetic graft.
  - A peak systolic velocity ratio (V_2/V_1) >2.0 indicates a hemodynamically significant stenosis (≥50%) involving the arterial inflow or venous outflow of an AVF.[7,10]
  - A peak systolic velocity ratio (V_2/V_1) >3.0 indicates a hemodynamically significant stenosis (≥50%) at the anastomosis of an AVF.[7,10]

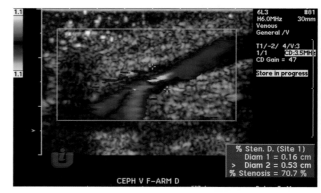

Significant lumenal reduction by color in an AVF

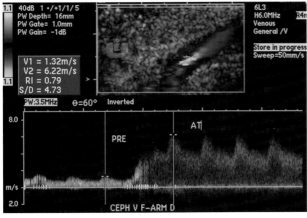

Significant stenosis by PW Doppler in
an AVF (pre and at stenosis)

- **Volume flow**: A volume flow less than 800 mL/min[11] may result in suboptimal dialysis graft performance. A volume flow less than 500 mL/min may result in suboptimal fistula performance.[7,12]

Access Occlusion

- An occlusion of the fistula/graft is present when no flow is detected by color or spectral Doppler.

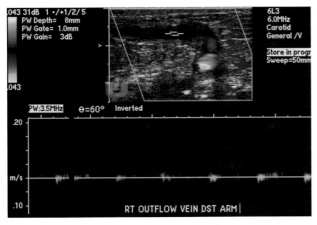

Occluded AVF by Doppler

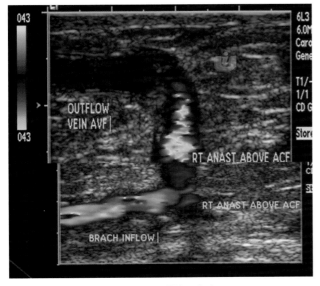

Occluded AVF by Color

Steal Syndrome

- When using PPG and digital pressures to evaluate the hand for steal syndrome, if there is a significant difference between the baseline digital *pressure* and amplitude of the PPG waveform compared to the post-compression pressure and PPG waveforms, there is an indication that the access is stealing flow from the hand.[15]

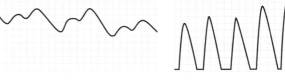

PPG at Rest
Pre-Compression
(50 mmHg/DBI = 0.47)

Repeat PPG after
AVF compression
(100 mmHg/DBI = 0.94)

- Flow reversal in the inflow artery distal to the anastomosis suggests the presence of arterial steal.
- A "side branch steal" is possible when an accessory branch of the outflow vein is at least one-third the diameter of the fistula. A significant reduction in velocity through the fistula after the branch and abnormal volume flows support the presence of a steal.[16] A large side branch may also prevent a fistula from maturing.[2]

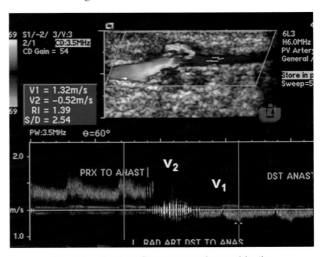

Steal by duplex: flow reversal noted in the
native artery distal to AVF anastomosis

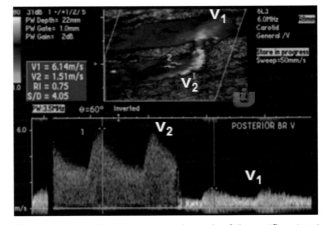

Elevated velocities in a venous branch of the outflow tract

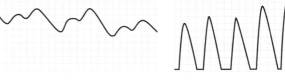

Additional Arterial Testing

Duplex of Arteriovenous Fistulas and Grafts for Hemodialysis Access

Other Pathology

- **Pseudoaneurysm**: A pseudoaneurysm is diagnosed when a pulsatile mass is identified by color and Doppler flow which is observed communicating with the access through a patent "neck". The neck/mass demonstrates a "to and fro" (pendulum) Doppler flow patterns to indicate a pseudoaneurysm. This may be difficult to assess due to the high flow states present in an arteriovenous fistula or graft. [17]

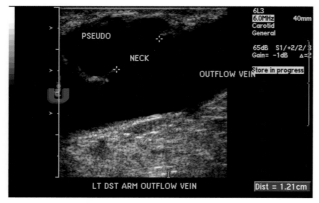

Pseudoaneurysmal dilatation of a dialysis graft

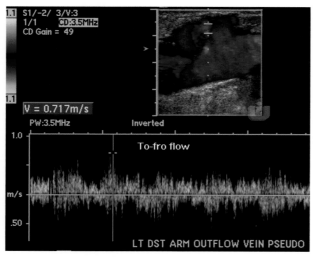

Spectral waveforms within the pseudoaneurysm of the graft

- **Aneurysm**: A focal enlargement with a diameter measurement that is at least twice the diameter of the proximal vessel indicates an aneurysmal dilatation. Aneurysms involving the arterial anastomosis of a fistula are a significant complication to be reported, as a surgical revision may be necessary. [8]

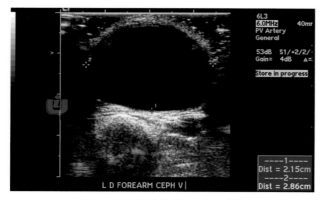

Aneurysmal dilatation of an AVF

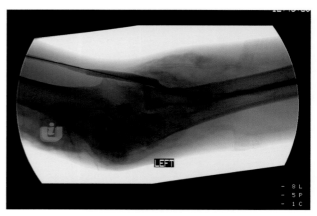

AVF fistulogram

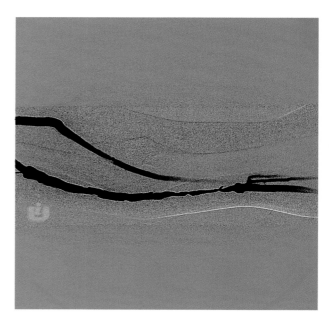

AVG shuntogram

Differential Diagnosis (for steal syndrome)

- Neuropathy
- Correlation
- Fistulogram/Shuntogram

Medical Treatment

- Modify risk factors (e.g., smoking cessation)
- Antiplatelet medication (e.g., aspirin)
- Anticoagulation (warfarin)
- Thrombolysis (acute blockage)
- Limb elevation

Surgical Treatment

- Open surgical thrombectomy
- Open surgical thrombectomy with patch angioplasty
- Pseudoaneurysm resection with interposition graft
- Bypass around a section of pseudoaneurysm
- Access revision (banding)
- Distal revascularization interval ligation (DRIL) procedure for vascular steal

Endovascular Treatment

- Intra-arterial directed thrombolysis
- High pressure balloon angioplasty
- Mechanical clot-removing endolumenal devices
- Stenting
- Patch angioplasty

Points to Remember

- The National Kidney Foundation has published the Kidney Disease Outcomes Quality Initiatives (KDOQI). These guidelines recommend that all dialysis patients receive regular monitoring and surveillance which can include duplex scanning to assess the anatomy and blood flow of the access.

- Obtain as much patient history as possible. This will make it easier locating the graft and is very helpful when multiple grafts are present. Many dialysis patients are good historians and they can usually tell you what conduit is currently being used during their dialysis session.

- Look for incisional scars on the extremity to give you a hint what type of access there is or where the anastomosis might be if a report of the operation is unavailable.

- AVF generally have a greater long term success rate when the pre-operative assessment has documented the absence of arterial disease (including a complete palmar arch) and superficial venous diameters >4.0 mm in the chosen extremity. [9]

- There is a maturation period of approximately 1-3 months before an access can be used for dialysis. [2,5,11,15]

- Studies indicate that the overall patency rate is higher for an AVF than it is for a prosthetic graft. [2-5,19]

- Studies indicate that there is a high success rate in AVF patency when the volume flow >500 mL/min and the outflow venous diameters >4 mm. [2,12]

- The most common sites for stenosis in a prosthetic graft are at the venous anastomosis [2-4] (>50%) or in the venous outflow tract (approximately 25%). Stenosis of the graft limbs, arterial anastomosis and central veins are less common. Multiple stenoses are possible.

- The calculation of volume flow assumes laminar flow was used. Significant error in calculation will occur if the segments used for measurement were aneurysmal, stenotic or exhibited turbulent flow patterns.

- Color Doppler can overestimate plaque and diameter reductions due to bleeding of the color flow. For increased accuracy, measure lumenal reduction in B-mode whenever possible.

- Pseudoaneurysms are linked with increased risk of graft thrombosis. They can also cause difficulty for the dialysis technician when accessing the graft. [4]

- Document potential fluid collections or "masses" around the access. Document pulsatility/non-pulsatility using color flow and PW Doppler with low scales. Measure anterior-posterior and transverse diameters of the "mass" and describe location and echogenicity (e.g., homogeneous, anechoic, etc.). No flow should be observed in a contained fluid collection. Noninfectious fluid collections include: hematoma, perigraft seroma or lymphocele. A typical location for a seroma is near the arterial anastomosis. [5]

- Venous hypertension can result if an access is placed in the same arm as a venous thrombosis, resulting in severe arm edema. [5]

- Duplex scanning of prosthetic grafts may be technically difficult 24-48 hours immediately post-op due to the presence of air within the walls of the graft, which ultrasound cannot penetrate.
- Some arterial steals can be asymptomatic. [2]
- Infection can occur at needle insertion sites. [5]

References

1. Pierre-Paul D, Gahtan V, Conte MS. (2005). Molecular biology and gene therapy in vascular disease. In Rutherford Vascular Surgery 6th edition. (172-192). Philadelphia. Elsevier Saunders.

2. Robbin ML, Lockhart ME. (2005). Ultrasound evaluation before and after hemodialysis access. In Zwiebel WJ, Pellerito JS (Eds.), Introduction to Vascular Ultrasonography 5th ed, (326-340). Philadelphia: Elsevier Saunders.

3. Lumsden AB, Bush RL, Lin PH, Peden EK. (2005). Management of thrombosed dialysis access. In Rutherford Vascular Surgery 6th edition. (1684-1692). Philadelphia. Elsevier Saunders.

4. Sidawy AN. (2005). Strategies of arteriovenous dialysis access. In Rutherford Vascular Surgery 6th edition. (1669-1676). Philadelphia. Elsevier Saunders.

5. Adams ED, Sidawy AN. (2005). Nonthrombotic complication of arteriovenous access for hemodialysis. In Rutherford Vascular Surgery 6th edition. (1692-1706). Philadelphia. Elsevier Saunders.

6. Hallett, JW, Brewster DC, Rasmussen TE (2001). Hemodialysis access. In Handbook of Patient Care in Vascular Diseases, 4th ed. (279-285). Philadelphia. Lippincott Williams and Wilkins.

7. Lockhart ME, Robbin ML. (2001). Hemodialysis access ultrasound. Ultrasound Quarterly. 17(3), 157-167.

8. NKF KDOQI Guidelines "Clinical Practice Guidelines and Clinical Practice Recommendations 2006 Updates Hemodialysis Adequacy, Peritoneal Dialysis Adequacy, Vascular Access". National Kidney Foundation. Retrieved from http://www.kidney.org/professionals/Kdoqi/guideline_upHD_PD_VA/va_guide1.htm. (12-7-2010).

9. Robbin ML, Oser RF, Allon M, Clements MW, Dockery J, Weber TM, Hamrick-Waller KM, Smith JK, Jones BC, Morgan DE, Saddekni S. (1998). Hemodialysis access graft stenosis: US detection. Radiology Sep 208(3), 655-661.

10. Grogan J, Castilla M, Lozanski L, Griffin A, Loth F, Bassiouny, H. (2005). Frequency of critical stenosis in primary arteriovenous fistulae prior to hemodialysis access: should duplex ultrasound surveillance be the standard of care? The Journal of Vascular Surgery, June 41(6), 1000-1006.

11. Back MR, Maynard M, Winkler A, Bandyk DF. (2008). Expected flow parameters within hemodialysis access and detection for remedial intervention of nonmaturing conduits. Vascular and Endovascular Surgery. 42(2), 150-158.

12. Robbin ML, Chamberlin NE, Lockhart ME, et al: Hemodialysis arteriovenous fistula maturity: US evaluation. Radiology 225(1):59-64,2002

13. Older RA, Gizienski TA, Wilkowski MJ, Angle JF, Cote DA. (1998). Hemodialysis access stenosis: early detection with color Doppler ultrasound. Radiology 207, 161-164.

14. Dumars MC, Thompson WE, Bluth EI, Lindberg JS, Yoselevitz M, Merritt CR. (2002). Management of suspected hemodialysis graft dysfunction: usefulness of diagnostic ultrasound. Radiology 222, 103-107.

15. White JG, Kim A, Josephs LG, Menzoian JO. (1999). The hemodynamics of steal syndrome and its treatment. Ann Vasc Surg. May;13(3):308-12.

16. Beathard GA: (2003). Aggressive treatment of early fistula failure in hemodialysis patients. Kidney Int 63(1):346-352.

17. Arshad FH, Sutijono D, Moore CL. (2010). Emergency ultrasound diagnosis of a pseudoaneurysm associated with an arteriovenous fistula. Acad Emerg Med. Jun;17(6):e43-5. Epub 2010 May 14

18. Bohannon WT, Silva MB. (2005). Venous transposition in the creation of arteriovenous access. In Rutherford Vascular Surgery 6th edition. (1677-1683). Philadelphia. Elsevier Saunders.

19. Voormolen EH, Jahrome AK, Bartels LW, Moll FL, Mali WP, Blankestijn PJ (2009.) Nonmaturation of arm arteriovenous fistulas for hemodialysis access: A systematic review of risk factors and results of early treatment. Vasc Surg. May;49(5):1325-36.

Definition

The combination of real time B-mode imaging with pulsed wave and color flow Doppler and/or systolic blood pressures to evaluate the penile arterial system.

Etiology (of erectile dysfunction)

- Psychogenic
- Neurogenic /neurologic
- Arterial insufficiency
- Hormonal imbalance
- Cavernosal venous leak/ venous insufficiency/ impaired venous occlusion

Risk Factors

- Hypertension
- Hypercholesteremia
- Diabetes
- Peripheral arterial occlusive disease
- Smoking
- Prostatectomy
- Hypogonadism
- Vascular surgery (e.g., aortoiliac bypass, etc.)
- Coronary artery disease
- Peyronie's disease (calcified plaque or fibrosis affecting the tunica albuginea)
- Spinal surgery
- Pelvic surgery

Indications for Exam

- Impotence
- Peyronie's disease
- Penile ischemia/pain

Contraindications/Limitations

- Duplex imaging is often difficult for a single technologist to perform without assistance to work machine controls due to the small arteries involved.

- Calipers for measurement must be placed quickly. Even slight movements of the probe can skew measurements during the process.

Penile Anatomy

- The penis is comprised of three chambers of spongy tissue:
  - The paired corpora cavernosa (a.k.a. corpus cavernosum) contains sinusoidal chambers comprised of smooth muscle which is partially responsible for changes in resistance within the penis. The spongy tissue in these chambers fills with blood during an erection.
  - A single corpus spongiosum is located on the dorsal plantar side of the penis. It surrounds the urethra.

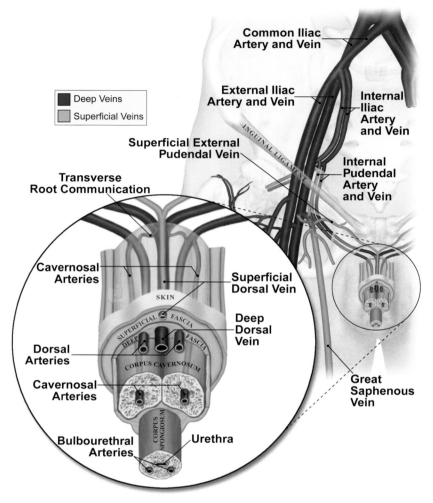

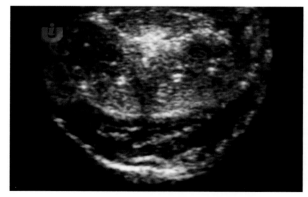

Penile anatomy: Transverse duplex image illustrates the three chambers of the penis

Arteries of the Penis

- The internal iliac artery (a.k.a. hypogastric artery) and internal pudendal arteries supply blood to the groin.
- The internal pudendal artery becomes the penile artery bilaterally. There are several terminal branches:
  - **Cavernosal artery**: responsible for transporting blood to the main erectile tissues of the penis (corpora cavernosa).
    - Right cavernosal artery
    - Left cavernosal artery
  - **Dorsal artery (a.k.a. superficial dorsal artery)**: responsible for supplying blood to the skin, corpus spongiosum and glans penis.
  - **Urethral artery** (a.k.a. spongiosal): responsible for transporting blood to the corpus spongiosum (urethral) and the Cowper's gland (bulbar).

Veins of the Penis

- **Superficial dorsal vein**: drain the blood from the skin
- The cavernosa is drained by the following veins:
  - Emissary veins
  - Deep dorsal veins
  - Internal pudendal vein
  - Hypogastric vein
  - Circumflex veins

Normal Fluid Dynamics

Normal flow in the penis differs depending on the physiological state.

- In a non-erectile state (flaccid), there is low resistance to arterial inflow because blood flows from the arteries to the veins of the penis through a series of pre-cavernosal AV shunts. Arterioles within the cavernosa are constricted at this point.
- As the penis approaches an erectile state:
  - Arterioles dilate within each cavernosum, so that resistance decreases.
  - Arterial inflow increases, resulting in a low resistance Doppler waveforms.
  - AV shunts start to close, resulting in an increased perfusion pressure to the penis.
  - Flow resistance in the corpora cavernosa increases and venous outflow drops.
  - There is an increase in arterial flow and a decrease in venous outflow.
  - Eventually the arterial inflow decreases, indicated by a high resistance Doppler waveform.

> *Increased resistance is needed to maintain an erectile state.*

Mechanism of disease

There are several mechanisms that may contribute to erectile dysfunction (ED); anatomical, vascular, neurogenic or hormonal. [1,2]

- Failure of the AV shunts to close negatively affects flow resistance. Incompetent veins allow blood flow to leak out of the penis, reducing rigidity. [1]
- Failure to maintain adequate arterial flow results in the inability to obtain or maintain an erection. This may be due to lack of inflow by the arteries, extrinsic compression or narrowing. [1]
- Lack of psycho-erotic stimulation, heavy smoking, the use of antihypertensive drugs, etc. may fail to produce the neurochemical reaction or parasympathetic innervations needed to produce erection. [1,2]

Location of Disease

- Cavernosal arteries

Patient History/Symptoms

- Impotence
- Penile pain

Physical Examination

- Palpation of pulses at the groin to identify the possible presence of PAD (poor pulses at groin may indicate poor arterial inflow/vascular dysfunction)

Penile Testing Protocol

There are several techniques used to evaluate the penile vasculature. They include penile pressures, VPR tracings and duplex imaging. One or more of these techniques may be used during an evaluation and may include the injection of a vasodilator.

Penile Arterial Duplex Protocol (with and without injection)

- Obtain a patient history to include symptoms and risk factors.
- Room temperature should be kept warm (21-24º C).
- The patient is examined a supine manner with the penis in a cephalad position.
- High-frequency (5-7 MHz) (8-15 MHz) linear transducers are used for imaging.

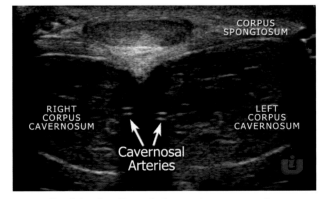

Pre-injection B-mode image-transverse view

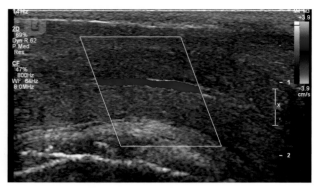

Pre-injection cavernosal artery by color flow

Pre-Injection Duplex

- Locate the two corpora cavernosa of the penis in the transverse (short axis) plane with B-mode imaging. The corpus spongiosum will be along the ventral side of the penis.

> *To help hold the penis still, you can drape a folded towel across to maintain stability.*

- Identify echogenicity of the tissue, looking for areas of high echogenicity, as the penile tissue less hyperechoic that the arterial walls.
- Record grayscale images in the transverse plane of the corpora cavernosa and the corpus spongiosum. Observe for similar size between the corpora cavernosa.
- Record grayscale images in the longitudinal (sagittal) plane of the corpora cavernosa and the corpus spongiosum.

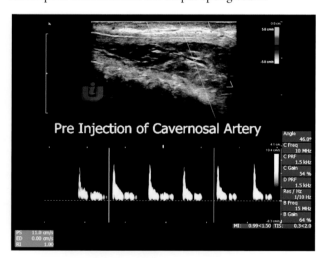

Cavernosal artery Doppler waveform pre-injection

- Record and measure the peak systolic velocity (PSV) and end-diastolic velocity (EDV) at the base of the shaft using pulsed wave Doppler (≤60º Doppler angle, with the angle cursor parallel to the vessel walls in the center of the flow stream) in the longitudinal plane of the:
  - Proximal right and left cavernosal arteries
- Transverse diameter measurements should be taken of the cavernosal arteries at the base of the shaft. Measurements should be taken near or at systole.

Duplex with Injection

- After intracavernosal injection of a vasodilator, (e.g., papaverine or proglastin E) the penis should be massaged by the patient to create an erection or place a 2-2.5 cm penile pressure cuff or band on the penis for 2-3 minutes after injection and then remove.

> *Normal erection time (duration) should be approximately 30 minutes.*

> *Response to the injection is enhanced if the dorsal vein at the base of the penis is compressed during the injection. If a poor erection is achieved, try placing rubber band oe penile pressure cuff at base of penis. If improvement is seen, a venous leak is suspected.*

- The physician will inject a potent vasodilatory agent into the cavernosum (e.g., 30 mg papaverine). [1] Only one side of the cavernosum will require injection due to communications across the intercavernosal septum.
- Record the PSV and EDV of the right and left cavernosal arteries for 20 minutes post injection in five minute increments (e.g., at 5 minutes, at 10 minutes, etc.). Color flow may be a useful tool to locate these arteries.
- The inter-cavernosal arteries which balance the flows to the cavernosa are the helicine arteries and are seen most clearly during the immediate post-injection phase.
- Transverse diameter measurements should be taken of the cavernosal arteries at the base of the shaft. Measurements should be taken at systole and compared to pre-injection values.

TABLE 73: **Penile Artery Duplex Protocol Summary**

- Record gray sale images of the corpora cavernosa and corpus spongiosum in transverse and longitudinal planes. Observe echogenicity of the tissues. Measure transverse diameter measurements of the cavernosal arteries.

- Record and measure the peak systolic velocity (PSV) and end diastolic velocity (EDV) in the right and left proximal cavernosal arteries.

If using intracavernosal injection:
- Penis should be massaged by the patient to create an erection or wrap a tourniquet or penile pressure cuff around the base of the penis. Inject vasodilator agent. Remove cuff or tourniquet after 2-3 minutes, post-injection.

- Measure transverse diameter measurements of the cavernosal arteries, post injection for comparison to pre-injection values.

- Record and measure the peak systolic velocity (PSV) and end diastolic velocity (EDV) in the cavernosal arteries post-injection.

- Determine classification of disease according to laboratory diagnostic criteria.

TABLE 75: Penile Pressures Protocol Summary

- Wrap an arterial cuff around the arm and obtain bilateral brachial artery blood pressures.
- Apply 2-2.5 cm pressure cuff around the base of the penis.
- Using a high frequency 8 MHz CW probe, locate the cavernosal artery.
- Inflate the penile cuff until the Doppler signal is obliterated, about 20-30 mmHg beyond the last audible arterial signal.
- Slowly decrease the pressure in the penile cuff at a rate of 2-4 mmHg per second. The pressure is recorded as soon as the first audible arterial Doppler signal returns.
- Calculate the penile-brachial index.
- Determine classification of disease according to laboratory diagnostic criteria

Penile Artery Pressures Protocol

- Obtain a patient history to include symptoms and risk factors.
- The patient is examined in a supine position.
- Appropriately wrap a blood pressure cuff around the base of the penis. Also wrap pressure cuffs around the arm for brachial pressures. Cuffs should be placed "straight" rather than angled. All cuffs should fit snugly so that inflation of the bladder transmits the head of pressure into the tissue rather than into space between the bladder and the limb, producing falsely elevated readings.
- Locate the right and left proximal cavernosal arterial signals using a high frequency (8 MHz) CW Doppler probe. (Use a lower frequency probe (e.g., 4 MHz) when needed).
- Angle between 45-60°, pointing the probe towards the heart.
- Manipulate the probe slightly to obtain the strongest arterial signal.
- Record several representative cavernosal artery waveforms.
- The following instructions can be used when testing with an automatic cuff inflator or standard manometer:
- Inflate the pressure cuffs 20-30 mmHg above the last audible arterial signal heard using the Doppler probe.

  - Deflate the cuff slowly (at a rate of 2-4 mmHg per second). The systolic pressure is recorded as soon as the first audible arterial Doppler signal returns. The Doppler pulse must continue after hearing the first pulse to assure there is an actual pulse rather than motion artifact.

    > *For patients with irregular heart beats, decrease deflation speeds.*

  - Obtain penile pressures using the right and left cavernosal arteries. Obtain bilateral brachial artery (BrA) pressures
  - Divide the highest cavernosal artery pressure by the highest brachial pressure to determine the penile-brachial index (PBI).
  - Determine severity of disease according to laboratory diagnostic criteria

Penile VPR

- Patient is examined in the supine position.
- Cuffs should be placed "straight" rather than angled. Choose appropriately sized pneumatic cuffs for each section of the limb:
  - 12 cm width; arm (some labs prefer a 10 cm cuff)
  - 2-2.5 cm width; base of penis

- Inflate the penile cuffs to approximately 60 mmHg.
- Record VPR waveforms using the appropriate gain settings. (Consider the factory recommended settings of the VPR equipment being used).

TABLE 76: Penile VPR Protocol Summary

- Apply a 10-12 cm arterial cuff around the arm and a 2-2.5 cm pressure cuff around the base of the penis.
- Inflate the cuffs to approximately 60 mmHg.
- Record VPR waveforms using the appropriate gain settings. (Consider the factory recommended settings of the VPR equipment being used.)

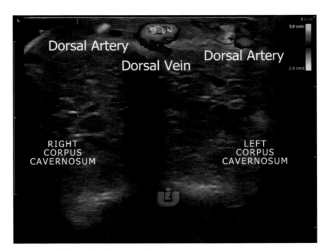

Dorsal artery and veins: transverse view

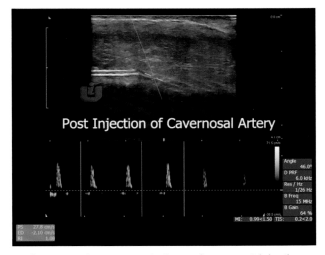

Cavernosal artery spectral waveforms post-injection

Interpretation

Normal

- **PBI:** A normal penile-brachial index is >0.75. [2,8]
- **Doppler waveforms and flow velocities:**
  - Cavernosal artery PSV >29 cm/s (post-injection) indicates normal arterial inflow adequate for an erection. [2,3,4]
  - EDV when penis is fully erect should be very low (<5 cm/s) or reversed due to the increased resistance during erection. [3,4]

– A difference in PSV of <10-15 cm/s between the right and left cavernosal arteries is normal. [4]

– Low systolic velocities and high resistant waveform patterns demonstrating absent or reversed diastolic flow should be observed in the flaccid state. [6]

– Biphasic waveforms (sharp systolic upstroke with diminished or absent diastolic flow) are normally observed after injection of a vasodilatory agent.[1,4,6] Waveforms may exhibit low resistant wave characteristics if full erection is not achieved.

– **Normal response to a cavernosal injection:** A low resistance waveform can be expected immediately post injection and may persist for 5 minutes. The diastolic component should exhibit increasing resistance to flow after about 5 minutes until blood velocities are <5 cm/s.

– **Diameters:** Arterial diameters should increase at a minimum 70-75% post-injection in the cavernosal arteries. [2,4]

• **General grayscale characteristics:** Normal cavernosal tissue echogenicity is relatively homogeneous. All areas of increased focal echogenicity should be noted. [4] The injection site will be echogenic.

• **Venous flow:** Venous flow in the dorsal vein is not normally observed during erection. [1,6]

Abnormal

• **PBI**

– Penile-brachial indices between 0.60-0.74 are considered marginally reduced.

– An abnormal penile-brachial index is <0.60. [2,8]

• **General grayscale characteristics**: Areas of increased focal echogenicity in the cavernosal tissue can indicate scarring or tunical plaques. [6]

• **Doppler waveforms and flow velocities**

– Peak systolic velocity (PSV) <29 cm/s (post-injection) indicates arterial disease, especially when the PSV <25 cm/s. [3,4]

> *PSV should not be used for diagnosis in men with duplicated cavernosal arteries; the normal PSV may be <30 cm/s.*[6]

– A difference in PSV of >10-15 cm/s between the right and left cavernosal arteries also suggests underlying arterial disease. [4]

• **Diameters**: An arterial diameter increase less than 70-75% post-injection in the cavernosal arteries indicates inadequate vessel compliance. [2,4]

Other Pathology

• **Arteriovenous malformation (AVM):** An arteriovenous malformation such as an AV fistula can occur between any artery and an adjacent vein and is characterized by color bruit on duplex image along with high velocity, low-resistant spectral waveforms at the same site by pulsed wave Doppler. [1,4]

• **Venous leak**: Venous flow observation by duplex during an erection suggests venous leakage and failure of AV shunts to close. Abnormal EDV published in the literature ranges between 4.5-8 cm/s. [1,4,5,6]

• **Venous thrombosis**: Intralumenal echoes are visualized within the dorsal vein due to thrombus and the venous diameters may appear dilated in an acute event. Confirm the absence of venous flow with pulse-wave (PW) Doppler when suspected.

• **Peyronie's disease:** Multiple bright echoes seen in both cavernosa is compatible with this condition. When echoes are limited to a single cavernosum, trauma may have been the cause instead.

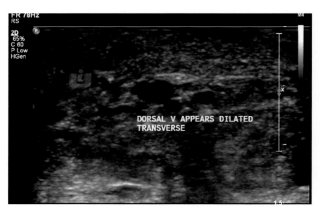

Acute occlusion suspected in the dorsal vein by B-mode image

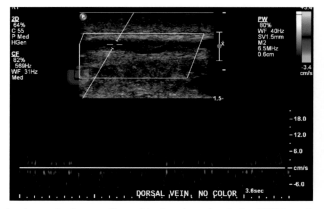

Acute occlusion confirmed in the dorsal vein by PW Doppler

TABLE 77: **Diagnostic Criteria for Penile Brachial Index**

• **Normal**: ≥0.75
• **Marginal**: 0.60-0.74
• **Abnormal**: <0.60

Source: Modified from Zierler RE, Sumner DS. (2005). Physiologic assessment of peripheral arterial occlusive disease. In *Rutherford Vascular Surgery 6th edition*. (197-222). Philadelphia. Elsevier Saunders.

Penile VPR Tracings [7]

The volume pulse waveform is primarily interpreted by its contour (shape) and amplitude (height).

- **Normal** tracings demonstrate:
  - Sharp upstroke
  - Sharp systolic peak
  - Gradual downslope bowing towards baseline
  - Dicrotic notch, however some patients may have inward bowing on the downslope
- **Abnormal** tracings demonstrate:
  - Rounded systolic peak
  - Loss of dicrotic notch [2]
  - Downslope bends slightly away from the baseline
  - Very low amplitude or flat, non-pulsatile tracing

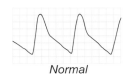

Normal

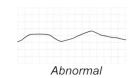

Abnormal

Differential Diagnosis

- Arterial occlusive disease (ipsilateral)
- Pelvic steal
- Arterial vasospasm
- Neurological/nerve damage (e.g. spinal cord injury, CVA, diabetic neuropathy, Alzheimer's or Parkinson's disease)
- Endocrine disorders
- Hormone deficiency (e.g., hypogonadism, thyroid disease)
- Psychogenic (e.g., anxiety, depression, schizophrenia, stress)

Correlation

- Angiography
- Cavernosometry
- Cavernosography

Pharmacology

- Vasodilators
  - Sildenafil (Viagra)
  - Tadalafil (Cialis)
  - Vardenafil (Levitra)
  - Alprostadil
  - Yohimbine

Points to Remember

- Successful erections have been documented with peak systolic velocities of <29 cm/s, and diastolic values at zero.
- **Priapism** is a painful condition of sustained persistent erection unaccompanied by sexual excitement. [9]
  - Priapism is a potential complication post injection.
  - Priapism is also a complication in sickle cell patients.
  - Types include:
    - **Ischemic** (venoocclusive, low-flow): Ischemic is the most common type and can be caused by pelvic vascular thrombosis, dorsal penile vein thrombosis, drug therapy, or may be idiopathic.
    - **Non-ischemic** (arterial, high flow): Non-ischemic priapism is caused by unregulated arterial inflow, such as an AV fistula. This may be due to a recent trauma to the vasculature of the penis. Non-ischemic priapism does not usually present with penile pain as a symptom.
  - While both types may lead to erectile dysfunction if untreated, ischemic priapism can be painful and lead to penile necrosis or gangrene.
  - Corrective actions for priapism vary by type. Ischemic treatment can include ice packs, walking, and decompression of the corpora via large bore needle aspiration. In more severe cases, a temporary shunt from the cavernosa to the spongiosum may be placed to provide a reduction in swelling.
- In erectile dysfunction cases that do not respond to pharmaceutical therapy, a vacuum device and constriction ring may be prescribed as a medical treatment. Surgical treatment may include an implantation of a penile prosthesis.
- Warm compressions applied to the penis can enhance visualization of the cavernosal artery.
- Cavernosometry in conjunction with injection of a vasodilatory agent is the preferred method for diagnosing penile venous insufficiency. [6]
- In patients with Peyronie's disease, scar tissue forms inside the penis causing pain in both the flaccid and erect states.
- Duplex and penile pressures are appropriate exams for impotency testing. Duplex imaging is the appropriate test for Peyronie's disease. Penile pressures are appropriate for ischemia and pain.
- Arterial duplex may also be used to help identify causes of priapism due to trauma.

References

1. Kornic AL, Villemarette PY, Baum N, Hower Jr. JF. (1990). Vasculogenic impotence: diagnostic application of color flow Doppler. *The Journal of Vascular Technology.* 14(4) 173-179.
2. DePalma RG. (2005). Vasculogenic erectile dysfunction. In *Rutherford Vascular Surgery 6th edition.* (1261-1270). Philadelphia. Elsevier Saunders.
3. DePalma RG, Schwab FJ, Emsellem HA, et al. (1990) Non-invasive assessment of impotence. *Surg Clinics N America.* Feb: 70(1) (119-132).
4. Hattery RR, King BF, Lewis RW, James M, McKusick MA. (1991). Vasculogenic impotence. *Contemporary Uroradiology.* 29(3). (629-645).
5. Bassiouny HB, Levine LA. (1991). Penile duplex sonography in the diagnosis of venogenic impotence. *The Journal of Vascular Surgery.* 13 (75-83).
6. Zwiebel WJ, Benson CB, Doubilet PM. Duplex ultrasound evaluation of the male genitalia. In Zwiebel WJ, Pellerito JS (Eds.), *Introduction to Vascular Ultrasonography 5th ed.* (659-684). Philadelphia: Elsevier Saunder
7. Kempczinski RF. (1982). Segmental volume plethysmography: The pulse volume recorder. In: Kempczinski RF and Yao SJS. Practical Non-invasive Vascular Diagnosis. (105--117). Chicago: Yearbook Medical.
8. Zierler RE, Sumner DS. (2005). Physiologic assessment of peripheral arterial occlusive disease. In Rutherford Vascular Surgery 6th edition. (197-222). Philadelphia. Elsevier Saunders.
9. Bassett J, Rajfer J. (2010). Diagnostic and therapeutic options for the management of ischemic and nonischemic priapism *Rev Urol.* 12(1): (56–63).

Venous Testing
Lower Extremity Venous Duplex Ultrasound

The combination of real time B-mode ultrasonography with pulsed wave Doppler and color flow to evaluate the lower extremity veins for evidence of thrombus

Etiology (of venous thrombosis)
- The theory of Virchow's Triad states that venous thrombosis is caused by venous stasis, vein wall (intimal) injury or a hypercoaguable state.
- Varicose veins
- Extrinsic compression

Risk Factors
- Age (greater with advanced age)
- Immobilization
- Genetic prothrombotic conditions (clotting disorders, such as Factor V Leiden)
- Post-operative phase (especially after orthopedic surgery)
- Central venous or femoral catheters
- Female
- Pregnancy
- Oral contraceptives
- Estrogen replacement
- Cancer/malignancy
- Previous DVT
- Heart complications (MI, CHF, etc.)
- Obesity

Family history
- Smoking
- COPD
- Blood type (highest risk with type-A lowest risk with type-O)
- Trauma
- Antiphospholipid antibodies (lupus, etc.)
- Occupations requiring long period of standing or sitting
- Varicose veins
- Congenital abnormalities (Klippel-Trenaunay)
- Inflammatory bowel disease
- Drug abuse
- Cerebrovascular events (stroke, TIA)
- May-Thurner syndrome

Indications for Exam
- Edema/swelling (especially when unilateral)
- Limb pain/tenderness
- Symptoms of pulmonary embolism (PE) (shortness of breath, chest pain, hemoptysis)
- Ulceration (esp., gaiter area)
- Discoloration at the gaiter area
- Varicose veins
- Hypercoaguable state

- Pallor (phlegmasia alba dolens)
- Cyanosis (phlegmasia cerulea dolens)
- Positive D-dimer test result

Contraindications/Limitations
- Poor visualization due to vessel depth because of obesity or severe edema
- Open wounds prohibiting access by the ultrasound probe
- Casts that cannot be removed or traction that limits access to the scan areas
- Patients who cannot be adequately positioned

Mechanism of disease [1,2]
There are three factors responsible for the formation of venous thrombosis, as outlined in Virchow's Triad: (vein wall injury, hypercoagulability and stasis of blood flow). A combination of any of these events may increase the risk of venous thrombosis.

- There is a balance between coagulation (process to prevent excessive bleeding after injury) and anticoagulation (process to prevent spontaneous intravascular clotting) in normal blood flow.
- The venous endothelial layer is normally antithrombotic. In response to endothelial injury, leukocytes (white blood cells) attach to the vessel wall. A plasma protein known as prothrombin is activated. Prothrombin activator catalyzes conversion of prothrombin into thrombin. Thrombin acts as an enzyme to convert fibrinogen into fibrin threads, forming a clot.
- Hypercoaguable states result from genetic mutation or acquired deficiencies that accompany certain diseases (e.g., liver disease). In such cases, naturally occurring anticoagulants (antithrombin, protein C, protein S, etc.) are deficient. For example, the genetic mutation, factor V Leiden, causes resistance to the natural anticoagulant protein C.
- Non-movement of blood flow (stasis) permits coagulation. Platelets are thought to become trapped due to flow recirculation behind the valve cusps. Platelets adhere to the subendothelial (collagen) layer of the venous wall and may aggregate depending on the amount of coagulation and thrombolysis occurring in the body at that time.
- Increased activation of coagulation factors in those suffering from cancer is thought to lead to formation of venous thrombosis. In addition, the levels of coagulation inhibitors normally found in the blood (e.g., proteins C or S) are thought to be reduced in these patients.
- Thrombosis in pregnancy is attributed to a prothrombotic state along with decreased venous outflow by the weight of the fetus. The use of estrogen (in replacement therapy or contraceptives) alters coagulation and may predispose an individual to thrombosis.
- Venous aneurysms are a rare condition. Research suggests several possible causes; either an increase or decrease in the fibrous connective tissue and elastic fibers or decreased smooth muscle cells and an increase in fibrous connective tissue. [3]

- Once thrombus is formed, it can:
  - **Stabilize**: Stabilization includes adherence of the thrombus to the vessel wall without changing location or propagating. If thrombus has formed, the most favorable occurrence would be to stabilize. This reduces the risk of embolization and PE for the patient.
  - **Propagate**: Propagation includes "growth of the thrombus" in size or location. Examples of propagation include a thrombus that extends from the superficial system into the deep system or from a calf vein into the popliteal vein.
  - **Shed/Embolize**: A portion of the thrombus breaks free and travels elsewhere in the vascular system. The greatest risk to the patient is that the thrombus travels to the lungs and results in a pulmonary embolus.

Location of Disease

> Thrombus located within the deep veins is known as deep venous thrombosis (DVT). Thrombus located within the superficial veins is known as superficial thrombosis.

- Although any venous site can develop thrombus, common origins include:
  - Muscular veins (gastrocnemius and soleal sinus)
  - Valve sites
  - Venous confluences
  - Deep venous system (common femoral, deep femoral, femoral, popliteal, peroneal, posterior tibial, inferior vena cava and iliac veins)
  - Superficial venous system (great and small saphenous)
  - Perforators

Patient History

- Acute onset of leg pain
- Acute onset of swelling
- Persistent leg/calf swelling (usually unilateral, but can be bilateral)
- Symptoms of PE (e.g., shortness of breath, chest pain, hemoptysis)
- Previous DVT
- Clotting issues (including problems regulating anticoagulation therapy, malignant cancer)

- Recent periods of immobilization (e.g., bed rest, long plane or car ride)
- Post-operative; orthopedic or neurosurgery for example, (can occur anytime during surgery or for 6 months thereafter)

Physical Examination

- Edema or swelling
- Tenderness
- Limb redness or warmth (superficial thrombophlebitis)
- Varicose veins
- Hyperpigmentation, hardened tissue around the ankles
- Ulceration (esp., gaiter area)
- Pallor (phlegmasia alba dolens)
- Cyanosis (phlegmasia cerulea dolens)

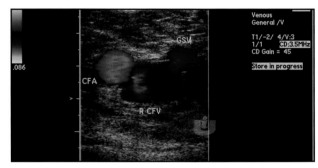

Partially occlusive thrombus in the common femoral vein at the saphenofemoral junction

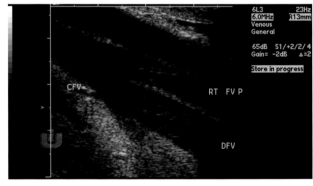

Femoral bifurcation with free-floating thrombus in both the proximal femoral and deep femoral veins

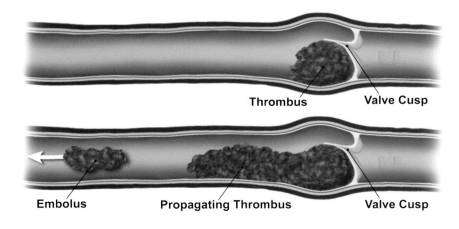

Thrombosis of vein. Should any of a thrombus "shed" itself upstream, an embolism may result.

Thrombus   Valve Cusp

Embolus   Propagating Thrombus   Valve Cusp

Dual Screen Vein Compression

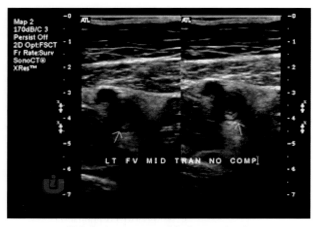

Totally incompressible femoral vein

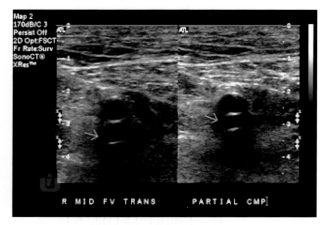

Partially compressible femoral vein

Lower Extremity Venous Duplex Protocol

- Obtain a patient history to include symptoms and risk factors.
- The patient is examined in the supine position with the head elevated. Placing the bed in reverse Trendelenburg position may optimize the exam by increasing the size of the calf veins when visualization is difficult.
- Some patients may require the use of a range of transducers, including high-frequency (5-7 MHz) (8-15 MHz) transducers and a lower frequency (1-4 MHz) transducer.

> *Keep the probe at a 90° angle to the skin for the best grayscale images.*

Transverse Scan and Images

- Locate the common femoral vein and artery at the groin above the saphenofemoral junction in the transverse (short axis) plane. The vein should collapse with light to moderate probe pressure, while the artery remains open. Observe for complete collapse of the vein walls upon compression.

> *Vein compression at the distal thigh is sometimes difficult. Try placing one hand under the thigh while compressing the vein with the probe or push your hand up against the probe to compress the veins.*

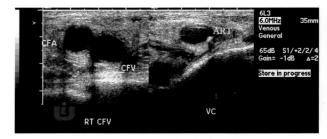

Dual screen: normal vein wall collapse

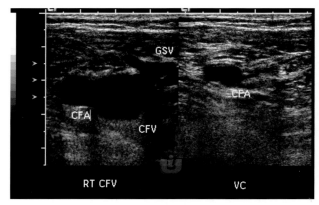

Dual screen: saphenofemoral junction compression

- Veins can usually be imaged from a medial view. Move the probe distally performing venous compression in the transverse plane every 2-4 cm along the limb while watching for full coaptation of the vein walls.
- Record transverse images using "dual-screen" on the duplex scanner. Obtain and freeze an image without vein compression on the left side of the screen. Capture an image with vein compression on the right side of the screen. Document transverse images of the following veins with and without compressions as described above:
  - Common femoral vein-*above the saphenofemoral junction*
  - Saphenofemoral junction-image *includes the common femoral and proximal great saphenous veins*
  - Proximal deep femoral vein
  - Proximal femoral vein
  - Mid femoral vein

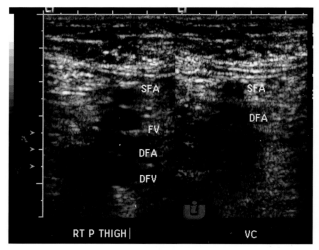

Dual screen: femoral bifurcation with compression

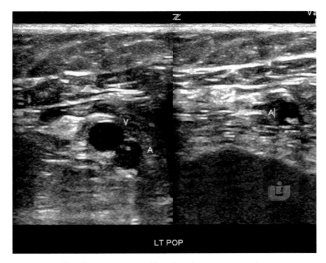

Dual screen: popliteal vein compression

– **Distal femoral vein**: try a medial to posterior approach if visualization is difficult or change to a lower frequency probe.

– **Popliteal vein**: move the probe behind the knee using a posterior approach to best visualize this vein. It is often best to start at the mid popliteal, at the crease of the knee and move proximally to the femoral vein and then distally to the tibial-peroneal confluence to cover the entire popliteal vein.

– **Posterior tibial veins**: place the probe posterior to the medial malleolus and use color flow as a guide to locate these veins alongside their artery.

– **Peroneal veins**: the peroneal veins can be seen using a medial view superficial to the fibula and deep to the posterior tibial veins. They can also be visualized using a posterolateral approach alongside the fibula.

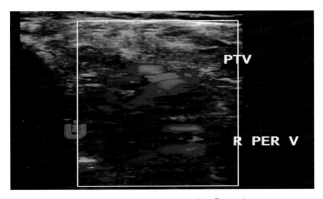

Patent tibial veins by color Doppler

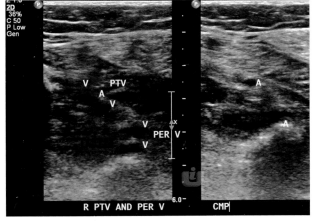

Dual screen: tibial vein compressions

– Additional documentation of venous compression can be performed of the common and external iliac, great and small saphenous, gastrocnemius, soleal or anterior tibial veins when appropriate.

Longitudinal Scan and Images

> *Use venous presets on the duplex scanner. Low color flow and Doppler scales will be needed to detect flow.*

- Return the probe to the groin and rotate onto the common femoral vein (CFV) in the longitudinal (sagittal) plane. Record images using color Doppler of the following veins:
  – Common femoral vein
  – Saphenofemoral junction
  – Deep femoral vein
  – Femoral vein
  – Popliteal vein

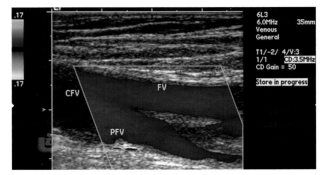

Femoral vein bifurcation

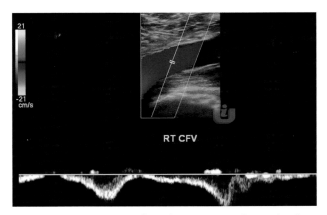

Normal spectral waveform in a common femoral vein

> *Some labs record venous PW Doppler waveforms without setting an angle since actual velocities are usually not important in a venous exam. If your lab chooses to set an angle, use a ≤60° Doppler angle with the cursor placed parallel to the vessel walls in the center of the flow stream.*

- Record images of the veins in longitudinal view along with pulsed wave (PW) Doppler. Spectral documentation should illustrate spontaneity, respiratory variation and augmentation. Document venous flow in the following segments:

– Common femoral vein: either above or at the saphenofemoral junction.

– Deep femoral vein (DFV): begin at the distal CFV and move the probe distally to observe the DFV deep to the femoral vein from a medial approach (patient's leg is turned outward).

– Femoral vein: the femoral vein courses superficial to the DFV from a medial approach. Capture an image in the proximal thigh or with the DFV at the femoral bifurcation.

– Popliteal vein: move the probe behind the knee and use a posterior approach.

– When necessary, additional documentation of patency can be performed of the inferior vena cava, common and external iliac veins, great saphenous, small saphenous or tibial veins.

– If veins are duplicated, PW spectral Doppler waveforms need to be assessed in each vein individually.

– Use PW Doppler to analyze absence of flow by placing the Doppler sample volume in any vein segment suspected to be thrombosed. Doppler flow or lack of flow, compliments compression, color flow and B-mode images. Use the adjacent artery as a guide to identify an occluded vein when possible.

– Repeat for the contralateral extremity if a bilateral exam was ordered.

• If a unilateral exam was requested, documentation of the contralateral common femoral vein with and without compression, as well as a venous Doppler spectral waveform, must be recorded for comparison.

TABLE 78: Lower Extremity Venous Protocol Summary

Scan transverse (short axis) with and without compression in grayscale and color flow	Scan longitudinal (sagittal axis) with PW Doppler
• CFV	• CFV
• Saphenofemoral junction	• DFV
• Proximal DFV	• FV
• Proximal FV	• PopV
• Mid FV	
• Distal FV	
• PopV	
• PTV	
• PerV	

• Additional documentation of compression and PW Doppler waveforms may be recorded in segments other than those listed.

• If venous compressions are contraindicated due to anatomy or patient discomfort, document patency with color flow and PW spectral waveforms.

• Document additional PW Doppler waveforms in all veins when dual (or more) venous systems are present.

Interpretation[9]

General grayscale and color characteristics

• Determine if the vein collapses completely with light probe pressure.

• Determine whether echogenic material is observed within the lumen of the vein.

Normal

• **Compressibility:** The vein is free of thrombus if it compresses completely and is free of intralumenal echoes.

• **Color Doppler:** Wall-to-wall color flow will fill the vein spontaneously or upon distal limb compression.

Color Flow Doppler

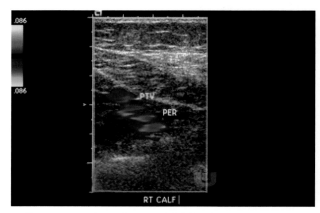

Transverse view of normal tibial veins with color flow

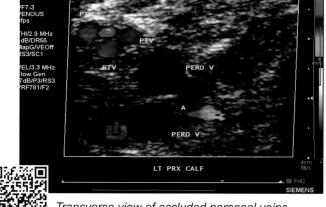

Transverse view of occluded peroneal veins with absent color flow

Abnormal

• **Compressibility:** Intralumenal echoes are visualized within the vein and full coaptation of the vein on manual compression is absent or limited due to thrombus. Compression of the artery with probe pressure can be a confirmation of an incompressible venous segment.

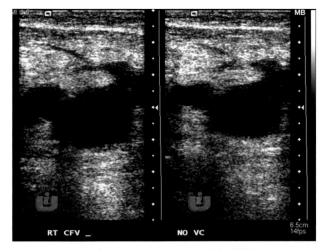

Dual screen: incompressible CFV

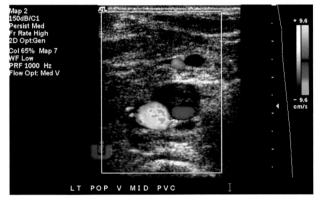

Partially occlusive thrombus in the popliteal vein by color flow

Color Doppler

> *Color flow can obscure a partially occlusive thrombus if the color gain is set too high.*

- If partially occlusive thrombus is present, color flow will be seen flowing around echogenic material in the vein, spontaneously or with distal limb compression.
- If totally occlusive thrombus is present, no color flow will be observed even with distal limb compression.

> *Use flow in the adjacent artery as a guide to identify an occluded vein. But always confirm absence of flow by placing the Doppler sample volume in the vessel.*

- It is possible for only one vein of a pair to be thrombosed. For this reason it is important to make sure all veins are studied carefully.

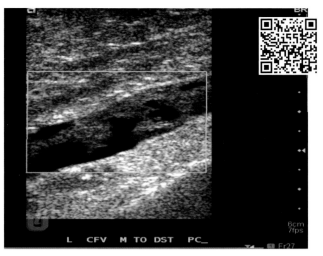

Partially occlusive venous thrombosis by B-mode

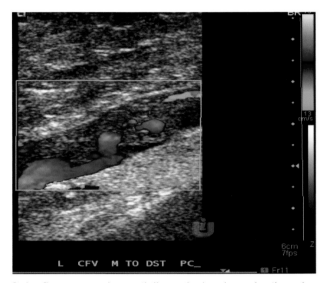

Color flows around a partially occlusive, irregular thrombus

- **Thrombus**: If thrombus is present, determine whether the thrombus is partially or totally occlusive, its location, as well as the extent and the characteristics of the thrombus [5,6]
  - **Acute thrombus**: Characteristics include medium to lightly echogenic or anechoic, spongy texture upon compression, poor attachment to the vein wall or "free floating" within the lumen. A moving tail may be seen at the end of the thrombus. When a vein is fully thrombosed, the vein is often dilated (in an acute event), especially compared to the adjacent artery. [1,3,7]

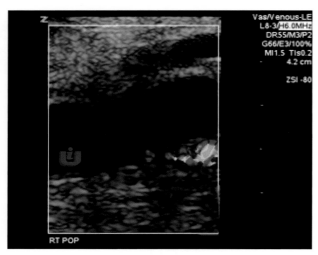

*Totally occlusive acute DVT documented
in the longitudinal plane*

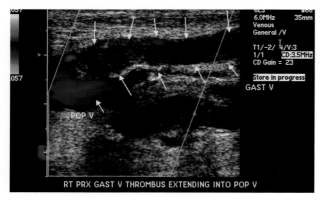

*Acute gastrocnemius vein thrombus
extending into the popliteal vein*

– **Chronic thrombus**: Characteristics include brightly
echogenic or heterogeneous echoes, irregular surface texture
and thrombus which is attached to the venous wall. The
vein can stay the same size as the artery, but often contracts
in diameter over time. Collateral veins may be observed
adjacent to the affected vein(s) and small irregular flow
channels within the thrombus can sometimes be seen
with color.

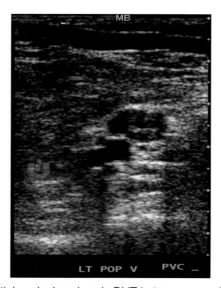

Partial occlusive chronic DVT in transverse plane

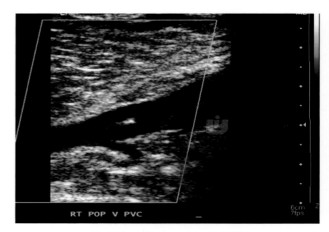

*Partial occlusive chronic DVT
in longitudinal plane*

– **Indeterminate age**: Characteristics of both acute and
chronic stages may be present, making age difficult to
determine. It is best not to guess.

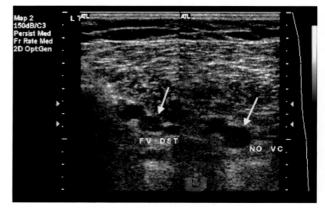

Dual screen: totally occlusive indeterminate age DVT

TABLE 79: **Thrombosis Descriptions and Characteristics**	
Acute	**Chronic**
• Light to medium echogenic/anechoic	• Bright/heterogeneous echoes
• Spongy texture on compression (homogeneous)	• Irregular texture (Heterogeneous)
• Poorly attached or free floating	• Attached
• Dilated vein (if totally occluded)	• Same size as artery or vein is contracted
	• Collateral veins may be noted

• Veins can be partially or totally incompressible in both
acute and chronic stages.
• Combination of events can occur (e.g., acute on top of
chronic thrombus).
• Chronic thrombus with partial recanalization is seen as
small color flow channels within thrombus.
• Age of thrombus is sometimes indeterminate.

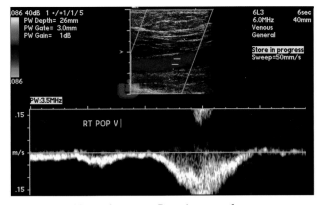

Normal venous Doppler waveform

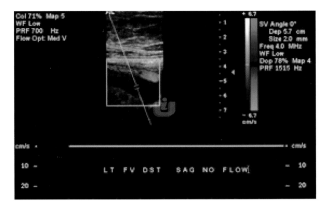

Occluded venous segment with absent color and PW Doppler

Venous Doppler observations

- Determine whether venous flow is:

  - Spontaneous (automatically heard with Doppler)
  - Phasic (flow increases and decreases with respiration)
  - Augmenting (increases) with distal compression
  - Pulsatile

Normal

- **Spontaneity:** The vein demonstrates spontaneous flow, especially in the large veins above the knee. In the calf veins, the absence of spontaneous flow can be a normal finding.
- **Phasicity:** Venous signals are phasic and vary with respiration and the cardiac cycle. During deep inhalation, venous signals decrease/discontinue and increase during exhalation due to changes in intrathoracic pressures during the respiratory cycle. In the calf veins, the absence of phasic flow is a normal finding.
- **Augmentation:** Compression of the limb distal to the probe augments or increases venous flow.
- **Pulsatility:** is absent in the lower extremity veins.

Pulsed Wave Doppler

- **Spontaneity:** Absence of flow indicates venous obstruction, except in the calf veins.
- **Phasicity:** Continuous venous flow suggests either obstruction from DVT in a proximal venous segment or extrinsic compression of a proximal vein.

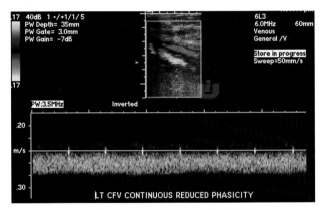

Continuous venous signal of CFV

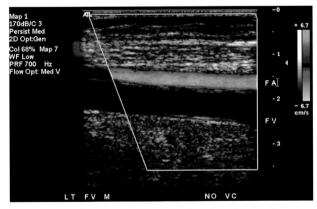

Occluded venous segment with absent color flow

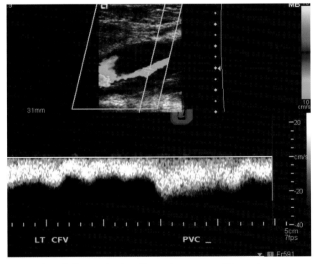

Partially occlusive thrombus can still produce spontaneous, phasic signal with augmentation

- **Augmentation:** If distal compression does not produce augmentation of the venous signal, a total obstruction distal to the probe is suspected. A weak or dampened augmentation also suggests venous obstruction distal to the probe. It may be helpful to change the patient's position and/or try compressing a more muscular area of the leg after giving time for venous refill.

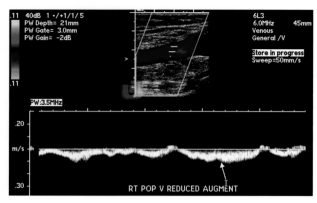

No flow augmentation

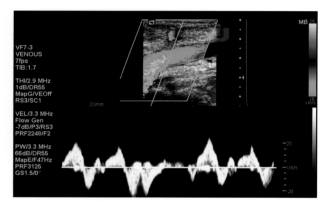

Pulsatile venous flow

- **Pulsatility**: Pulsatile venous flow is present when CHF, distal fistula and/or a hypervolemic state is present.
- A normal Doppler signal can be elicited proximal to a dual venous system when only one vein is thrombosed or if large collateral veins are present.

Other Pathology

- **Extrinsic compression**: Continuous venous flow suggests either obstruction in a proximal venous segment or extrinsic compression of a vein.
- **Venous aneurysm**: is diagnosed when there is an area of significant venous dilatation compared to the proximal venous segment.[3]

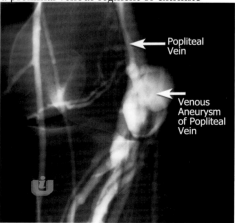

Popliteal vein aneurysm by venography

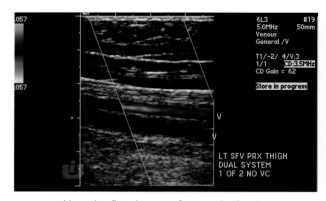

No color flow in one of two paired veins

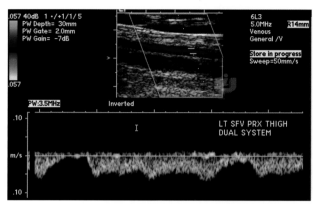

Doppler flow in only one of two veins of dual venous system

Differential Diagnosis

- Arterial disease
- Lymphedema
- Cellulitis
- Cysts (popliteal, Baker's, etc.)
- Extrinsic compression
- Hematoma
- Muscle tear
- Joint effusion

- Adenopathy
- Arteriovenous fistula
- Heart failure (edema)
- Direct injury to extremity
- Vascularized mass
- Collagen vasculitis
- Abscess

Correlation

- Venogram
- MRI
- CT scan

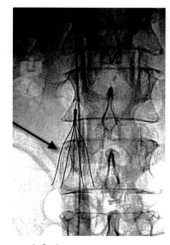

Inferior vena cavagram showing an IVC filter

Illinois State Medical Society

Are You at Risk for DVT?

FOR PATIENTS — Complete this risk assessment tool to find out.

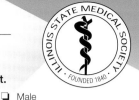

❏ Male
❏ Female — Today's Date _____

Name _____

Only your doctor can determine if you are at risk for Deep Vein Thrombosis (DVT), a blood clot that forms in one of the deep veins of your legs. A review of your personal history and current health may determine if you are at risk for developing this condition. Take a moment to complete this form for yourself (or complete it for a loved one). Then be sure to talk with your doctor about your risk for DVT and what you can do to help protect against it. Your doctor may want to keep a copy in your file for future reference.

Directions:
1. Check all statements that apply to you.
2. Enter the number of points for each of your checked statements in the space at right.
3. Add up all points to reach your total DVT Risk Score.

   Then, share your completed form with your doctor.

Add 1 point for each of the following statements that apply now or within the past month:

❏ Age 41– 60 years _____
❏ Minor surgery (less than 45 minutes) is planned _____
❏ Past major surgery (more than 45 minutes) within the last month _____
❏ Visible varicose veins _____
❏ A history of Inflammatory Bowel Disease (IBD) (for example, Crohn's disease or ulcerative colitis) _____
❏ Swollen legs (current) _____
❏ Overweight or obese (Body Mass Index above 25) _____
❏ Heart attack _____
❏ Congestive heart failure _____
❏ Serious infection (for example, pneumonia) _____
❏ Lung disease (for example, emphysema or COPD) _____
❏ On bed rest or restricted mobility, including a removable leg brace for less than 72 hours _____
❏ Other risk factors (1 point each)*** _____

*** Additional risk factors not tested in the validation studies but shown in the literature to be associated with thrombosis include BMI above 40, smoking, diabetes requiring insulin, chemotherapy, blood transfusions, and length of surgery over 2 hours.

For women only: Add 1 point for each of the following statements that apply:

❏ Current use of birth control or Hormone Replacement Therapy (HRT) _____
❏ Pregnant or had a baby within the last month _____
❏ History of unexplained stillborn infant, recurrent spontaneous abortion (more than 3), premature birth with toxemia or growth restricted infant. _____

Add 2 points for each of the following statements that apply:

❏ Age 61–74 years _____
❏ Current or past malignancies (excluding skin cancer, but not melanoma) _____
❏ Planned major surgery lasting longer than 45 minutes (including laparoscopic and arthroscopic) _____
❏ Non-removable plaster cast or mold that has kept you from moving your leg within the last month _____
❏ Tube in blood vessel in neck or chest that delivers blood or medicine directly to heart within the last month (also called central venous access, PICC line, or port) _____
❏ Confined to a bed for 72 hours or more _____

Add 3 points for each of the following statements that apply:

❏ Age 75 or over _____
❏ History of blood clots, either Deep Vein Thrombosis (DVT) or Pulmonary Embolism (PE) _____
❏ Family history of blood clots (thrombosis) _____
❏ Personal or family history of positive blood test indicating an increased risk of blood clotting _____

Add 5 points for each of the following statements that apply now or within the past month:

❏ Elective hip or knee joint replacement surgery _____
❏ Broken hip, pelvis or leg _____
❏ Serious trauma (for example, multiple broken bones due to a fall or car accident) _____
❏ Spinal cord injury resulting in paralysis _____
❏ Experienced a stroke _____

Add up all your points to get your total Caprini DVT Risk Score [_____]

What does your Caprini DVT Risk Score mean?
- Risk scores may indicate your odds of developing a DVT during major surgery or while being hospitalized for a serious illness.
- Airplane passengers who fly more than five hours may also be at risk for DVT.

- Studies have shown if you have 0-2 risk factors, your DVT risk is small. This risk increases with the presence of more risk factors.
- Please share this information with your doctor who can determine your DVT risk by evaluating all of these factors.

For more information call ISMS at 1-800-782-4767, ext. 1678

www.isms.org

Adapted with permission. Our thanks to ISMS member, J. A. Caprini, MD, associated with NorthShore University HealthSystem
February 2013

Venous Testing

Lower Extremity Venous Duplex Ultrasound

Medical Treatment and Prevention

- Anticoagulation therapy (e.g., heparin, warfarin)
- DVT prophylaxis (e.g., intermittent pneumatic cuff compression)
- Limit long periods of inactivity
- Promote venous return (e.g., elevate legs, wear elastic stockings/support hose)
- Compression bandaging (for ulceration)

Surgical Treatment

- IVC filter (acute DVT)
- Iliofemoral venous thrombectomy
- Bypass grafting (caval occlusion)
- Surgical ligation/excision/bypass (aneurysms)

Endovascular Treatment

- Catheter-directed thrombolysis with Urokinase, etc. (acute DVT)
- Balloon venoplasty and stenting (chronic iliofemoral DVT)
- Mechanical thrombectomy-such as Angiojet (acute DVT)

TABLE 81: Diagnostic Criteria for Venous Duplex	
Normal	**Abnormal**
• Complete coaptation of vein walls with light probe pressure	• Lack of complete vein compression
• Absent intralumenal thrombus	• Intralumenal echoes present (acute thrombus can be echolucent)
• Color flow fills the lumen completely	• Decrease or absence of color flow
• Normal venous Doppler spontaneity, phasicity and augmentation	• Abnormal venous Doppler spontaneity, phasicity or augmentation
• No venous dilatation	• Dilated or contracted veins noted

Points to Remember

- Venous duplex ultrasound can identify the presence, exact location and extent of venous thrombosis. The course of the veins, collaterals and thrombus can be visualized using B-mode and color while the analysis of Doppler waveform changes can estimate the severity of obstructions.
- The left leg has a higher incidence of DVT than the right leg. Since the left common iliac vein crosses under the right common iliac artery, it sometimes becomes thrombosed. This is known as May-Thurner syndrome. [11]
- Femoral and popliteal veins are commonly duplicated.
- Compressions should always be performed in the transverse plane to ensure full compression and so that duplicated veins are not missed.
- Dilatation of the lower extremity venous system can be due to venous or portal hypertension.

- Another patient position for scanning the popliteal vein is prone.
- The size of the vessels can also be affected by the position of the bed or the room temperature.
- Putting a patient in the reverse Trendelenburg position can improve visibility of small veins (e.g., calf veins).
- Upper extremity venous aneurysm are reported to be more common than lower extremity venous aneurysms. [9]
- Incidental findings such as superficial tissue edema or enlarged lymph nodes may be helpful in the report for the clinicians to understand swelling/edema in the absence of thrombus.

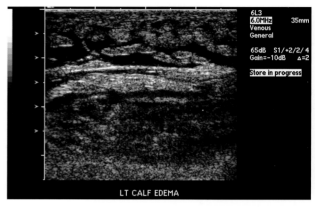

Lower extremity superficial tissue edema by B-mode image

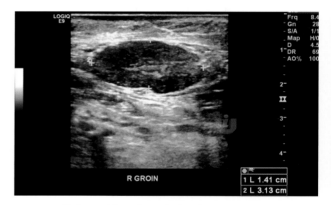

Enlarged lymph node by B-mode image

References

1. Wakefield TW. (2005). Bleeding and clotting: fundamental considerations. In Rutherford Vascular Surgery 6th edition. (493-511). Philadelphia. Elsevier Saunders.

2. Guyton AC. (1986). Hemostasis and blood coagulation. In Textbook of Medical Physiology 7th edition. (76-86). Philadelphia: WB Saunders.

3. Gillespie DL, Villavicencio JL, Gallagher C, Chang A, Hamelink JK, Fiala LA, O'Donnell SD, Jackson MR, Pikoulis E, Rich, NM. (1997). Presentation and management of venous aneurysms. *J Vasc Surg.* Nov;26(5):845-52.

4. Thrush A, Hartshorne T. (2005). Duplex assessment of deep venous thrombosis and upper limb venous disorders. In Peripheral Vascular Ultrasound, How Why and When, 2nd ed. (189-206). Edinburgh: Elsevier Churchill Livingstone.

5. Zwiebel, WJ (2005). Ultrasound Diagnosis of Venous Thrombosis. In Zwiebel WJ, Pellerito JS (Eds.), *Introduction to Vascular Ultrasonography 5th ed*, (449-465). Philadelphia: Elsevier Saunders.

6. Meissner MH. (2005). Venous duplex scanning. In Rutherford Vascular Surgery 6th edition. (254-270). Philadelphia. Elsevier Saunders.

7. Myers K, Clough A. (2004). Venous thrombosis in the lower limbs. In Making sense of vascular ultrasound: A hands on guide. (181-197). London: Hodder Arnold.

8. Dawson DL, Beals H. (2010). Acute lower extremity deep venous thrombosis. In Zierler RE (Ed.), Strandess's duplex scanning disorders in vascular diagnosis 4th ed. (179-198).Philadelphia Wolters Kluwer Lippincott Williams & Wilkins.

9. Sumner DS, Mattos MA. (1993). Diagnosis of deep vein thrombosis with real-time color and duplex scanning. In Vascular Diagnosis 4th edition. (785-800). St. Louis. Mosby.

10. Gloviczki P, Yao, JST (Eds.) (2001). Handbook of Venous Disorders, 2nd ed. (p. 38) London: Arnold.

11. Gloviczki P, Cho JS. (2005) Surgical treatment of chronic occlusions of the iliac veins and the superior vena cava. In Rutherford Vascular Surgery 6th edition. (2303-2320). Philadelphia. Elsevier Saunders.

Definition

The combination of real time B-mode ultrasonography, pulsed wave Doppler and color flow to evaluate the lower extremity veins for evidence of valvular incompetence. Chronic venous insufficiency (CVI) is caused by incompetent valves in the superficial and/or deep venous system and can result in venous hypertension and stasis.

Rationale

Reflux means to "flow backward". Venous reflux is venous flow moving in the wrong direction, either away from the heart or from the deep to the superficial system through the perforating veins. Duplex ultrasound can identify the presence, exact location, extent, and severity of venous reflux.

Etiology (of chronic venous insufficiency)

- Genetic
- History of venous thrombosis
- Venous hypertension, caused by valve damage or dysfunction

Risk Factors

- Age (greater with advanced age)
- Previous deep vein thrombosis (DVT)
- Female
- Pregnancy
- Obesity
- Family history
- Occupations requiring long period of standing or sitting
- Congenital abnormalities (e.g., Klippel-Trenaunay)

Indications for Exam

- Varicose veins
- Chronic edema/swelling which worsens at the end of the day (especially when unilateral)
- Pain, which may be localized to a specific varix or described as a "dull ache"
- Discoloration at the gaiter area
- Ulceration (gaiter area)
- Worsening pain on walking (with evidence of any chronic changes noted above) may be venous claudication.
- Restless leg syndrome

Contraindications/Limitations

- Poor visualization due to vessel depth because of obesity or severe edema
- Ulcerations prohibiting access by the ultrasound probe
- Patients with extensive bandages or casts
- Patient's inability to stand for an extended period of time or the inability to place the patient in a extreme reversed Trendelenburg position with available equipment

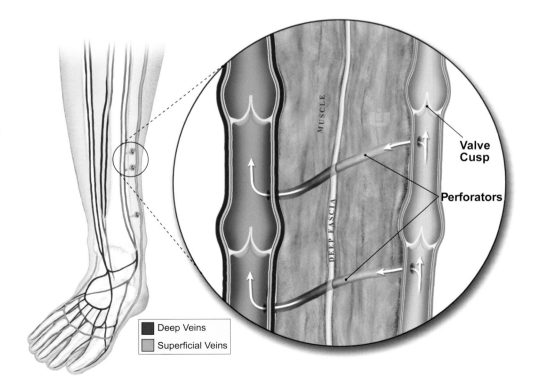

Venous Perforators

Perforator Venous System Anatomy (connection between the deep and superficial systems)

MUSCLE

DEEP FASCIA

Valve Cusp

Perforators

Deep Veins
Superficial Veins

> *Venous claudication is pain upon walking,
> which is relieved with leg elevation.*

Mechanism of disease

Venous Flow with Normal Valve Function [1]

- The direction of normal blood flow in the deep and superficial veins is toward the heart. In the perforating (communicating) veins, blood normally flows from the superficial to the deep veins.

- At various times, the blood may encounter pressure to move backwards away from the heart, for example in response to gravity. Normally, flow reversal is prevented by the venous valves which close in response to the pressure from the reversed flow.

- Upon exercise, the action of the calf muscles normally sends blood up the leg away from the calf. This action empties the calf veins, reduces the blood volume and reduces venous pressure.

Venous Flow with Abnormal Valve Function

- Valvular damage and dysfunction (valvular incompetence) result in *venous reflux*, which is venous flow in the wrong direction, away from the heart.

- In the perforating veins, blood flows in the wrong direction from the deep to the superficial system.

- Venous reflux creates a high blood volume in the veins distal to the incompetent valve(s).[1] High blood volume in a vein causes increased venous pressure (*venous hypertension*).[1] Hypertension will be greatest upon standing due to the effect of hydrostatic pressure from gravity, adding to the increased pressure from volume.[1]

- Normally, venous blood volume and venous pressure are reduced by activation of the calf muscle pump upon walking. When the valves are not working, the venous volume and resulting pressure do not reduce sufficiently and the patient suffers from *ambulatory venous hypertension*.[1]

- Venous hypertension also increases pressure within the venules and capillaries. This high pressure system encourages fluids to escape into the tissues causing edema. [1]

- Local edema results in a decrease in fluid and protein reabsorption. Fibrinogen and red blood cells (RBC) in the capillaries escape into the tissues. Proteins organize and form tissue fibrosis (hardening of the skin). The RBC's break down and cause hyperpigmentation (dark tissue discoloration). Oxygen intake is decreased in the tissues, causing tissue malnutrition/hypoxia. Ulceration may follow.[4]

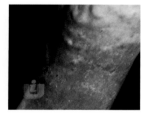

*Hyperpigmentation
of the distal leg*

Varicose Veins

- The pathogenesis of primary varicose veins remains unclear. Initially it was thought that varicose veins are due to valvular incompetence. [5,6] However, a current hypothesis states that alterations in vein wall structure (cells and extracellular matrix) cause weakness and altered tone, leading to valvular dysfunction.

– There is a decrease in the elastin content of varicose vein walls. There is also a change in the ratio of type I to type III collagen with an increase in type I (rigid, provides tensile strength) and a decrease in type III (compliant, increases elasticity). These changes undoubtedly contribute to the weakening of the varicose vein wall.

– The degradation of the extracellular matrix (ECM) is a function of matrix metalloproteinases and their inhibitors. An increase in matrix degradation would weaken the wall, while a decrease could promote ECM accumulation. Reports have varied on whether their levels remain the same, increase or decrease in varicose vein. [18]

– Interspersed in varicose veins are thick (two-fold thicker than normal veins) and thin regions (two-fold thinner than normal veins). [19] In the thick regions, smooth muscle cells are no longer organized in circumferential and longitudinal bundles but disrupted by an increased amount of fibrous tissue. The intima is thickened with an increase in smooth muscle cells. In the thin regions, there is a decrease in cell number. The adventitia is thin and lacks vasa vasorum. These regions correspond to areas of dilatation.

- Tributaries of the great saphenous vein (GSV) are thought to varicose before the main trunk of the GSV because they contain fewer smooth muscle cells in their vessel walls and lack support in the subcutaneous fat layer under the skin where they are commonly located. [1]

Pregnancy

- Pregnancy increases the amount of blood circulating in your system and causes veins to enlarge. The pressure of the fetus on the veins can decrease the blood flow back through the pelvic venous system.[1,6,7]

Location of Disease

Incompetent valves may be located at any segment of the deep, perforating, or superficial veins, but are more commonly found in the superficial venous tributaries. [2]

- Perforating veins in the gaiter area-medial aspect of the leg, just above the medial malleolus (most common)
- Saphenofemoral junction (SFJ)

Patient History

- Persistent leg/calf swelling (usually unilateral)
- Previous DVT
- Localized pain, burning or itching
- Tired, heavy legs after prolonged standing
- Symptoms can increase for women around menstruation.

Physical Examination

- Edema
- Tenderness
- Tenderness, warmth or redness along the course of a superficial vein or varicosity
- Varicose veins
- Hyperpigmentation, hardened tissue around the ankles
- Ulceration (gaiter area)
- Dermatitis
- Noticeable telangiectasia
- Severe, chronic swelling and symptoms of CVI (listed above) with pain/aching that worsens when walking and is relieved by elevation (venous claudication)

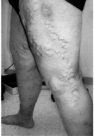
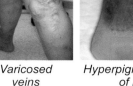
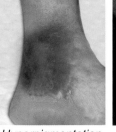
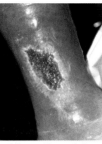

| *Varicosed veins* | *Hyperpigmentation of leg* | *Ulceration of the gaiter area* |

Images courtesy of Joseph Caprini MD, MS, FACS, RVT and Claudia Benge RPhS, RVS, RVT, RDMS, RDCS, FSVU

> *Superficial veins course within the superficial compartment, above the deep muscular fascia. A vein located outside of the saphenous compartment is known as a tributary and is not a main vein. It is important for the physician to know whether the vein in question is a tributary or within the saphenous compartment.*

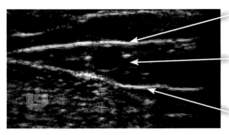

Saphenous fascia

Great saphenous vein

Investing fascia of the thigh

Fascial components of the saphenous compartment [8]

Lower Extremity Venous Insufficiency Duplex Protocol

- Obtain a patient history to include symptoms and risk factors.
- Patient is examined to rule out venous obstruction in the supine position with the head elevated or in a reversed Trendelenburg position.

> *Use "low-flow" machine settings to study the veins (low wall filter, color scale and gain sensitive for blood flow 5-10 cm/s).*

- Higher-frequency transducers (5-7 MHz) (8-15 MHz) should work well for visualization of the superficial and perforating veins, including their connection to the deep veins. Some patients may require the use of a range of transducers including a lower frequency (1-4 MHz) transducer for the deep veins.
- Before the assessment for reflux, a standard venous exam to rule out thrombosis is typically performed (see chapter on *Lower Extremity Venous Duplex Ultrasound*).
- The patient must be examined for insufficiency while standing or with the bed in an extreme reverse Trendelenburg position.
  - When standing the patient, use a stool or platform with a handrail. Have the patient hold the handrail and slightly rotate the leg outward. Then have the patient transfer weight onto the opposite leg.

> *Standing the patient on a stool makes it easier for the technologist to reach the machine.*

- The calf veins can be examined for reflux while the patient sits with their legs dangling over the side of the bed.

> *The superficial veins do not have a corresponding artery, which makes them easy to distinguish from deep veins.*

> *Deep inspiration followed by "bearing down" (Valsalva maneuver) creates an abrupt cessation of blood flow when valves close properly.*

- The *Valsalva maneuver* may be used during testing in order to increase intra-abdominal pressure and interrogate proximal venous valves for competency. This maneuver involves asking the patient to inhale deeply. While holding this breath, the patient will need to contract the abdomen. Ask the patient to release the breath and relax the abdomen after 1-2 seconds.

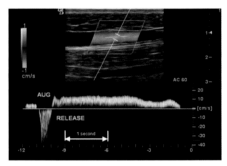

Venous reflux by PW Doppler
Image courtesy of GE Healthcare

> *Most ultrasound machines have a mechanism to measure time in seconds for the purpose of assessing the significance of reflux.*

- Record venous flow with color and pulsed wave (PW) Doppler spectral waveforms in longitudinal (sagittal axis) view at the following locations: (use the Valsalva maneuver and manual distal leg compressions to try to elicit reflux if it is present. Some laboratories use an automatic cuff inflator to further standardize the distal compression). [5]

> *Some labs record venous PW Doppler waveforms without setting an angle since actual velocities are usually not important in a venous exam. If your lab chooses to set an angle, use a ≤60° Doppler angle with the cursor placed parallel to the vessel walls in the center of the flow stream.*

  - Proximal common femoral vein (above SFJ)
  - Saphenofemoral junction (SFJ)
  - Distal common femoral vein (below SFJ)
  - Proximal great saphenous vein
  - Proximal femoral vein in the proximal thigh (*Note: there is often a valve just distal to the femoral bifurcation*)
  - Multiple levels of the great saphenous vein in the proximal, mid, distal thigh, at knee and proximal, mid, distal calf
  - Popliteal vein
  - Saphenopopliteal junction (SPJ)
  - Multiple levels of the small saphenous vein (SSV)
  - Giacomini vein (when visualized)
  - Any visualized perforating veins

> *You may turn the patient prone while scanning behind the knee. Use a pillow under the shin to put a bend in the knee and reduce pressure on the PopV.*

- Additional documentation of reflux can be performed as necessary of the tibial or other veins.
- Report the connection between the vein of Giacomini and the deep system when visualized.
- Report the location of any varicosed tributaries and where they connect to the great or small saphenous veins when indicated.

> *Saphenous diameters help physicians choose between various treatment options.*

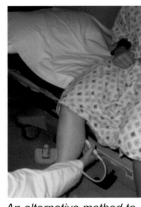

An alternative method to image the calf veins is to sit the patient on the side of the bed. Make sure the back of the leg or knee is not compressed against the bed.

- Measure several diameters of the main GSV trunk from the groin to the knee (e.g. proximal thigh, mid thigh and at the knee). A diameter at the saphenofemoral junction may also be a requested measurement. If a diameter measurement of the SSV is required, document this about 3 cm from either the popliteal crease or the SPJ.
- Physicians may request depth measurements between the main trunk of the GSV and the skin (top of screen) when considering certain treatments, such as radiofrequency ablation.
- Repeat for the contralateral extremity if a bilateral exam was ordered.

Alternative Testing Method

- Using pressure cuffs, a rapid cuff inflator and air source. Cuffs are inflate at various levels for 3 seconds while continuously recording a spectral waveform using a duplex scanner:
  - A 24cm width cuff is wrapped around the thigh and inflated for 3 seconds at 80 mmHg to test for reflux while imaging in the CFV, proximal FV and at the SFJ.
  - A 12 cm width cuff is wrapped around the calf and inflated for 3 seconds at 100 mmHg to test for reflux in the GSV, mid/distal FV, PopV, perforators and at the SPJ. This cuff is then moved to the ankle level and reinflated for 3 seconds at the same pressure while duplex is used to detect reflux in the PerV, PTV and SSV.
  - A 7 cm width cuff is wrapped around the transmetatarsal portion of the foot and inflated for 3 sec at 120mmHg to test for reflux in the PTV, PERV, distal GSV and any perforators.
- The normal response would be no flow detected during cuff deflation.
- An abnormal response would be retrograde flow during cuff deflation due to valvular incompetence.

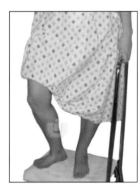

Instruct the patient to stand on a stool with their leg rotated outward and ask the patient to shift their weight onto the contralateral leg while the veins are evaluated for reflux.

- The reflux times of 1 second, 0.5 second and 0.35 seconds are typically used as diagnostic criteria.
- If the sum of venous closure time in the FV and PopV is > 4 seconds, severe reflux us suggested. [3]

Interpretation

Venous Doppler observations

- Determine whether venous blood is flowing exclusively back to the heart (normal direction).

Normal: No Venous Reflux

- Venous flow should be directed towards the heart (negative deflection of the Doppler tracing)
  - both during and after compression of the leg below the probe
  - during the Valsalva maneuver
  - during manual compression above the probe
- A brief period of reflux (<0.5 sec) immediately after maneuvers is most likely the normal amount of time for a valve to fully close. [2,9]

Abnormal Venous Reflux

- Abnormal, incompetent valves allow both antegrade and retrograde flow direction (negative and positive deflection of the Doppler tracing). Venous reflux (reversed flow direction) may be seen:
  - during manual leg compressions above the probe
  - upon release of compression below the probe
  - during the Valsalva maneuver, indicating reflux

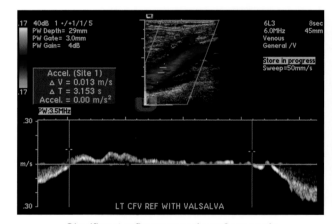

Significant reflux measuring >3 seconds

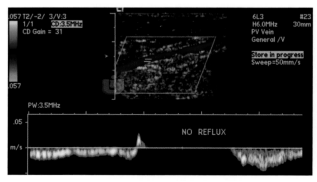

Normal valve closure results in a brief period of flow reversal

– Reflux is considered to be clinically significant when it lasts for more than: [2,8,10,11]

- 1 second in the deep veins (CFV, FV, POPV)
- 0.5 second in the tibial veins
- 0.5 second in the superficial veins
- 0.35 second in a perforating vein

> Some labs report reflux in milliseconds instead of seconds.

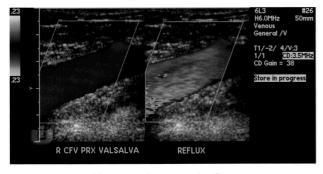

Venous reflux by color flow

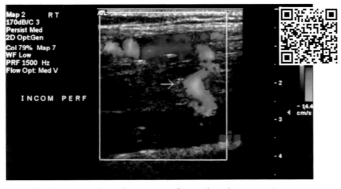

Perforator reflux-flow away from the deep system

TABLE 82: Lower Extremity Venous Insufficiency Examination Protocol Summary

Scan longitudinal (sagittal axis) with color and PW Doppler

- Proximal and distal CFV segments
- Proximal FV
- Saphenofemoral junction
- Proximal, mid, distal thigh and at knee GSV
- Proximal, mid and distal calf GSV
- PopV
- Saphenopopliteal junction
- Giacomini vein (when visualized)
- Proximal, mid and distal calf SSV
- Tibial veins (PTV, PerV) (when appropriate)
- Perforator veins (when visualized)
- Note location where varicose tributaries connect with saphenous veins.
- Measure necessary superficial venous diameters according to lab protocol.
- Additional documentation may be recorded as necessary in segments other than those listed above.

TABLE 83: Diagnostic Criteria for Venous Reflux

Venous System Reflux Criteria [2,8,10,11]

	Deep	Superficial	Perforator
Normal	<1 sec	<0.5 sec	<0.35 sec
Abnormal	>1 sec	>0.5 sec	>0.35 sec

Differential Diagnosis

- Lymphedema
- Cellulitis
- Deep venous thrombosis
- Adenopathy
- Arteriovenous fistula
- Direct injury to extremity
- Mass (including vascularized mass)
- Arteriovenous malformation (AVM)
- Collagen vasculitis
- Abscess
- Peripheral neuritis
- Stasis dermatitis
- Klippel-Trenaunay
- Skin cancer
- Arterial disease

Correlation

- Photoplethysmography for reflux testing
- Continuous-wave Doppler reflux testing
- Descending venography

Medical Treatment

- Promote venous drainage (e.g., elevate legs, wear elastic stockings/support hose)
- Limit long periods of inactivity
- Compression bandaging (for ulceration)
- Injection sclerotherapy
- Ultrasound-guided sclerotherapy
- Laser therapy
- Proper skin care

Surgical Treatment

- Ligation (e.g., of saphenofemoral junction)
- Venous ablation
- Stab avulsion phlebectomy
- Vein stripping
- Subfascial endoscopic perforator vein surgery
- Transverse repair of incompetent valves
- Subfascial ligation of perforators
- Ambulatory phlebectomy

Endovascular Treatment

- Radiofrequency ablation
- Transilluminated power phlebectomy (TIPP)
- Laser-thermal ablation

Points to Remember

- Approximately 25% of American women and 15% of American men suffer from some type of varicose veins (VV). Higher estimates have also been reported.[12,13]
- Approximately 50% of those over 50 years of age have VV. [7]
- Approximately 2-5% of Americans suffer from venous insufficiency.[14]
- Approximately 500,000 Americans suffer from venous ulceration. [10]

- If both parents had VV, there are estimates that there is a 90% chance of developing them. If you are male and only one parent had VV, the chances of developing VV is 25%. If you are female the chances of developing VV is 62%. Even if neither parent had VV, there is still a 20% chance of developing VV. [15]
- Varicose veins can occur anywhere in the body, though are most often located in the legs.
- There are several terms used to describe venous issues which are sometimes used incorrectly. *Thrombophlebitis* is defined as inflammation of a vein associated with a blood clot. *Phlebitis* simply means inflammation of a vein and can exist without thrombus.
- Superficial venous thrombosis can occur with or without inflammation.
- Studies estimate than 69% of patients with a history of DVT will develop chronic venous insufficiency within 1 year. [2]
- Radiofrequency ablation may not be a treatment option for saphenous vein diameters >14 mm in the thigh. Saphenous diameters <6 mm may not be amenable to radiofrequency or laser probes. [10]
- The distance from the vein to the skin should be 8–10 mm to prevent thermal damage during certain treatments. [10]
- Studies have shown that a perforator diameter greater than 3-4 mm is indicative of venous incompetence. [10]
- Dilatation of the lower extremity venous system can be due to venous or portal hypertension.
- **Klippel-Trenaunay** syndrome is a congenital condition characterized by port-wine stains on the skin, varicosed veins and excessive limb growth. Either one limb or multiple limbs may be affected. In some cases, deep veins are abnormal (e.g., absent segments, lack of venous valves and either smaller diameters or dilated veins). [16,17]
- A congenital absence of valves (as in Klippel Trenaunay syndrome) is extremely rare. When it does occur, it can affect the entire body or just the extremities (legs > arms).
- The American Venous Forum has developed a classification system for chronic venous disease called **CEAP** which categorizes clinical class (C), etiology (E), anatomic location (A) and pathological mechanism (P). Classification examples include: [2,11]
  - Category "C1" related to telangectasias
  - Category "C2" related to varicose veins
  - Category "C3" related to edema
  - Category "C4" related to skin changes, such as eczema
  - Category "C5" related to healed ulceration and "C4" skin changes
  - Category "C6" related to active ulceration and "C4" skin changes
- Birth control pills can increase the risk of varicose/spider veins. [7]
- Spider veins are not true varicose veins and are oftentimes thought to be related to hormonal changes.
- The number and severity of varicose veins can increase with each additional pregnancy. Varicose veins can improve postpartum.
- Putting a patient in the reverse Trendelenburg position can improve visibility of smaller veins (e.g., calf veins).
- The size of the superficial veins can be affected by the position of the bed or the room temperature.

- *"Outward flow"* may be another term used for reflux.
- *Lipodermatosclerosis* refers to a condition involving chronic inflammation and scarring of the skin and fat tissue due to chronic venous hypertension. The skin become darkened, smooth and often tender. [1,4]

References

1. Sumner DS, Zierler RE. (2005). Vascular physiology: essential hemodynamic principles. In Rutherford *Vascular Surgery 6th edition*. (75-123). Philadelphia. Elsevier Saunders.
2. Labropoulos N, Leon LR. (2005). Evaluation of chronic venous disease. In Mansour MA, Labropoulos N. (Eds.), Vascular Diagnosis, (447-461). Philadelphia: Elsevier Saunders
3. Zwiebel, WJ (2005). Ultrasound diagnosis of venous insufficiency. In Zwiebel WJ, Pellerito JS (Eds.), Introduction to Vascular Ultrasonography 5th ed, (479-499). Philadelphia: Elsevier Saunders.
4. Meissner MH. (2010). Chronic venous disorders. In Zierler RE (Ed.), Strandess's duplex scanning disorders in vascular diagnosis 4th ed. (223-229).Philadelphia Wolters Kluwer Lippincott Williams & Wilkins. Oklu et al. (2012). J Vasc Interv Radiol; 23:33–39.
5. Browse NL, Burnand, KG, Thomas, ML (1988). Disease of the Veins; Pathology, Diagnosis and Treatment, Edward Arnold, a division of Hodder & Stoughton.
6. Meissner MH, Strandess DE. (2005). Pathophysiology and natural history of acute deep venous thrombosis. In *Rutherford Vascular Surgery 6th edition*. (2124-2142). Philadelphia. Elsevier Saunders.
7. Min RJ, Rosenblatt M. US Department of Health and Human Services, Office on Women's Health (2010). Varicose Veins and Spider Veins. Retrieved from http://www.womenshealth.gov/faq/varicose-spider-veins.cfm. (7-7-2010).
8. Coleridge-Smith P, Labropoulos N, Partsch H, Myers K, Nicolaides A, Cavezzi A. (2006). Duplex ultrasound investigation of the veins in chronic venous disease of the lower limbs: UIP consensus document. Part I. Basic principles. Eur J Vasc Endovasc Surg 31, 83–92
9. Meissner MH. (2005). Venous duplex scanning. In *Rutherford Vascular Surgery 6th edition*. (254-270). Philadelphia. Elsevier Saunders.
10. Cina A, Pedicelli A, Di Stasi C, Pocelli A, Fiorentino A, Cina G, Rulli F, Bonomo L. (2005). Color Doppler sonography in chronic venous insufficiency: what the radiologist should know. *Curr Probl Diagn Radiol*, 34; 51-62.
11. Pascarella L, Mekenas, L (2006). Ultrasound examination of the patient with primary venous insufficiency. In *The Vein Book*, Philadelphia: Elsevier 171-181.
12. Callam MJ. (1994). Epidemiology of varicose veins. *British Journal of Surgery*, 81:167-173.
13. Varicose veins and venous insufficiency: Interventional radiology nonsurgical outpatient procedure treats varicose veins. (2010). Society of Interventional Radiologists. http://www.scvir.org/patients/varicose-veins/. (12-9-2010).
14. Tessier DJ, Williams RA. (10-5-2006). "Chronic venous insufficiency" Emedicine. Retrieved from: http://emedicine.medscape.com/article/461449-overview (date viewed).
15. Cornu-Thenard A, Boivin P, Baud JM, De Vincenzi I, Carperntier PH. (1994). Importance of the familiar factor in varicose disease. Clinical study of 134 families. *J Dermatol Surg*. 20:318-326.
16. Janniger CK. (3-17-2010). Klippel-Trenaunay-Weber Syndrome. *eMedicine*. Retrieved from http://www.emedicine.com/article/1084257-overview. (12-5-2010).
17. Connors JP, Mulliken JB. (2005). Vascular tumors and malformations in childhood. In *Rutherford Vascular Surgery 6th edition*. (1626-1645). Philadelphia. Elsevier Saunders
18. Lim and Davies. (2009) Pathogenesis of primary varicose veins British Journal of Surgery; 96: 1231–1242).
19. Badier-Commander et al. (2001). Smooth muscle cell modulation and cytokine overproduction in varicose veins. An in situ study. J Pathol; 193: 398-407.

Definition

The combination of real time B-mode imaging with pulsed wave and color flow Doppler (duplex scanning) used during the procedure for vein mapping, vein access, catheter placement and the infusion of perivenous anesthetic.

Rationale

Venous duplex ultrasound is the primary diagnostic imaging modality utilized for identifying patients with chronic venous insufficiency (CVI). Duplex ultrasound not only determines the presence of reflux in both deep and superficial veins, but it also identifies venous obstruction which might affect decisions regarding interventional procedures. B-mode ultrasound also is the primary imaging modality to guide venous access and ablative treatment in the lower extremities.

Etiology *(of conditions treated using thermal ablation)*

- Congenital
- Primary venous insufficiency
- History of venous thrombosis
  - Secondary venous insufficiency to valve injury, usually due to venous thrombosis
- Venous hypertension, caused by valve damage or dysfunction

Risk Factors

- Genetics (complex and involving many genes)
- Age (greater with advancing age)
- Obesity
- Female gender
- Pregnancy (greater with each pregnancy)
- Previous venous thrombosis
- Occupations requiring long period of standing or sitting

Indications *(for venous ablation procedure)*

- Significant volume of reflux in the saphenous venous system with documented valve closure time greater than 500 ms (Most pathologic reflux is over 1000 ms) in the great saphenous vein, contributing to the development of:
  - Retrograde flow
  - Varicose veins
  - Soft tissue pain or tenderness
  - Edema
  - Venous stasis dermatitis
  - Venous ulceration. [38]
  - Leg fatigue

Contraindications/Limitations

- Pregnancy or breast feeing
- Tortuous veins which cannot be traversed with endovenous glidewire/catheter techniques (rare)
- Obstructed deep venous system resulting in the saphenous veins becoming major outflow collateral
- Close proximity of the target vein to a nerve
- Obstructed deep venous system (e.g., acute)
- Anesthetic allergy
- Coagulopathy
- Patient immobility

Location of Veins *(treated with chemical or thermal ablation)*

- Great saphenous vein (GSV): most commonly affected
- Small saphenous vein (SSV): second most commonly treated
- Anterior accessory saphenous vein (AASV)
- Posterior accessory saphenous vein (PASV)
- Thigh extension of the small saphenous vein
- Perforators: (rare) including, but not limited to:
  - Posterior tibial
  - Paratibial perforators
  - Perforators in the thigh, buttock and lateral calf may also be treated if clinically indicated.

Patient History

- Leg discomfort, fatigue, heaviness, burning, stinging, pruritus
- Soft tissue leg pain or tenderness
- Lower extremity swelling
- Enlarging varicose veins
- Spontaneous venous hemorrhage
- Symptoms often are worse with dependency or perimenstrual

Physical Examination

- Varicose veins
- Tenderness in soft tissue
- Edema
- Hyperpigmentation near the ankles or foot
- Stasis dermatitis
- Superficial thrombophlebitis
- Venous stasis ulceration
- Lipodermatosclerosis
- Corona Phlebectasia
- Venous ulceration
- Active or healed ulcer

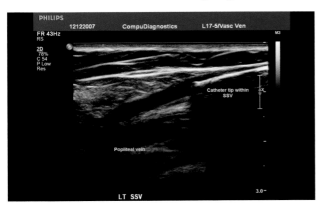

Catheter tip position Image courtesy of Diana L. Neuhardt, BS MBA RVT

Lower Extremity Venous Duplex Protocol for Pre and Post Venous Ablation

See chapter on Lower Extremity Venous Insufficiency Duplex for full venous reflux exam protocol.

Pre-procedure Vein Mapping Duplex Protocol

- Prior to the ablation procedure, the vein to be treated is mapped with skin markings. Essential elements of the mapping include an assessment of:
  - Location of the vein to be treated
  - Maximum diameter (with patient supine)
  - Depth of vein from skin surface (vein segments less than 8-10 mm below the surface of the skin may develop a tender, palpable cord with hyperpigmentation which slowly resolves and treatment of superficial veins may result in thermal burns of the skin)
  - Tributaries
  - Aneurysmal segments
  - Duplicate vein segments
  - Evidence of challenges to catheterization e.g., obstruction, webs, tortuosity, large tributary veins, the catheter may want to feed into the perforating veins.
  - Areas of hypoplasia and aplasia
  - Determination of the intended vein access site

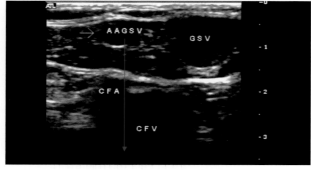

The arrow demonstrates the anatomical landmark of the Alignment Sign. The AASV is aligned with the femoral artery and vein. Note the vessels are within the saphenous compartment

Image courtesy of Jean White, Quality Vascular Imaging, Inc.

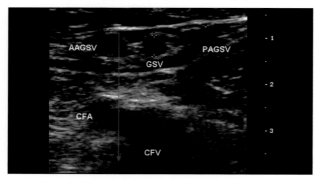

Unusual variant of the Alignment Sign, the AAGSV is on the left, GSV in the middle and PAGSV on the right. Note the vessels still are within the saphenous compartment.

Image courtesy of Jean White, Quality Vascular Imaging, Inc.

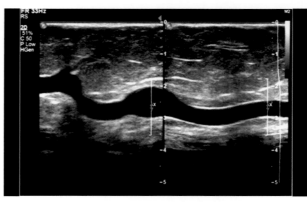

Tortuous venous segment

Image courtesy of Paula Heggerick BS RVT RDMS RPhS FSVU

- Patient positioning (GSV)
  - The exam is best performed with the bed in the reverse Trendelenburg position.
  - Leg is externally rotated and slightly bent at the knee.
  - Using a straw (or a pencil capable of marking the skin while the gel is still on the skin), the sonographer can make skin depressions while mapping vein.
  - Depressions will stay visible after gel is removed from the skin.
    - Remove any remaining gel.
    - Use a permanent marker to map the venous pathway and include any areas of interest such as:
      - Large perforators
      - Tortuous segments
      - Chronic disease
  - Two access sites should be indentified in case one is not able to be used (e.g., due to venous spasm).

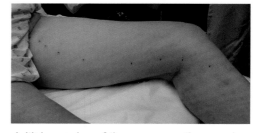

Initial mapping of the venous pathway using the "straw method"

Image courtesy of Paula Heggerick BS RVT RDMS RPhS FSVU

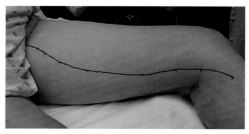

Final mapping of the venous pathway and areas of interest

Image courtesy of Paula Heggerick BS RVT RDMS RPhS FSVU

Peri-procedural Ultrasound

- During the procedure, B-mode ultrasound is used to:
  - Obtain percutaneous vein access.
  - Assess for adequate tumescent fluid within the saphenous compartment around the vein being treated (a halo of fluid should completely surround the vein prior to thermal ablation).
  - Assure that the vein being treated is >1 cm from the skin surface (to prevent skin burn)
  - Observe the immediate affect of the heat on the treated vein.

Procedural Ultrasound

- During the procedure, ultrasound is used to:
  - Guide needle access to the vein.
  - Guide placement of glidewire and sheath.
  - Guide positioning of the LASER fiber tip or the radiofrequency catheter tip in the great saphenous vein (GSV), usually 2 ½ cm below the deep venous junction.
  - Guide infusion of perivenous anesthetic to create a halo of fluid surrounding the target vein.
  - Assure that the target vein is at least 8-10 mm below the surface of the skin to reduce the likelihood of a palpable visible cord or skin burn post-operatively.
  - Observe the immediate effect of the heat upon the target vein.

Post-procedural Ultrasound

- Most centers evaluate the target vein and the associated deep vein, i.e., great saphenous and common femoral veins or the small saphenous and the popliteal veins 1 to 7 days post-treatment.
- Following endovenous treatment, duplex ultrasound is used to evaluate:
  - Occlusion of the targeted vein segment
  - Secondary thrombosis of associated tributary veins and the target vein above or below the targeted segment
  - Endovenous Heat Induced Thrombus (EHIT) described for the great saphenous vein in:
    - EHIT I confined to the great saphenous vein near the saphenofemoral junction
    - EHIT II great saphenous vein thrombus extending into the common femoral vein, less than 50% diameter compromise of the CFV
    - EHIT III great saphenous vein thrombus extending into the common femoral vein, more than 50% diameter compromise of the CFV
    - EHIT IV occlusion of the common femoral vein

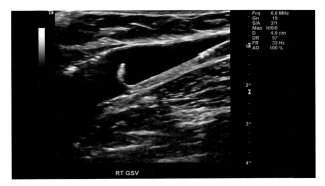

J-wire placed in the GSV to be treated
Image courtesy of Patrick Washko, BS RT RDMS RVT

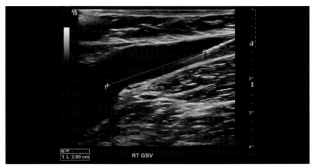

Wire placed 2 cm distal to SFJ
Image courtesy of Patrick Washko, BS RT RDMS RVT

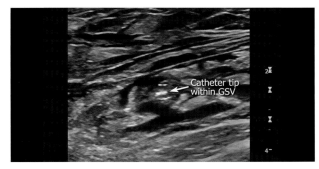

Tumescent fluid within the saphenous compartment
Image courtesy of Patrick Washko, BS RT RDMS RVT

Below are post-operative images illustrating absence of flow within the GSV   *Images courtesy of Paula Heggerick BS RVT RDMS RPhS FSVU*

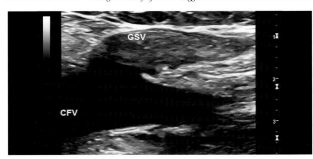

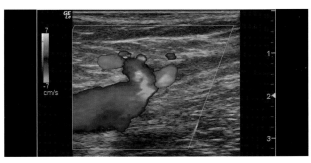

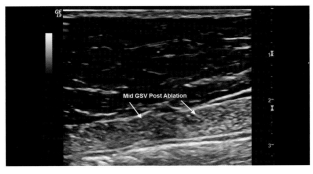

TABLE 84: Duplex Imaging for Venous Ablation Protocol Summary

Scan pre, peri and post-procedure with B-mode US, PW Doppler and color duplex are complementary

Position the patient in the supine position, with the leg externally rotated and the knee slightly bent. The bed should be in a slight reverse Trendelenburg position.

Pre-procedure

- Determine the source, presence and extent of deep and superficial venous reflux.
- Document the maximum diameter of any superficial veins to be treated.
- Document the depth of any superficial veins to be treated.
- Document location and size of all significant tributaries off any veins to be treated.
- Identify 2 access sites (in case one site is unusable, in the event of venous spasm).
- Document any additional clinically significant observations, including but not limited to aneurysmal segments, duplicated veins, evidence of venous obstruction, etc.

Peri-procedure

- Provide guidance for the physician during wire/catheter placement and make observations to ensure procedure's success:
    - Confirm the catheter tip is distal to the deep system by 1-2.5 cm; it should also be distal to the superficial inferior epigastric vein if possible.
    - Assess for adequate perivenous tumescent anesthesia within the saphenous compartment around the treated venous segment (Observe for a halo of fluid surrounding the vein prior to thermal ablation).
    - Assure treated venous segment is >1 cm from skin surface.
    - Observe for abnormalities after heat is administered during ablation.

Post-procedure

- Document vein sclerosis/fibrosis of the treated venous segment (non-compressible vein with thickened vein walls and absence of flow by duplex).
- Document absence or presence of deep venous thrombosis in the surrounding venous segments.
- Additional documentation may be recorded as necessary in segments other than those listed above.

Interpretation at a Glance

TABLE 85: Diagnostic Criteria for Post-Venous Ablation Venous Duplex

Normal

- Complete vein sclerosis/fibrosis of the treated venous segment by B-mode image, PW Doppler and color flow
- Absence of deep vein thrombosis:
    - Absent intralumenal deep vein thrombus
    - Color flow fills lumen completely
    - Normal venous Doppler spontaneity, phasicity and augmentation of the deep venous system

Abnormal

- Lack of complete vein ablation
- Presence of deep vein thrombosis:
    - Intralumenal echoes (although acute thrombus can be echolucent)
    - Decrease or absence of color flow
    - Abnormal venous Doppler spontaneity, phasicity or augmentation

Interpretation *(to determine success of treatment)*

- Expectations from the ultrasound evaluation of the treated vein segment immediate post-procedure include:
    - The vein should be non-compressible
    - Vein walls should appear thickened
    - Absence of flow by color and PW Doppler in the treated venous segment
    - Documented absence of deep venous thrombosis

Correlation

- Venogram
- MR venography
- CT venography

Endovascular Treatment

- Sclerotherapy, with or without US guidance

Surgical Treatment

- Ligation, with or without stripping
- Phlebectomy
- Transilluminated power phlebectomy (Trivex)
- Superficial perforator ligation surgery (SEPS)

Points to Remember

- True DVT is a rare finding. Endovenous Heat Induced Thrombosis (EHIT) post-ablation can occur as an extension of the thrombus from the treated area and would typically be limited to the femoral or popliteal regions.

- Trendelenburg positioning of the bed will facilitate emptying of the veins.

- Duplex ultrasound at 9-12 months post-procedure ultimately determines the success (sono absent) of the procedure.

- Most labs schedule 45-90 minutes for each venous ablation procedure.

- There is a high success rate for healing of venous ulceration, post procedure.

- Obese patients may have a higher rate of failure. The cause may be due to a higher central venous pressure.

- Most recanalization will occur between 6-12 months post-procedure.

- *Tumescent* is a term which describes a fluid mixture that serves as an anesthetic during the ablation procedure. When the tumescence is injected into the tissue, the area becomes swollen and firm or "tumescent".

References

1. American College of Phlebology (ACP) www.phlebology.org
2. American Registry for Diagnostic Medical Sonography (ARDMS) www.ardms.org
3. Cardiovascular Credentialing (CCI) www.cci-online.org
4. American Venous Forum (AVF) www.venous-info.com
5. Intersocietal Commission for the Accreditation of Vascular Laboratories (ICAVL) www.icavl.org
6. Society of Vascular Ultrasound (SVU) www.svunet.org

Books

7. Bergan J. (2006). The Vein Book. Elsevier.
8. Gloviczki P. (2009). Handbook of Venous Disorders 3rd edition, Hodder Arnold.
9. Fronek H, Fundamental of Phlebology: Venous disease for clinicians. 2nd edition. Royal Society of Medicine Press 2008
10. Goldman M, Bergan J, Guex JJ. (2007). Sclerotherapy: Treatment of Varicose and Telangiectatic Leg Veins. Mosby.
11. Ricci S, Georgiev M, Goldman, M. (2005). Ambulatory Phlebectomy. 2nd edition. Taylor & Francis Group.
12. Weiss R. (2001). Vein Diagnosis and Treatment. McGraw-Hill.

Articles

13. Khilani NM, Elston DM, Khan S, Butler DF, Miller JJ, Crawford GH. (2010). Varicose Vein Treatment with Endovenous Laser Therapy. www.emedicine.medscape.com (accessed 12/4/2011).

Definition

The combination of real time B-mode ultrasonography with pulsed wave Doppler and color flow to evaluate the upper extremity veins for evidence of thrombus

Etiology (of venous disease)

- The theory of Virchow's triad states that venous thrombosis is caused by: venous stasis, vein wall (intimal) injury or a hypercoaguable state.
- Extrinsic compression

Risk Factors

- Age (greater with advanced age)
- Central venous catheters
- Repetitive arm activities (e.g., weight lifting)
- Immobilization
- Genetic prothrombotic conditions (clotting disorders, such as Factor V Leiden)
- Post-operative phase (especially after orthopedic surgery)
- Pregnancy
- Oral contraceptives
- Estrogen replacement
- Cancer/malignancy
- Previous DVT
- Heart complications (e.g., MI, CHF)
- Obesity
- Family history
- Smoking
- COPD
- Blood type (highest risk with type-A, lowest risk with type-O)
- Trauma
- Antiphospholipid antibodies (e.g., lupus)
- Congenital abnormalities
- Drug use
- Cerebrovascular events (stroke, TIA)

Indications for Exam

- Edema/swelling (especially when unilateral)
- Limb pain/tenderness
- Limb redness
- Suspected injury after venous puncture/catheterization, especially of the IJV
- Symptoms of pulmonary embolism (PE) (e.g., shortness of breath, chest pain, hemoptysis)

Contraindications/Limitations

- Anatomical limitations (clavicle and ribs)
- Open wounds prohibiting access by the ultrasound probe
- Casts that cannot be removed or traction that limits access to the scan areas
- Poor visualization due to vessel depth because of obesity or severe edema
- Patients who cannot be adequately positioned

Mechanism of disease [1,2]

There are three factors responsible for the formation of venous thrombosis, as outlined in Virchow's Triad: (vein wall injury, hypercoagulability and stasis of blood flow). A combination of any of these events may increase the risk of venous thrombosis.

- There is a balance between coagulation (process to prevent excessive bleeding after injury) and anticoagulation (process to prevent spontaneous intravascular clotting) in normal blood flow.

- The venous endothelial layer is normally antithrombotic. In response to endothelial injury, leukocytes (white blood cells) attach to the vessel wall. A plasma protein known as prothrombin is activated. Prothrombin activator catalyzes conversion of prothrombin into thrombin. Thrombin acts as an enzyme to convert fibrinogen into fibrin threads, forming a clot.

- Hypercoaguable states result from genetic mutation or acquired deficiencies that accompany certain diseases (e.g., liver disease). In such cases, naturally occurring anticoagulants (antithrombin, protein C, protein S, etc.) are deficient. For example, genetic mutation, factor V Leiden, causes resistance to the natural anticoagulant protein C.

- Non-movement of blood flow (stasis) permits coagulation. Platelets are thought to become trapped by low shear stress (flow) at valve cusps. Platelets adhere to the subendothelial (collagen) layer of the venous wall and may aggregate depending on the amount of coagulation and thrombolysis occurring in the body at that time.

- Increased activation of coagulation factors in those suffering from cancer is thought to lead to formation of venous thrombosis. In addition, the levels of coagulation inhibitors normally found in the blood (e.g., proteins C or S), are thought to be reduced in these patients.

- The use of estrogen (in replacement therapy or birth control) alters coagulation and may predispose individuals to thrombosis.

- Venous aneurysms are a rare condition. Research suggests several possible causes; decreased smooth muscle cells and an increase in fibrous connective tissue or either an increase or decrease in the fibrous connective tissue and elastic fibers.[3]

- Once thrombus is formed, it can:

  - **Stabilize:** Stabilization includes adherence of the thrombus to the vessel wall without changing location or propagating. If thrombus has formed, the most favorable occurrence would be to stabilize. This reduces the risk to the patient.

  - **Propagate:** Propagation includes "growth of the thrombus" in size or location. Examples of propagation may include a thrombus that extends from the superficial system into the deep system.

  - **Embolize:** During embolization, a portion of a thrombus breaks free and travels downstream in the vascular system. The greatest risk to the patient is that the thrombus travels to the lungs and results in a pulmonary embolus.

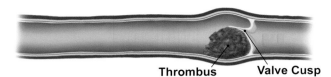

Thrombus   **Valve Cusp**

Thrombosis of vein

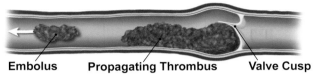

Embolus   **Propagating Thrombus**   **Valve Cusp**

Embolization of thrombus

> *Thrombus located within the deep veins is known as deep venous thrombosis (DVT). Thrombus located within the superficial veins is known as superficial thrombosis (SVT). Some labs may call this thrombosis.*

Location of Disease

Although any venous site can develop thrombus, common origins include:

- Valve sites
- Venous confluences
- Superficial venous system (basilic, cephalic, median cubital)
- Deep venous system:
  - "Central veins" typically refer to the jugular, innominate, subclavian and sometimes axillary veins Brachial, radial, ulnar veins

Patient History

- Previous DVT
- Post-operative; orthopedic or neurosurgery for example, (can occur anytime during surgery or for 6 months thereafter)
- Persistent swelling (usually unilateral, but can be bilateral)
- Clotting issues (including problems regulating anticoagulation therapy, malignant cancer)
- Localized pain, burning or itching
- Symptoms of pulmonary embolism (PE) (e.g., shortness of breath, chest pain, hemoptysis)

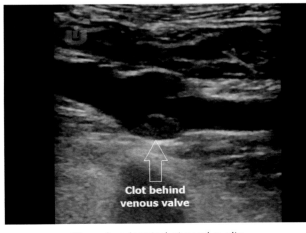

Thrombus located at a valve site

Physical Examination

- Edema or swelling
- Tenderness
- Limb redness or warmth
- Dark pigmentation, hardened tissue
- Cyanosis (superior vena cava syndrome)
- Excessive collaterals around area of concern

Upper Extremity Venous Duplex Protocol

- Obtain a patient history to include symptoms and risk factors.
- The patient is examined in the supine position with the head turned slightly to the side and the chin slightly raised.

> *Use venous presets on the duplex scanner; low color flow and Doppler scales will be needed to detect venous flow.*

- Some patients may require the use of a range of transducers; including high-frequency (5-7 MHz) (8-15 MHz) transducers and a lower frequency (1-4 MHz) transducer may be useful around the clavicle.

> *Use the deep probe to aid visualization around the clavicle.*

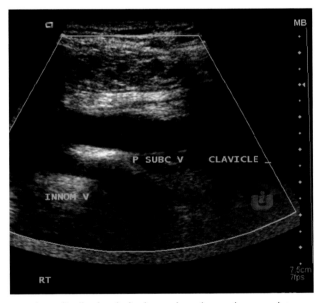

Longitudinal subclavian vein using a deep probe

Transverse Scan and Images

> *Asking the patient to "sniff" will cause compression of the SCV and sometimes results in flow augmentation.*

- Perform venous compression in the transverse plane (short axis) every 2-4 cm along the limb. This is anatomically difficult and may not be possible near the clavicle. Instead of compressions, have the patient inhale or ask the patient to "sniff, like you're going to sniff a flower".

Dual Screen Vein Compression

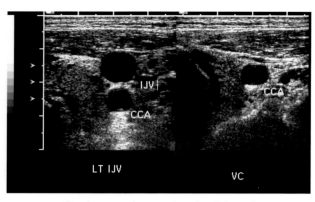

Dual screen image showing internal jugular vein compressibility

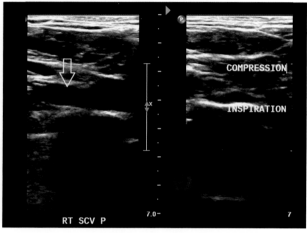

Dual screen image showing subclavian vein compressibility (demonstrated using the "sniff" technique)

- Record transverse images using "dual-screen" on the duplex scanner. Obtain and freeze an image without vein compression on the left side of the screen. Capture and an image with vein compression on the right side of the screen. Document transverse images of the following veins with and without compressions as described above:

  – Internal jugular vein (IJV)
  – Subclavian vein (if possible)
  – Axillary vein
  – Brachial vein
  – Basilic vein
  – Cephalic vein

> Keep the probe at a 90° degree angle to the skin for the best grayscale images.

- Additional documentation of compressions can be performed when indicated and anatomically possible to include the subclavian vein junction, brachiocephalic (innominate), radial, ulnar or median cubital veins.

Dual Screen Image Showing Venous Compressibility

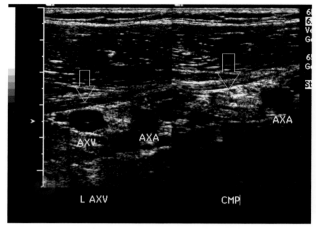

Dual screen showing axillary vein compressibility

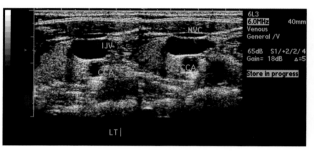

Dual screen showing internal jugular vein partial compressibility

Longitudinal Scan and Images

- Record pulsed wave venous spectral waveforms with color Doppler in the longitudinal (sagittal axis) view.
- Observe for augmentation of venous flow.
- Documentation should illustrate spontaneity, phasicity, augmentation. Pulsatility should be documented in all but the brachial and superficial veins. Record at the following locations:

  – Internal jugular vein
  – Subclavian vein
  – Axillary vein(s)
  – Brachial vein
  – Cephalic vein
  – Basilic vein
  – Document spectral waveforms of paired veins individually.
  – Additional

> Some labs record venous PW Doppler waveforms without setting an angle since actual velocities are usually not important in a venous exam. If your lab chooses to set an angle, use a ≤60° Doppler angle with the cursor placed parallel to the vessel walls in the center of the flow stream.

  documentation of patency can be performed when necessary of the distal brachiocephalic, jugular-subclavian junction, radial, ulnar or median cubital veins.

- Use PW Doppler to analyze absence of flow by placing the Doppler sample volume in any vein segment suspected to be thrombosed. Doppler flow or lack of flow, compliments compression, color flow and B-mode images. Use the adjacent artery as a guide to identify an occluded vein when possible.
- Repeat for the contralateral extremity if a bilateral exam was ordered.

TABLE 86: **Upper Extremity Venous Protocol Summary**	
Scan transverse (short axis) with and without color compression	**Scan longitudinal (sagittal axis) in grayscale and PW Doppler (color Doppler can be used intermediately)**
• Internal jugular vein (IJV)	• Internal jugular vein (IJV)
• Subclavian vein (SCV)	• Subclavian vein (SCV)
• Axillary vein (AXV)	• Distal brachiocephalic (BCV)
• Brachial vein (BRV)	• Axillary vein (AXV)
• Basilic vein (BSV)	• Brachial vein (BRV)
• Cephalic vein (CV)	• Cephalic vein (CV)
• Subclavian-jugular confluence (optional)	• Basilic vein (BSV)
• Distal BCV (optional)	• Subclavian-jugular confluence (optional)
• Radial vein (RV) (optional)	• Radial vein (RV) (optional)
• Ulnar vein (UV) (optional)	• Ulnar vein (UV) (optional)
• Median cubital vein (MCV) (optional)	• Median cubital vein (MCV) (optional)

- Additional documentation of compression may be recorded in segments other than those listed during evaluation for thrombus as necessary. (Compressions may be anatomically contraindicated, especially near the clavicle. If so, document patency with color flow and PW spectral waveforms.)
- Document additional PW Doppler waveforms in all veins when dual (or more) venous systems are present.

- If only a unilateral exam was requested, documentation of the contralateral subclavian venous spectral waveform is performed for comparison.

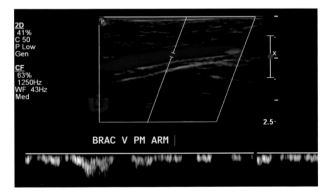

Normal brachial vein spectral waveform

> *The transverse or oblique plane to the body may be better for recording flow in the distal brachiocephalic (innominate) vein.*

General grayscale and color characteristics

Normal

- **Compressibility:** The vein is free of thrombus if it compresses completely and is free of intralumenal echoes.
- **Color Doppler:** Wall to wall color flow will fill the vein spontaneously or upon distal limb compression.

Abnormal

- **Compressibility:** Intralumenal echoes are visualized within the vein and full coaptation of the vein on manual compression is absent or limited due to thrombus.
  - Compression of the artery with probe pressure can be a confirmation of an incompressible venous segment.
- **Color Doppler:**
  - If partially occlusive thrombus is present, color flow will be seen flowing around echogenic material in the vein, spontaneously or with distal limb compression.

    > *Color flow can obscure a partially occlusive thrombus if the color gain is set too high.*

  - If totally occlusive thrombus is present, no color flow will be observed even with distal limb compression.

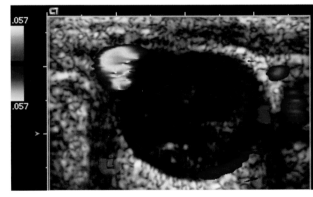

Transverse vein with color flow around thrombus

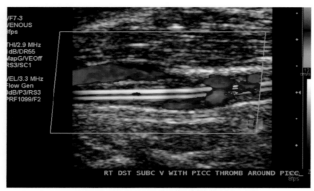

Longitudinal subclavian vein with color flowing around PICC line thrombus

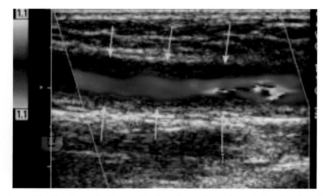

Longitudinal-partially occlusive thrombus (partial color flow)

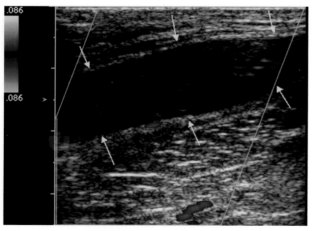

Longitudinal-totally occlusive thrombus (no color flow, low color scale)

- It is possible for only one vein of a pair to be thrombosed. For this reason it is important to make sure all veins are studied carefully.

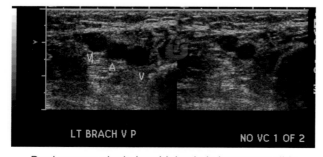

Dual screen: single brachial vein is incompressible

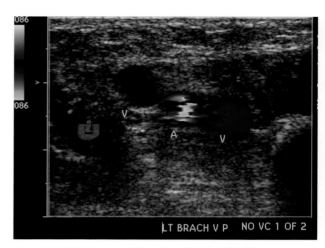

Single brachial vein without color flow in transverse plane

- **Thrombus:** If thrombus is present, determine whether the thrombus is partially or totally occlusive, its location and the extent and the characteristics of the thrombus.
  - **Acute thrombus:** Characteristics include medium to lightly echogenic or anechoic, spongy texture upon compression, poor attachment to the venous wall or "free floating" within the lumen. A moving tail may be seen at the end of the thrombus. When a vein is fully thrombosed, the vein is often dilated, especially compared to the adjacent artery.

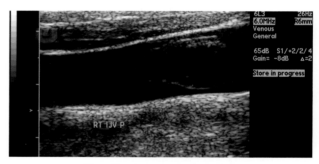

Free floating, acute thrombus

  - **Chronic thrombus:** Characteristics include brightly echogenic or heterogeneous echoes, irregular surface texture and thrombus which is attached to the venous wall. The vein can stay the same size as the artery, but often contracts in diameter over time. Collateral veins may be observed adjacent to the affected vein(s) and small irregular flow channels within the thrombus can sometimes be seen with color.

  - **Indeterminate age:** Characteristics of both acute and chronic stages may be present, making age difficult to determine. It is best not to guess.

Stages of Thrombus

*Comparison of Typical Venous Diameter
During the Different Stages*

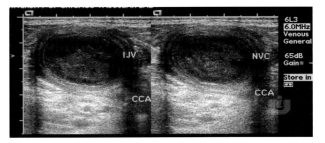

Acute IJV DVT

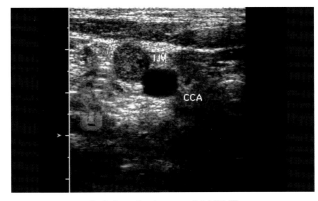

Indeterminate age: IJV DVT

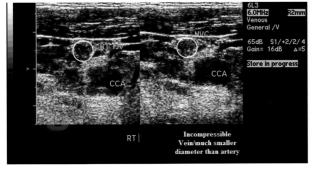

Chronic IJV DVT

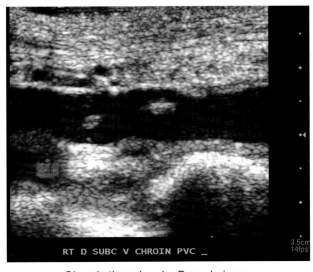

Chronic thrombus by B-mode image

TABLE 87: **Thrombosis Descriptions and Characteristics**	
Acute	**Chronic**
• Light to medium echogenic/anechoic	• Bright/heterogeneous echoes
• Spongy texture on compression (homogeneous)	• Irregular texture (heterogeneous)
• Poorly attached or free floating	• Attached
• Dilated vein (if totally occluded)	• Same size as artery or vein is contracted
	• Collateral veins may be noted

- Veins can be partially or totally incompressible in both acute and chronic stages.
- Combination of events can occurs (e.g., acute on top of chronic thrombus).
- Chronic thrombus with partial recanalization is seen as small color flow channels within thrombus.
- Age of thrombus is sometimes indeterminate.

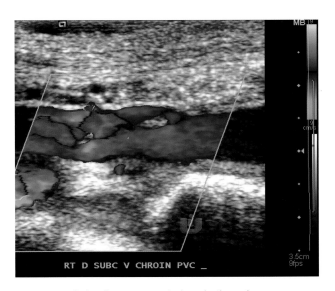

*Color flows around chronic thrombus
longitudinal view-irregular flow channel*

Venous Doppler observations

- Determine whether venous flow is:
  - Spontaneous (automatically heard with Doppler)
  - Pulsatile
  - Phasic (flow increases and decreases with respiration)
  - Able to augment (increases) with distal compression (or "sniff" technique)

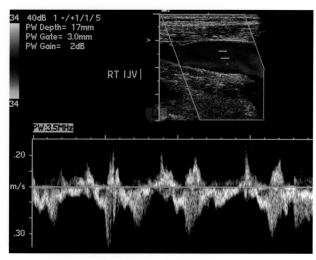

Normal spectral waveform-central veins (flow is normally spontaneous and pulsatile)

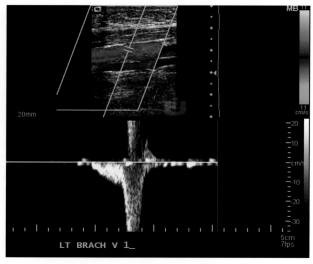

Normal spectral waveform-arm veins (normal for spontaneity and phasicity to be absent)

- **Spontaneity:** The vein demonstrates spontaneous flow, especially in the central veins (jugular, brachiocephalic (innominate), subclavian) and axillary vein. In the distal arm veins, the absence of spontaneous flow can be a normal finding.
- **Pulsatility**: Pulsatile venous flow should be present in the upper extremity, especially in the central veins. Compare pulsatility when evaluating the distal brachiocephalic (innominate), subclavian and internal jugular veins. Equally pulsatile BCV, SCV and IJV flow is expected.

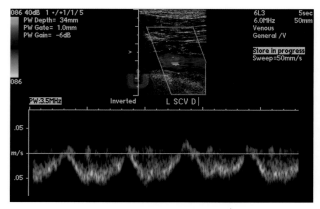

Normal, pulsatile subclavian spectral waveform

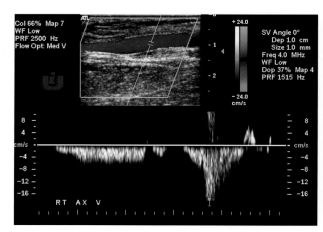

Normal, axillary spectral waveform (phasic, non-pulsatile flow which augments upon distal compression)

- **Phasicity:** Venous signals are phasic and vary with respiration and the cardiac cycle. Cardiac changes are more obvious in the central veins and respiratory changes are more obvious distally, in the axillary veins for example. During deep exhalation, venous signals typically decrease or discontinue and increase with inhalation due to changes in intrathoracic pressures during the respiratory cycle.
- **Augmentation:** Compression of the limb distal to the probe augments venous flow in the axillary and arm veins.

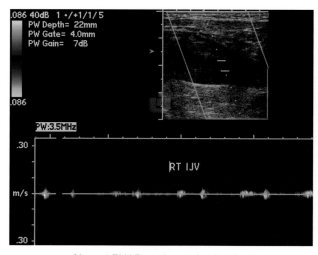

Absent PW Doppler and color flow

Abnormal

- **Spontaneity:** Absence of flow indicates venous obstruction. Use color flow in the adjacent artery as a guide to identify an occluded vein. But always confirm the absence of flow by placing sample volume in the vessel.

- **Pulsatility:** The absence of pulsatile venous flow suggests obstruction, especially in the central veins.

- **Phasicity:** Continuous venous flow (non-phasic flow) suggests either obstruction from DVT in a proximal venous segment or extrinsic compression of a proximal vein.

- **Augmentation:** If distal compression does not produce augmentation of the venous signal, a total obstruction distal to the probe is suspected. A weak or dampened augmentation also suggests venous obstruction distal to the probe. It may be helpful to change the patient's position and/or try compressing a more muscular area of the arm after giving time for venous refill.

> Normal Doppler signals may be present when thrombus is partially occlusive.

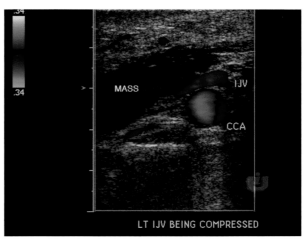

Extrinsic compression of vein suspected-transverse view

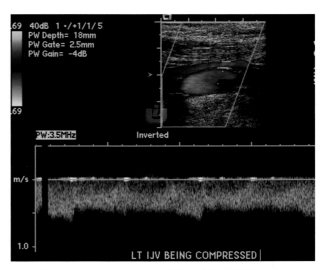

Venous compression confirmed by PW Doppler (continuous flow/lacks pulsatility)

TABLE 88: Diagnostic Criteria for Venous Duplex	
Normal	**Abnormal**
• Complete coaptation of vein walls with light probe pressure	• Lack of complete vein compression
• Absent intralumenal thrombus	• Intralumenal echoes present (acute thrombus can be echolucent)
• Color flow fills the lumen completely	• Decrease or absence of color flow
• Normal venous Doppler spontaneity, phasicity and augmentation	• Abnormal venous Doppler spontaneity, phasicity or augmentation
• No venous dilatation	• Dilated or contracted veins noted

Other Pathology

- **Extrinsic compression:** Continuous venous flow suggests either obstruction in a proximal venous segment or extrinsic compression of a vein.[11]

- **Venous stenosis:** When increased focal venous velocity is noted (compared to distal segments), with or without provocative positional maneuvers, a venous stenosis is suspected. This condition can occur secondary to thoracic outlet syndrome, dialysis access intervention or extrinsic compression. Some labs use a venous-velocity ratio of ≥2.5 (a velocity increase of at least 2.5 times the immediate distal venous segment) to diagnose a hemodynamically significant stenosis.[12]

- **Effort thrombosis:** *Effort thrombosis or Paget-Schroetter syndrome* usually involves the subclavian venous segment. In this syndrome, the subclavian vein (SCV) is compressed between the first rib and scalene muscle (the thoracic outlet), which results in formation of venous thrombus and flow obstruction.[11,13]

- **Superior vena cava syndrome versus BCV obstruction:** When comparing the distal brachiocephalic (innominate) veins, the absence of pulsatile flow on both sides suggests a proximal obstruction in both innominate veins or in the superior vena cava (SVC syndrome). If the decrease in pulsatility is unilateral, obstruction of that branchiocephalic vein proximally is suspected (BCV obstruction).[8]

- **Venous aneurysm:** is diagnosed when there is an area of significant venous dilatation compared to the adjacent venous segment. Common locations for upper extremity venous aneurysms include the internal jugular and axillary veins. Document the presence of any mural thrombus.[14]

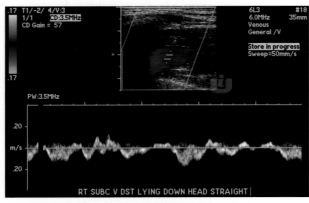

Normal SCV waveforms at rest

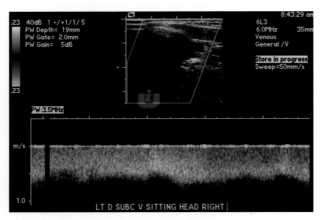

Increased venous flow with positional changes of the arm

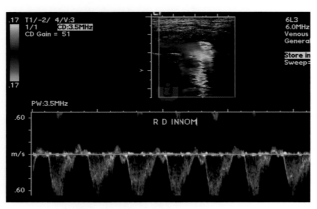

Normal innominate vein PW Doppler

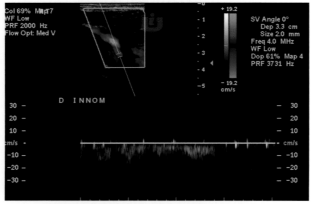

*Abnormal innominate vein: PW Doppler
with decreased pulsatility*

Differential Diagnosis

- Arterial disease
- Lymphedema
- Cellulitis
- Cysts
- Extrinsic compression
- Hematoma
- Muscle tear
- Joint effusion
- Adenopathy
- Arteriovenous fistula
- Heart failure
- Direct injury to extremity
- Vascularized mass
- Collagen vasculitis
- Abscess

Correlation

- CT scan
- MRI
- Venogram

Medical Treatment and Prevention

- Anticoagulation therapy (e.g., heparin, warfarin)
- Promote venous drainage (e.g., elevate arms, wear elastic/support sleeves)

Surgical Treatment

- IVC filter (acute DVT)
- SVC reconstruction (femoral, spiral saphenous vein, PTFE or cryopreserved grafts)

Endovascular Treatment

- Catheter-directed thrombolysis with urokinase, etc. (acute DVT)
- Mechanical thrombectomy such as Angiojet (acute DVT)
- Percutaneous translumenal angioplasty and stenting (SVC syndrome or axillo-subclavian issues

Points to Remember

- Venous duplex ultrasound can identify the presence, exact location, extent, and severity of venous thrombosis. The course of the veins, collaterals and thrombus can be visualized using B-mode and color while the analysis of Doppler flow patterns can yield further information regarding flow direction and both local and remote obstructions.
- Compressions should always be performed in the transverse plane to ensure full compression and so duplicated veins are not missed.
- The superficial veins of the upper extremity are the primary route of drainage for the arm.
- The upper extremity veins contain far fewer venous valves compared to the lower extremity.
- Upper extremity venous thrombosis is less likely to embolize and cause a symptomatic pulmonary embolism compared to DVT in the lower extremities. [8]
- Upper extremity AXV and SCV thrombosis is divided into two categories:
  - **Primary venous thrombosis** - also known as *Effort thrombosis or Paget-Schroetter syndrome,* results from compression and the repetitive trauma which occurs to the venous segment in the thoracic outlet.
  - **Secondary venous thrombosis:** occurs due to other causes (e.g., insertion of catheters, hemodialysis ports, pacemakers, immobilization, etc.). Secondary thrombosis is more common (80% of cases). [15]

- It is technically difficult to image the neck veins with the patient in a sitting position. The veins sometimes collapse due to compression by atmospheric pressure from the outside.

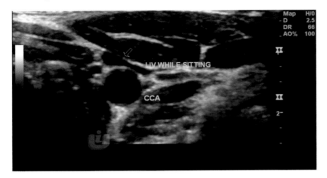

IJV collapses with patient sitting up

- Incidental findings, such as superficial tissue edema, may be helpful in the report for the clinicians to understand swelling/edema in the absence of thrombus.
- Upper extremity venous aneurysm are reported to be more common than lower extremity venous aneurysms, although both are rare. [14]

Central Venous Catheters [8]

- A central venous catheter is placed in one of the central veins and used to administer medication, nutrition, dialysis or chemotherapy treatments, etc. The use of central venous catheters has greatly increased in recent years. These lines increase the risk for venous thrombosis. [11]
- There are several different types of central venous catheters:
  - Tunneled catheters: A catheter that is "tunneled" under the skin makes it more discrete and keeps it in place before the catheter exits through the skin. Common tunneled catheters include *Hickman* and *Groshong* catheters.
  - Implanted ports remain under the skin and medications are injected through the skin into this type of catheter. Though these ports can be used for hemodialysis patients, they are primarily used for cancer treatment.
  - PICC line *(peripherally inserted central catheter)* is a line inserted in an arm vein with a tip that lies in one of the large veins in the chest. It can remain in position for up to six months.
- Observe the surface of any visualized intravenous catheters for thrombus development. It is possible for the thrombus that forms anywhere along these lines to extend into the more central veins.

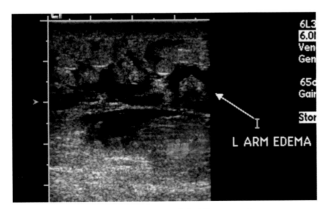

Upper extremity superficial tissue edema

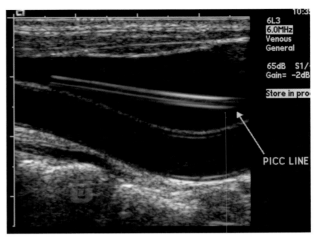

Upper extremity IJV PICC line without thrombus

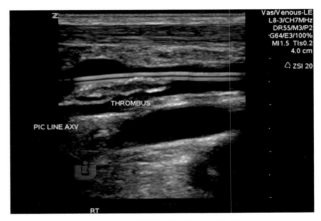

Upper extremity IJV PICC line with thrombus

References

1. Wakefield TW. (2005). Bleeding and clotting: fundamental considerations. In Rutherford Vascular Surgery 6th edition. (493-511). Philadelphia. Elsevier Saunders.
2. Guyton AC. (1986). Hemostasis and blood coagulation. In Textbook of Medical Physiology 7th edition. (76-86). Philadelphia: WB Saunders.
3. Gillespie DL, Villavicencio JL, Gallagher C, Chang A, Hamelink JK, Fiala LA, O'Donnell SD, Jackson MR, Pikoulis E, Rich, NM. (1997). Presentation and management of venous aneurysms. *J Vasc Surg*. Nov;26(5):845-52.
4. Thrush A, Hartshorne T. (2005). Duplex assessment of deep venous thrombosis and upper limb venous disorders. In Peripheral Vascular Ultrasound, How Why and When, 2nd ed. (189-206). Edinburgh: Elsevier Churchill Livingstone.
5. Zwiebel, WJ (2005). Ultrasound Diagnosis of Venous Thrombosis. In Zwiebel WJ, Pellerito JS (Eds.), *Introduction to Vascular Ultrasonography 5th ed*, (449-465). Philadelphia: Elsevier Saunders.
6. Meissner MH. (2005). Venous duplex scanning. In Rutherford Vascular Surgery 6th edition. (254-270). Philadelphia. Elsevier Saunders.
7. Myers K, Clough A. (2004). Venous thrombosis in the lower limbs. In Making sense of vascular ultrasound: A hands on guide. (181-197). London: Hodder Arnold.
8. Caps MT, Mraz BA. (2010). Upper extremity venous thrombosis. In Zierler RE (Ed.), Strandess's duplex scanning disorders in vascular diagnosis 4th ed. (199-221).Philadelphia Wolters Kluwer Lippincott Williams & Wilkins.
9. Sumner DS, Mattos MA. (1993). Diagnosis of deep vein thrombosis with real-time color and duplex scanning. In Vascular Diagnosis 4th edition. (785-800). St. Louis. Mosby.
10. Lohr, J (2005). Upper Extremity Venous Duplex Imaging. In Mansour MA, Labropoulos N. (Eds.), *Vascular Diagnosis*, (469-477). Philadelphia: Elsevier Saunders.
11. Green RM. (2005). Subclavian-axillary vein thrombosis. In *Rutherford Vascular Surgery 6th edition*. (1371-1392). Philadelphia. Elsevier Saunders.
12. Leon, LR, Labropoulos, N, Mansour MA. (2005). Hemodynamic principles as applied to diagnostic testing. In Mansour MA, Labropoulos N. (Eds.), *Vascular Diagnosis*, (7-21). Philadelphia: Elsevier Saunders.
13. Kreienberg PB, Shah, DM, Darling III, RC, Change BB, Paty SK, Roddy SP, Ozsvath KJ, Manish M. (2005) Thoracic outlet syndrome: In Mansour MA, Labropoulos N. (Eds.), *Vascular Diagnosis*, (517-522). Philadelphia: Elsevier Saunders.
14. Gillespie DL, Villavicencio JL, Gallagher C, Chang A, Hamelink JK, Fiala LA, O'Donnell SD, Jackson MR, Pikoulis E, Rich, NM. (1997). Presentation and management of venous aneurysms. *J Vasc Surg*. Nov;26(5):845-52.
15. Spiezia L, Simioni P. (2010). Upper extremity deep vein thrombosis. Intern Emerg Med. Apr;5(2):103-9. Epub 2009 Sep 26.

Definition

The combination of real time B-mode ultrasonography with pulsed wave Doppler and color flow to evaluate the inferior vena cava (IVC) and iliac veins for evidence of thrombus or external compression

Etiology

- Thrombosis; The theory of Virchow's triad states that venous thrombosis is caused by: venous stasis, vein wall (intimal) injury or a hypercoaguable state.
- Extrinsic compression (e.g., from renal or hepatocellular carcinomas or tumors that have spread to the paracaval lymph nodes for example)

Risk Factors

- Age (greater with advanced age)
- Immobilization
- Genetic prothrombotic conditions (clotting disorders, such as Factor V Leiden)
- Post-operative phase (especially after orthopedic surgery)
- Central venous or femoral catheters
- Female
  - Pregnancy
  - Oral contraceptives
  - Estrogen replacement
- Cancer/malignancy
- Previous DVT
- Heart complications (MI, CHF, etc)
- Obesity
- Family history
- Smoking
- COPD
- Blood type (highest risk with "type A," lowest risk with "type O")
- Trauma
- Antiphospholipid antibodies (lupus, etc.)
- Occupations requiring long periods of standing or sitting
- Varicose veins
- Congenital abnormalities (Klippel-Trenaunay)
- Inflammatory bowel disease
- Drug abuse
- Cerebrovascular events (stroke, TIA)
- May-Thurner syndrome

Indications for Exam

- Edema/swelling (especially when unilateral)
- Limb pain/tenderness
- Symptoms of pulmonary embolism (PE) (shortness of breath, chest pain, hemoptysis)
- Hypercoagulable state
- Duplex-guided filter insertion
- Pre-operative exam for patency prior to placement of caval filter
- Post-operative evaluation of filter device
- Pallor (phlegmasia alba dolens)
- Cyanosis (phlegmasia cerulea dolens- iliofemoral thrombosis)
- Positive D-dimer test result

Contraindications/Limitations

- Poor visualization due to vessel depth because of obesity, swelling or abdominal gas
- Compressibility of the IVC and iliac veins can be technically difficult due to the deep location of these veins.

Mechanism of Disease

There are three factors responsible for the formation of venous thrombosis, as outlined in Virchow's Triad (vein wall injury, hypercoagulability and stasis of blood flow). A combination of any of these events may increase the risk of venous thrombosis. [1]

- There is a balance between coagulation (process to prevent excessive bleeding after injury) and anticoagulation (process to prevent spontaneous intravascular clotting) in normal blood flow.
- The venous endothelial layer is normally antithrombotic. In response to endothelial injury, leukocytes (white blood cells) attach to the vessel wall. A plasma protein known as prothrombin is activated. Prothrombin activator catalyzes conversion of prothrombin into thrombin. Thrombin acts as an enzyme to convert fibrinogen into fibrin threads, forming a clot. [2,3]
- Hypercoaguable states result from genetic mutation or acquired deficiencies that accompany certain diseases (i.e., liver disease). In such cases, naturally occurring anticoagulants (antithrombin, protein C, protein S, etc.) are deficient. For example, the genetic mutation, factor V Leiden, causes resistance to the natural anticoagulant protein C. [4]
- Non-movement of blood flow (stasis) permits coagulation. Platelets are thought to become trapped by low shear stress (flow) at valve cusps. Platelets adhere to the subendothelial (collagen) layer of the venous wall, and may aggregate depending on the amount of coagulation and thrombolysis occurring in the body at that time.
- Increased activation of coagulation factors in those suffering from cancer is thought to lead to formation of venous thrombosis. In addition, the levels of coagulation inhibitors normally found in the blood (i.e., proteins C or S) are thought to be reduced in these patients. [4]
- Thrombosis in pregnancy is attributed to a prothrombotic state along with decreased venous outflow by the weight of the fetus. The use of estrogen (in replacement therapy or use of contraceptives) alters coagulation and may predispose an individual to thrombosis. [4]
- Once thrombus is formed, it can:
  - **Stabilize**: Stabilization includes adherence of the thrombus to the vessel wall without changing location or propagating. If thrombus has formed, the most favorable occurrence would be to stabilize. This reduces the risk of embolization or PE to the patient.
  - **Propagate:** Propagation includes "growth of thrombus" in size or location. The most notable importance of propagation is the possibility that a superficial system thrombus might propagate into the deep system.
  - **Embolize**: During embolization, a portion of the thrombus breaks free and travels elsewhere within the vascular system. The greatest risk to the patient is that the thrombus travels to the lungs and results in a pulmonary embolus. [2]
- Extrinsic compression from tumors, enlarged lymph nodes, etc. can result in stenosis or occlusion by placing enough pressure on venous walls to cause venous hypertension distal to the obstruction. [5]

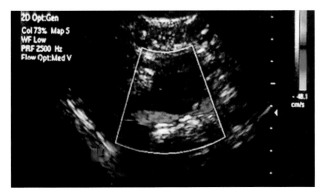

Extrinsic compression from a tumor which has narrowed the venous lumen by color flow

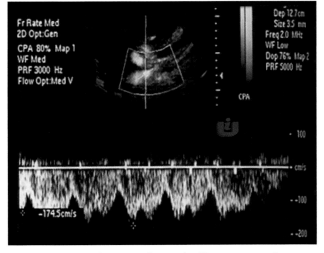

Increased venous flow velocities as a result of extrinsic compression from a tumor

Location of Disease

- IVC
- External or internal iliac veins

Patient History

- Acute onset of leg pain
- Acute onset of swelling
- Persistent leg swelling (usually unilateral, but can be bilateral)
- Symptoms of PE (shortness of breath, chest pain, hemoptysis)
- Previous DVT
- Clotting issues (including problems regulating anticoagulation therapy)

Physical Examination

- Edema or swelling
- Tenderness
- Pallor (phlegmasia alba dolens)
- Cyanosis (phlegmasia cerulea dolens)

IVC and Iliac Venous Duplex protocol

- Patients should be fasting for 6-12 hours to minimize the presence of air/bowel gas in the abdomen. A limited volume of clear liquids may be ingested prior to the examination (e.g., to swallow medications).

- Obtain a patient history to include symptoms and risk factors.
- Patient is examined in the supine position with the head slightly elevated.
- Use a lower frequency (1-4 MHz) curved or sector transducer for most patients. Thinner patients may require the use of a higher frequency (5-7 MHz) transducer.

Transverse IVC Scan and Images

> Scanning from the right flank is an alternative to the subxiphoid approach.

- Locate the IVC in the upper abdomen just below the xiphoid process in the transverse (short axis) plane. It may be possible to compress the vein wall with probe pressure, though color flow and spectral Doppler waveforms will be the main tools used during this evaluation in most patients.

- For the purposes of the ultrasound examination, the IVC is divided into three regions: [1]

  - **Suprahepatic**: superior to the liver

  - **Intrahepatic**: includes tributaries from the liver

  - **Infrahepatic**: inferior to the liver and to the level of the iliac bifurcation

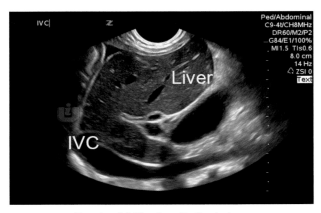

Proximal IVC—longitudinal plane

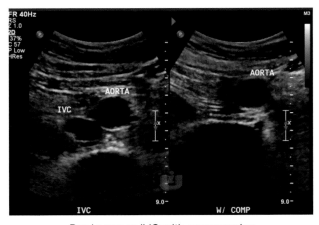

Dual screen: IVC with compression

> Keep the probe at a 90° angle to the skin for the best grayscale images.

- Image the IVC to the iliac bifurcation. Document transverse grayscale images of the IVC at the suprahepatic, intrahepatic and infrahepatic levels. Color flow can be added to demonstrate color filling of the vessel.

Longitudinal IVC Scan and Images

- Return the probe to the xiphoid process and rotate onto the IVC in the longitudinal (sagittal) plane. Record grayscale images of the IVC at the suprahepatic, intrahepatic and infrahepatic levels.

- Record images of the IVC using color Doppler at the suprahepatic, intrahepatic and infrahepatic levels.

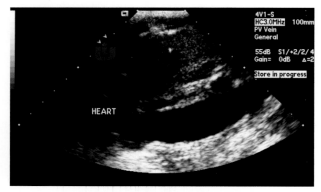

IVC in longitudinal plane by B-mode image

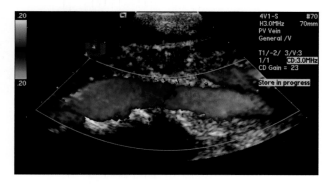

IVC in with longitudinal plane with color Doppler

- Document venous flow of the IVC in longitudinal view with pulsed wave (PW) Doppler. Some labs record venous PW Doppler flow without setting an angle since actual velocities are usually not important in a venous exam. (If your lab chooses to set an angle, use a ≤60º Doppler angle with the cursor placed parallel to the vessel walls in the center of the flow stream for spectral waveforms.) Spectral documentation should illustrate spontaneity, respiratory variation and phasicity. Record spectral waveform in the suprahepatic, intrahepatic and infrahepatic IVC segments.

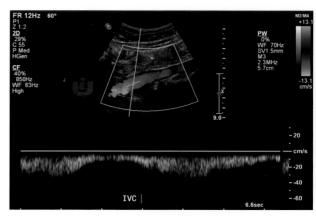

IVC spectral waveform by PW Doppler

> *Use abdominal and venous presets on the duplex scanner. Low color flow and Doppler scales will be needed to detect venous flow at these depths.*

Transverse Iliac Venous Scan and Images

- Reposition the probe in transverse at the infrahepatic IVC and scan distally to the common iliac venous bifurcation. Document a transverse grayscale image of the right and left common iliac veins (CIV) at the bifurcation near the umbilical level. Color flow can be added to demonstrate spontaneous color filling of the vessels.

- Continue distally, using color flow as a guide for the course of the vein. Document a transverse image of the right external (EIV) and internal iliac (IIV) veins at their bifurcation in the pelvis using color flow to demonstrate spontaneous color filling of the vessels.

Longitudinal Iliac Venous Scan and Images

- Return to the common iliac vein bifurcation and rotate onto the right common iliac vein in the longitudinal (sagittal) plane. Record venous flow in the proximal and mid/distal CIV with PW Doppler. Spectral documentation should illustrate spontaneity and respiratory variation.

- Continue distally, using color flow as a guide. Rotate onto the right EIV in the longitudinal (sagittal) plane. Record venous flow in the proximal and mid/distal EIV with PW Doppler. Compress the proximal thigh in attempt to elicit augmentation of venous flow. Spectral documentation should illustrate spontaneity, respiratory variation and possibly augmentation of the Doppler signal upon compression.

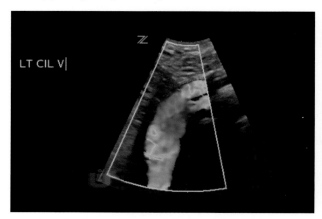

Longitudinal view of the common iliac vein as it bifurcates into the external and internal iliac veins

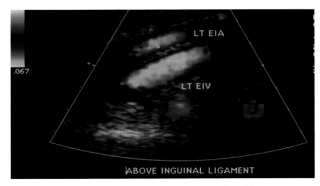

*External iliac vein and artery in with
longitudinal plane with color Doppler*

- Additional color and PW Doppler waveforms may be recorded in the internal iliac venous segment.
- Document any abnormal findings with grayscale and color imaging noted while scanning (e.g., thrombus, wall irregularity, extrinsic masses/tumors, etc.).
- Use PW Doppler to analyze absence of flow by placing the Doppler sample volume in any vein segment suspected to be thrombosed. Doppler flow or lack of flow, compliments compression, color flow and B-mode images. Use the adjacent artery as a guide to identify an occluded vein when possible.
- Repeat for the left common and external iliac venous system.
- Compare venous flow in the right and left external iliac veins to evaluate for obstruction at the common iliac level.

TABLE 89: **IVC and Iliac Venous Duplex Protocol Summary**	
Scan transverse (short axis) in grayscale and color	**Scan longitudinal (sagittal axis) with PW Doppler and color**

• IVC
  - Suprahepatic segment
  - Intrahepatic segment
  - Infrahepatic segment
• CIV
• EIV
• IIV (when visualized)
	• IVC
	• CIV (proximal and mid/distal segments)
	• EIV (proximal and mid/distal segments)
	• IIV (when visualized)

- Repeat the exam for the contralateral iliac segment when indicated.
- Additional documentation of compression and PW Doppler waveforms may be recorded in segments other than those listed during evaluation for thrombus as necessary.

Interpretation

General grayscale and color characteristics

- Determine whether echogenic material is observed within the lumen of the vein.
- Determine if the vein collapses completely with probe pressure (when possible).

Normal

- **Compressibility:** The vein is free of thrombus (intralumenal echoes) and compresses completely when technically possible. [6]

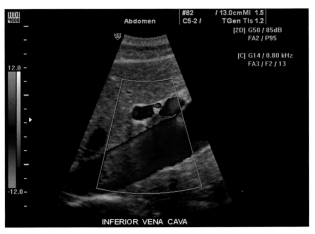

Wall to wall color fills a normal IVC
Image courtesy of Philips Healthcare

- **Color Doppler:** Wall to wall color flow will fill the vein spontaneously or upon distal limb compression. [6]
- **Diameter:** The average IVC diameter is 17.2 mm just below the renal veins during quiet respiration. The IVC diameter ranges between 5-29 mm at rest and increases approximately 10% with inspiration.[7]

> *Use flow in the adjacent artery as a guide to identify an occluded vein. Always confirm absence of flow by placing the sample volume within the vessel walls.*

TABLE 90: **Thrombosis Descriptions and Characteristics**	
Acute	**Chronic**
• Light to medium echogenic/anechoic	• Bright/heterogeneous echoes
• Spongy texture on compression (homogeneous)	• Irregular texture (heterogeneous)
• Poorly attached or free floating	• Attached
• Dilated vein (if totally occluded)	• Same size as artery or vein is contracted
	• Collateral veins may be noted

- Veins can be partially or totally incompressible in both acute and chronic stages.
- Combination of events can occurs (e.g., acute on top of chronic thrombus).
- Chronic thrombus with partial recanalization is seen as small color flow channels within thrombus.
- Age of thrombus is sometimes indeterminate.

- **General grayscale characteristics:** Intraluminal echoes are visualized within the vein.[8]
- **Compressibility:** Full coaptation of the vein on manual compression (when technically possible in the IVC-iliac segment) is absent or limited due to thrombus.[8] Compression of the artery but not the vein with probe pressure can be a confirmation of an incompressible venous segment.

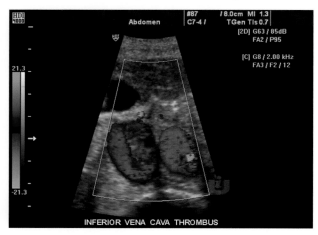

Partial thrombosis of the IVC by color flow in the transverse plane

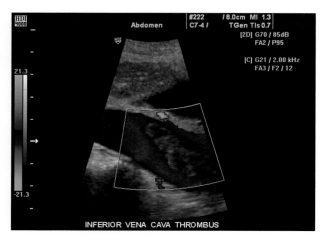

Partial thrombosis of the IVC by color flow in the longitudinal plane

Images courtesy of Philips Healthcare

> Color flow can obscure a partially occlusive thrombus if the color gain is set too high.

- **Color Doppler:**
  - If partially occlusive thrombus is present, color flow will be observed flowing around echogenic material in the vein spontaneously or with distal limb compression. [6,8]
  - If totally occlusive thrombus is present, no color flow will be observed spontaneously or with distal limb compression. [6,8]

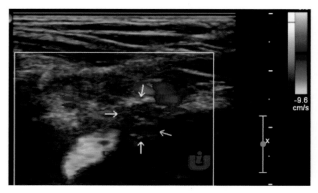

Total thrombosis of the external iliac vein by color flow in the transverse plane

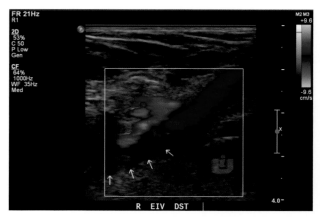

Total thrombosis of the external iliac vein by color flow in the longitudinal plane

Thrombus characteristics: If thrombus is present, determine whether the thrombus is partially or totally occlusive, its location, as well as the extent and characteristics of the thrombus.

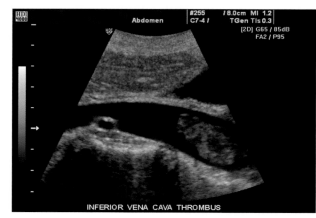

Acute IVC thrombus poorly attached to the wall

Image courtesy of Philips Healthcare

- **Acute thrombus**: Characteristics include lightly echogenic or anechoic clot, spongy texture and thrombus which is poorly attached to the venous wall or "free floating" within the lumen. A moving tail may be seen at the end of the thrombus. When a vein is fully thrombosed, the vein is often dilated in diameter. [7,8,9]

– **Chronic thrombus**: Characteristics include brightly echogenic or heterogeneous echoes, irregular surface texture and thrombus which is attached to the venous wall. The vein can stay the same size as the artery, but often contracts in diameter over time. Collateral veins may be observed adjacent to the affected vein(s) and small irregular flow channels can sometimes be seen with color. [8,9]

– **Indeterminate age**: Characteristics of both acute and chronic stages may be present (e.g., instead of acute venous dilatation or chronic venous constriction, the vein and artery are similar in size with mixed echogenicity). [9]

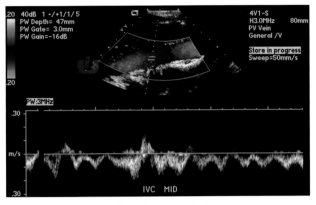

Normal venous Doppler recorded in the mid IVC

Venous Doppler Observations

• Determine whether venous flow is:

– Spontaneous (automatically heard with Doppler)
– Phasic- flow increases and decreases with respiration
– Augmentable (increases) with distal compression
– Pulsatile

Normal

– **Spontaneity:** The vein demonstrates spontaneous flow.

– **Phasicity:** Venous signals are phasic and vary with respiration/cardiac cycle in the distal IVC and iliac veins. During deep inhalation, venous signals decrease or discontinue and increase during exhalation due to changes in intrathoracic pressure during the respiratory cycle. [6,7]

– **Augmentation:** Compression of the limb distal to the probe can augment or increase venous flow in the external iliac veins. [6]

– **Pulsatility:** Pulsatility is often present in the proximal inferior vena cava due to its proximity to the heart. [6,7]

Abnormal

– **Spontaneity:** Absence of flow indicates venous obstruction. [8]

– **Phasicity:** Continuous venous flow (lack of respirophasicty) suggests either obstruction in a proximal venous segment or extrinsic compression of a proximal vein. [6,7]

– A comparable difference in external iliac venous signals between limbs suggests a common iliac venous obstruction on the side exhibiting decreased spontaneity or respirophasicty. [6]

– **Augmentation:** If distal compression does not produce augmentation of the venous signal, a total obstruction distal to the probe is suspected. A weak or dampened augmentation suggests a possible venous occlusion distal to the probe. [9]

> *Normal Doppler signals may be present when thrombus is partially occlusive.* [3]

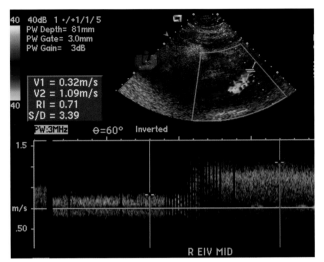

Extrinsic venous compression suspected by PW Doppler: increased venous velocities and visualization of a superficial mass

Other Pathology

• **IVC Filter:** IVC filters should be positioned below the level of the renal veins.

– Duplex documentation should depict patency of the IVC below the filter for a normal result.

– Thrombus visualized below the filter is an abnormal finding. [6,7]

• **Extrinsic compression:** IVC obstruction can result secondary to an extrinsic compression by a mass or intralumenal tumor. [7,11] Visualization of any echoic structures should be documented. Venous flow signals may be altered depending on the degree of compression.

– The IVC and iliac veins can become totally thrombosed secondary to the compression. The absence of color flow and PW Doppler signal using appropriate low-flow duplex settings indicates venous obstruction. [6]

– **Venous stenosis:** When continuous flow and increased venous velocities are noted (compared to proximal segments), a venous stenosis secondary to compression is suspected. [6]

• **Tumor invasion of the IVC:** On rare occasion, the lumen of the IVC can be invaded by a tumor. [6,7] On duplex image, the tumor appears moderately echogenic with diffuse color flow noted (typical characteristic of sarcomas or cancerous tumors). [6]

> *Since thrombus is non-vascularized, echogenic material with color flow is most likely a vascularized mass.*

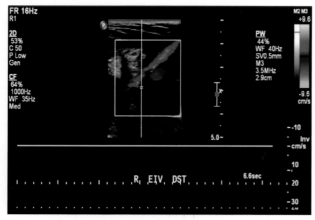

*Occluded external iliac venous segment
with absent color and PW Doppler*

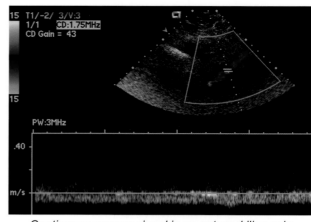

Continuous venous signal in an external iliac vein

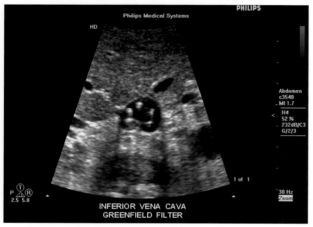

Transverse view of an IVC Greenfield filter

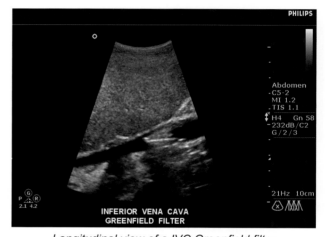

Longitudinal view of a IVC Greenfield filter

Images courtesy of Philips Healthcare

Differential Diagnosis

- Arterial disease
- Lymphedema
- Extrinsic compression
- Hematoma, cysts
- Adenopathy

- Arteriovenous fistula
- Heart failure (edema)
- Vascularized mass
- Abscess

Correlation

- CT scan
- MRI
- Venogram

Medical Treatment

- Anticoagulation therapy (e.g., heparin, warfarin)
- DVT prophylaxis (e.g., intermittent pneumatic cuff compression)
- Limit long periods of inactivity
- Promote venous return (e.g., elevate legs, wear elastic stockings/support hose)

Surgical Treatment

- IVC filter (acute DVT)
- Iliofemoral venous thrombectomy
- Iliocaval or IVC bypass (caval occlusion)

Endovascular Treatment

- Catheter directed thrombolysis with Urokinase, etc. (acute DVT)
- Balloon venoplasty and stenting for chronic iliofemoral DVT
- Mechanical thrombectomy, such as Angiojet (acute DVT)

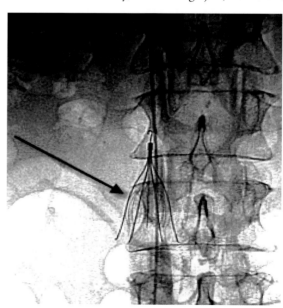

Inferior vena cavagram showing IVC filter

Venous Testing

IVC and Iliac Venous Duplex Ultrasound

Points to Remember

- Venous duplex ultrasound can identify the presence, location and extent of venous thrombosis or external compression. The course of the veins, collaterals and thrombus can be visualized using B-mode and color while the analysis of Doppler waveform changes can confirm occlusion and focal venous stenosis, or indirectly confirm proximal obstruction.

- The inferior vena cava and common iliac veins do not have valves.

- Perforation of the IVC in the presence of a filter is possible, though uncommon. [7]

- The left leg has a higher incidence of DVT than the right leg. Since the left common iliac vein crosses under the right common iliac artery, it sometimes becomes thrombosed. This is known as May-Thurner syndrome. [12]

- Free-floating thrombus in the iliofemoral veins has a higher risk of embolization (60%) than occlusive thrombus (5.5%). [8]

Anatomic Variations of the IVC

- The IVC can be duplicated, especially in the infrarenal portion of the vein. The iliac veins can continue from the pelvis without joining at an iliac venous bifurcation. Often the two IVC will join at the renal level and then follow a typical course. [6,7]

- Instead of its normal position to the right of the aorta, the IVC may be located on the left side. [13]

- There may be a congenital absence of the IVC at the intrahepatic level. The hepatic vein will be observed draining directly into the right atrium by duplex imaging. [7]

- Membranous obstruction of the IVC is a common cause of hepatic outflow obstruction. In these cases, a visible membrane is noted by ultrasound at the level of the diaphragm, with a reversal of blood flow and significant dilatation noted of the IVC. The right hepatic vein is most commonly obstructed and will appear dilated with slow, continuous flow. Portal hypertension and venous collateralization may also be noted. [7]

References

1. Gloviczki P. (2005). Introduction and general considerations. In *Rutherford Vascular Surgery 6th edition*. (2111-2123). Philadelphia. Elsevier Saunders.

2. Guyton AC. (1986). Hemostasis and blood coagulation. In *Textbook of Medical Physiology 7th edition*. (76-86). Philadelphia: WB Saunders.

3. Fareed J, Hoppensteadt DA, Iqbal O, Florian-Kujawski M, Tobu M, Bick, RL, Sheikh T, Jeske W. (2005). Normal and abnormal coagulation. In *Rutherford Vascular Sugery 6th edition*. (493-511). Philadelphia. Elsevier Saunders.

4. Henke PK, Schmaier A, Wakefield TW. (2005). Vascular thrombosis due to hypercoaguable states. In *Rutherford Vascular Sugery 6th edition*. (568-578). Philadelphia. Elsevier Saunders.

5. Sumner DS, Zierler RE. (2005). Vascular physiology: essential hemodynamic principles. In *Rutherford Vascular Sugery 6th edition*. (75-123). Philadelphia. Elsevier Saunders

6. Dawson DL, Beals H. (2010). Acute lower extremity deep venous thrombosis. In Zierler RE (Ed.), *Strandess's duplex scanning disorders in vascular diagnosis 4th ed*. (179-198). Philadelphia Wolters Kluwer Lippincott Williams & Wilkins

7. Zwiebel, WJ (2005). Ultrasound assessment of the aorta, iliac arteries and inferior vena cava. In Zwiebel WJ, Pellerito JS (Eds.), *Introduction to Vascular Ultrasonography 5th ed*, (530-552). Philadelphia: Elsevier Saunders.

8. Meissner MH. (2005). Venous duplex scanning. In *Rutherford Vascular Sugery 6th edition*. (254-270). Philadelphia. Elsevier Saunders.

9. Zwiebel, WJ (2005). Ultrasound Diagnosis of Venous Thrombosis. In Zwiebel WJ, Pellerito JS (Eds.), Introduction to Vascular Ultrasonography 5th ed, (449-465). Philadelphia: Elsevier Saunders.

10. Myers K, Clough A. (2004). Venous thrombosis in the lower limbs. In *Making sense of Vascular ultrasound: A Hands on Guide*. (181-197). London: Hodder Arnold.

11. Bower TC. (2005). Evaluation and management of malignant tumors of the inferior vena cava. In *Rutherford Vascular Sugery 6th edition*. (2245-2357). Philadelphia. El Sevier Saunders.

12. Gloviczki P, Cho JS. (2005) Surgical treatment of chronic occlusions of the iliac veins and the superior vena cava. In *Rutherford Vascular Sugery 6th edition*. (2303-2320). Philadelphia. El Sevier Saunders.

13. Sidawy AN. (2005) Embryology of the vascular system. In *Rutherford Vascular Sugery 6th edition*. (53-62). Philadelphia. El Sevier Saunders.v

Definition

The use of real time B-mode ultrasonography to evaluate the suitability of extremity veins for use in dialysis access creation or for bypass conduit

Risk Factors (requiring intervention using vein)

- Atherosclerosis
- Cardiac disease
- Renal failure
- Trauma
- Aneurysm

Risk Factors (for conditions that would affect venous suitability)

- Previous thrombosis
- Venous injury (e.g., intravenous lines or ports used for cancer treatment)
- Varicosities

Indications for Exam

- Severe ischemia of the upper or lower extremities which may require revascularization with autogenous conduit/bypass graft
- Severe ischemia of the heart which may require revascularization with autogenous conduit/bypass graft
- Renal failure requiring fistula placement for hemodialysis
- Request to identify patent veins for intravenous line placement

Contraindications/Limitations

- Open wounds prohibiting access by the ultrasound probe
- Casts that cannot be removed or traction that limits access to the scan areas
- Poor visualization due to vessel depth because of obesity or severe edema
- Patients who cannot be adequately positioned
- Anatomical limitations (clavicle and ribs)

Location of Disease

Location of disease can be focal or diffuse and affect any level or multiple levels. Common sites include:

- Valve sites
- The cephalic vein may demonstrate a venous stenosis at its junction with the subclavian vein.

Patient History

- Previous vein harvesting or history of vein stripping
- History of deep or superficial venous thrombosis

Physical Examination

Check for these possible contraindications to venous mapping prior to exam:

- Varicose veins
- Scars from previous vein harvesting (vein can be located proximal, distal, or near the scar)
- Palpable chord, redness or warmth along the superficial venous tract

Upper and Lower Extremity Venous Duplex Mapping Protocol

- The room and the patient should be warm and comfortable to prevent venous constriction.
- Obtain a patient history to include symptoms and risk factors.
- Patient position should be optimized so that gravity can help dilate the veins. Patient may be examined in one of several positions: while sitting, in the supine position with the head elevated and the arms dependent (upper extremity) or placed on a bed in a reverse Trendelenburg position (lower extremity).
- Some patients may require the use of a range of transducers for superficial vessels including high-frequency (5-7 MHz) (8-15 MHz) transducers. A lower frequency (1-4 MHz) transducer may be useful around the clavicle.
- Locate the superficial vein of interest in a transverse view (short axis) using B-mode imaging. A gentle tap of the veins, especially in the arm, can facilitate venous dilatation should the veins appear small in diameter. Hand exercises may also help dilate the arm veins.
- Perform venous compression every 2-4 cm along the superficial vein in the transverse plane to check for thrombosis. Thrombosed or phlebitic superficial venous segments should be documented since thrombosed veins are not suitable for bypass/access conduit.

> *Superficial veins run within the superficial compartment above the deep fascia and do not have a corresponding artery, which makes them easy to distinguish from the deep veins.*

- Document venous flow by recording a spectral tracing using pulsed wave Doppler in the longitudinal (sagittal) plane.
- Color flow imaging may also be used as additional documentation of patency.
- The anterior-posterior diameter of the vein is measured in the transverse plane with minimal, if any probe pressure. Measurements should be taken approximately every 2-3 inches or when a significant change in size is noted. Size changes are frequently seen near a tributary. Report the diameter measurements in millimeters.
- **Record measurements in duplicated systems, especially when diameters are sizable.**

Cephalic vein

Locate the cephalic vein (CV) at the "snuffbox" (the hollow on the radial aspect of the wrist when the thumb is extended fully). Follow the CV through the forearm. At the antecubital fossa, the CV continues into the (upper) arm. Follow the CV toward the shoulder to the junction with the axillary and subclavian veins, near the clavicle at the deltopectoral groove. Note the presence of any double cephalic venous systems. Record diameter measurements at the following levels:

- At wrist
- Distal forearm
- Mid forearm
- Proximal forearm
- Antecubital fossa
- Distal arm
- Mid arm
- Proximal arm
- Cephalic-subclavian vein confluence

Basilic vein

Locate the basilic vein (BSV) medially in the arm, near the elbow. Follow the BSV superiorly along the medial arm, toward its junction with the axillary or brachial vein. Go back and follow the BSV posteriomedially through the forearm. Note the presence of any double basilic venous systems. Record diameter measurements at the following levels:

- At wrist
- Distal forearm
- Mid forearm
- Proximal forearm
- Antecubital fossa
- Distal arm
- Mid arm
- Proximal arm
- Basilic-brachial-axillary vein confluence

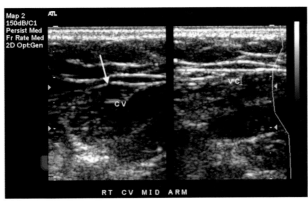

Dual screen image showing a compressible cephalic vein

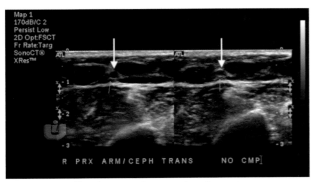

Dual screen image showing an incompressible cephalic vein

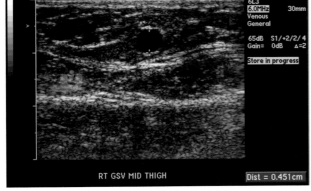

Lower extremity transverse diameter measurement

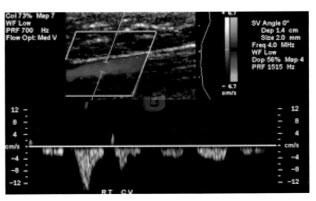

Normal cephalic vein Doppler waveforms

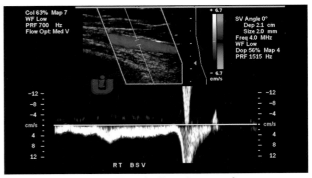

Normal basilic vein Doppler waveforms

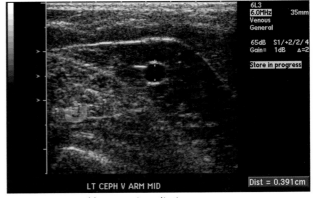

Upper extremity transverse diameter measurement

Typical Anatomic Variations of the Veins at the Antecubital Fossa

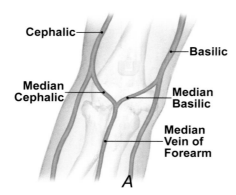

A

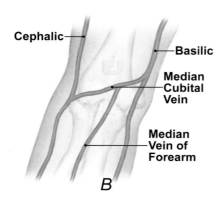

B

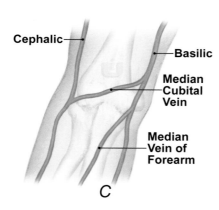

C

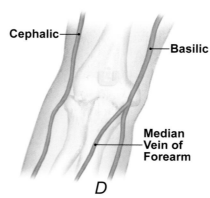

D

Anatomical variations of the superficial veins in the cubital fossa.(A) M-shaped configuration, (B and C) N-shaped configurations with the MCV terminating in CV and BSV, respectively, (D) no communication between the CV and BSV.

Median cubital vein

Only one diameter measurement of the median cubital vein (MCV) in the antecubital fossa is usually recorded, since this vein is very short. When indicated, determine the anatomical connections of the MCV and note potential variations in this area, which are common:

Lower Extremity Superficial Veins

Great saphenous vein

- Locate the great saphenous vein (GSV) at the saphenofemoral junction. Follow the vein along the medial aspect of the thigh, calf and ankle. Note the presence of any large great saphenous accessory tributaries. Record diameter measurements at the following levels:

  - Groin (just distal to the saphenofemoral junction)
  - Proximal thigh
  - Mid thigh
  - Distal thigh
  - At knee
  - Proximal calf
  - Mid calf
  - Distal calf
  - At ankle

Small saphenous vein

- Locate the small saphenous vein (SSV) at the saphenopopliteal junction (or its alternative origin). Follow the vein along the posterior aspect of the calf to the ankle. Note the presence of any large small saphenous accessory tributaries. Record diameter measurements at the following levels:

  - Just distal to the saphenopopliteal junction (or at origin in the distal thigh, etc.)
  - Proximal calf
  - Mid calf
  - Distal calf
  - At ankle

> *A vein located outside of the saphenous compartment is known as a tributary and is not a main vein. It is important to note this distinction for the surgeon since most expect reported veins to run in the saphenous compartment.*

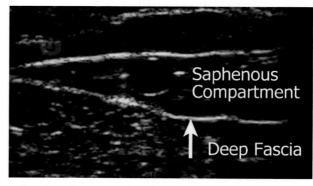

Great saphenous vein within saphenous compartment

- Large GSV or SSV tributaries may be present and confused with the main venous trunk being examined. It is often helpful to move to the most distal point of the vein and scan proximally. For example, the GSV often has large tributaries just below the knee that may be confused with the main trunk of the GSV. It is helpful to move to the anterior-medial malleolar area (ankle) to identify the GSV and map the vein proximally from that point to the knee.

TABLE 91: **Upper and Lower Extremity Venous Duplex Mapping Protocol Summary**

Scan transverse (short axis) with and without compression in grayscale (to check for thrombus) and measure (anterior-posterior) venous diameters (in millimeters) as appropriate at the following levels:

Upper Extremity-Cephalic (CV), Basilic (BSV), Median Cubital (MCV)	Lower Extremity-great saphenous (GSV) Small Saphenous (SSV)
• Proximal arm (CV/BSV)	• Saphenofemoral junction (GSV)
• Mid arm (CV/BSV)	• Proximal thigh (GSV)
• Distal arm (CV/BSV)	• Mid thigh (GSV)
• Antecubital fossa (CV/BSV/MCV)	• Distal thigh (GSV)
• Proximal forearm (CV/BSV)	• Origin SSV (e.g., saphenopopliteal junction)
• Mid forearm (CV/BSV)	• At knee (GSV/SSV)
• Distal forearm (CV/BSV)	• Proximal calf (GSV/SSV)
• At wrist (CV/BSV)	• Mid calf (GSV/SSV)
• Origin CV, BSV and MCV veins	• Distal calf (GSV/SSV)
	• At ankle (GSV/SSV)

- Document venous flow using PW Doppler or color flow imaging.
- Measure length of entire continuous venous segment(s) in centimeters (cm).
- Map the vein course using indelible marker when instructed.
- Repeat for the contralateral extremity if necessary.

- Comment on the continuity of all venous segments studied and measure the length of suitable vein in centimeters (cm).

- Mark the course of the vein with an indelible marker if indicated. Marking may help in cases of unusual anatomy or to mark major tributaries and double systems.

  - Keep the probe perpendicular to the surface of the skin.
  - Keep the visualized vein in the middle of the ultrasound screen in transverse view and place a small mark in the middle and just above the transducer. Continue with this method along the extremity.
  - At the end of the exam, "connect-the-dots" to represent the course of the visualized vein.

Interpretation

> Interpretation as to the suitable nature of a vein is left to the surgeon's discretion. In general, patent veins 3 mm in diameter can usually dilate to >4 mm diameter under arterial pressure for use as dialysis conduit or a bypass graft.[3]

- Criteria for suitable venous diameter differs among surgeons and according to the procedure planned. The basic interpretation of a venous mapping exam analyzes:

  - Diameter ranges
  - Health of the vein
  - Continuity of the vein

2-D Image Observations
General Grayscale and Color Characteristics

- Determine whether echogenic material is observed within the lumen of the vein.

- Determine if the vein collapses completely with light probe pressure.

Normal

- **Compressibility:** The vein is free of thrombus if it compresses completely and is free of echogenic material within its lumen. [8]

> Check each vein of a duplicated or bifed system.

- **Color Doppler:** Color flow will fill the vein completely upon distal limb compression. [5,6]

Abnormal [5]

- **Compressibility:** Echogenic material is visualized within the vein and full coaptation of the vein on manual compression is absent or limited due to thrombus. [6,8]

  - If the vein is sclerosed, its walls will appear very thickened, although the lumen may be collapsible. [1]

- **Color Doppler:**

  - Color flow can be observed moving around echogenic material within the vein upon distal limb compression if partially occlusive thrombus is present. [8]
  - Color flow cannot be observed upon distal limb compression if totally occlusive thrombus is present using appropriate low-flow machine settings. [6,8]

- **Varicosed segments** are not suitable for operative use and should be reported. [1]

- **Thrombus:** If thrombus is present, determine whether the thrombus is partial or totally occlusive, its location, as well as the extent and the characteristics of the thrombus.

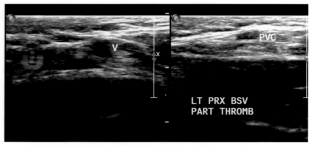

Partially incompressible/partially occlusive thrombus

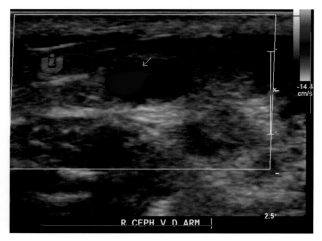

Acute, partially occlusive thrombus

- **Acute thrombus**: Characteristics include lightly echogenic or anechoic clot, spongy texture and thrombus, which is poorly attached to the venous wall or "free floating" within the lumen. A moving tail may be seen at the end of the thrombus. The vein is often dilated in diameter. [5,7]
- **Chronic thrombus**: Characteristics include brightly echogenic or heterogeneous echoes, irregular surface texture and thrombus, which is attached to the venous wall. The vein often contracts in diameter over time. Collateral veins may be observed adjacent to the affected vein(s). [5,7]
- **Indeterminate age**: Characteristics of both acute and chronic stages may be present. [5,7]

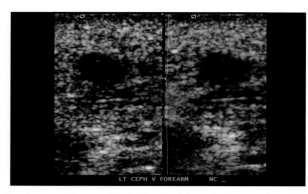

Dual screen image illustrating indeterminate age thrombus

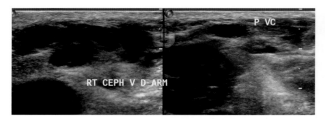

Dual screen image illustrating chronic thrombus in a cephalic vein

TABLE 92: **Thrombosis Descriptions and Characteristics**	
Acute	**Chronic**
• Light to medium echogenic/anechoic	• Bright/heterogeneous echoes
• Spongy texture on compression (homogeneous)	• Irregular texture (heterogeneous)
• Poorly attached or free floating	• Attached
• Dilated vein (if totally occluded)	• Same size as artery or vein is contracted
	• Collateral veins may be noted

- Veins can be partially or totally incompressible in both acute and chronic stages.
- Combination of events can occurs (e.g., acute on top of chronic thrombus).
- Chronic thrombus with partial recanalization is seen as small color flow channels within thrombus.
- Age of thrombus is sometimes indeterminate.

Venous Doppler observations

> *Normal Doppler signals may be present when thrombus is partially occlusive.*[5]

- Observe venous flow for:
  - Spontaneity-signal automatically heard with Doppler
  - Phasicity-flow increases and decreases with respiration
  - Augmentation-increase with distal compression

Normal

- **Spontaneity and phasicity:** *Note-* In the superficial veins, the absence of spontaneous and phasic flow can be a normal finding.
- **Augmentation:** Compression of the limb distal to the probe augments venous flow. [6,8]

Abnormal

- **Spontaneity:** Absence of flow indicates venous obstruction. [8]
- **Phasicity:** Continuous venous flow suggests either obstruction in a proximal venous segment or extrinsic compression on the vein. [7]

- **Augmentation:** If distal compression does not produce augmentation of the venous signal, an obstruction distal to the probe is suspected. A weak or dampened augmentation suggests a partial or total occlusion distal to the probe and may be caused by poor filling of the vein.[7]

TABLE 93: Diagnostic Criteria for Venous Duplex	
Normal	**Abnormal**
• Complete coaptation of vein walls with light probe pressure	• Lack of complete vein compression
• Absent intralumenal thrombus	• Intralumenal echoes present (acute thrombus can be echolucent)
• Color flow fills the lumen completely	• Decrease or absence of color flow
• Normal venous Doppler spontaneity, phasicity and augmentation	• Abnormal venous Doppler spontaneity, phasicity or augmentation
• No venous dilatation	• Dilated or contracted veins noted

Correlation

- Venogram

Points to Remember

- The GSV has many tributaries and is commonly used as conduit for cardiac and vascular bypass surgeries.

- The GSV is often the first choice for an autogenous graft. [3] In some cases, the GSV may be absent, previously used as a bypass, stripped if it was varicosed, not continuous/long enough for the required bypass or unsuitable because of thrombophlebitis. In the absence of great saphenous veins, arm veins become an alternative for autogenous bypass grafts. [1]

- An anastomosis to either the cephalic or basilic veins may be used in the upper extremities to create an arteriovenous fistula for dialysis. [9]

- Placing a tourniquet around the upper arm may help to dilate the veins while imaging. [9]

- A drawing or diagram may be provided by the technologist to aid the surgeon regarding diameter or course of the vessels.

- When marking the vein on the skin, a probe cover may be used to minimize damage by the waterproof markers to the transducer membrane.

- Another technique to mark the vein uses a straw placed vertically on the skin over the site of the vein, which can be rotated back and forth to create a round mark on the skin. After the gel and the transducer are removed, the circular marks on the skin can be connected, using an indelible marker, indicating the course of the vein. [1]

- The location of valve sinuses need not be noted unless they are stenotic or otherwise abnormal. If valve leaflets are visualized, they should appear thin and freely moving within the lumen. If the valve leaflet is rigid, brightly echoic and fixed in the lumen, report this as an abnormality.

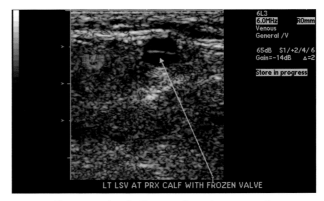

Frozen valve in the small saphenous vein

- In cases of DVT, the superficial system can act as the primary pathway for venous return. Documentation of the deep veins can also be part of a venous mapping exam. The surgeon may want to confirm there is no evidence of DVT before removing superficial veins.

- Complex and small venous systems can take as long as one hour to map completely.

- Marking venous tributaries on the skin for the surgeon helps direct incisions directly over the vein to avoid skin flaps, wound complications and ultimately improves post-operative healing. [3]

References

1. Gibson KD, Ebert A. (2010). Preoperative vein mapping. In Zierler RE (Ed.). Strandess's duplex scanning disorders in vascular diagnosis 4th ed. (231-234).Philadelphia Wolters Kluwer Lippincott Williams & Wilkins.

2. Patel, ST, Mills JL. (2005). The preoperative, intraoperative, and post-operative non-invasive evaluation of infrainguinal vein bypass grafts. In Mansour MA, Labropoulos N. (Eds.), *Vascular Diagnosis*, (277-292). Philadelphia. Elsevier Saunders.

3. Mills, JL. (2005). Infrainguinal bypass. In *Rutherford Vascular Surgery 6th edition*. (1154-1174). Philadelphia. Elsevier Saunders.

4. Dawson DL, Beals H. (2010). Acute lower extremity deep venous thrombosis. In Zierler RE (Ed.), *Strandess's duplex scanning disorders in vascular diagnosis 4th ed*. (179-198).Philadelphia Wolters Kluwer Lippincott Williams & Wilkins.

5. Myers K, Clough A. (2004). Venous thrombosis in the lower limbs. In *Making sense of vascular ultrasound: A hands on guide*. (181-197). London: Hodder Arnold.

6. Myers K, Clough A. (2004). Diseases of vessels to the upper limb. In *Making sense of vascular ultrasound: A hands on guide*. (227-254). London: Hodder Arnold.

7. Zwiebel, WJ (2005). Ultrasound Diagnosis of Venous Thrombosis. In Zwiebel WJ, Pellerito JS (Eds.), *Introduction to Vascular Ultrasonography 5th ed*, (449-465). Philadelphia. Elsevier Saunders.

8. Meissner MH. (2005). Venous duplex scanning. In *Rutherford Vascular Surgery 6th edition*. (254-270). Philadelphia. Elsevier Saunders.

9. Robbin ML, Lockhart ME. (2005). Ultrasound evaluation before and after hemodialysis access. In Zwiebel WJ, Pellerito JS (Eds.), *Introduction to Vascular Ultrasonography 5th ed*. (325-340). Philadelphia: Elsevier Saunders.

Definition

Venous photoplethysmography (PPG) is a tool used to evaluate the lower extremity veins for evidence of valvular incompetence. Venous PPG can also help differentiate between primary and secondary venous insufficiency in order to plan treatment options.

Chronic venous insufficiency (CVI) is caused by incompetent valves in the superficial and/or deep venous systems that can result in venous hypertension and stasis.

Venous PPG testing involves exercise or manual calf compressions to cause contraction of the calf muscles. These contractions empty the blood out of the veins in the lower leg.

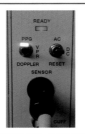

The venous or DC mode on the PPG instrument is used to monitor slow venous changes. The arterial or AC mode is used to monitor the faster volume changes that occur with arterial pulsations.

Principle

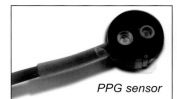

PPG sensor

PPG equipment can monitor and display blood volume changes over time.

A PPG sensor consists of an infrared light and a receiver that is attached to the skin in the gaiter area with double-sided tape or a Velcro strap. Infrared light is transmitted into the superficial tissues and the reflected light is received by the sensor. The reflected signal relates to the quantity of red blood cells in the cutaneous circulation.

Normally while being tested, the calf muscles compress the veins during exercise or manual compression, and there is a rapid decrease in venous blood volume followed by a slow refilling of the veins via the arteries and capillaries.

After setting a baseline for the PPG tracing, the calf veins are emptied through exercise or manual compression and the leg is rested so that veins can refill.

The PPG tracing demonstrates the volume changes during this venous emptying and filling. From this tracing the venous refill time (a.k.a., venous recover time or VRT) can be calculated.

Valvular incompetence results in a faster VRT than normal, since veins refill via immediate back flow of venous blood, past the incompetent valves rather than through the normal course; artery, arteriole, capillary, and then vein.

Mechanism of Disease

Calf Muscle Pump

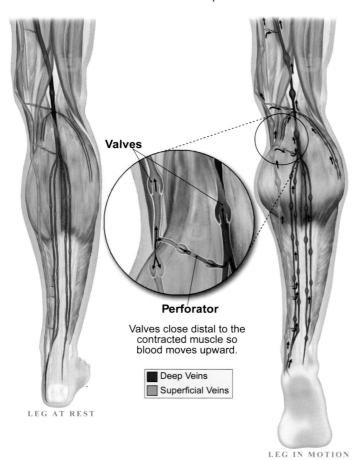

Valves

Perforator

Valves close distal to the contracted muscle so blood moves upward.

- Deep Veins
- Superficial Veins

LEG AT REST

LEG IN MOTION

When the leg is in motion (walking), muscle contractions squeeze the veins, forcing blood past the open valves of the deep, superficial and perforating veins upward towards the heart. After the muscle relaxes, valves close to prevent backflow (reflux).

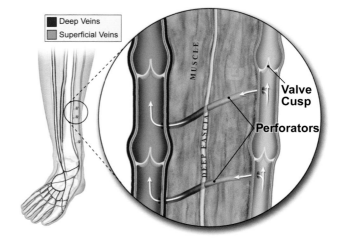

- Deep Veins
- Superficial Veins

MUSCLE

DEEP FASCIA

Valve Cusp

Perforators

Blood flows normally from the superficial to deep veins via perforators.

Venous Flow with Normal Valve Function

- The direction of normal blood flow in the deep and superficial veins is toward the heart. In the perforating (communicating) veins, blood normally flows from the superficial to the deep veins. [1]

- At various times, the blood may encounter pressure to move backwards away from the heart, in response to gravity, for example. Normally, flow reversal is prevented by the venous valves which close in response to pressure from the reversed flow. [1]

- Upon exercise, the action of the calf muscles normally sends blood up the leg away from the calf. This action empties the calf veins, reduces the blood volume and reduces venous pressure. [1]

Venous Flow with Abnormal Valve Function

- Valvular damage and dysfunction (valvular incompetence) result in *venous reflux*, which is venous flow in the wrong (or opposite) direction, away from the heart and back into the leg.

- In the perforating veins, blood flows in the wrong direction from the deep to the superficial system.

- Venous reflux creates a high blood volume in the veins distal to the incompetent valve(s). [1]

- High blood volume in a vein causes increased venous pressure or *venous hypertension*. [1]

- The hypertension will be greatest upon standing due to the effect of hydrostatic pressure from gravity, adding to the increased pressure from volume. [1]

- Normally venous blood volume and venous pressure are reduced by activation of the calf muscle pump upon walking. When the valves are not working, the venous volume and resulting pressure do not decrease sufficiently and the patient suffers from *ambulatory venous hypertension*. [1]

- Venous hypertension also increases pressure within the venules and capillaries. This high pressure system encourages fluids to escape into the tissues causing edema. [1]

- Local edema results in a decrease in fluid and protein reabsorption. Fibrinogen and red blood cells (RBC) in the capillaries escape back into the tissues. Proteins organize and form tissue fibrosis (causing hardening of the skin). The RBCs break down and cause hyperpigmentation (dark tissue discoloration). Oxygen intake is decreased in the tissues, causing tissue malnutrition/hypoxia. Ulceration may follow. [1,2,3,4]

Varicose Veins

- Histological studies describe an increase in collagen and fibrous tissue within the layers of the venous wall in varicose vein patients. Collagen bundles disrupt the typical, orderly configuration of smooth muscles cells (SMC) in the medial layer. These SMC are thought to contain an excessive amount of granules, which may secrete collagenase and elastase, resulting in weakening of the venous wall and dilatation. Weakened venous walls allow for dilatation and elongation. [5]

- Varicose veins demonstrate decreased ability to contract normally and the valves of varicosed veins become stretched. [1]

- Tributaries of the great saphenous vein (GSV) are thought to varicose before the main trunk of the GSV because they contain less muscle in their vessel walls and lack support in the subcutaneous fat layer under the skin where they are commonly located. [1]

PREGNANCY

- Pregnancy increases the amount of blood circulating in the body and causes veins to enlarge. The pressure of the fetus on the veins can decrease the blood flow back through the pelvic venous system. [1,6,7]

Location of Disease

Incompetent valves may be located at any segment of the deep, perforating, or superficial veins, but are more commonly found in the superficial venous tributaries. [2]

- Most common location for incompetent perforating veins is the gaiter area- just above the medial malleolus.

- Saphenofemoral junction (SFJ)

Patient History

- Persistent leg/calf swelling (usually unilateral)
- Previous DVT
- Localized pain, burning or itching
- Tired, heavy legs after prolonged standing
- Varicose veins
- Skin changes and skin ulcers

Physical Examination

- Edema
- Tenderness, warmth or redness along the course of a superficial vein or varicosity
- Varicose veins
- Hyperpigmentation, hardened tissue around the ankles
- Ulceration (esp., gaiter area)
- Dermatitis in the gaiter area or area along the course of a superficial vein
- Noticeable telangiectasia
- Venous claudication- severe symptoms of CVI (including those listed above) with pain/aching that worsens when walking and is relieved by elevation of the leg.

Indications for Exam

- Varicose veins
- Chronic edema/swelling which worsens at the end of the day (especially when unilateral)
- Pain, which may be localized to a specific varix or described as a "dull ache"
- Discoloration at the gaiter area
- Ulceration (esp., gaiter area)
- Venous claudication

Contraindications/Limitations

- PPG testing is a subjective test. Although an actual number is calculated (VRT), it is an overall measurement and not specific to a certain vein.
- Patient's inability to maximally point/flex their foot (manual compression can be used in such cases).
- Patient's inability to sit and hang their limb over the bedside.
- Ulcerations and lack of intact skin, prohibiting placement of the PPG sensor.
- Patients with extensive bandages or casts

Venous PPG Protocol

- Obtain a patient history to include symptoms and risk factors.
- Ensure that the patient is not vasoconstricted (cold).
- Explain the procedure to the patient and make sure they understand their role during the examination.
- The patient is positioned at the edge of the bed/stretcher with their legs dangling over the side in a non-weight bearing position. Be sure that the bed is not compressing the back of the calf.

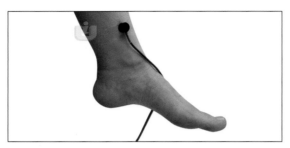

Resting venous PPG position

- The PPG monitor is set in the DC (venous) mode.
- The PPG sensor is firmly adhered to the ankle about 2 to 5 cm above the medial malleolus (gaiter area) with double stick transparent tape or a Velcro strap. Try not to touch the tape surface that is under the probe since fingerprints can degrade the skin/probe coupling and reduce the amplitude of the signal. Ensure that there will be no movement between the PPG sensor and the skin during the exercise.

> *Skin integrity must be checked before placing the PPG sensor. Choose a location that is free of ulceration or hardened skin. Do not place sensor directly on a varicosed vein.*

- Turn on the PPG strip chart recorder at a speed of 5 mm/sec. Adjust the PPG gain to the machines midpoint and set the tracing near the top portion of the chart.
- Ask the patient to begin cycles of plantarflexion (where they point their foot upward) and dorsiflexion (where they point their foot downward). This type of exercise causes contraction of the calf muscles and empties the blood out of the veins in the lower leg.

> *Demonstrating the exercise for the patient often helps to obtain maximum flexion and correct timing.*

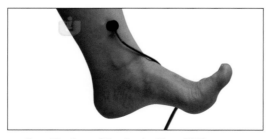

Dorsiflexion of the foot with a PPG sensor

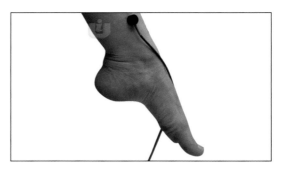

Plantarflexion of the foot with a PPG sensor

- If the tracing starts to drift off the page during exercise, readjust the gain and position of the trace.

> *As an alternate to dorsi- and plantarflexions, manual compressions of the gastrocnemius muscle will empty the blood out of the calf veins. With the patient's legs dangling off the bed, place your thumbs along each side of the tibia and squeeze the back of the patient's calf upward with your remaining fingers. Compress the calf for 1 second, then release the compression for 1 second. Five of these compressions are typically performed.*

- The PPG tracing should drop with exercise and then slope slowly upwards once the exercise is completed.
- Let the patient know they can relax while the recording is being taken and analyzed.
- On the tracing, note when the PPG slope either stabilizes by flattening out for at least 5 seconds or peaks and falls slightly. If the tracing is still rising after 30 seconds, you can stop the recording since this is far past the threshold for reflux.

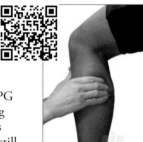

Manual compressions

> *Remember to keep the speed of the PPG strip chart recorder at 5 mm/sec.*

- Determine the VRT by calculating the amount of time between the end of the exercise or manual compressions and the peak or beginning of the plateau.

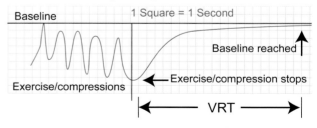

Calculation of the VRT

- Repeat the exam several times on each leg, with a 1 minute rest period between each attempt. Report the average or *mean* VRT. The author suggests collecting VRT from three exercises, calculating the sum, dividing this value by 3 and reporting the number as the mean VRT.

Additional testing based on initial VRT results:

- **If the VRT is ≥20 seconds:** Valvular function is normal and testing is complete.

- **If the VRT is <20 seconds:** Apply a 10-12 cm straight pressure cuff (or tourniquet) to the distal thigh to be used to occlude the superficial venous system.

- Inflate the pressure cuff to approximately 50 mmHg. This should occlude the GSV in the sitting position, while the deep system remains patent.

  - Repeat the exercise and recalculate the VRT.
    - **If the VRT is ≥20 sec:** testing is complete.
    - **If the VRT is <20 sec:** use duplex scanning to further evaluate for reflux or apply a 10-12 cm straight pressure cuff (or tourniquet) just below the knee to occlude the small saphenous venous system. Repeat the exercise and recalculate the VRT.

TABLE 94: Photoplethysmography Protocol Summary

- Hang the leg over the bedside in a non-weight bearing position. Keep the calf from touching the bed.

- Place the PPG transducer about 2 inches above the medial malleolus using double-stick transparent tape or a velcro strap.

- Turn the recorder on DC (venous) mode and run the PPG tracing at a speed of 5 mm/sec.

- Ask the patient to perform 5 cycles of the plantarflexion/dorsiflexion exercise, resting about 1 minute between cycles. (Or perform manual compressions if the patient is unable to exercise independently.)

- Wait for the tracing to either plateau, peak, or run for 30 seconds, whichever comes first.

- Calculate the VRT on the recorded trace by counting from the end of the exercise/compression cycle until the tracing reaches a stable baseline or 30 seconds.

- Repeat the exam several times on each leg in order to calculate a mean VRT.

The exam is finished if the mean VRT is ≥20 sec.

Continue with additional testing or use duplex imaging to further evaluate reflux if the mean VRT is <20 sec.

- Inflate a pressure cuff placed on the distal thigh to 50 mmHg.

- Repeat the exercise/compression several times and calculate the mean VRT.

The exam is completed if the mean VRT is ≥20 sec. Continue with additional testing or use duplex imaging to further evaluate reflux if the mean VRT is <20 sec.

- Inflate a pressure cuff placed on the proximal calf to 50 mmHg.

- Repeat the exercise/compression several times and calculate the mean VRT.

Interpretation

VRT without use of a cuff

- VRT ≥20 sec is considered normal; the venous refill time via the arterial system is within normal limits.

- VRT <20 sec is associated with chronic venous insufficiency (CVI). The calf veins do not empty properly due to venous obstruction and/or incompetent venous valves allowing for retrograde flow (back flow).

VRT with use of a thigh cuff

- If the mean VRT is <20 seconds without a tourniquet and ≥20 seconds after application of a pressure cuff on the thigh, the diagnosis is primary venous insufficiency or incompetence of the great saphenous system.

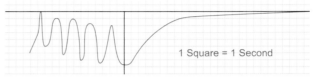

Abnormal initial VRT (7 sec) normalizes with placement of a thigh cuff (20 sec)

- If the mean VRT remains abnormal (<20 seconds) with the application of a pressure cuff on the thigh, the diagnosis is secondary venous insufficiency or incompetence of the superficial and deep systems.

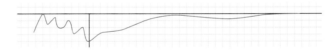

Abnormal initial VRT (8 sec) remains abnormal with placement of a thigh cuff (10 sec)

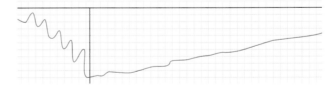

Abnormal initial VRT normalizes after placement of a proximal calf cuff (22 sec)

VRT with use of a cuff below the knee

- If the mean VRT <20 seconds with the tourniquet below the knee but ≥20 seconds with the tourniquet above the knee, this finding suggests reflux in the small saphenous vein.

- If the mean VRT <20 seconds with the tourniquet above AND below the knee; deep venous, great saphenous and small saphenous venous incompetence is present.

> Some labs may use normal VRT values as low as 17.

Interpretation at a glance

	TABLE 95: **Diagnostic Criteria for PPG**	
Cuff Position	**Mean VRT**	**Location of venous incompetence**
No tourniquet	≥20 sec	None
	<20 sec	Incompetence present (*further testing needed to determine if superficial or deep)
Distal thigh tourniquet	≥20 sec	Great saphenous
	<20 sec	Deep and superficial venous system
Proximal calf tourniquet	≥20 sec	Small saphenous
	<20 sec	Deep and superficial venous systems

Differential Diagnosis for CVI

- Lymphedema
- Cellulitis
- Deep venous thrombosis
- Adenopathy
- Arteriovenous fistula
- Direct injury to extremity
- Mass (including vascularized mass)
- Arteriovenous malformation (AVM)
- Collagen vasculitis
- Abscess
- Peripheral neuritis
- Stasis dermatitis
- Klippel-Trenaunay
- Skin cancer
- Arterial disease

Correlation

- Lower extremity venous insufficiency duplex scan
- Continuous-wave Doppler reflux testing
- Descending venography

Medical Treatment for CVI

- Promote venous drainage (e.g., elevate legs, wear elastic stockings/support hose)
- Limit long periods of inactivity
- Compression bandaging (for ulceration)
- Injection sclerotherapy
- Ultrasound-guided sclerotherapy
- Laser therapy
- Proper skin care

Surgical Treatment for CVI

- Venous ablation
- Phlebectomy
  - Stab avulsion phlebectomy
  - Ambulatory phlebectomy
  - Transilluminated power phlebectomy (Trivex or TIPP)
- Vein stripping
- Subfascial endoscopic perforator vein surgery
- Transverse repair of incompetent valves
- Subfascial ligation of perforators
- Superficial perforator ligation surgery (SEPS)

Endovascular Treatment for CVI

- Radiofrequency ablation
- Laser-thermal ablation

Points to Remember

- If the trace does not decrease during testing, let the patient rest for about 1 minute and try increasing the gain settings, while repeating the exercise.
- Primary venous insufficiency is thought to have a congenital etiology and involves the superficial more than the deep venous system.
- Secondary venous insufficiency is typically an acquired condition (e.g., after venous thrombosis) and can involve the superficial, perforating and deep venous systems. [8]

References

1. Sumner DS, Zierler RE. (2005). Vascular physiology: essential hemodynamic principles. In Rutherford *Vascular Surgery 6th edition*. (75-123). Philadelphia. Elsevier Saunders.
2. Labropoulos N, Leon LR. (2005). Evaluation of chronic venous disease. In Mansour MA, Labropoulos N. (Eds.), Vascular Diagnosis, (447-461). Philadelphia: Elsevier Saunders
3. Zwiebel, WJ (2005). Ultrasound diagnosis of venous insufficiency. In Zwiebel WJ, Pellerito JS (Eds.), Introduction to Vascular Ultrasonography 5th ed, (479-499). Philadelphia: Elsevier Saunders.
4. Meissner MH. (2010). Chronic venous disorders. In Zierler RE (Ed.), Strandess's duplex scanning disorders in vascular diagnosis 4th ed. (223-229).Philadelphia Wolters Kluwer Lippincott Williams & Wilkins.
5. Browse NL, Burnand, KG, Thomas, ML (1988). Disease of the Veins; Pathology, Diagnosis and Treatment, Edward Arnold, a division of Hodder & Stoughton.
6. Meissner MH, Strandess DE. (2005). Pathophysiology and natural history of acute deep venous thrombosis. In *Rutherford Vascular Surgery 6th edition*. (2124-2142). Philadelphia. Elsevier Saunders.
7. Min RJ, Rosenblatt M. US Department of Health and Human Services, Office on Women's Health (2010). Varicose Veins and Spider Veins. Retrieved from http://www.womenshealth.gov/faq/varicose-spider-veins.cfm. (7-7-2010).
8. Eberhardt RT, Raffetto JD. (2005). Contemporary Reviews in Cardiovascular Medicine. Circulation. 111: 2398-2409.

Additional References

Barnes RW, Garrett WV, Hummel BA, et al: (AAMI 13th Annual Meeting, March 1978) Photoplethysmographic assessment of altered cutaneous circulation in the post-phlebitic syndrome. In Technology in Diagnosis and Therapy. (25). Washington, DC,

Abramowitz HB, Queral LA, Flinn WR, et al: The use of photoplethysmography in the assessment of venous insufficiency: a comparison to venous pressure measurements. Surgery 86:434-441, 1979.

Li JM, Anderson FA, Wheeler HB: Non-invasive testing for venous reflux using photoplethysmography: standardization of technique and evaluation of interpretation criteria. Bruit [J Vasc Technol] 7:25-29, 1983.

Needham TN, Jury P, Hoare M: Photoplethysmographic refilling time: the relationship between the initial rate of refilling and venous incompetence. Bruit [J Vasc Technol] 7:18-21, 1983.

Definition

Air plethysmography (APG)® quantifies the physiological components of chronic venous disease including; chronic obstruction, valvular reflux, calf muscle pump function and venous hypertension.

Rationale

APG® uses a calibrated air chamber to measure small volumetric changes of the calf in response to positional changes and exercise by measuring absolute volume changes of blood in milliliters (ml). Lower extremity venous function is measured by quantitating venous valve reflux and the efficiency of the calf muscle pump function by measuring venous filling (measured as the patient stands from a supine position), calf ejection (following one tip-toe exercise) and residual volume (following a series of tip-toe exercises).

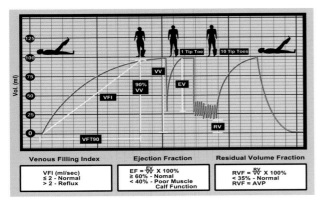

Graph displays volume changes during the standard testing procedure

Etiology

- Previous deep vein thrombosis
- Superficial vein thrombosis
- Venous hypertension
- Calf muscle pump failure
- Lymphedema
- Congenital AV fistula

Risk Factors

- Age (greater with advanced age)
- Previous deep vein thrombosis
- Female
- Pregnancy
- Obesity
- Family history
- Occupations requiring long period of standing or sitting
- Congenital abnormalities (e.g., Klippel-Trenaunay)

Indications for Exam

- Venous insufficiency
- Varicose veins
- Muscle pump evaluation
- Venous ulcerations
- Post treatment, follow-ups

Contraindication/Limitations

- Patients with acute venous thrombosis
- Excessive bandaging or casts
- Patients must be able to stand
- Patients must be able to follow directions for exercise

Mechanism of Disease

Normal Venous Flow

- Normally, venous blood volume and venous pressure are reduced by activation of the calf muscle pump upon walking. When the valves are not working, the venous volume and resulting pressure do not reduce sufficiently and the patient suffers from *ambulatory venous hypertension*.
- Normally, blood is propelled from the superficial veins via perforators to the deep venous system and toward the heart.
- Venous outflow in the lower extremities depends upon:
  - Vein patency
  - Valve competence
  - Adequate calf muscle function

Abnormal Venous Flow, Abnormal Valve Function and the Calf Pump

- Severe chronic venous insufficiency is often caused by calf muscle pump failure.
- Calf muscle pump failure is common in patients with venous leg ulcers.
- Valvular damage and dysfunction (valvular incompetence) result in *venous reflux*, which is venous flow in the wrong direction, away from the heart.
- In the perforating veins, blood flows in the wrong direction from the deep to the superficial system.
- Venous reflux creates a high blood volume in the veins distal to the incompetent valve(s).
- High blood volume in a vein causes increased venous pressure (venous hypertension). [1]
- The hypertension will be greatest upon standing due to the effect of hydrostatic pressure from gravity, adding to the increased pressure from volume. [1]
- Venous hypertension also increases pressure within the venules and capillaries.
- This high pressure system encourages fluids to escape into the tissues causing edema. [1]

Location of Disease

- Incompetent valves may be located at any segment of the deep, perforating or superficial veins, but are more commonly found in the superficial venous tributaries. [2]
- Perforating veins in the gaiter area medial aspect of the leg, just above the medial malleolus (most common location)
- Areas affected by calf muscle pump failure

Calf Muscle Pump

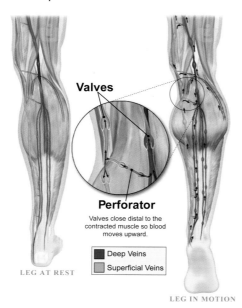

Valves

Perforator

Valves close distal to the
contracted muscle so blood
moves upward.

■ Deep Veins
□ Superficial Veins

LEG AT REST

LEG IN MOTION

*When the leg is in motion (walking), muscle
contractions squeeze the veins, forcing blood past the
open valves of the deep, superficial and perforating
veins upward towards the heart. After the muscle
relaxes, valves close to prevent backflow (reflux)*

Patient History

- Leg edema or swelling
- Varicose veins
- Pain
- Itching
- Aching

- Throbbing
- Tired, heavy legs
- Fatigue
- Restlessness
- Night cramps

Physical Exam

- Leg edema or swelling
- Tenderness
- Varicose veins

- Venous hyperpigmentation
- Venous ulceration
- Venous claudication

Air Plethysmography Protocol

(for reflux, calf pump function and venous hypertension testing)

- Obtain a patient history to include symptoms and risk factors.
- Patient is placed in the supine position; the leg is externally rotated resting on a foam foot support.
- The sensing cuff is placed around the calf, ensuring that the cuff only touches the leg.
- The cuff is attached to a pressure transducer, amplifier, and recorder and is calibrated.
- The patient is asked to rest for approximately 3-5 minutes so the cuff can be stabilized and there is equilibration of arterial inflow.

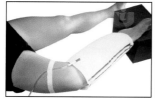
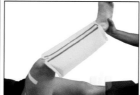

*Patient resting with calibrated cuff and elevation
of the leg to empty the venous system*

Reflux

- Elevate the leg 45° with your hand for approximately 15 seconds, making sure the patient's leg is relaxed while being held.

- After a stable zero baseline is obtained, while ensuring no disturbance to the cuff, ask the patient to stand and hold onto a frame for support. The purpose is to examine the limb while it is non-weight bearing.

> *Hint: You will need to demonstrate the testing sequencing
> a few times to ensure maneuvers are understood.*

- Ask the patient to remain standing with no weight bearing on the leg being examined. Obtain a stable baseline trace while standing. The leg begins filling with resting arterial inflow and venous flow if reflux if present. This change in volume is called the *venous volume* (VV). The normal VV is 80-150 ml.

- The *venous filling index* (VFI) is calculated using the VV. The VFI is the average filling rate of the veins to 90% of the VV. A normal VFI is <2 ml/sec. with slow filling from the arterial supply.

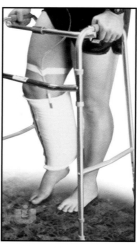

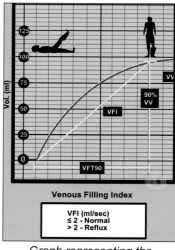

Venous Filling Index

VFI (ml/sec)
≤ 2 - Normal
> 2 - Reflux

*As the patient stands,
the leg fills with resting
arterial inflow and
venous flow
(if reflux is present)*

*Graph representing the
increase in leg volume upon
standing (venous volume, VV).
The VFI is then calculated
from this maneuver*

Calf Muscle Pump Function

- After obtaining a stable plateau, the patient is asked to stand on both feet and perform one tip-toe maneuver. A decrease in volume (ml) is observed during the exercise due to venous emptying from calf muscle contraction. This volume change from one tip toe is the *ejection volume* (EV).

  - This maneuver can be repeated until two or three consistent calf EV are obtained.

- The *ejection fraction* (EF) is calculated from this EV and the VV.

$$EF = EV/VV \times 100$$

- A normal EF is 60% or greater.

Venous Hypertension

- The patient is asked to stand on both feet once again and perform a series of 10 rapid tip-toe exercises at a rate of one per second. The patient then returns to the original position with no weight bearing on the leg being examined. A diminishing calf volume is recorded with the exercises.

- Once a plateau in the tracing is obtained from the 10 tip toe maneuvers, the patient is returned to the supine position, ensuring no weight bearing on the leg being examined. The leg is once again elevated. A new zero baseline is obtained, which will be used to measure *residual volume* (RV).

- The value of the *residual volume fraction* (RVF) has been shown to correlate directly to *ambulatory venous pressure* (AVP). The RVF is calculated as follows:

$$RVF = RV/VV \times 100$$

- This entire exam can be repeated with a tourniquet, cuff or stockings.

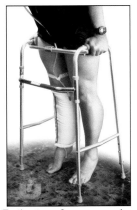

Patient performs a series of ten tip toe maneuvers. As the patient stands, the leg fills with resting arterial inflow and venous flow (if reflux is present)

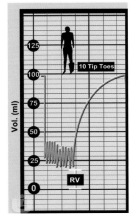

Graph representing diminished calf volume (RV) from the 10 tip toes

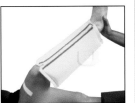

Elevating the leg to empty the venous system

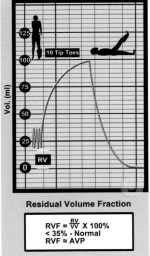

Residual Volume Fraction

$$RVF = \frac{RV}{VV} \times 100\%$$
$$< 35\% \text{ - Normal}$$
$$RVF \approx AVP$$

Graph representing re-establishing the zero functional venous volume

---

Reflux

1. The patient's leg is elevated to empty the veins.

2. The patient stands and the leg begins fill to their venous volume (VV) with resting arterial inflow and reflux, if present.

   - The Venous Filling Index (VFI) is the average filling rate of the veins to 90% of Venous Volume.

   - Normal legs fill with less that 2 ml/sec.

   - This measurement can be repeated with a tourniquet occluding the superficial veins to quantify deep versus superficial reflux or with compression stockings.

Calf Muscle Pump Function

3. The patient performs one tip-toe movement. The Ejected Volume (EV) is the amount of blood in ml expelled by the calf muscle pump. Ejection Fraction is calculated as EF = EV/VV x 100%. A normal leg exhibits 60% or greater ejection fractions.

Venous Hypertension

4. The patient performs 10 tip-toe measurements

5. The patient goes back to the supine position with the leg elevated to reestablish the zero functional venous volume upon which the residual volume is measured.

Residual Volume Fraction (RVF) is calculated as RVF= RV//VV x 100% and has been shown to correlate directly to Ambulatory Venous Pressure (AVP)

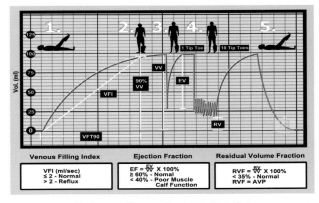

Reflux, calf muscle pump function and venous hypertension

Interpretation

Changes in calf volume which occur during the examination provide quantitative information regarding the venous system. A series of direct and derived measurements are calculated and recorded. The non-invasive equivalent of venous reflux, calf muscle pump function and ambulatory venous pressure are determined.

TABLE 97: Air Plethysmography Normal Values

Direct Measurements	Normal Values
Functional Venous Volume (VV) *(the increase in leg volume on standing)*	100-150 ml
Venous Filling Time (VFT$_{90}$) *(time taken to reach 90% of VV)*	70-170 sec
Ejected Volume (EV) *(decrease in leg volume from one tiptoe movement)*	60-150 ml
Residual Volume (RV) *(volume of blood left in the veins after 10 tiptoe movements)*	2-45 ml
Derived Measurements	**Units**
Venous Filling Index *(VFI)* *(average filling rate: 90%VV/VFT$_{90}$)*	ml/sec
Ejection Fraction *(EF=(EV/VV)x 100)*	%
Residual Volume Fraction	%

TABLE 98: Diagnostic Criteria for Venous Filling Index

VFI (ml/sec)	Interpretation
≤2	Normal
>2-5	Mild reflux
>5-10	Moderate reflux
>10	Severe reflux

- The venous filling index (VFI) indicates the degree of valvular insufficiency.
  - The VFI represents the increased volume changes from the supine position to the standing position.
  - The VFI is the average, gravity induced filling rate defined as the ratio of 90% of the venous volume (VV) divided by the time taken to achieve 90% of venous filling. This measures average filling rate and is expressed in milliliters per second (ml/sec).
  - Venous filling should produce an increase in the leg venous volume of 100-150 ml in normal limbs and 100 to 350 ml in limbs with chronic venous insufficiency.

- A VFI of 2 ml/sec or less indicates absence of significant venous reflux and normal slow filling of the veins from the arterial inflow circulation.
- A VFI greater than 7 ml/sec is associated with a high incidence of skin changes, chronic swelling and ulceration.

TABLE 99: Diagnostic Criteria for Ejection Fraction (EF)

EF (%)	Interpretation
>60%	Normal
30-55%	Primary varicose veins (average 50%)
20-55%	Deep venous insufficiency (average 40%)
18-50%	Deep venous obstruction (average 35%)

- The ejection fraction (EF) is a measure of calf muscle pump function and is measured as a percentage (%) of functional calf volume.
  - EF is calculated by dividing the volume of blood ejected (EV) by the calf during one tip-toe exercise and dividing it by the functional venous volume (VV):

$$EF = EV/VV \times 100$$

  - Normal ejection fractions are greater than 60%.
  - Venous valvular insufficiency results in lower ejection fractions, usually due to reflux in the deep venous system.

Higher VV and low EF are associated with a greater incidence of ulceration.

- Possible causes of poor calf muscle pump are:
  - Non-venous related problems, including arthritis
  - Proximal obstruction that prevents blood flow from traveling out of the calf
  - Incompetent calf perforator veins
  - Calf varicosities that retain a large venous volume not expelled with calf muscle contraction.

TABLE 100: Diagnostic Criteria for Residual Volume Fraction (RVF)

RVF (%)	Interpretation
<35	No incidence of ulceration
>35	Venous hypertension

The greater the RVF % the greater the incidence of CVI and ulceration

RVF % is equivalent to the ambulatory venous pressure in mmHg

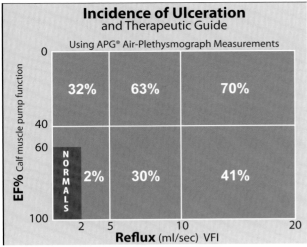

Incidence of Ulceration
and Therapeutic Guide
Using APG® Air-Plethysmograph Measurements

EF% Calf muscle pump function			
0	32%	63%	70%
40			
60	NORMALS 2%	30%	41%
100			

Reflux (ml/sec) VFI

Plotting the VFI and EF can predict the likelihood of ulceration Source: Christopoulous and Nicolaides, St Mary's Vascular Laboratory, London, England

- The residual volume fraction (RVF) indicates the overall efficiency of the calf muscle pump.

  - The RVF compares the volume changes between the 10 tip-toe exercises and the zero baseline. It is reported as a percentage of the functional calf volume.

  - There is a good linear correlation between RVF and ambulatory venous pressure (AVP).

  - RVF is calculated by dividing the residual volume (RV) by the functional venous volume (VV).

    RVF = RV/VV x 100

    > *Higher ending baseline values are typically the result of exercise hyperemia and an outflow obstruction.*

  - Because most of the blood in the calf will be ejected during exercise, normal extremities will have a RVF of 35% or less.

  - A RVF >35 mmHg indicates venous hypertension. Extremities with chronic venous insufficiency usually have reflux and have less efficient calf muscle pumps, creating a RVF >35%.

- The ending baseline (after the RVF test) may be higher or lower than the baseline value at the beginning of the VFI test.

> *In cases of venous obstruction, arterial inflow may be greater than the obstructed vein's capacity for outflow and the calf cannot be completely emptied. The RVF is not reliable in these cases since it will be an artificially low "normal" value due to the obstruction-related elevated baseline.*

- The beginning baseline from the VFI test could be used to get a more accurate RVF measurement when poor outflows exist.
- Not elevating the leg high enough for an adequate ending baseline will cause false results.

Differential Diagnosis *(for obstruction, abnormal valve and calf pump function)*

- Deep venous thrombosis
- Lymphedema
- Cellulitis
- Arteriovenous fistula
- Arterio-venous malformation

Correlation
- Venous photoplethysmography for reflux testing
- Descending venography

Medical Treatment
- Promote venous drainage (e.g., elevate legs, wear elastic stockings/support hose)
- Limit long periods of inactivity
- Compression bandaging (for ulceration)
- Injection sclerotherapy
- Ultrasound guided sclerotherapy

Surgical treatment
- Ligation (e.g., of saphenofemoral junction)
- Venous ablation
- Stab avulsion phlebectomy
- Vein stripping
- Subfascial endoscopic perforator vein surgery
- Transverse repair of incompetent valves
- Subfascial ligation of perforators
- Ambulatory phlebectomy

Endovascular Treatment
- Radiofrequency ablation
- Laser thermal ablation

Points to Remember
- APG® provides a global measurement of venous function.
- The more efficient the calf muscle pump, the lower level of pressure in the venous system.
- Failure of the calf muscle pump interferes with healing.
- Failure of the calf muscle pump in some patients is related to decreased mobility of the ankle joint due to painful venous ulceration in this area.
- The EF can be >100%, suggesting exercise empties more blood than does gravity, indicating an excellent calf pump function.
- APG® can be used to monitor pre and post-op venous changes.
- Negative ending baseline values may be due to cuff slippage during the ten toe-up exercises.
- Selecting the zero volume too early in the trace will result in underestimated VFI values.
- The differential diagnosis of peripheral edema discriminates venous insufficiency from cardiac disease, lymphedema and cellulitis.
- The VFT 90 or the amount of time required to fill 90% of the venous volume is more accurate to use than the VV.

References

1. Nicolaides, A. et al. Investigation of Patients with Deep Venous Thrombosis and Chronic Venous Insufficiency. Med-Orion Publishing Co. Los Angeles CA.
2. Christopoulous DG, Nicolaides AN, Szendro G: Air-plethysmography and the effect of elastic compression on venous hemodynamics of the leg. J Vasc Surg 5:148-159, 1987.
3. Christopoulous DG, Nicolaides AN, Galloway JMD: Objective non-invasive evaluation of venous surgical results. J Vasc Surg 8:683-687, 1988.
4. Katz M, Comerota A, Kerr R: Air-plethysmography (APG): a new technique to evaluate patients with chronic venous insufficiency. J Vasc Technol 15:23-27, 1991.
5. Nicolaides, A. et al. How Air Plethysmography (APG) Influences Patient Management. ACI Medical, 1993.

Definition

The use of real time B-mode imaging with pulsed wave and color flow Doppler to assess the abdominal aorta and iliac arteries for stenosis, occlusion or the presence, location and size of any aneurysm. This examination is also used to monitor any change in aneurysm size from previous exams.

Etiology

- Atherosclerosis
- Infectious aortitis (e.g., mycotic, syphilis)
- Vasculitis
- Congenital abnormalities
- Connective tissue disorders (e.g., Marfan's syndrome or Ehler-Danlos syndrome)
- Trauma

Risk Factors

- Age (increases with age)
- Smoking
- Hypertension
- Atherosclerosis
- Male gender
- Caucasian
- Immediate relative with an abdominal aortic aneurysm (AAA) history
- Trauma

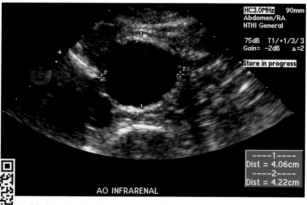

Abdominal aortic aneurysm by B-mode imaging

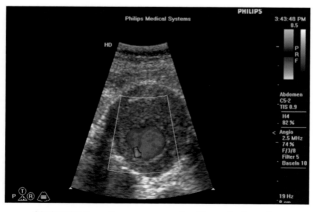

Abdominal aortic aneurysm by B-mode imaging
Image courtesy of Philips Healthcare

Indications for Exam

- Surveillance of known AAA or iliac artery aneurysm
- Abdominal bruit (abnormal sound heard through auscultation caused by vibrations from turbulent flow)
- Abdominal pain
- Pulsatile aorta or mass on physical examination
- Immediate family member with a history of AAA
- History of hypertension, age >50 years with a family history of AAA
- Presence of an aneurysm at another location (e.g., iliac, femoral, popliteal)
- Aortic coarctation
- Evidence of lower extremity arterial inflow disease
- Evidence of distal emboli in the absence of a femoral-popliteal artery or cardiac source

Contraindications/Limitations

- Obesity may cause poor visualization due to vessel depth.
- Abdominal gas may prohibit visualization of any or all vessels.

Abdominal Aortic Aneurysm Types

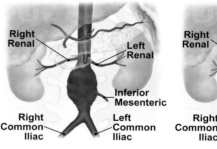

Fusiform type aneurysm

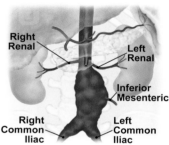

Fusiform type aneurysm with iliac artery involvement

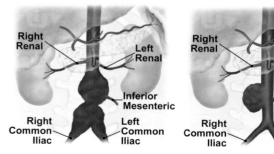

Bi-lobed fusiform type aneurysm　　　*Saccular type aneurysm*

Stent Location

Stents can be located within any vessel. Stents are often placed in the common or external iliac arteries.

Graft Location

Bypass grafts connect two arteries to direct flow around an obstruction or an aneurysm in the aorta and/or iliac arteries. The bypass grafts can be placed between any two vessels. The infrarenal aorta is typically used for the proximal anastomosis if the aorta is the inflow artery. Examples of typical aortoiliac-arterial grafts encountered in the vascular lab for surveillance include:

> See "Arterial Bypass" chapter for more on graft/stent location and types

- Aortobifemoral (abdominal aorta to bilateral femoral arteries)

- Aortoiliac (abdominal aorta to one or both iliac arteries)

- Iliofemoral-Renal artery

- Iliac artery-Femoral artery

- Femoral-Femoral (cross-femoral or "x-fem" bypass)

- Axillo-femoral (axillary artery to a femoral artery)

- A bypass may be anastomosed to another bypass (e.g., aorto-femoral-popliteal bypass)

Mechanism of disease

- **Atherosclerosis** is the most common arterial disease. Atherosclerotic plaque forms in the artery to block flow by either narrowing it *(arterial stenosis)* or totally blocking the artery *(arterial occlusion)*. The term "hemodynamically significant obstruction" refers to either a stenosis or an occlusion that results in a decrease in blood pressure or flow distal to the obstruction. Typically, a stenosis must narrow the diameter of the artery by at least 50% to decrease pressure and flow distally. An arterial occlusion is typically seen from one major branch to the next. [1]

- **Emboli** may occur as contents of a plaque or fragments of an organized thrombus from the heart or aneurysm loosen and flow downstream. Emboli become lodged in a distant blood vessel, causing arterial occlusion and reduction of flow.[2]

- **Extrinsic compression** from tumors, musculo-skeletal configuration, hematoma, etc. can result in stenosis or occlusion by placing enough pressure on arterial walls to compromise blood flow. [1]

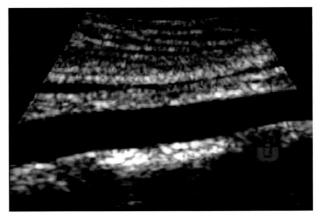

Normal abdominal aorta in the longitudinal plane

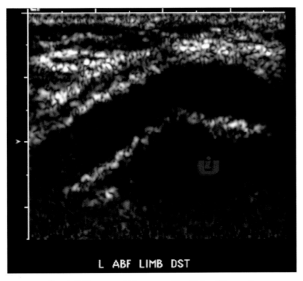

L ABF LIMB DST

Aortobifemoral Bypass Graft by B-mode

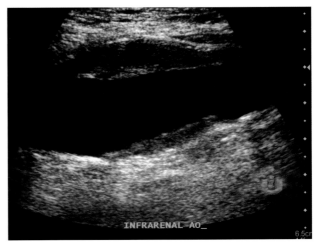

INFRARENAL AO_

Aneurysm of the abdominal aorta in the longitudinal plane with mural thrombus

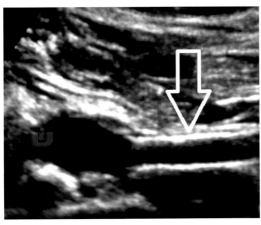

Common Iliac Artery Stent by B-mode

Abdominal Aorto-Iliac Duplex Ultrasound

Abdominal Arterial Testing

- **Aneurysmal disease**
  - Aneurysms are most commonly caused by atherosclerotic or inflammatory processes. Aneurysms are caused by the breakdown of the vessel wall by a multifactorial process involving: connective tissue metabolism, nutrient and oxygen levels, chronic inflammation and biomechanical wall stress.
  - There is increased degradation of elastin and collagen in aneurysmal arteries.
  - Elastin degradation plays a key role in aneurysmal dilatation whereas the degradation of collagen leads to rupture.
  - It has been suggested that the infrarenal abdominal aorta is at greater risk for aneurysm compared to the thoracic aorta because the infrarenal abdominal aorta has fewer vasa vasorum per medial lamellar unit. Vasa vasorum are the primary source of nutrients and oxygen for media smooth muscle cells
  - Localized destruction of the arterial wall may also be caused by an infectious agent which infiltrates the adventitial layer through the vasa vasorum (mycotic aneurysm). [6]
  - **Arterial thrombosis** forms as an abdominal aortic aneurysm expands. Stagnant blood in areas of the aneurysm (stasis) permits coagulation within the artery causing mural thrombosis.

- **Aortic dissection** begins with a tear in the intimal layer of the artery, allowing blood flow to access the medial layer. A dissection between the intimal and medial layers results in true and false lumens. [7] Pulsatile flow and high blood pressure may cause propagation of a dissection into multiple arteries. Blood flows through the tear in the intimal layer and may clot, flow in and out of the tear, or flow further downstream to enter the true lumen through a second tear distally.

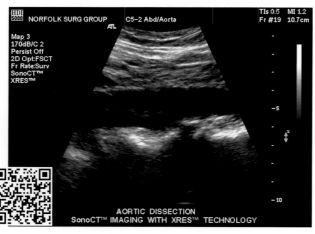

Dissection of abdominal aorta by B-mode image
Image courtesy of Philips Healthcare

- A **pseudoaneurysm** (PA) or "false aneurysm" forms due to trauma to all three layers of the arterial wall. A PA is a hematoma receiving its blood supply via communication with an artery through a patent "neck."
  - One cause of PA is trauma to the aortoiliac segment (e.g., puncture for catheterization, gunshot wound, etc.).[8]
  - PA can develop at the femoral anastomosis of a aortobifemoral graft due to degeneration of the native artery.[9]

Graft Complications

- **Technical errors** can result in failure of a bypass or stent. Kinking or twisting of the graft limb is one possible cause.[9] Early failure of either can occur even without an identifiable mechanical defect or cause.
- **Graft thrombosis** is the most frequent complication of aortofemoral bypass, usually affecting one of the limbs. [9]
  - Failure resulting from atherosclerotic progression in the inflow/outflow beds often occurs in grafts. [9]
  - Some patients have an undiagnosed hypercoaguable disorder which causes thrombosis or occlusion of the graft. [9]
- Additional mechanisms of complication include graft infections and trauma to the graft. [9]

Location of Disease

- Location of disease can be focal or diffuse and affect any level or multiple levels.
- For aneurysm:
  - Infrarenal abdominal aorta (most common site)
  - Abdominal aorta plus iliac
  - Thoracoabdominal
  - Isolated iliac
- For dissection:
  - Aorta (beginning at the subclavian)
  - Ascending aorta
- Common location of graft obstruction:
  - Graft anastomotic sites
  - Inflow arterial tract
  - Outflow arterial tract
  - Graft kink
- Arterial stenting often involves the iliac arteries.

Patient History

- Many aneurysm cases are asymptomatic.
- Aneurysm found unexpectedly during physical exam, radiological or CT exams that were performed for unrelated reasons
- Sense of fullness in the epigastrium
- Previous therapeutic procedure (e.g., bypass, stenting)

Physical Examination

- Pulsatile abdominal mass
- Lower back pain
- Systolic murmur in the region of the aneurysm
- Bruit in aorto-iliac region
- Pulselessness
- Cyanosis

Abdominal Aorto-Iliac Duplex Ultrasound Protocol

- Patients should be fasting for 6-12 hours to minimize the presence of air in the abdomen. A limited volume of clear liquids may be ingested prior to the examination (e.g., to swallow medications).
- Obtain a patient history to include symptoms, risk factors and past vascular interventions and general dates if available.
- Patient is supine with arms and legs adequately supported. The patient may bend their knees up to aid in relaxation of the abdominal wall and decrease lumbar pain.

- Acoustic windows used to image the abdominal aorta include: midline of the upper abdomen, left flank with patient supine or right lateral decubitus.
- Most patients require a low frequency (1-4 MHz) transducer to image these deeper abdominal structures, though some patients may require the use of a range of transducers, including a higher-frequency (5-7 MHz) probe.

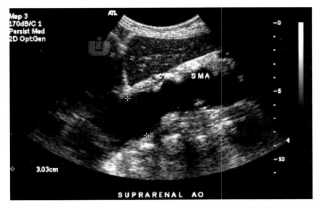

Suprarenal aorta diameter measured longitudinally

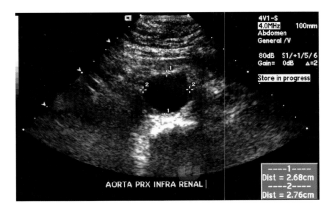

Infrarenal aorta diameter measured in transverse

- The aortic lumen is measured from outer wall to outer wall in both the longitudinal (sagittal) and transverse (short-axis) planes.

Transverse (Short-Axis) Scan

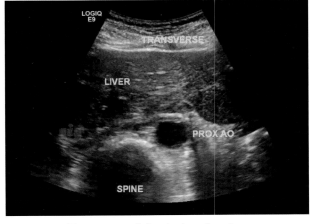

Transverse abdominal aorta artery

- Place the transducer at the midline below the xyphoid process in the transverse (sagittal) plane (the liver should be on the left of the display screen). Move the transducer slowly, inferiorly towards the umbilicus with intermittent color flow Doppler. Evaluate the aorta for atherosclerotic plaque, aneurysm, calcification, thrombus, dissection and tortuosity during the scan.
- At the aortic bifurcation (near the umbilicus), the right and left common iliac arteries should be clearly demonstrated.

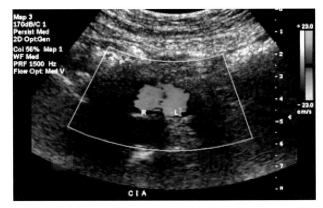

Transverse iliac artery bifurcation

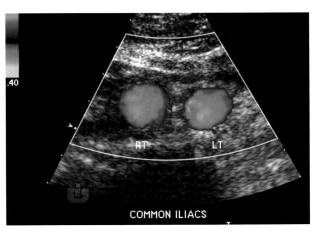

Transverse proximal common iliac arteries

- The maximum anterior-posterior and medial-lateral (transverse) diameters of the aorta should be measured at the following levels:
  - Suprarenal aorta, at or above the celiac trunk
  - Juxtarenal aorta, at the level the renal arteries
  - Infrarenal aorta, below the renals, but above the iliac bifurcation
  - Proximal common iliac arteries

> *Place calipers parallel to the axis of flow when measuring diameters.*

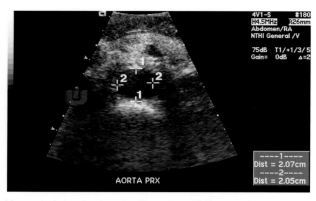

Normal abdominal aorta diameters (#1's anterior-posterior measurement, #2's transverse measurement)

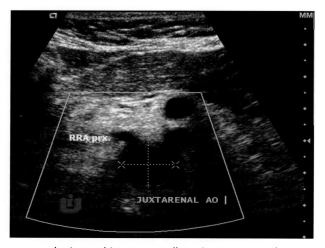

Juxtarenal transverse diameters measured

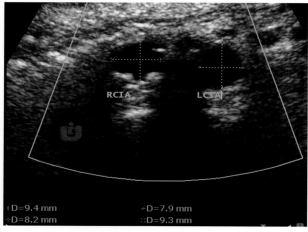

Proximal common iliac artery transverse diameters

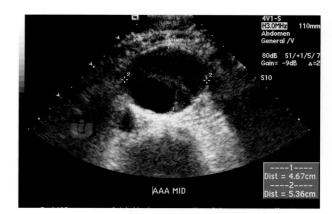

Abnormal abdominal aorta diameters-aneurysm

- A transverse aortic aneurysm evaluation should include:
  - Maximum anterior-posterior and transverse diameters of the true lumen
  - Location of the aneurysm (level)
  - Documentation regarding presence and location of thrombus and attempt to classify the type of aneurysm (e.g., fusiform, saccular)
  - Use of B-mode and color flow Doppler to identify the residual vessel lumen if present

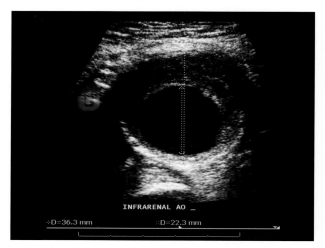

Residual lumen of an aneurysm by B-mode

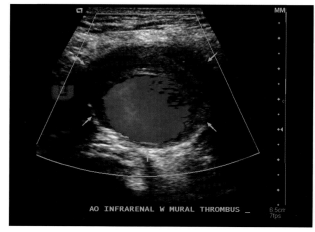

Residual lumen of an aneurysm with color flow

Longitudinal (Sagittal) Scan and Images

- Place the transducer at the midline below the xyphoid process and turn the probe longitudinally. The grayscale image of the abdominal aorta from the diaphragm to the aorta-common iliac bifurcation is evaluated for the presence of atherosclerotic plaque, aneurysm, calcification, thrombus, dissection or tortuosity.

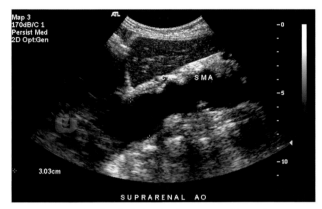

Longitudinal abdominal aorta on B-mode
(Note: diffuse plaque)

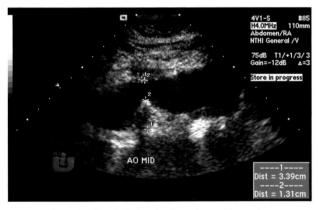

Longitudinal abdominal aorta on B-mode
with lumenal reduction measurement

- Document the maximum longitudinal diameter from outer wall to outer wall on axis at the following levels:
  - Suprarenal aorta, at or above the celiac trunk
  - Juxtarenal aorta, at the level the renal arteries
  - Infrarenal aorta, below the level the renal arteries, but above the iliac bifurcation
- Longitudinal aortic aneurysm evaluation should include:
  - Maximum longitudinal diameters
  - Location of the aneurysm (level)
  - Length of aneurysm
  - Use of color flow Doppler to identify true vessel lumen
  - Documentation regarding presence and location of thrombus, atherosclerotic plaque and/or calcification

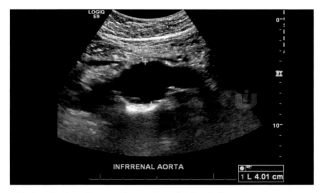

Abdominal aorta: maximum longitudinal diameter measured

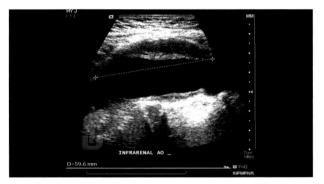

Abdominal aorta: length of aneurysm measured

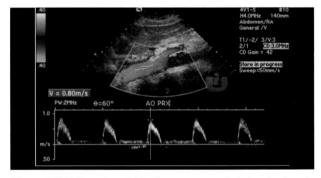

Normal PW Doppler within the suprarenal abdominal aorta

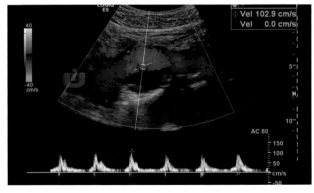

PW Doppler within an abdominal aortic aneurysm

- Determine the peak systolic velocities (PSV), and end-diastolic velocities (EDV) using pulsed wave Doppler (≤60° Doppler angle with the angle cursor parallel to the vessel walls and sample volume within the center of the flow stream) at the following levels:

  – Suprarenal aorta, at or above the celiac trunk

  – Juxtarenal aorta, at the level the renal arteries

  – Infrarenal aorta, below the renal arteries but above the iliac bifurcation

  – Right common iliac artery and left common iliac artery

  – Document the highest obtainable velocity through any stenotic area(s) by moving the sample gate through the area of stenosis and obtain representative waveforms. Record velocities and waveforms just proximal to the stenosis and just distal to the stenosis. Document post-stenotic turbulence and color bruit when present.

TABLE 101: **Abdominal Aortolliac Duplex Protocol Summary**

Transverse (Short-Axis) Scan

- Measure the anterior-posterior (AP) and transverse diameters of the abdominal aorta in grayscale at the following levels:

  - Suprarenal aorta, at or above the celiac artery

  - Juxtarenal aorta, at the level of the renal arteries

  - Infrarenal aorta, below the renal arteries, but above the iliac bifurcation

  - Right and left common iliac arteries

Longitudinal (Sagittal) Scan

- Measure peak systolic and end diastolic velocities with PW Doppler and measure the longitudinal diameters of the abdominal aorta in grayscale at the following levels:

  - Suprarenal aorta, at or above the celiac artery

  - Juxtarenal aorta, at the level of the renal arteries

  - Infrarenal aorta, below the renal arteries, but above the iliac bifurcation

  - Right and left common iliac arteries

- When an area of stenosis is identified, "walk" the sample gate through the area of stenosis and obtain representative waveforms at the point of highest velocity within the stenosis, as well as just proximal and distal to the stenosis.

Aortoiliac Bypass Graft/Stent Surveillance Protocol

- Obtain a patient history to include symptoms and risk factors.

- Obtain past surgical reports and records including type of bypass graft or stent placement and general date of surgery.

- Patient is typically examined in the supine position for grafts and stents.

- Obtain bilateral ABIs. (Never put a blood pressure cuff over a bypass graft or stent without first consulting the Medical Director of the lab or lab protocol.)

- Some patients may require the use of a range of transducers; including high-frequency (5-7 MHz) transducer and a lower frequency (1-4 MHz) transducer.

- Evaluate for graft or stent abnormalities while scanning (e.g., anastomotic pseudoaneurysm, thrombosis, stenosis, intimal hyperplasia, perigraft fluid).

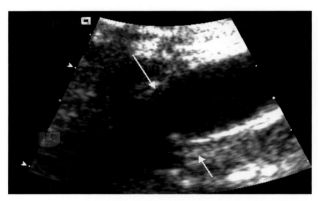

Proximal anastomosis of aortobifemoral bypass graft (AFB)

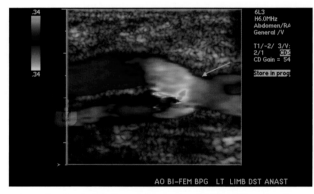

Longitudinal distal anastomosis of AFB with color flow

- Record transverse and longitudinal images with and without color flow of the:

  – Inflow/proximal native artery

  – Proximal anastomosis or stent origin

  – Proximal graft or stent

  – Mid graft or stent

  – Distal graft or stent

  – Distal anastomosis or end of stent

  – Outflow/distal native artery

  – Any areas where a lumenal reduction or color bruit are noted

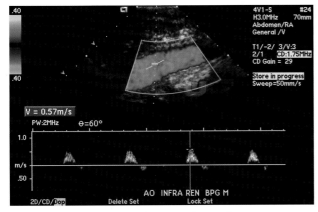

Mid-AFB graft spectral waveform

- Record and measure the peak systolic velocity (PSV) in the longitudinal plane using pulsed wave Doppler (≤60° Doppler angle with the angle cursor parallel to the vessel walls and sample volume within the center of the flow stream) at the following levels:

  - Inflow/proximal native artery
  - Proximal anastomosis or stent origin
  - Proximal graft or stent
  - Mid graft or stent
  - Distal graft or stent
  - Distal anastomosis or end of stent
  - Outflow/distal native artery

> Early post-operative flow patterns (within the 1st month) in a bypass graft may have increased diastolic flow (post-operative reactive hyperemia) and may not have a triphasic waveform.

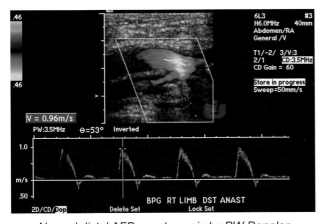

Normal distal AFB anastomosis by PW Doppler

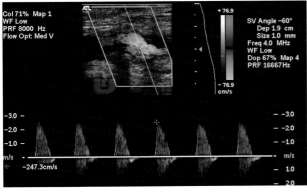

Stenotic distal AFB anastomosis by PW Doppler

- When an area of stenosis is identified, "walk" the sample gate through the area of stenosis and obtain representative waveforms proximal, at and distal to the stenosis. Post-stenotic turbulence and color bruit should be documented when present.

- Determine classification of stenosis according to laboratory diagnostic criteria.

- Repeat protocol for other grafts as necessary.

Interpretation

- Determine:
  - Arterial diameters
  - If there is any change in spectral waveform analysis (e.g., triphasic to biphasic to monophasic)
  - Peak systolic velocity (PSV) and flow direction
  - V_2/V_1 peak systolic velocity ratio (Vr); where V_2 represents the maximum PSV of a stenosis and V_1 is the PSV of the proximal normal segment
  - Location and characteristics of any plaque or thrombus identified

Normal

- **Arterial diameters:** The mean diameter of a normal infrarenal aorta is approximately 2.0 cm.[5]
- **Flow velocities:** Normal flow velocities should be >40 cm/s.[10] PSV and Vr are essentially uniform throughout the sampled arterial segment.
- **Doppler waveforms:** Normal abdominal arterial waveforms are triphasic. A triphasic signal is demonstrated by strong forward flow in late systole (sharp upstroke), followed by flow reversal in early diastole (below baseline), plus a late diastolic component.[11]
- **General grayscale and color characteristics:** The artery is free of intralumenal echoes. When utilized, color Doppler fills the entire arterial lumen.

Abnormal

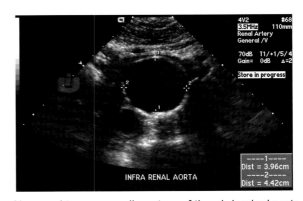

Abnormal transverse diameters of the abdominal aorta

- **Arterial diameters:**
  - Mild dilatation of the aorta >2.0 and <3.0 cm is describe as *ectatic*.[3]
  - A moderate aortic aneurysm is 3-5 cm in diameter.[5]
  - Severe aneurysmal disease is present when diameters are >5.0 cm.[12]

- **Flow velocities:** A hemodynamically significant lesion (>50%) will result in a focal velocity increase (at least double the velocity in the proximal arterial segment).[13] There will be a velocity ratio >2.0 between segments.

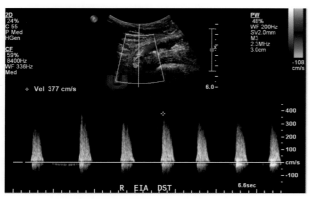

External iliac artery stenosis by PW Doppler

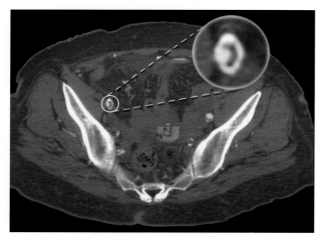

Same external iliac artery stenosis by CT scan

- **Doppler waveforms:**
  - Flow through an aneurysm can exhibit systolic dampening and a prominent diastolic reversal associated with the swirling of blood within the dilated lumen.[13]
  - When waveforms demonstrate post-stenotic turbulence and accompany a velocity ratio >2.0 (PSV at-stenosis/ PSV pre-stenosis) through a region, a hemodynamically significant stenosis is suspected. A change in spectral waveform (from triphasic to biphasic or monophasic) will support this finding. [14]
- **General grayscale and color characteristics:**
  - Visualization of mural thrombus is possible within an aneurysm. Observed echoes are often heterogeneous in nature and create a residual lumen. [3]

> *Diameter reduction measurements should only be used in conjunction with peak systolic velocity measurements.*

  - Intralumenal echoes are visualized in cases of atherosclerotic disease within the artery resulting in a measurable lumenal reduction.
  - When utilized, color Doppler does not fill the entire arterial lumen. A color bruit may be observed, suggesting a hemodynamically significant lesion.[13]

> *Color is never diagnostic without PW Doppler confirmation.*

- **Occlusion:** An occlusion is recognized in a native artery or stent/bypass graft by the absence of both color saturation and confirmed by the lack of an audible Doppler signal in the artery.[13]

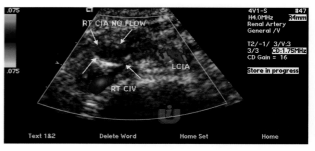

Right common iliac artery occlusion is suspected by color flow in the transverse plane

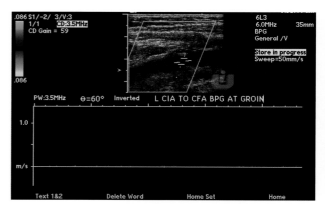

Absent Doppler signal in the common iliac artery confirms common femoral bypass graft-occlusion **Other Pathology**

- **Arteriomegaly** is the term used to describe uniform arterial dilation throughout an artery greater than 50% of its typical diameter. [15] The artery can also be described as "ectatic" in some vascular laboratories.
- **Pseudoaneurysm** A pseudoaneurysm is diagnosed in the aortoiliac segment when a pulsatile mass is identified by color and Doppler flow communicating with the native artery or an anastomotic site through a patent "neck".[16] The neck must demonstrate to and fro (pendulum) Doppler flow patterns to indicate a pseudoaneurysm.
- **Dissection:** A dissection of the arterial lumen is recognized as two distinct flow channels by B-mode and/or color Doppler. One lumen is known as the "true lumen" while the other is referred to as the "false lumen". An intimal flap may be seen within the arterial lumen by B-mode image.[7]

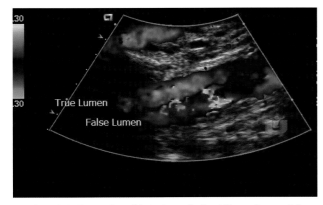

Arterial dissection (Note two distinct flow channels)

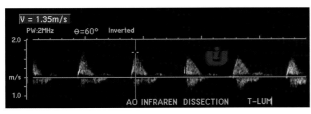

PW Doppler within true lumen

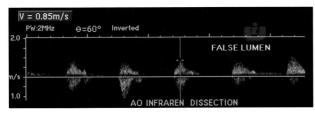

PW Doppler within false lumen

Plaque and Lesion Descriptions/Characteristics

- **Diffuse**: long segment of the artery lined with plaque, but <50% at any point
- **Stenotic**: lumen is narrowed and velocity increases with post-stenotic turbulence. Hemodynamically significant stenosis typically occurs when narrowing results in a >50% diameter reduction (75% area reduction). A stenosis can be focal or long segment.
- **Calcific**: highly reflective plaque(s) with acoustic shadowing
- **Occluded**: complete occlusion of the vessel
- **"Moving"/"Mobile"**: debris within the lumen is poorly adhered to the vessel wall, i.e., moving thrombus

TABLE 102: Normal Arterial Dimensions and Peak Systolic Velocities

Arterial Vessel	Average Diameter ± SD* (cm)	Velocity + SD* (cm/s)
Infrarenal aorta	2.0 ± 0.3	65 ± 15
Common iliac artery	1.6 ± 2	95 ± 20
External iliac artery	0.79 ± 0.13	119 ± 22
Common femoral artery	0.82 ± 0.14	114 ± 25
* SD, *standard deviation*		

Source: Armstrong PA, Bandyk DF. (2007). Duplex scanning for lower extremity arterial disease. In AbuRahma AF, Bergan JJ (Eds.). Non-invasive Vascular Diagnosis: A Practical Guide to Therapy 2nd ed. (253-261). London:Springer Verlag.

TABLE 103: Diagnostic Criteria for Abdominal Aortic Aneurysm and Dissection

Condition	Diameter (cm)
Ectasia	2.0-3.0
Aneurysm	>3.0
– Moderate	3.0 -5.0
– Severe	>5.0
Dissection	True and false lumen present

Source: Internally validated at the University of Chicago Medical Center Vascular Laboratory.

Aortoiliac Bypass Graft/Iliac Stent Interpretation

- Analyze all of the following data from the physiologic and duplex exams:
  - Ankle-brachial indices (ABI)
  - Peak systolic velocity (PSV) and flow direction
  - Velocity ratios (Vr), where highest peak systolic velocity at stenosis (V_2) is divided by the PSV of the proximal normal segment (V_1)
  - Waveform configurations and changes through the inflow, bypass/stent and outflow arteries including flow direction
  - B-mode image information (e.g., plaque, diameter of vessel or other pathology)
  - Reasons image and velocity data may not agree (e.g., size mismatch between stent/graft and native artery)
- Use the exam data listed above to determine if the graft or stent is normal or abnormal.

Normal (absence of a hemodynamically significant stenosis, <50%)

- **General grayscale and color characteristics**
  - Synthetic aortic bypass grafts have a characteristic "textured" appearance on B-mode image.[17]
  - Normally, there is no echogenic material within the arterial lumen of an aortic bypass. Color fills the lumen from wall to wall in transverse and longitudinal views with appropriate settings.[17]
  - Stents can typically be seen within the lumen of clearly visualized arteries. Deeper stents may be difficult to identify with certainty.
- **Inflow artery**: A normal arterial inflow waveform is triphasic. Velocity ratios (Vr) are <2.0 in the inflow tract.[17,18]

- **Proximal anastomosis**: Normal Vr are <2.0. Waveforms may demonstrate the typical disturbed flow patterns seen at bifurcations/branches or areas of angulation. These changes are focal at the anastomosis and normalize distally. A large inflow artery feeding a small diameter graft may result in a higher velocity ratio due to the size change. The image should be scrutinized for the presence of intralumenal echoes. [17,18]
- **Body of graft/stent**
  - Velocity ratios are <2.0 throughout the graft/stent body. [17,18]
  - Waveform configurations remain essentially the same as in the inflow artery throughout a non-obstructed conduit.
- **Distal anastomosis**: There is often a size change between the wider bypass graft and smaller diameter native artery resulting in a velocity increase. A normal distal anastomosis demonstrates a Vr <3.4. The image should be scrutinized for the presence of intralumenal echoes. Waveform configuration may be disturbed due to vessel angulation and size change.
- **Outflow artery**: Velocities remain fairly constant with Vr <2.0. Outflow arterial waveforms are similar to those in the graft body.[17,18] Flow direction may be retrograde in the native artery proximal to the distal anastomosis.

Abnormal

> *Definitive criterion for abdominal aortoiliac bypass stenosis have not been widely addressed in the literature so it varies across institutions. Some labs use the same criterion used for the lower extremities.*

Generally in any arterial intervention, findings of a decrease in ABI >0.15 on serial exam is indicative of significant disease progression in the inflow, graft or outflow arteries. [19]

- **Inflow artery**
  - Velocity ratios >2.0 within the native artery associated with post-stenotic turbulence and waveform changes (from triphasic to biphasic to monophasic) indicate a hemodynamically significant stenosis (≥50%).[14,17,20]
  - Low resistance waveform patterns at least 2 cm proximal to the anastomosis indicate a significant inflow artery obstruction.

- **Proximal anastomosis**
  - Velocity ratios >2.0 (or >3.0 if the graft has a much smaller diameter than the inflow vessel) with elevated velocities, stenotic waveform patterns, spectral broadening and post-stenotic turbulence indicate a hemodynamically significant stenosis (≥50%).
  - Image demonstrates echogenic material at the point of highest velocity.

- **Body of graft/stent**
  - Velocity >300 cm/s and a Vr >2.0 within an iliac stent indicate a hemodynamically significant stenosis (≥50%). [21]

  - Monophasic waveforms throughout the graft can indicate an obstruction in the inflow tract. Graft waveforms that demonstrate high-resistance, with no end diastolic velocity or a staccato pattern, indicate a distal anastomotic or outflow tract obstruction.

- **Distal anastomosis**: A velocity ratio >3.4 is indicative of a hemodynamically significant stenosis (≥50%), particularly if post-stenotic turbulence is present and the waveform pattern changes distally compared to the pre-anastomotic waveform pattern.

> *It is important to look at the images for intralumenal defects at the anastomosis or marked diameter changes that may account for velocity increases.*

Other Pathology

- **Graft occlusion**: An occlusion of the graft or stent is present when echogenic material is observed within the graft/stent lumen **and** no flow is detected by spectral Doppler, and color in transverse and longitudinal views. [17]

> *An occlusion suspected by color is never diagnostic without PW Doppler confirmation.*

- A **pseudoaneurysm** is diagnosed when a pulsatile mass is identified by color and Doppler flow (often near an anastomotic site) which is observed communicating with the bypass or native artery through a patent "neck". The neck must demonstrate to and fro (pendulum) Doppler flow patterns to indicate a pseudoaneurysm. [17]
- **Perigraft fluid** is suspected when anechoic, fluid-filled structures surround the bypass conduit. Ultrasound cannot determine the exact fluid substance which may be related to infection, hematoma, etc. [17]

Differential Diagnosis

- Acute appendicitis
- Myocardial infarction
- Chronic diseases of the digestive tract
- Urinary tract infections
- Pancreatitis
- Renal calculi (kidney stones)

Correlation

- Spiral CT scan
- MRI
- Aortography

Medical Treatment

- Treat underlying cause (e.g., systemic hypertension)
- Serial imaging exams to monitor changes in diameter

Surgical Treatment

- Open repair for aneurysm diameter >5.0 cm and/or for aneurysms rapidly increasing in size (>1.0 cm per year)
- Aortic rupture is a surgical emergency

Endovascular Treatment

- Endolumenal graft
- Stent (e.g., iliac artery stenosis)

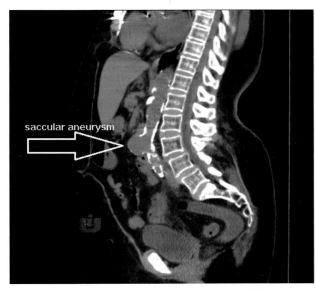

Saccular abdominal aortic aneurysm by CT scan

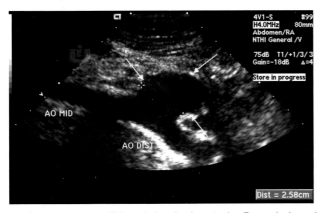

Saccular aneurysm off the abdominal aorta by B-mode imaging

Points to Remember

- Patients may be given Simethicone (e.g., Gas-X, Mylanta, etc.) before the exam to reduce abdominal gas.
- Since it is perpendicular to the flow channel, the anterior-posterior arterial diameter measurement is more reliable than the transverse arterial diameter. [5,17]
- Studies estimate the prevalence of AAA discovered through ultrasound screening ranges from 4.2–8.8% for men, and 0.6–1.4% in women. [22]
- A family history of AAA increases AAA development risk four-fold.[23] The risk can increase twelve-fold if an immediate family member was an AAA patient.[5]
- The majority of AAA are atherosclerotic and infrarenal (below the renal arteries). [5]
- The predicted expansion rate of AAA is 0.2-0.5 cm per year.[5]
- The primary complication of AAA is rupture (in excess of 80% mortality rate). [24]
- Symptoms of impending rupture or rupture include:[5]
  - severe abdominal pain radiating through to the back
  - temporary loss of consciousness
  - hypotension
  - shock
  - sudden death (rupture)

- Over 50% of patients with a femoral artery aneurysm also have an AAA. Concurrent iliac artery aneurysms are much less frequent. [25]
- Embolization is associated with abdominal aortic aneurysm due to thrombus or atherosclerotic plaque. A patient presenting with "blue toe syndrome" should be worked up for AAA. [5]
- The Deficit Reduction Act (DRA) of 2005 calls for Medicare coverage for a one-time abdominal aortic aneurysm ultrasound screening test for men ages 65-75 with a history of smoking, as well as men and women ages 65-75 with a family history of AAA. Reimbursement began January 1, 2007. [26]
- Extremely low flow states are possible both above and below occlusions. Color Doppler parameters must be adjusted to detect low velocities. If this is not done, the length of the occlusion could be overestimated.

References

1. Sumner DS, Zierler RE. (2005). Vascular physiology: essential hemodynamic principles. In *Rutherford Vascular Surgery 6th edition*. (75-123). Philadelphia. Elsevier Saunders.
2. Fecteau SR, Darling III RC, Roddy SP. (2005). Arterial thomboembolism. In *Rutherford Vascular Surgery 6th edition*. (971-986). Philadelphia. Elsevier Saunders.
3. Dawson DL, Lee ES, Lindholm K. (2010). Aortic and peripheral aneurysms. In Zierler RE (Ed.), Strandess's duplex scanning disorders in vascular diagnosis 4th ed. (157-168). Philadelphia Wolters Kluwer Lippincott Williams & Wilkins
4. Stary HC, Chandler AB, Dinsmore RE, Fuster V, Glagov S, Insull W, Rosenfeld ME, Schwartz CJ, Wagner WD, Wissler RW. A definition of advanced types of atherosclerotic lesions and histological classification of atherosclerosis. *Atherosclerosis, Thrombosis and Vascular Biology*. 1995; 15; 1521-1531.
5. Schermerhorn ML, Cronenwett JL. (2005). Abdominal aortic and iliac aneurysms. In *Rutherford Vascular Surgery 6th edition*. (1408-1452). Philadelphia. Elsevier Saunders.
6. Reddy DJ, Weaver MR. (2005). Infected aneurysms. In *Rutherford Vascular Surgery 6th edition*. (1581-1596). Philadelphia. Elsevier Saunders.
7. Black III JH, Cambria RP. (2005). Aortic dissection: perspectives for the vascular/endovascular surgeon. In *Rutherford Vascular Surgery 6th edition*. (1512-1533). Philadelphia. Elsevier Saunders.
8. Coimbra R, Hoyt DB. (2005). Epidemiology and natural history of vascular trauma. In *Rutherford Vascular Surgery 6th edition*. (1001-1006). Philadelphia. Elsevier Saunders.
9. Brewster DC. (2005). Direct reconstruction for aortoiliac occlusive disease. In *Rutherford Vascular Surgery 6th edition*. (1106-1136). Philadelphia. Elsevier Saunders.
10. Myers K, Clogh A. (2004) Renovascular diseases. In *Making Sense of Vascular Ultrasound*. (255-282). London: Hodder Arnold.
11. Zierler RE, Olmstead KA. (2010). Renal duplex scanning. In Zierler RE (Ed.), *Strandess's duplex scanning disorders in vascular diagnosis 4th ed.* (283-310).Philadelphia Wolters Kluwer Lippincott Williams & Wilkins.
12. Hallett JW, Brewster DC, Rasmussen TE. (2001). Aneurysms and aortic dissection. In: *Handbook of Patient Care in Vascular Diseases*. (204-221). Philadelphia Lippincott Williams & Wilkins
13. Burns PN. (1993). Principles of deep Doppler ultrasonography. In Bernstein EF (Ed.). *Vascular Diagnosis 4th ed.* (249-268). St. Louis: Mosby Yearbook Inc.
14. Rzucidlo EM, Zwolak RM. (2005). Arterial duplex scanning. In *Rutherford Vascular Surgery 6th edition*. (233-253). Philadelphia. Elsevier Saunders.
15. Cronenwett JL. (2005). Arterial aneurysms. In *Rutherford Vascular Surgery 6th edition*. (1403-1408). Philadelphia. Elsevier Saunders.
16. Brewster DC. (2005). Direct reconstruction for aortoiliac occlusive disease. In *Rutherford Vascular Surgery 6th edition*. (1106-1136). Philadelphia. Elsevier Saunders.
17. Zwiebel, WJ (2005). Ultrasound assessment of the aorta, iliac arteries and inferior vena cava. In Zwiebel WJ, Pellerito JS (Eds.), Introduction to Vascular Ultrasonography 5th ed, (530-552). Philadelphia. Elsevier Saunders.
18. Zierler RE. (2005). Ultrasound assessment of lower extremity arteries. In Zwiebel WJ, Pellerito JS (Eds.), Introduction to Vascular Ultrasonography 5th ed, (341-356). Philadelphia: Elsevier Saunders.
19. Bandyk, DF, (2005). Ultrasound assessment during and after peripheral intervention. In Zwiebel WJ, Pellerito JS (Eds.), *Introduction to Vascular Ultrasonography 5th ed*, (357-379). Philadelphia: Elsevier Saunders.
20. Hallett, JW, Brewster DC, Rasmussen TE, (2001) Non-invasive Vascular Testing, In Handbook of Patient Care in Vascular Diseases, (29-49), Philadelphia: Lippincott Williams & Wilkins
21. Back MR, Novotney M, Roth SM, Elkins D, Farber S, Cuthbertson D, Johnson BL, Bandyk DF. (2001). Utility of duplex surveillance following iliac artery angioplasty and primary stenting *J Endovasc Ther*. Dec;8(6):629-37.
22. Primary care screening for abdominal aortic aneurysm (2/2005). U.S. Preventive Services Task Force Evidence Syntheses, formerly Systematic Evidence Reviews. *Retrieved from*: http://www.ncbi.nlm.nih.gov/bookshelf/br.fcgi?book=es35&part=A30099.
23. Gerhard-Herman M, Gardin JM, Jaff M, Mohler E, Roman M, Naqvi TZ. (2006). Guidelines for non-invasive vascular laboratory testing: a report from the american society of echocardiography and the society of vascular medicine and biology. J Am Soc Echocardiogr 19:955-972.
24. Nordon IM, Hinchliffe RJ, Loftus IM, Thompson MM. (2010). Pathophysiology and epidemiology of abdominal aortic aneurysms *Nat Rev Cardiol*. Nov 16.
25. Van Bockel JH, Hamming JF. (2005). Lower extremity aneurysms. In Rutherford Vascular Surgery 6th edition. (1534-1551). Philadelphia. El Sevier Saunders.
26. Centers for medicare and medicaid services. (09/20/2010 1:09:09 PM). *Retrieved from* https://www.cms.gov/deficitreductionact.

Definition

The combination of real time B-mode ultrasonography with pulsed-wave and color flow Doppler to assess an aortic endograft for the presence of possible endoleak, stenosis or occlusion and to monitor any changes in size of a previously documented aneurysm sac

Etiology (of endograft complications)

- Endoleak
- Graft migration
- Graft infection
- Graft-limb external compression or kinking
- Embolization
- Thrombosis
- Technical error (graft misplacement)
- Limb separation
- Graft material complications (tears)
- Atherosclerosis

Risk Factors (for endograft complications)

- Age (increases with age)
- Smoking
- Hypertension
- Atherosclerosis
- Male gender
- Caucasian
- Immediate relative with an abdominal aortic aneurysm (AAA) history
- Trauma

Indications for Exam

- Post-operative surveillance of endovascular repair
- Hip/buttock claudication or impotence in patients post-operative for endovascular repair.

Contraindications/Limitations

- Obesity may cause poor visualization due to vessel depth
- Abdominal gas may prohibit visualization of any or all vessels

Endograft Configurations

- Bifurcated aortoiliac
- Aorto uni-iliac
- Straight aortic tube graft

Mechanism of Endograft Complications

- **Embolization** can occur when introducing an endograft into the sac of an AAA, especially when there is intramural thrombus.[1] Renal failure (from renal obstruction) and distal embolization to the legs are concerns.

> *Anytime the aneurysm sac is still receiving flow, pre-operative concerns of aneurysm enlargement and rupture remain.*

- **Endoleaks** may originate from these sources:[2]
  - Poor attachment of the graft to the vessel wall (**Type I**)
  - Patent arterial branches communicate with the aneurysm sac. Multiple patent branches can supply an inflow/outflow channel to the sac (**Type II**). Sources include the lumbar, inferior mesenteric, accessory renal arteries, etc.
  - A separation between the graft-limb modules (**Type III**).
  - Abnormal porosity of the graft material (**Type IV**)

- **Stent migration** occurs when displacement forces exceed the strength of fixation at the proximal/distal attachment site. Movement of the endograft can cause an endoleak, kink or graft-limb thrombosis.

Patient History

- Endovascular repair of an abdominal aortic aneurysm
- Complication found unexpectedly during physical exam, radiological or CT exams
- Many complications of endovascular repair present without symptoms

Physical Examination

- Pulsatile abdominal mass
- Lower back pain
- Systolic murmur in the region of the aneurysm
- Peripheral edema due to obstruction of the inferior vena cava

Abdominal Aortic Stent Graft Examination

- Patients should be fasting for 6-12 hours to minimize the presence of air in the abdomen. A limited volume of clear liquids may be ingested prior to the examination (e.g., to swallow medications).
- Patient is supine with arms and legs adequately supported. The patient may bend their knees up to aid in relaxation of the abdominal wall and decrease lumbar pain.
- Acoustic windows for imaging the abdominal aorta include: midline of the upper abdomen, left flank with patient supine or right lateral decubitus.
- A low frequency (1-4 MHz) transducer should be used for imaging these deep structures.
- To detect flow within the aneurysm sac, use program settings sensitive for low-color flow and Doppler velocities.

Transverse (Short-Axis) Scan

- The transducer is placed at the midline, below the xyphoid process and moved slowly, inferior toward the umbilicus during exam. Image the abdominal aorta (intra-aneurysm sac portion) in grayscale from the diaphragm to the aortic bifurcation with intermittent color flow Doppler. Scan the iliac arteries to the inguinal ligament. Document any areas of graft compression, lumenal defect, separation of modular junctions or areas of color flow or echolucency within the sac.
- The aneurysm sac is measured from outer wall to outer wall in both the anterior-posterior and transverse planes, perpendicular to the flow axis. Document the maximum cross sectional diameter to assess for enlargement. Note the anatomic level of the image.

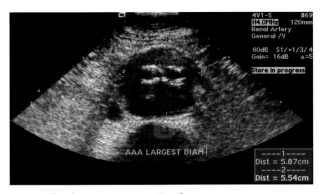

*Duplex measurements of an aneurysm sac
(#1's anterior-posterior measurement,
#2's transverse measurement)*

- During serial examination, measure and document the circumference of the aneurysm sac at its greatest diameter using the "area calculation" function of the duplex scanner. Document any noticeable changes regarding clot formation within the aneurysm sac.
- Determine the proximal fixation site between the stent and vessel wall. B-mode imaging without color is recommended in most cases. In transverse, record the aortic diameter at this site.

Longitudinal (Sagittal) Scan

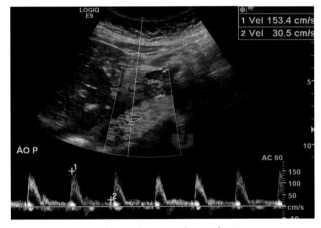

*PW Doppler waveforms from
abdominal aorta above stent*

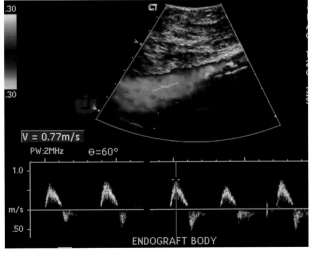

PW Doppler waveforms from body of the endograft

- Turn the probe longitudinally. Using pulsed wave Doppler (≤60° Doppler angle, with the angle cursor parallel to the vessel walls in the center of the flow stream) record a spectral waveform in the abdominal aorta above the stent (typically suprarenal aortic segment). Observe for dissection or evidence of intimal flap at this level.
- Document a B-mode image of the proximal fixation site. Record peak systolic velocity (PSV) and end diastolic velocity (EDV) at this point. Turn color flow on and observe for evidence of endoleak within the aneurysm sac at this level.

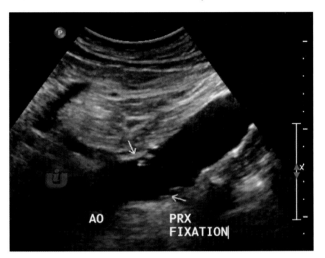

Proximal fixation site of stent-longitudinal B-mode view

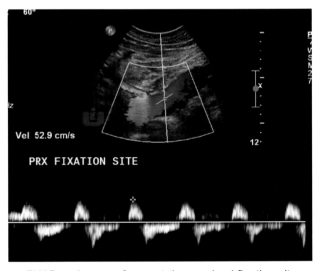

PW Doppler waveforms at the proximal fixation site

- Analyze the body of the endovascular graft using color flow and spectral Doppler to look for any flow abnormalities or intralumenal defects. Record a peak systolic velocity (PSV) and end diastolic velocity (EDV) from the body of the graft. Special attention should be given to any areas of kinking within the graft that may display increased velocities or stenosis and a decrease in distal flow. Record additional velocities pre and post any stenotic areas.
- The aneurysm sac is measured from outer wall to outer wall in the longitudinal plane. Remember to keep the probe perpendicular to the axis of the aorta. Document the maximum diameter to assess for enlargement. Note anatomic level of image taken for accurate comparison to previous exams.

- Using color Doppler, sweep the Doppler cursor through the aneurysm sac to detect any areas of extrastent flow. An area of leak will generate uniform, reproducible color flow which should persist through diastole.

> *Care should be taken to differentiate between color-bleeding and artifact (due to low scales) versus a true endoleak.*

- Confirm the absence or presence of flow outside the stent in multiple scanning planes. Document waveform, velocity and flow direction in any areas of extrastent flow. Note anatomic location.

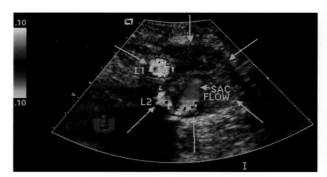

Color Doppler recorded in the transverse plane indicates evidence of endoleak

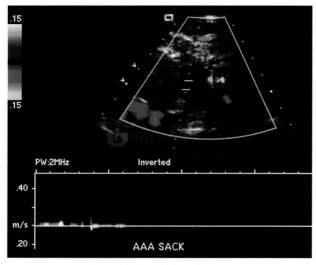

PW Doppler recorded in the transverse plane; no evidence of endoleak

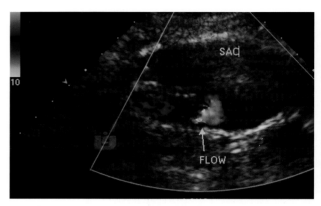

Color flow image indicates evidence of endoleak

- If no color is noted within the sac with the patient supine, have the patient assume a right lateral decubitus position and scan again (from the back of the patient), as this position may uncover a leak not previously seen.

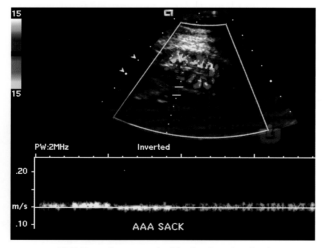

PW Doppler recorded in the longitudinal plane; no evidence of endoleak

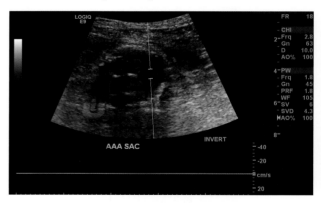

No leak evident by PW Doppler when patient is in supine position

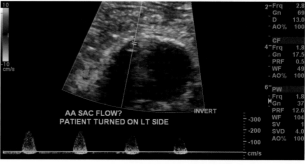

Evidence of leak in the same patient when scanned in the lateral decubitus position

- If an endoleak is present, determine the source (e.g., at a fixation site, from a branch or at junction between graft modules). Typical spectral waveform patterns will be "to-and-fro". Observe for small jets of flow in real time, filling the aneurysm sac.

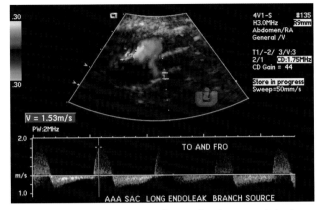

To-and-fro Doppler waveforms due to an endoleak

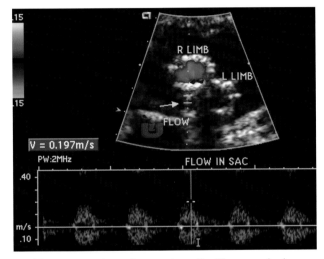

Transverse view of an endograft with an occlusion of the left graft limb and evidence of an endoleak

- Assess velocity and waveforms from each graft-limb to detect stenosis due to graft compression or occlusion. Calculate the velocity ratios (Vr), where the highest peak systolic velocity at stenosis (V_2) is divided by the PSV of the proximal normal segment (V_1).

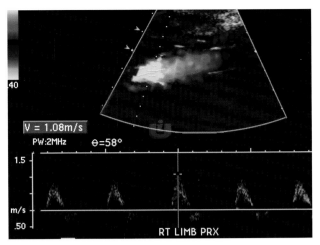

PW Doppler waveforms from the right graft limb

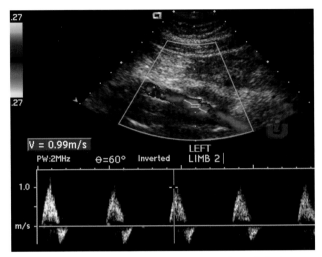

PW Doppler waveforms from the left graft limb

- Determine the distal fixation site between the stent and vessel wall. Note the anatomic location. Turn color flow on and observe for evidence of endoleak at this level.
- Assess velocity and waveforms from the outflow artery, inferior to the distal attachment site. Calculate the velocity ratio in any areas of increased velocity.
- Analyze the bilateral common femoral waveforms to document aortoiliac inflow to the legs.

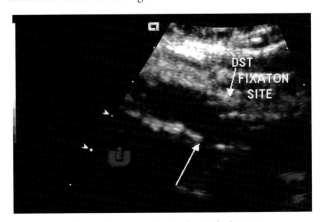

Distal fixation site on B-mode image

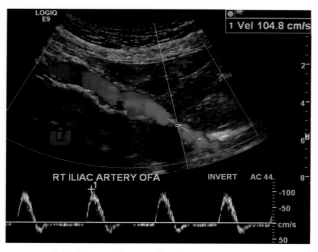

Arterial waveforms distal to the endograft

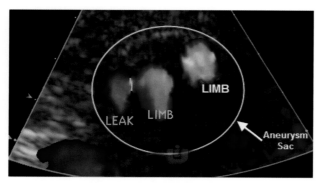

Transverse view of endoleak with color flow

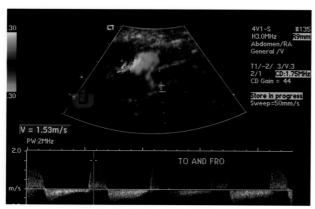

*Endoleak PW Doppler waveforms
(to-and-fro waveform pattern)*

TABLE 104: Abdominal Aortic Stent Graft Protocol Summary

Scan in longitudinal (sagittal) and transverse (short-axis) planes with grayscale, low color and PW Doppler velocity scales.

- Measure aneurysm sac from outer wall to outer wall in both anterior-posterior and transverse planes in both transverse and long views. Keep perpendicular to the vessel axis when measuring. Document maximum cross sectional diameter.

- Determine the proximal fixation site.

- Record peak systolic velocity (PSV), end diastolic velocity (EDV) and waveforms in the abdominal aorta above the stent.

- Observe body of the endograft in transverse and long views using low scale color flow and spectral Doppler to look for any flow abnormalities/intralumenal defects*. Record PSV, EDV and waveform from the body of the stent.

- Sweep the Doppler cursor throughout the aneurysm sac to detect any areas of extrastent flow and document any waveforms.

- Determine source of any endoleaks present.

- Record PSV, EDV and waveforms from each graft-limb.

- Determine the distal fixation site.

- Record outflow PSV, EDV and waveforms.

- Record bilateral common femoral PSV, EDV and waveforms.

  * Observe for and document any areas of graft compression, luminal defect or separation of modular junctions.

Interpretation

Normal

- **Aneurysm size:** Expect the aneurysm size to decrease or remain stable post-operatively after exclusion from circulation. No flow by color or Doppler is expected in the aneurysm sac.[3,4]

- **General grayscale and color characteristics:** There are no areas of echolucency within the aneurysm sac by B-mode image. There is no evidence of color flow within the aneurysm sac with appropriate low-flow settings.

- **Doppler waveforms and velocities:** The body and limbs of the endograft should be widely patent with no evidence of significant velocity increase (e.g., Vr <2.0).

> *Color is never diagnostic without PW Doppler confirmation.*

Abnormal

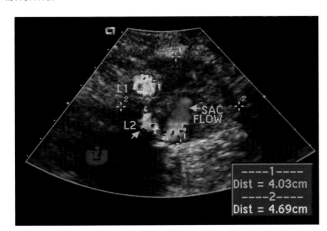

Duplex Measurement of aneurysm sac-endoleak

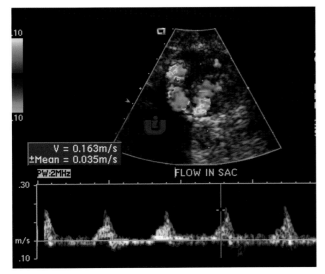

PW Doppler from aneurysm sac-endoleak

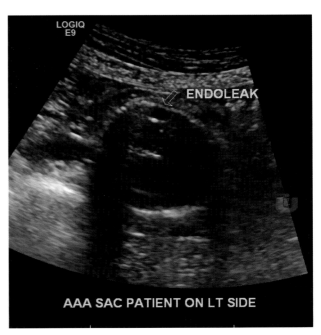

Endoleak suspected by an area of
echolucency on B-mode image

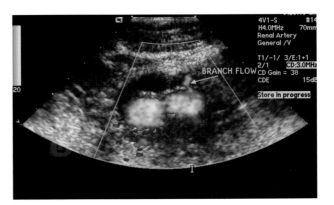

Endoleak documented with power Doppler

- **Aneurysm size**: A >0.5 cm increase in the diameter
  of the aneurysm sac on B-mode image is suggestive of
  endoleak.[2,4] Further imaging (e.g., CT scan) may be needed
  to confirm such findings.[3,4]

- **General grayscale and color characteristics**: An area of
  endoleak is recognized in the B-mode image by echolucency or
  pulsation within the aneurysm sac and confirmed by color and
  spectral Doppler waveforms.[3-5] Always attempt to reproduce
  evidence of an endoleak to reduce false-positive reports.[4]

- **Doppler waveforms and velocities**
  - **Stenosis**: A limb stenosis is recognized by color aliasing
    and confirmed by increased velocities.[4,7] Compare velocities
    at the level of the stenosis to the velocities in the proximal
    normal segment. A velocity ratio >2.0 and the presence
    of post-stenotic turbulence indicate a hemodynamically
    significant stenosis. Diameter reduction measurements
    should only be used in conjunction with peak systolic
    velocity measurements.
  - **Endoleak**: True endoleaks create reproducible uniform color
    Doppler data, including waveforms in sync with the patient's
    cardiac cycle.[4] Doppler waveforms of the endoleak should
    differ from the waveform characteristics in the endograft.[6]

  - Typically, the inferior mesenteric and lumbar arteries
    occlude after endovascular repair.[4] If they remain
    patent, determine flow direction in these side vessels
    and analyze carefully for possible endoleak.[7]
  - The direction of flow will be used to determine
    the afferent (inflow) and efferent (outflow) sources
    communicating with the aneurysm.[4] Depending on
    the source of the endoleak, biphasic, monophasic or
    bidirectional waveforms may be recorded.[3,4,6]
  - In a small research series, biphasic waveforms suggested
    that the endoleak had an inflow and outflow source.
    Endoleaks with monophasic and bidirectional waveforms
    are more likely to spontaneously thrombose.[6]

- **Endotension** is indicated when an increase in the aneurysm's
  size is measured, without any endoleak detected by duplex.[2]

- **Occlusion:** An occlusion is recognized by the absence of color
  saturation confirmed by the lack of an audible PW Doppler
  signal in the endograft or native artery.

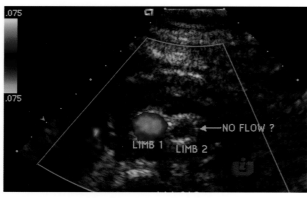

*Occlusion of a graft limb suspected
in transverse view by color flow*

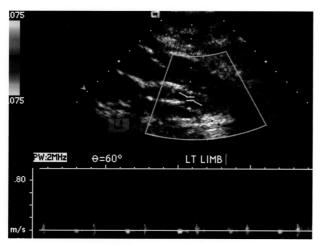

PW Doppler confirms occlusion of the graft limb

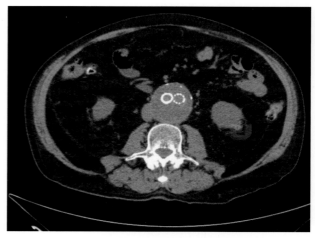

CT scan of endograft limbs in transverse

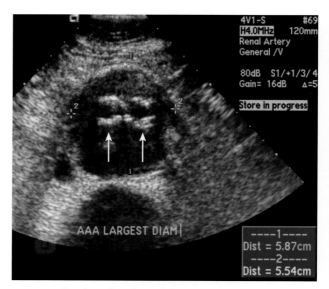

Duplex of endograft limbs in transverse

TABLE 105: Endoleak Classification

Type	Source of Endoleak
Type I	Attachment site (either proximal or distal)
Type II	Branch site (such as; lumbar, inferior mesenteric, intercostal, internal iliac, hypogastric or accessory renal arteries)
Type III	Modular disconnection, fabric tear
Type IV	Porosity

Correlation

- CT scan
- MRI
- Aortography

Surgical Treatment

- Open repair of aortic aneurysm

Endovascular Treatment

- Balloon dilatation of the involved graft component (to treat a leak or stenosis)
- Placement of supportive stenting or endograft extension pieces

Points to Remember

- Post-operative surveillance is generally performed at 1, 6, 12 and 18 months. Annual surveillance is recommended thereafter.
- When the source of a true endoleak cannot be determined, reporting should indicate that the inflow/outflow source is indeterminate.
- During follow-up exams, the location of the graft is compared to previous studies for evidence of graft migration.
- Post-operatively, the movement of non-clotted blood within the aneurysm sac may be seen moving due to pulsatility from the adjacent endovascular graft.
- Wall calcification and patient movement may produce flashes of color within the aneurysm sac.

Reference

1. Sumner DS, Zierler RE. (2005). Vascular physiology: essential hemodynamic principles. In Rutherford Vascular Surgery 6th edition. (75-123). Philadelphia. Elsevier Saunders.

2. Fecteau SR, Darling III RC, Roddy SP. (2005). Arterial thomboembolism. In Rutherford Vascular Surgery 6th edition. (971-986). Philadelphia. Elsevier Saunders.

3. Dawson DL, Lee ES, Lindholm K. (2010). Aortic and peripheral aneurysms. In Zierler RE (Ed.), Strandess's duplex scanning disorders in vascular diagnosis 4th ed. (157-168). Philadelphia Wolters Kluwer Lippincott Williams & Wilkins

4. Stary HC, Chandler AB, Dinsmore RE, Fuster V, Glagov S, Insull W, Rosenfeld ME, Schwartz CJ, Wagner WD, Wissler RW. A definition of advanced types of atherosclerotic lesions and histological classification of atherosclerosis. Atherosclerosis, Thrombosis and Vascular Biology. 1995; 15; 1521-1531.

5. Schermerhorn ML, Cronenwett JL. (2005). Abdominal aortic and iliac aneurysms. In Rutherford Vascular Surgery 6th edition. (1408-1452). Philadelphia. Elsevier Saunders.

6. Reddy DJ, Weaver MR. (2005). Infected aneurysms. In Rutherford Vascular Surgery 6th edition. (1581-1596). Philadelphia. Elsevier Saunders.

7. Black III JH, Cambria RP. (2005). Aortic dissection: perspectives for the vascular/endovascular surgeon. In Rutherford Vascular Surgery 6th edition. (1512-1533). Philadelphia. Elsevier Saunders.

8. Coimbra R, Hoyt DB. (2005). Epidemiology and natural history of vascular trauma. In Rutherford Vascular Surgery 6th edition. (1001-1006). Philadelphia. Elsevier Saunders.

9. Brewster DC. (2005). Direct reconstruction for aortoiliac occlusive disease. In Rutherford Vascular Surgery 6th edition. (1106-1136). Philadelphia. Elsevier Saunders.

10. Myers K, Clogh A. (2004) Renovascular diseases. In Making Sense of Vascular Ultrasound. (255-282). London: Hodder Arnold.

11. Zierler RE, Olmstead KA. (2010). Renal duplex scanning. In Zierler RE (Ed.), Strandess's duplex scanning disorders in vascular diagnosis 4th ed. (283-310).Philadelphia Wolters Kluwer Lippincott Williams & Wilkins.

12. Hallett JW, Brewster DC, Rasmussen TE. (2001). Aneurysms and aortic dissection. In: Handbook of Patient Care in Vascular Diseases. (204-221). Philadelphia Lippincott Williams & Wilkins

13. Burns PN. (1993). Principles of deep Doppler ultrasonography. In Bernstein EF (Ed.). Vascular Diagnosis 4th ed. (249-268). St. Louis: Mosby Yearbook Inc.

14. Rzucidlo EM, Zwolak RM. (2005). Arterial duplex scanning. In Rutherford Vascular Surgery 6th edition. (233-253). Philadelphia. Elsevier Saunders.

15. Cronenwett JL. (2005). Arterial aneurysms. In Rutherford Vascular Surgery 6th edition. (1403-1408). Philadelphia. Elsevier Saunders.

16. Brewster DC. (2005). Direct reconstruction for aortoiliac occlusive disease. In Rutherford Vascular Surgery 6th edition. (1106-1136). Philadelphia. Elsevier Saunders.

17. Zwiebel, WJ (2005). Ultrasound assessment of the aorta, iliac arteries and inferior vena cava. In Zwiebel WJ, Pellerito JS (Eds.), Introduction to Vascular Ultrasonography 5th ed, (530-552). Philadelphia: Elsevier Saunders.

18. Zierler RE. (2005). Ultrasound assessment of lower extremity arteries. In Zwiebel WJ, Pellerito JS (Eds.), Introduction to Vascular Ultrasonography 5th ed, (341-356). Philadelphia: Elsevier Saunders.

19. Bandyk, DF, (2005). Ultrasound assessment during and after peripheral intervention. In Zwiebel WJ, Pellerito JS (Eds.), Introduction to Vascular Ultrasonography 5th ed, (357-379). Philadelphia: Elsevier Saunders.

20. Hallett, JW, Brewster DC, Rasmussen TE, (2001) Non-invasive Vascular Testing, In Handbook of Patient Care in Vascular Diseases, (29-49), Philadelphia: Lippincott Williams & Wilkins

21. 21 Back MR, Novotney M, Roth SM, Elkins D, Farber S, Cuthbertson D, Johnson BL, Bandyk DF. (2001). Utility of duplex surveillance following iliac artery angioplasty and primary stenting

22. J Endovasc Ther. Dec;8(6):629-37.

23. Primary care screening for abdominal aortic aneurysm (2/2005). U.S. Preventive Services Task Force Evidence Syntheses, formerly Systematic Evidence Reviews. Retrieved from: http://www.ncbi.nlm.nih.gov/bookshelf/br.fcgi?book=es35&part=A30099.

24. Gerhard-Herman M, Gardin JM, Jaff M, Mohler E, Roman M, Naqvi TZ. (2006). Guidelines for non-invasive vascular laboratory testing: a report from the american society of echocardiography and the society of vascular medicine and biology. J Am Soc Echocardiogr 19:955-972.

25. Nordon IM, Hinchliffe RJ, Loftus IM, Thompson MM. (2010). Pathophysiology and epidemiology of abdominal aortic aneurysms Nat Rev Cardiol. Nov 16.

26. 25 Van Bockel JH, Hamming JF. (2005). Lower extremity aneurysms. In Rutherford Vascular Surgery 6th edition. (1534-1551). Philadelphia. El Sevier Saunders.

27. Centers for medicare and medicaid services. (09/20/2010 1:09:09 PM). Retrieved from https://www.cms.gov/deficitreductionact.

Definition

The combination of real time B-mode ultrasonography with pulsed wave and color flow Doppler to assess the renal arteries for the presence of stenosis/occlusion or other disease states such as fibromuscular dysplasia. Doppler and color flow are also used to evaluate the renal veins for evidence of thrombus.

Etiology (of renal vessel disease)

- Atherosclerosis, resulting in stenosis or occlusion
- Fibromuscular dysplasia (FMD)
- Embolus
- Vasculitis
- Occlusion
- External compression
- Thrombosis
- Aneurysm
- Arteriovenous fistula
- Trauma

Risk Factors

- Age (increased risk with age)
- Hypertension
- Race (African-Americans having the highest risk)
- Diabetes
- Kidney disease
- Family history of kidney disease
- Smoking
- Hyperlipidemia
- Obesity
- Coronary artery disease
- Young, middle-aged Caucasian women (highest risk for fibromuscular dysplasia)

Indications for Exam

- Hypertension (HTN)
  - of unknown origin (essential hypertension)
  - malignant, benign or secondary types of types of HTN
  - changes in previously controlled HTN
- Elevated blood-urea-nitrogen (BUN) levels (*azotemia*)
- Known atherosclerosis of the aortoiliac segment, especially accompanied by HTN
- Unilateral, small (atrophic) kidney
- Cystic kidney disease
- Aneurysm/pseudoaneurysm
- Pre and post-operative surgical intervention, revascularization, endovascular procedure or percutaneous translumenal dilatation of the renal arteries

Contraindications/Limitations

- Obesity may cause poor visualization due to vessel depth.
- Abdominal gas may prohibit visualization of any or all vessels.

Anatomy

- The right and left main renal arteries (RA) originate laterally from the abdominal aorta, immediately inferior to the superior mesenteric artery.

> The right kidney is lower than the left kidney due to the R-lobe of the liver.

- The right and left renal veins (RV) originate from the inferior vena cava.
- The right RA is longer than the left and is posterior to the inferior vena cava and right RV.
- The left RV runs between the abdominal aorta and superior mesenteric artery.
- The left RA lies posterior to the left renal vein.
- The segmental arteries originate before or immediately after entering the kidney.
- The interlobar arteries evaluated within the kidney parenchyma are branches of the segmental arteries. The medulla is adjacent to the renal sinus and pyramids.
- The arcuate arteries evaluated within the kidney parenchyma are branches of the interlobar arteries as they pass around the pyramids giving rise to the interlubar arterioles. The cortex is the most peripheral portion of the parenchyma, located between the medulla and renal capsule.

Anatomic Variations of the Kidney and Renal Arteries

- A "horseshoe kidney" is a congenital abnormality which results in the fusion of both kidneys. Beginning the scan with a midline abdominal approach is suggested for this situation.
- In 20-30% of patients, one to three accessory renal arteries may be present, especially on the left side. They usually originate from the aorta below the main renal artery and often enter the kidney directly.
- A renal artery may also branch anywhere before entering the kidney.

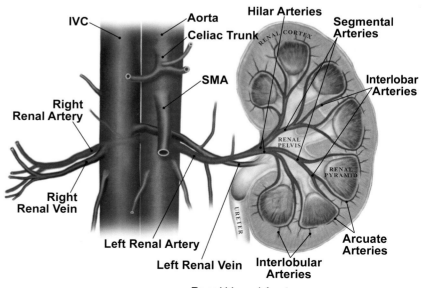

Renal Vessel Anatomy

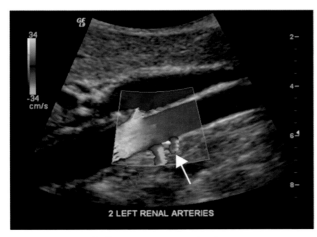

Left accessory renal artery
(Note second left-sided branch off the aorta)
Image courtesy of GE Healthcare-Ultrasound Division

Mechanism of disease

- Renal arterial stenotic or occlusive disease results in decreased renal blood flow to the kidney. [1]
  - When baroreceptors detect a decrease in blood flow, the enzyme, renin is released.

> *The kidney maintains blood pressure by regulating the balance of sodium and water retention.* [1]

  - The renin-angiotensin system is activated, which increases angiotensin II levels. Sodium and water retention ensues. If the contralateral kidney is healthy, it can compensate by increasing its urine output to prevent volume expansion.
  - Angiotensin II increases blood pressure and causes peripheral vasoconstriction.
  - A sustained increase in hypertension results.
  - When there is only single kidney function, if that renal artery is obstructed, the kidney cannot rely on increased urine output from the contralateral kidney to prevent sodium and water retention. The volume expansion which results causes elevated blood pressure and suppresses renin production by the stenotic kidney.
- **Atherosclerosis** is the most common arterial disease. Atherosclerotic plaque forms in the artery to block flow by either narrowing it (arterial stenosis) or totally blocking the artery (arterial occlusion). The term "hemodynamically significant obstruction" refers to either a stenosis or an occlusion that results in a decrease in blood pressure or flow distal to the obstruction. Typically, a stenosis must narrow the diameter of the artery by at least 50% to decrease pressure and flow distally. An arterial occlusion is typically seen from one major branch to the next.[2]
- **Emboli** may occur as contents of a plaque or fragments of an organized thrombus from the left-side of the heart, suprarenal aneurysm or ulcerative aortic plaque loosen and flow downstream.[3] Emboli become lodged in a distant blood vessel, causing an arterial obstruction which reduces flow.[4] Sources for renal emboli include renal artery dissection, traumatic renal artery occlusion or cardiac sources.[1]
- **Fibromuscular dysplagia** is a non-atherosclerotic arterial disease which affects the distal renal arteries. Multiple, focal stenoses are present, resembling a "string of beads" on imaging studies. The exact mechanism of disease is unclear.

- **Renal artery thrombosis** can occur when there is advanced atherosclerosis of the aorta and its branches.[3]
- **Renal vein thrombosis** can occur in adults in one or both renal veins due to cancer (especially renal cell carcinoma), hypercoaguable states, pregnancy, use of contraceptive medications, trauma or sickle cell anemia. Neonates are also at risk for renal vein thrombosis. [3]
- **Nutcracker syndrome (or "left renal vein entrapment")**: Compression of the left distal renal vein between the aorta and superior mesenteric artery can occur in rare cases. Nutcracker syndrome is also known as "renal vein entrapment syndrome". [5]
- **Aneurysmal disease** results from atherosclerosis or congenital defect. [6]
- **Arterial dissection** of the renal artery can occur spontaneously with atherosclerosis, trauma or dysplastic renovascular disease as the underlying cause. [6]

Location of Disease

- In atherosclerosis, the ostial or proximal renal arterial segments is affected.
- In fibromuscular lesions, the mid-distal arterial segments are affected.
- In nutcracker syndrome, venous dilatation occurs distal (upstream) to the compression.

Patient History

- Systemic hypertension
- Unexplained hypokalemia
- Renal failure
- Abnormal urinalysis (e.g., serum potassium, creatinine)
- Unexplained episodes of congestive heart failure (CHF)
- Flash pulmonary edema
- Left flank abdominal pain radiating to the buttocks (nutcracker syndrome)
- Hematuria
- Anemia

Physical Examination

- Abdominal bruit-abnormal sound heard through auscultation caused by turbulent flow.

Duplex Examination of the Renal Arteries

- Patient should be fasting for 6-12 hours to minimize the presence of air and fluids in the abdomen. A limited volume of clear liquids may be ingested prior to the examination to swallow medications.
- Obtain any past surgical reports or records of bypass graft or stent placement and general date of surgery if available.
- Patient should be supine with arms and legs adequately supported. The patient may bend their knees up to aid in relaxation of the abdominal wall and decrease lumbar pain.
- A low frequency transducer (2.0-4.0 MHz) should be used for imaging deep renal structures.

> *A 0° angle is used in the kidney parenchyma since waveform morphology is the only concern, not velocities.*

- Pulsed wave (PW) Doppler should be at a ≤60° angle in the renal arteries. The sample volume should be parallel to the vessel walls and within the center of the flow stream. In the kidney parenchyma, the Doppler angle should be set to 0° (zero).

- Imaging of the renal arteries can be accomplished using the following approaches. (Transverse (short-axis) plane is the most common approach.)
  - The origin and proximal portion of the renal arteries can be visualized with the patient in the supine position and the transducer oriented to obtain a transverse view. The right RA arises from the lateral aspect of the abdominal aorta at approximately 10-o'clock. The right renal vein is anterior to the right RA. The left RA, originating from the aorta at approximately the 3- 4-o'clock position, lies inferior to the left renal vein and can be more difficult to image than the right RA.

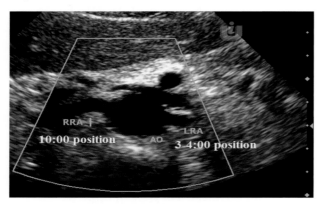

*Renal artery origins off the abdominal aorta
(transverse, gray-scale view)*

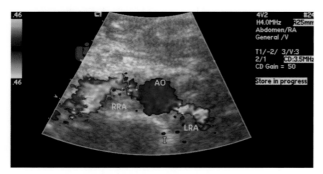

Right and left renal artery origins off the abdominal aorta

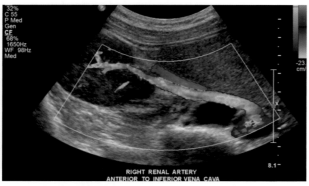

*Right renal artery coursing from the
abdominal aorta to the kidney*
Image courtesy of Philips Healthcare

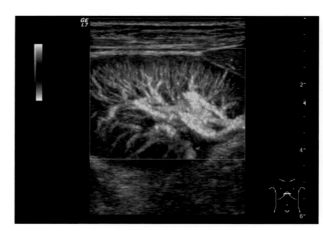

Kidney parenchyma with color flow
Image courtesy of GE Healthcare-Ultrasound Division

"Banana Peel" View

- The patient is placed in a left lateral decubital position. The right RA can be seen peeling off the aorta upward and the left RA can be seen peeling away from the aorta.
- Views of the liver, inferior vena cava and abdominal aorta can be accessed from this window.

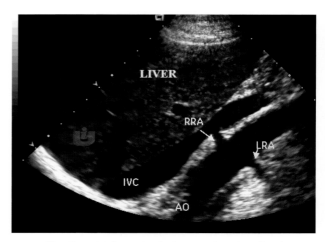

*The liver and renal arteries can be visualized
using the "banana peel" view.*

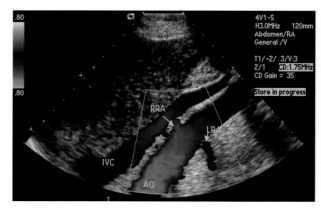

Right and left renal artery origins off the aorta with color flow

Using the Liver as a Window

– The patient is turned to a right-side-up-decubitus position and the liver is used as a window to visualize the origin of the right RA.

Spleen as a Window

– The patient is placed in a left lateral decubital position. The spleen and the left kidney are used as acoustic windows to visualize the left renal artery.

Renal Artery Scanning Protocol

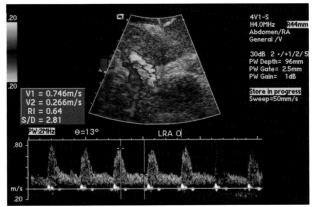

Normal renal artery waveforms

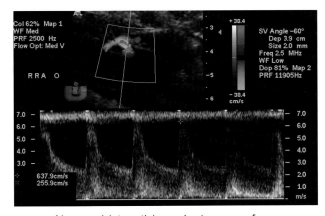

Abnormal (stenotic) renal artery waveforms

Abdominal aorta

- Examine the abdominal aorta for aneurysm, plaque, thrombus, dissection, tortuosity and/or other abnormalities.
- Record a PW Doppler peak systolic velocity (PSV) in the suprarenal abdominal aorta, at or above the superior mesenteric artery, to be used in the renal artery/aortic ratio (RAR) calculation.
- Observe for important variants of the renal arteries (e.g., renal artery duplication).

> Color flow Doppler and power Doppler may aid in locating the arteries and areas of interest.

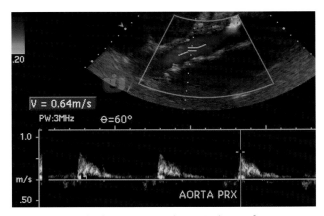

Abdominal aorta normal spectral waveforms

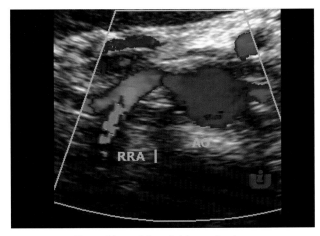

Branching of the right renal artery

Right Renal Artery

- Locate the superior mesenteric artery in a transverse view and then move the transducer slightly distal to image the right RA.
- Measure the PSV and EDV at the origin, proximal, mid and distal portions of the right RA. A transverse probe orientation is often best when recording from the ostia and proximal segments, while a longitudinal (sagittal) orientation works for the mid and distal segments. Attempt to sample as far distal as possible.
- Document the highest PSV and EDV through any stenotic area(s) and document post-stenotic turbulence.
- Examine the renal artery for aneurysm, plaque, thrombus, dissection and/or other abnormalities.
- Image the right kidney, with and without color flow, and examine the kidney for anomalies such as cysts, dilated collection systems and/or tumors.
- Obtain a long-axis image of the right kidney and measure kidney length, pole-to-pole. A difference between both kidneys of >2 cm calls for re-measurement of the smaller kidney to confirm the discrepancy.

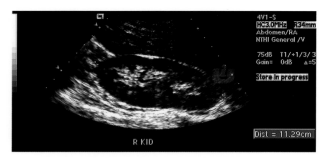

Pole-to-pole diameter measurement of the kidney

- Calculate the RAR by dividing the highest PSV of the renal artery by the highest PSV in the suprarenal abdominal aortic segment.

Right Renal Vein

- Place the transducer in the right lower quadrant over the kidney and angle medially. Use color flow as a guide to locate the right renal vein.

- Document patency of the right RV using color flow and PW Doppler.

> *Even with RV occlusion, you may observe venous flow within the kidney from hilar collaterals.*[7]

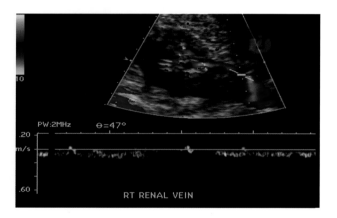

> *The left renal vein can be a useful landmark when it crosses over the aorta near the origin of the right RA.*

Right Renal Parenchyma

- Record PSV, EDV and Doppler spectral waveforms from the upper and/or lower poles of the kidney in the medullary and cortical regions of the organ. Use a 1.5-2 mm sample volume and a 0^0 (zero) Doppler angle for these measurements. Since parenchymal vessels are not easily imaged, color flow is a useful tool to guide placement of the Doppler sample volume. Waveforms with the highest amplitude and velocity should be documented from the parenchyma.

> *Asking the patient to take a deep breath in and hold it may improve kidney visualization.*

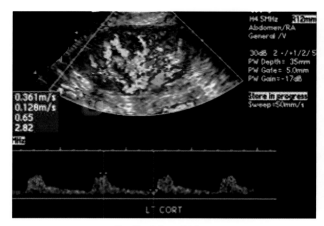

Cortical flow-kidney

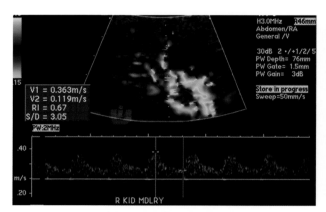

Medullary flow-kidney

- Calculate the resistive index (RI) of the medullary and cortical arteries. The formula for RI is (1 - [EDV/maximum systolic velocity] x 100) or (PSV-EDV)/PSV. (Many duplex scanners will automatically calculate RI from the spectral tracings during the exam.)

- Determine classification of stenosis according to laboratory diagnostic criteria.

- Repeat for the left RA, RV and parenchyma.

Renal Bypass Graft/Stent Surveillance Protocol

- Evaluate for graft or stent abnormalities while scanning (e.g., thrombosis, stenosis, residual valves, aneurysm, kinks, intimal hyperplasia, perigraft fluid, arteriovenous fistula).

- Record images in a longitudinal view with and without color flow of the:
  - Inflow/proximal native artery
  - Proximal anastomosis
  - Proximal graft or stent
  - Mid graft or stent
  - Distal graft or stent
  - Distal anastomosis
  - Outflow/distal native artery

- Scroll or "walk" the Doppler sample volume through the bypass graft/stent checking for focal changes in velocity and waveform configuration.

- Record and measure the peak systolic velocity (PSV) in longitudinal using pulsed wave Doppler (≤60° Doppler angle with the angle cursor parallel to the vessel walls and sample volume within the center of the flow stream) at the following levels:

  - Inflow/proximal native artery, at least 2 cm proximal to the anastomosis
  - Proximal anastomosis
  - Proximal graft or stent
  - Mid graft or stent
  - Distal graft or stent
  - Distal anastomosis
  - Outflow/distal native artery

- Determine classification of stenosis according to laboratory diagnostic criteria.

TABLE 106: Renal Duplex Protocol Summary

Abdominal Aorta
- Evaluate the abdominal aorta for aneurysm, plaque, thrombus, dissection, and/or tortuosity.
- Obtain a PW Doppler peak systolic velocity (PSV) in the abdominal aorta, at or above the superior mesenteric artery, for use in the renal artery/aortic ratio (RAR).

Right Renal Artery
- Record PSV and EDV at the origin, proximal, mid and distal portions of the right renal artery.

Left Renal Artery
- Record PSV and EDV at the origin, proximal, mid and distal portions of the left renal artery.

Right Kidney
- Image the right kidney in the long-axis and measure its diameter.
- Identify the cortical and medullary arteries using color flow. Record PSV and EDV in the upper and/or lower poles of the kidney according to lab criteria.

Left Kidney
- Image the left kidney in the long-axis and measure its diameter.
- Identify the cortical and medullary arteries using color flow. Record PSV and EDV in the upper and/or lower poles of the kidney according to lab criteria.

Renal Veins
- Identify the left and right RV using color flow and record spectral waveforms of these veins.

Calculations
- Calculate the renal artery/aortic ratio (RAR) (bilaterally) and determine the classification of disease.

  The highest renal artery PSV ÷ the highest PSV in the suprarenal abdominal aortic segment

- Calculate the resistive indices (RI) (bilaterally) using cortical and medullary flow to determine the presence of intrinsic disease.

  Resistive index= 1 - [EDV/PSV] x 100
  or (PSV - EDV)/ PSV x 100

Interpretation

Normal

> *The RAR is only reliable when abdominal aortic velocities are normal. Base interpretation on absolute velocities instead of RAR when the aortic PSV is <45 cm/s or >100 cm/s.[12,13]*

- **Waveform characteristics and flow velocities:**
  - The normal renal artery waveform is a low resistance flow pattern (forward flow in diastole). [8,9]
  - Normal peak systolic arterial velocities are <180-200 cm/s. [8,10]
- **Renal-aortic ratio**: A normal renal-aortic ratio (RAR) is <3.5. [10,11]
- **Kidney diameter**: A normal kidney length is 10-12 cm with a 4.5-6 cm width. [13,14]
- **Kidney parenchyma:**
  - Normal parenchymal arterial flow will appear similar to the distal renal artery; a low resistance waveform (forward flow in diastole) with an average peak systolic velocity between 20-30 cm/s in the cortex and 30-40 cm/s in the medullary region at a 0° angle. [14]
  - Normal RI values are <0.70. [13]
- **General grayscale and color characteristics**:
  - No echogenic material should be observed within the lumen of the native artery, vein, graft or stent by B-mode and color flow.
  - Two separate areas of the kidney parenchyma around the renal sinus should be evident by B-mode image: the medulla and cortex. The echogenic characteristics of a normal cortex are similar to the liver or spleen at a similar depth. The cortex should have a "scalloped" or "notched" appearance. [14]
- **Venous flow**: The renal veins are normally pulsatile near their origins by PW Doppler. Venous signals recorded near the renal hilum will be more phasic with respiration.[14]

Abnormal

- **Waveform characteristics and flow velocities:**
  - A hemodynamically significant arterial stenosis is recognized by color aliasing, and confirmed by increased PSV >180-200 cm/s. [8,10]
  - The presence of post-stenotic turbulence and color bruit support the diagnosis of an arterial stenosis. [9,10]
  - Severely abnormal, monophasic arterial Doppler waveforms are characterized by a slow upstroke, low amplitude, and broad peak with no evidence of the reversed flow component in late systole. The upstroke has a general direction of being tipped to the right. Continuous forward flow is typical in diastole, but diastolic flow may be absent if there is distal resistance from an additional high-grade distal obstruction, for example.
    - Monophasic waveforms are typically present distal to an occlusion or a very high grade stenosis.
    - An alternate term for severely abnormal waveforms found in the kidney beyond a hemodynamically significant renal artery stenosis is "parvus tardus".[9,10,15] Parvus tardus means "low and late" or "low and slow", referring to the slow upstroke and low amplitude of this waveform.
    - Diameter reduction measurements should only be used in conjunction with peak systolic velocity measurements.

- **Renal-aortic ratio**: An abnormal renal-aortic ratio (RAR) is >3.5.[8,10,11]
- **Kidney diameter**: A kidney length under 9 cm is highly suspicious for decreased blood flow.[9,15] Bilateral kidney diameters should be within 2 cm of each other.[14]
- **Kidney parenchyma:**
  - Abnormal parenchymal arterial flow will exhibit increased pulsatility and decreased diastolic flow.[8,9]
  - An RI >0.80 is abnormal. [8-10,15]
- **General grayscale and color characteristics:**
  - Echogenic material is observed within the lumen of native artery, graft or stent by B-mode. Color flow does not fill the arterial lumen completely.
  - Incidental findings on B-mode imaging include renal calculi (kidney stones), tumors, etc. Renal cysts are a common finding. Single or multiple cysts may be observed in any part of the kidney. These cysts are typically round or oval, anaechoic and smooth in appearance.[14]
- **Venous flow**: Pulsatile flow through the entire renal vein from the origin to the renal hilum suggests increased central venous pressure due to congestive heart failure, pulmonary edema, etc.[14]

> *Renal vein thrombosis may be secondary to a tumor or other source of extrinsic compression.*[13]

- **Renal vein thrombosis:**[13,14] Echogenic material may or may not be observed with the lumen of the RV by B-mode image depending on the age of the thrombus. Color flow will be observed flowing around echogenic material or be absent, depending on whether the clot is partially or totally occlusive. Confirm any suspected occlusion by PW Doppler.
  - Dilatation of the vein proximal to the occlusion and an enlarged kidney may be observed in an acute event. The thrombus may be echolucent in acute cases.
  - Echogenic material within the lumen of the vein suggests a chronic event. Continuous venous flow signals may be observed if the vein has recanalized.[14]

Other Pathology

> *An occlusion should never be based on color alone. Always confirm flow by placing the Doppler sample volume in the vessel lumen.*

- **Occlusion**: An arterial occlusion is present when no flow is detected by spectral Doppler and color. [9,10,13,15]
- **Fibromuscular dysplasia:** When a series of hemodynamically significant velocity increases are noted in the mid/distal segment of the renal artery along with significant turbulence, FMD is suspected.[9] A "string of beads" is the classic appearance on B-mode and color Doppler images (where segments of the artery can be seen narrowing and then widening in series). [6,16]
- **Nutcracker syndrome:** Increased venous velocities (up to 5 times greater than the velocities at the hilum of the kidney) are observed at the point of entrapment. The renal vein is typically enlarged about five times the measured diameter at the point of entrapment.[5] Doppler waveforms will exhibit either decreased spontaneity, phasicity and continuous renal vein flow or an absent Doppler signal in nutcracker syndrome. [5]

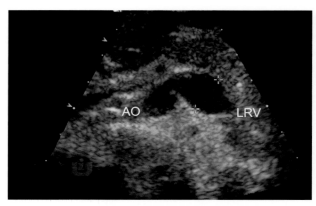

"Nutcracker syndrome": increased renal vein diameter distal to the compression of the vein

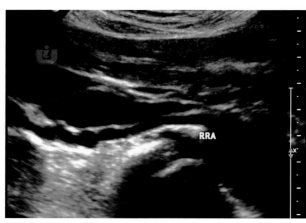

Fibromuscular dysplasia of the renal artery: "string of beads"

- **Aneurysmal disease**: Renal artery aneurysms usually occur before the artery reaches the parenchyma and are often saccular. Aneurysm diameters between 5-9 cm have been reported.[6] Fusiform aneurysms are less common with diameters <2 cm.[6] PSV may decrease proximal to the dilatation and normalize distally.[9]
- **Arterial dissection**: A dissection of the arterial lumen is recognized by two distinct flow channels by B-mode and/or color Doppler separated by an intimal echo. One lumen is known as the "true lumen" while the other is referred to as the "false lumen". One of the lumens may demonstrate increased velocities and stenotic waveforms. [9]

TABLE 107: Normal Renal-Aortic Peak Systolic Velocities

Arterial Vessel	Peak Systolic Velocity
Aorta	80-100 cm/s
Renal artery	<180 cm/s
Medullary artery	30-40 cm/s (at 0° angle)
Cortical artery	20-30 cm/s (at 0° angle)

Source:: Zierler RE, Olmstead KA. (2004). Renal Duplex Scanning: in Strandess's Duplex Scanning of Vascular Disorders, (283-310). Philadelphia: Lippincott Williams and Wilkins.

TABLE 108: Diagnostic Criteria for Significant Renovascular Resistance Within the Kidney

- Normal low renovascular resistance: RI <0.70
- Borderline increased renovascular resistance: RI between 0.70-0.80
- Increased renovascular resistance: RI >0.80

Source: Internally validated at the University of Chicago Medical Center Vascular Laboratory.

Differential Diagnosis

- Hypotension, due to ACE inhibitors

Correlation

- Spiral CT scan
- MRA
- Renal arteriography

Medical Treatment

- Vasodilator therapy (e.g., ACE inhibitors)

Surgical Treatment

- Endarterectomy
- Bypass grafting (aorto-renal, splachno-renal)
- Renal artery reimplantation
- Ex-vivo reconstruction

Endovascular Treatment

- Balloon angioplasty, with or without stenting

TABLE 109: Diagnostic Criteria of Renal Artery Stenosis

Normal: no detectable renal artery stenosis

- Low resistance waveform
- No focal velocity increase
- RAR <3.5
- Peak systolic velocity <180-200 cm/s

<60% diameter reduction: mild narrowing; no hemodynamic significance

- Low resistance waveform
- Focal velocity increase with possible post-stenotic turbulence
- RAR >2.0 but <3.5
- Peak systolic velocity <180-200 cm/s

>60% diameter reduction: hemodynamically significant stenosis

- Post-stenotic turbulence (mosaic flow pattern by color flow Doppler) with focal velocity increases
- RAR >3.5
- Peak systolic velocity >180-200 cm/s

Occlusion: complete obstruction of renal artery

- No detectable renal artery signal by color or PW Doppler
- Kidney length <9 cm (when occlusion is chronic)

Source: Rzucidlo EM, Zwolak RM. (2005). Arterial duplex scanning. In *Rutherford Vascular Surgery 6th edition*. (233-253). Philadelphia. Elsevier Saunders.

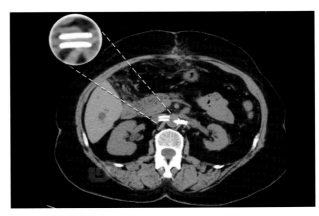

Bilateral renal artery stents by CT scan

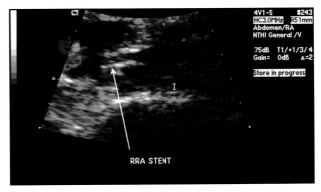

Right renal artery stent by duplex scan

Points to Remember

- Renal artery scanning is a difficult exam which requires time, patience and a long learning curve.
- Patient inability to hold their breath or suspend breathing for short periods of time may make it difficult to obtain accurate Doppler recordings.
- To minimize technical difficulties due to bowel gas, renal exams are best performed in the morning after the patient has fasted overnight. Encourage the patient not to smoke or chew gum before the exam.
- Patient may be given Simethicone (Gas-X, Mylanta, etc.) before the exam to reduce abdominal gas.
- Intercostal views may be necessary to visualize the kidneys.
- Atherosclerosis is the most common cause of renovascular hypertension (RVH). [17] FMD accounts for a smaller percentage of all RVH cases.
- When fibromuscular dysplasia (FMD) is detected in the renal arteries, you may be asked to scan the carotid and mesenteric arteries since the disease commonly coexists in these vessels. FMD can be either unilateral or bilateral.
- Stenosis of the renal artery may be unilateral, although bilateral renal stenoses are possible, especially when atherosclerotic disease is the cause.
- The same diagnostic criteria used for native renal arteries has shown to be accurate in the diagnosis of post-intervention (e.g., renal bypass) duplex data. [8,10]
- Measuring hilar acceleration time or acceleration index (AI) (also known as acceleration time (AT)) is an indirect method of renal duplex testing used in some labs. An AT >0.100 seconds is indicative of proximal arterial stenosis. [10] AT/AI values show low-sensitivity for detecting disease and cannot differentiate between renal artery stenosis and occlusion. [13]
- Blood in the urine (*hematuria*) and abdominal pain are signs of acute renal vein thrombosis. In cases of acute renal vein occlusion, an enlarged kidney and atypical echogenicity of the renal parenchyma may be noted including: [7]
  - Hypoechoic cortex, with or without usual separation of the cortical/medullary regions
  - Loss of typical intrarenal echogenicity and observation of linear "streaks" through the parenchyma
- Slow-moving venous flow in the renal vein suggests proximal obstruction in the absence of observed thrombus. [7]
- Report any incidental findings so additional diagnostic studies may be obtained if necessary. [14]

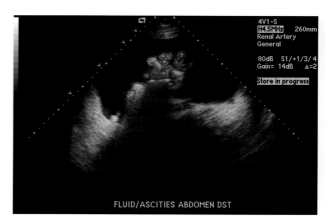

Ascites noted in the abdomen

Image courtesy of Philips Healthcare

References

1. Hansen KJ, Pearce JD. (2005). Renal complication. In *Rutherford Vascular Surgery 6th edition*. (863-874). Philadelphia. Elsevier Saunders.
2. Sumner DS, Zierler RE. (2005). Vascular physiology: essential hemodynamic principles. In *Rutherford Vascular Surgery 6th edition*. (75-123). Philadelphia. Elsevier Saunders.
3. Desai TR, Gupta N, Gewertz BL. (2005). Acute renovascular occlusive events. In *Rutherford Vascular Surgery 6th edition*. (1871-1877). Philadelphia. Elsevier Saunders.
4. Fecteau SR, Darling III RC, Roddy SP. (2005). Arterial thromboembolism. In *Rutherford Vascular Surgery 6th edition*. (971-986). Philadelphia. Elsevier Saunders.
5. Alimi YS, Hartung O. (2010). Iliocaval venous obstruction. In Cronenwett JL. Johnston KW (Eds.), *Rutherford Vascular Surgery 7th edition*. (Chapter 59) Philadelphia: Saunders Elsevier.
6. Calligaro KD, Dougherty MJ. (2005). Renal artery aneurysms and arteriovenous fistulae. In *Rutherford Vascular Surgery 6th edition*. (1861-1870). Philadelphia. Elsevier Saunders
7. Pellerito JS, Zwiebel, WJ (2005). Ultrasound assessment of native renal vessels and renal allografts. In Zwiebel WJ, Pellerito JS (Eds.), *Introduction to Vascular Ultrasonography 5th ed*. (611-636). Philadelphia: Elsevier Saunders.
8. Zierler RE. (2005). Vascular diagnosis of renovascular disease. In Mansour MA, Labropoulos N. (Eds.), *Vascular Diagnosis*, (333-340). Philadelphia: Elsevier Saunders.
9. Neumyer MM, Isaacson J. (1995). Direct and indirect renal arterial duplex and Doppler color flow evaluations. *J Vasc Technol*, 19(5-6):309-316.
10. Rzucidlo EM, Zwolak RM. (2005). Arterial duplex scanning. In *Rutherford Vascular Surgery 6th edition*. (233-253). Philadelphia. Elsevier Saunders.
11. Kohler TR, Zierler RE, Martin RL, et al. (1986). Non-invasive diagnosis of renal artery stenosis by ultrasonic duplex scanning. *J Vasc Surg* 4:450-456.
12. Armstrong PA, Bandyk DF. (2010). Arterial duplex scanning. In Cronenwett JL. Johnston KW (Eds.), *Rutherford Vascular Surgery 7th edition*. (Chapter 15). Philadelphia: Elsevier Saunders.
13. Myers K, Clogh A (2004) Renovascular diseases. In *Making Sense of Vascular Ultrasound*. (255-282). London: Hodder Arnold.
14. Zierler RE, Olmstead KA. (2004). Renal Duplex Scanning: in *Strandess's Duplex Scanning of Vascular Disorders*, (283-310). Philadelphia: Lippincott Williams and Wilkins.
15. Cairols M. (2005). Renal artery color-flow scanning: technique and applications. In Mansour MA, Labropoulos N. (Eds.), *Vascular Diagnosis*, (341-349). Philadelphia: Elsevier Saunders.
16. Stanley JC, Wakefield TW. (2005). Arterial fibrodysplagia. In *Rutherford Vascular Surgery 6th edition*. (431-452). Philadelphia. Elsevier Saunders.
17. DeLoach SS, Mohler III E. Atherosclerotic risk factors. In Cronenwett JL. Johnston KW (Eds.), *Rutherford Vascular Surgery 7th edition*. (Chapter 29). Philadelphia: Saunders Elsevier.

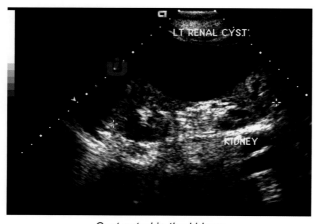

Cyst noted in the kidney

Definition

The combination of real time B-mode ultrasonography with pulsed wave and color flow Doppler to evaluate the celiac and mesenteric arteries for the presence and severity of stenosis or occlusion, as well as other disease states and to assess hemodynamics after vascular reconstruction.

Etiology

- Atherosclerosis
- Median arcuate ligament syndrome
- Fibromuscular dysplagia
- Embolus (acute ischemia)
- Thrombosis (acute ischemia)
- Occlusion
- Aneurysm
- Arteriovenous fistula
- Trauma
- Status post-angioplasty/stent
- Aortic dissections
- Neurofibromatosis
- Takayasu's arteritis
- Radiation injury
- Systemic lupus
- Drug use

Risk Factors

- Hypertension
- Diabetes
- Obesity
- Hypercholesterolemia
- Smoking
- Age
  - Patients with median arcuate ligament syndrome are typically young.
  - Patients with chronic mesenteric ischemia are typically elderly.
- Female

Indications for Exam

- Abdominal pain and cramping, associated with eating
- Significant unexplained weight loss
- Abdominal bruit
- Suspected visceral artery aneurysm
- Unexplained gastrointestinal symptoms
- Post-operative evaluation of a mesenteric vascular reconstruction

Contraindications/Limitations

- Obesity may cause poor visualization due to vessel depth.
- Abdominal gas may prohibit visualization of any or all vessels.
- Recent abdominal surgery (tenderness and staples may limit visualization).
- Breathing difficulties may limit evaluation (e.g., shortness of breath, rapid breathing, etc.).

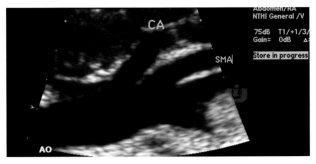

Celiac and superior mesenteric arteries-origin off the proximal aorta with B-mode

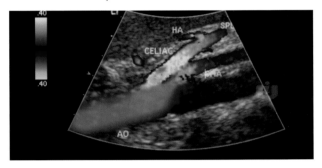

Anatomy

- The celiac artery (CA) and the superior mesenteric artery (SMA) originate from the anterior wall of the suprarenal aorta. The CA is the first branch off the abdominal aorta with the SMA following 1-2 cm distally.

> The term "splanchnic" is sometimes used to refer to the visceral arteries.

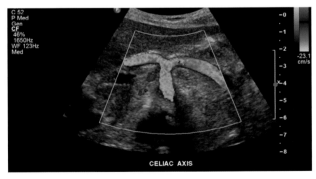

Transverse celiac trunk with common hepatic and splenic arterial branches

Image courtesy of Philips Healthcare

- The celiac trunk (CA) divides into the common hepatic (HA) and the splenic (SA) arteries. This division occurs 1-2 cm from the celiac artery origin. A third branch, the left gastric artery, is usually too small to visualize on duplex, but may be documented if noted.

- The inferior mesenteric artery (IMA) originates below the renal arteries at the left anteriolateral abdominal aorta, 3-5 cm above the iliac bifurcation.

- The CA and SMA supply blood to the duodenum and small bowel.
- The SMA and IMA supply blood to the colon and proximal rectum.
- There is normally an extensive network of collaterals between the mesenteric vessels which enlarge when there is a stenosis or occlusion present.
  - The main collateral channel between the CA and SMA is the gastroduodenal artery to the pancreaticoduodenal arteries.
  - The Arc of Riolan can connect the SMA and IMA and is an important pathway when there is a stenosis or occlusion in either artery.
  - The IMA has multiple collateral pathways: middle colic branch of the SMA to the marginal artery of Drummond or the middle hemorrhoidal artery (branch of the internal iliac).

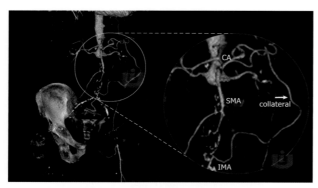

Collateral pathway: marginal artery of Drummond

Anatomic Variations of the Celiac/Mesenteric Arteries

- The CA and SMA may share a common origin or trunk.
- Hepatic artery origin off the SMA
- Hepatic artery originating off the abdominal aorta

Mechanism of Disease

- Mesenteric blood flow is regulated by several mechanisms: intrinsic (metabolic) and extrinsic (neural and hormonal).[1]
  - A lack of oxygen to the mesenteric organs causes cellular injury and mucosal ischemia within the intestines. Tissue necrosis and metabolic acidosis are significant consequences. [1,2]
  - Extracellular volume decreases. The renin-angiotensin system is activated, releasing renin which increases angiotensin II levels, causing vasoconstriction. [1]
  - Blood volume is lost and an abnormal increase in the concentration of fluids results in the release of vasopressin (antidiuretic hormone) from the pituitary gland, causing mesenteric vasoconstriction and venorelaxation. [1]
- **Atherosclerosis** can significantly narrow the arterial supply to the intestinal organs. Atherosclerotic plaque forms in the artery to block flow by either narrowing it (arterial stenosis) or totally blocking the artery (arterial occlusion). The term "hemodynamically significant obstruction" refers to either a stenosis or an occlusion that results in a decrease in blood pressure or flow distal to the obstruction. Typically, a stenosis must narrow the diameter of the artery by at least 50% to decrease pressure and flow distally. [3]

- **Vasospasm**, usually affecting the SMA, occurs as a result of neurohormonal triggers. Mesenteric vasospasms occur while the body releases vasopressin and angiotensin to help correct hypervolemic states or cardiogenic shock. [2]
- Compression of the celiac trunk by the median arcuate ligament of the diaphragm is another mechanism for mesenteric ischemia. [1] Lumenal stenosis is thought to be caused by intimal fibrosis from the compression. Compression increases during expiration. [4]
- **Thrombosis** may result from low-flow states. [5]
- Mesenteric ischemia is categorized as acute or chronic:

Chronic Mesenteric Ischemia [6]
  - Most commonly caused by progression of atherosclerotic disease (stenosis or occlusion) in the aorta, celiac or proximal mesenteric arteries.
  - Less common causes include arteritis, aneurysm, mesenteric artery dissection or hypercoaguable conditions.

Acute Mesenteric Ischemia [5]
  - Caused by arterial occlusion usually due to an cardiac embolism, occurring most frequently in the SMA due to its smaller size.
  - Caused by arterial occlusion due to thrombosis of the SMA.
  - Caused by small vessel insufficiency (e.g., poor collateral circulation).

> *The condition of acute mesenteric ischemia has a high mortality rate, (70%).*

Location of Disease

- Typical at the ostia (opening) of proximal celiac or mesenteric arterial segments

Graft Location

Typical arterial grafts encountered for surveillance include:

- Abdominal aorta-Celiac artery
- Abdominal aorta-Superior mesenteric artery (SMA)
- Abdominal aorta-Celiac and SMA

Graft Type

- PTFE (Polytetrafluoroethylene)

Patient History

- Significant weight loss
- Abdominal pain 30-60 minutes after eating
- Complaints of bloating, nausea, vomiting, or diarrhea

Physical Examination

- Abdominal bruit (abnormal sound heard through auscultation caused by turbulent flow)
- Abdominal tenderness
- Ischemic symptoms include: fever, abdominal distention, dehydration, shock, gastrointestinal bleeding and peritoneal signs (rebound tenderness, guarding).

Celiac and Mesenteric Artery Duplex Protocol

- Patient should fast 6-12 hours before examination to minimize the presence of air in the abdomen. A limited volume of clear liquids may be ingested prior to the examination (e.g., to swallow medications). Studies are usually performed in the morning.

- Patient is studied while supine with the head slightly elevated and the arms and legs adequately supported. The patient may bend their knees up to aid in relaxation of the abdominal wall and decrease lumbar pain.

- Some patients may require the use of a range of transducers; including high-frequency (5-7 MHz) and low frequency transducers (2.0-4.0 MHz for imaging deeper structures).

- Pulsed-wave (PW) Doppler angle should be ≤60° with the angle cursor parallel to the vessel walls and the sample volume within the center of the flow stream.

> Doppler angles greater than 60° result in falsely elevated velocities.

Evaluation of Abdominal Aorta

- Place the transducer just beneath the xyphoid process. Orient the transducer to obtain a transverse view of the abdominal aorta. Examine the abdominal aorta for aneurysm, plaque, thrombus, dissection, tortuosity and other abnormalities.

- Record grayscale images in longitudinal (sagittal) view of the supraceliac abdominal aorta. Document additional images using color flow as needed.

- Record a PW Doppler peak systolic velocity (PSV) and end diastolic velocity (EDV) of the supraceliac aorta in the longitudinal plane.

- Document grayscale and color images in areas of suspected stenosis. Measure diameter reduction, especially in hemodynamically significant lesions. Document any post stenotic turbulence or color bruit.

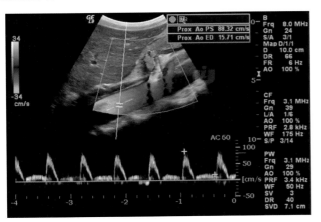

Normal abdominal aorta spectral tracing

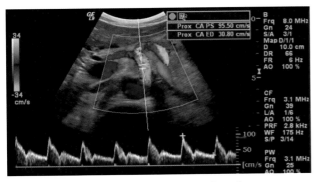

Normal celiac trunk spectral tracing

Images courtesy of GE Healthcare Ultrasound Division

Evaluation of Celiac Artery

- Orient the transducer to obtain a longitudinal view of the celiac trunk and its ostia. Record grayscale images in a longitudinal view. Document additional images using color flow as needed. Examine for tortuosity or abnormalities such as plaque, aneurysm or thrombus. In some cases, a transverse orientation will provide a better axis for evaluation.

- Measure the PSV and EDV from the origin, proximal, and distal portions of the celiac trunk/artery. Note direction of flow.

- Measure PSV and EDV in the branches of the celiac trunk: the common hepatic (HA) and the splenic (SA) arteries. Note direction of flow.

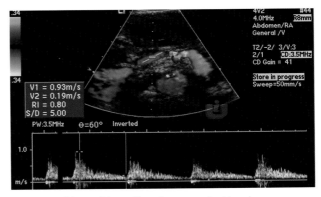

Normal hepatic artery spectral tracing

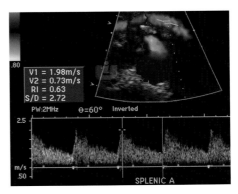

Normal splenic artery spectral tracing

- Document PSV and EDV with PW Doppler through any area(s) of stenoses. Document post stenotic turbulence.

- Determine the classification of disease according to laboratory diagnostic criteria.

> When instructed to "image arteries in transverse," because of the angulation of visceral arteries it may look like you are holding the probe longitudinally while the arteries appear transverse on the monitor. Image abdominal arteries transverse to the axis of the vessel and not transverse to the body.

> Color flow Doppler and power Doppler may aid in locating these arteries.

Duplex Evaluation for Median Arcuate Ligament Syndrome (MALS)

- In each and every patient that has an increased PSV in the celiac artery, ask the patient to take a deep breath and record the PSV again. If the celiac artery PSV normalizes, there is evidence of the CA being compressed by the median arcuate ligament.

Median Arcuate Ligament Syndrome

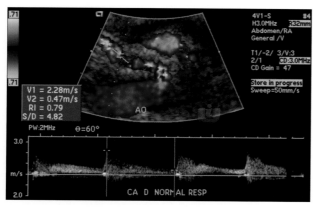

Abnormal celiac artery PSV during quiet respiration

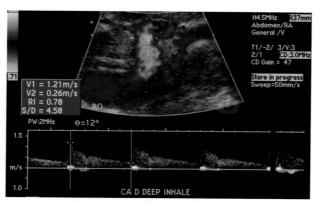

Normal celiac artery PSV while patient takes a deep breath

Evaluation of Superior Mesenteric Artery

- Slide the transducer distally 1-2 cm down the aorta from the celiac origin. Orient the transducer to obtain a longitudinal view of the superior mesenteric artery at its ostia. Examine for tortuosity or abnormalities such as plaque, aneurysm or thrombus.
- Record PSV and EDV with PW Doppler from the origin, proximal, mid and distal portions of the SMA. Note direction of flow.
- Record grayscale images in a longitudinal view of the SMA, especially near its origin. Document additional images using color flow as needed.
- Document the highest PSV and EDV through any area(s) of stenoses. Document post-stenotic turbulence.
- Document grayscale and color images in areas of suspected stenosis. Measure diameter reduction, especially in hemodynamically significant lesions.
- Determine the classification of disease according to laboratory diagnostic criteria.

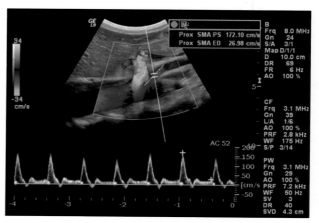

Normal superior mesenteric artery spectral tracing
Image courtesy of GE Healthcare-Ultrasound Division

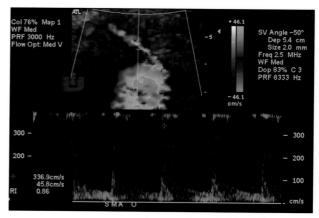

Abnormal (stenotic) superior mesenteric artery spectral tracing

Evaluation of Inferior Mesenteric Artery

- The inferior mesenteric artery originates off the aorta and lies superior to the common iliac arteries, 3-5 cm above the iliac bifurcation. In transverse, the artery comes off at approximately the 1–2 o'clock position. This artery is sometimes difficult to visualize due to abdominal gas at this level.

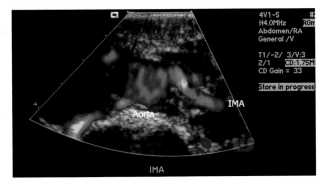

Transverse inferior mesenteric artery

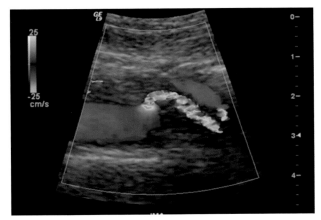

Inferior mesenteric artery (longitudinal)
Image courtesy of GE Healthcare-Ultrasound Division

- Orient the transducer to obtain a longitudinal view of the inferior mesenteric artery at its ostia. Examine for tortuosity or abnormalities such as plaque, aneurysm or thrombus.

- Record grayscale images of the IMA in longitudinal view. Document additional images using color flow as needed. In some cases, a transverse orientation will provide a better axis for documentation.

- Record PSV and EDV from the origin and proximal segment of the IMA. Note direction of flow. Record additional velocities from the mid/distal artery as necessary.

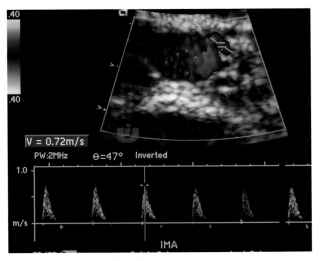

Normal inferior mesenteric artery

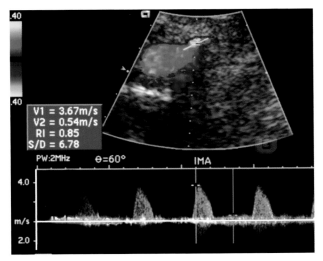

Abnormal (stenotic) inferior mesenteric artery

- Document the highest PSV and EDV through any area(s) of stenoses. Document post-stenotic turbulence.

- Document grayscale and color images in areas of suspected stenosis. Measure diameter reduction, especially in hemodynamically significant lesions.

- Determine the classification of disease according to laboratory diagnostic criteria.

TABLE 110: Celiac and Mesenteric Artery Duplex Protocol Summary

Abdominal Aorta

- Evaluate the abdominal aorta for aneurysm, plaque, thrombus, dissection and/or tortuosity. Document a longitudinal (sagittal) grayscale image of the artery.
- Obtain a PW Doppler peak systolic velocity (PSV) and end diastolic velocity (EDV) of the abdominal aorta, superior to the celiac (CA) and superior mesenteric (SMA) arteries.

Celiac Trunk

- Document a grayscale image of the proximal CA (either in longitudinal (sagittal) or transverse view, depending on the course of the vessel).
- Record the highest PSV and EDV of the celiac trunk at the following levels:
  - Celiac trunk ostia
  - Proximal celiac artery
  - Distal celiac artery.

Hepatic and Splenic Arteries

- Document a transverse image of the proximal hepatic and splenic arteries.
- Record the highest PSV and EDV in each artery.

Superior Mesenteric Artery

- Document a longitudinal (sagittal) grayscale image of the superior mesenteric artery.
- Record the highest PSV and EDV of the SMA at the following levels:
  - SMA ostia
  - Proximal SMA
  - Mid SMA
  - Distal SMA.

Inferior Mesenteric Artery

- Document a longitudinal (sagittal) or transverse grayscale image of the inferior mesenteric artery, depending on the course of the vessel.
- Record PSV and EDV of the ostial and proximal portion of the IMA.
- Document grayscale and color images in areas of suspected stenosis. Measure diameter reduction, especially in hemodynamically significant lesions.
- Determine the classification of disease according to laboratory diagnostic criteria.

Post-operative Duplex Evaluation of Splanchnic Bypass or Stent

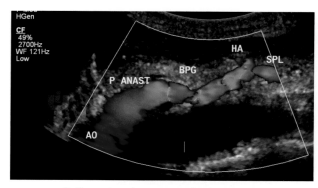

Celiac artery bypass graft off the aorta

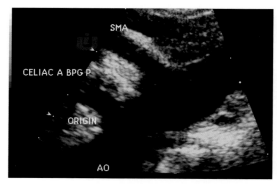

Celiac and SMA bypass grafts off the aorta

- Record images in a longitudinal view with and without color flow Doppler of the:
  - Inflow/proximal native artery
  - Proximal anastomosis
  - Proximal graft or stent
  - Mid graft or stent
  - Distal graft or stent
  - Distal anastomosis
  - Outflow/distal native artery.

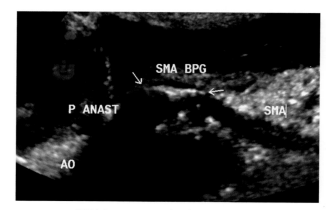

SMA bypass-proximal anastomosis

- Record the PSV in longitudinal using pulsed wave Doppler (≤60° Doppler angle with the angle cursor parallel to the vessel walls and sample volume within the center of the flow stream) at the following levels:
  - Inflow/proximal native artery

- Proximal anastomosis
- Proximal graft or stent
- Mid graft or stent
- Distal graft or stent
- Distal anastomosis
- Outflow/distal native artery

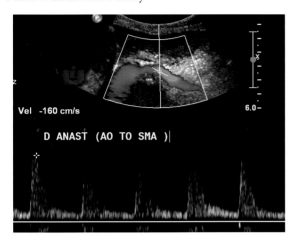

SMA bypass: distal anastomosis spectral waveforms

Interpretation

Normal: Fasting

- **Doppler waveforms and flow velocities**: Normal, fasting superior and inferior mesenteric arterial flow is represented by a high resistance waveform. There is a reverse flow component in early diastole and the waveform is similar to a triphasic peripheral arterial signal. The peak systolic velocity will be <275 cm/s.[7]

Normal: Non-Fasting

- **Doppler waveforms and flow velocities**: Normal celiac, hepatic and splenic arterial flow is represented by a low resistance waveform (slow acceleration, slow deceleration and continuous diastolic forward flow) with a peak systolic velocity <200 cm/s. [7]
- **General grayscale and color characteristics**: The artery is free of intralumenal echoes. When utilized, color Doppler fills the entire arterial lumen.

Abnormal

- **Doppler waveforms and flow velocities**
  - **Stenosis**: A hemodynamically significant stenosis is initially recognized by color aliasing and confirmed by increased peak systolic velocities. The presence of post-stenotic turbulence supports the presence of a stenosis. [8]
    - **Celiac artery**
      - PSV >200 cm/s in the celiac artery suggests a stenosis greater than 70%. [7]
      - An EDV ≥55 cm/s in the celiac artery suggests a stenosis greater than 50%. [9]
      - Retrograde common hepatic artery flow suggests a hemodynamically significant stenosis or occlusion of the celiac artery. [10]
    - **Superior or inferior mesenteric arteries**
      - PSV >275 cm/s in the SMA or IMA suggests a stenosis greater than 70%. [7]

- An end diastolic velocity of >45 cm/s is used to diagnose a hemodynamically significant stenosis greater than 50% in the SMA. [11]
  - **Occlusion**: An occlusion of the artery is present when no flow is detected by spectral Doppler. The extent of the occlusion can often be determined by identifying a large collateral at the proximal and distal end of the occlusion. [8] These collaterals often exit or enter the artery at 90º to the vessel.

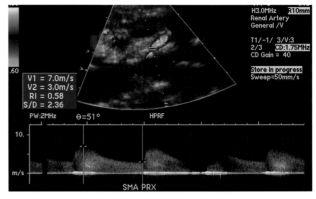

Significant SMA stenosis

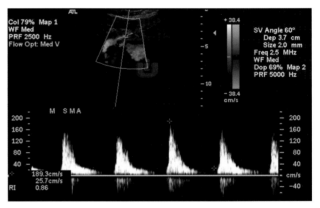

Post-stenotic turbulence in a mid SMA

- **General grayscale and color characteristics**
  - Lumenal reduction or wall irregularities may be observed by B-mode image. [8] Diameter reduction measurements should only be used in conjunction with peak systolic velocity measurements.
  - Color Doppler does not fill the entire arterial lumen, instead a color jet can be visualized through the narrowed lumen. [8]
  - An occlusion of the artery is present when no flow is detected by color flow. [8]

> *Always confirm lack of flow by using PW Doppler, placing the Doppler sample gate in the artery.*

  - Retrograde color flow in a mesenteric artery suggests hemodynamically significant stenosis or occlusion (e.g., retrograde SMA flow can be present with an occlusion at the origin of the SMA). [8]
- **Post-intervention restenosis**: The same criterion is often used to categorize initial stenosis and post-intervention restenosis. Comparison of PSV recorded during a baseline duplex evaluation soon after the procedure and follow-up studies is another method to diagnose disease progression.

- **Median arcuate ligament syndrome**: If the celiac artery PSV increases with expiration and normalizes with inspiration, this suggests that the CA is being compressed by the median arcuate ligament. [8]

TABLE 111: Normal Celiac and Mesenteric Peak Systolic Velocities (PSV)

Artery	PSV (cm/s)
Celiac artery	98-105
Superior mesenteric artery	97-142
Inferior mesenteric artery	93-189

Source: Pellerito JS. (2005). Ultrasound assessment of the splanchnic (mesenteric) arteries. In Zwiebel WJ, Pellerito JS (Eds.), In *Introduction to Vascular Ultrasonography 5th ed*, (571-583). Philadelphia: Elsevier Saunders.

TABLE 112: Normal Celiac and Mesenteric Waveforms

- Normal CA, HA and SA waveforms are typically biphasic in nature as they feed low resistance outflow beds.
- Normal SMA waveforms are triphasic in the fasting state. This high resistance waveform will change to a low resistance waveform after ingestion of a meal.

TABLE 113: Diagnostic Criteria of Celiac for Mesenteric Artery Stenosis

<70% diameter reduction

- Low resistance waveform CA, HA and SA
- An end diastolic velocity >45 cm/s in the SMA suggests a >50% stenosis.
- An end diastolic velocity >55 cm/s in the CA suggests a >50% stenosis.

**≥70% diameter reduction:
Hemodynamically significant stenosis**

- Peak systolic velocity >200 cm/s in the celiac arteries
- Retrograde common hepatic artery flow suggests significant celiac disease.
- Peak systolic velocity >275 cm/s in the mesenteric arteries
- Mosaic color flow pattern and a focal velocity increase and evidence of post-stenotic turbulence by PW Doppler distal to the increase

Occlusion: Complete obstruction of celiac/mesenteric arteries

- No detectable CA, SMA and/or IMA color flow and PW Doppler signal.

Sources: Moneta GL, Lee RW, Yeager RA et al. (1991). Duplex ultrasound criteria for diagnosis of splanchnic artery stenosis or occlusion. *J Vasc Surg* 14:511: 520.
Moneta GL, Lee RW, Yeager RA et al. (1993). Mesenteric duplex scanning: A blinded prospective study. *J Vasc Surg* 17:79: 86

Differential Diagnosis

- Cholecystitis
- Diverticulitis
- Appendicitis
- Intestinal obstruction
- Cancer
- Peptic ulcer disease
- Pancreatitis
- Inflammatory bowel disease

Correlation

- Spiral CT scan
- Barium study of the upper/lower GI tract
- Endoscopy
- Arteriography

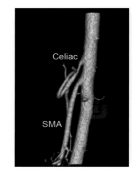

Medical Treatment

- Vasodilator therapy (e.g., papaverine)

Surgical Treatment

- Endarterectomy
- Bypass grafting (supraceliac or infrarenal aorto-mesenteric)
- Vein patch
- Arteriotomy/thromboembolectomy
- Decompression of the median arcuate ligament and diaphragmatic crura with/without bypass grafting
  - Laparoscopic surgery
  - Celiac endarterectomy/patch angioplasty

Endovascular Treatment

- Angioplasty

Celiac artery peak systolic velocities; pre and post surgical decompression of the median arcuate ligament (shown in two photos below)

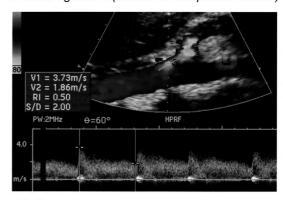

Celiac artery pre-operative spectral waveforms

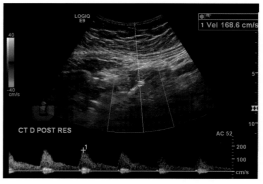

Celiac artery intra-operative spectral waveforms

Points to Remember

- Patients may be given Simethicone (Gas-X, Mylanta, etc.) before the exam to reduce abdominal gas.

- Celiac/mesenteric artery scanning is a difficult exam which requires time, patience and a long learning curve.

- Patient's inability to hold his/her breath for short periods of time, shortness of breath or rapid breathing may make it difficult to obtain accurate Doppler recordings.

- Patients usually describe pain about 30 minutes after eating that can last for several hours. This experience can result in a patient's "fear of food" and they may skip meals to avoid the pain, resulting in weight loss.

- Typically, at least two of the three mesenteric arteries (CA, SMA, IMA) have significant disease before symptoms of severe or chronic mesenteric ischemia are noted. The SMA is almost always one of the arteries involved. [1,6,12]

- Normal IMA PSV range from 93-189 cm/s. [8] When aortic or mesenteric disease is present, the PSV is thought to be closer to the higher end of this range depending on how much collateral flow is present through the IMA. [13]

- The celiac and superior mesenteric arteries can be stented.

- Duplex may not demonstrate elevated flow velocities in elderly patients or those with low cardiac output even when hemodynamically significant disease is present. [8]

- Flow velocities may be elevated in younger patients without mesenteric disease being present. [8]

- Intestinal collaterals are able to compensate for ischemia to some extent for up to about 12 hours before substantial injury occurs.

- Emergent surgical/interventional treatment is often required for acute mesenteric ischemia.

- Research suggests that there is no significant benefit from post-prandial evaluation (rescanning after ingestion of a meal) for the diagnosis of ≥70% stenosis. PSV will be significantly elevated either fasting or nonfasting. [9]

References

1. Wyers MC, Zwolak RM. (2005). Physiology and diagnosis of splachnic arterial occlusion. In *Rutherford Vascular Surgery 6th edition*. (1707-1717). Philadelphia. Elsevier Saunders.

2. Desai TR, Bassiouny HS. (2005). Diagnosis and treatment of nonocclusive mesenteric ischemia. In Rutherford Vascular Surgery 6th edition. (1728-1731). Philadelphia. Elsevier Saunders.

3. Sumner DS, Zierler RE. (2005). Vascular physiology: essential hemodynamic principles. In Rutherford Vascular Surgery 6th edition. (75-123). Philadelphia. Elsevier Saunders.

4. Aziz F, Comerota AJ. (12-3-2009). Abdominal Angina. eMedicine. Retrieved from http://emedicine. medscape.com/article/188618-overview. (12-11-2010).

5. Moore EM, Endean ED. (2005). Treatment of acute intestinal ischemia caused by arterial occlusions. In Rutherford Vascular Surgery 6th edition. (1718-1728). Philadelphia. Elsevier Saunders.

6. Huber TS, Lee WA, Seeger JM. (2005). Chronic mesenteric ischemia. In Rutherford Vascular Surgery 6th edition. (1732-1747). Philadelphia. Elsevier Saunders.

7. Moneta GL, Lee RW, Yeager RA et al. (1991). Duplex ultrasound criteria for diagnosis of splachnic artery stenosis or occlusion. J Vasc Surg 14:511-520.

8. Pellerito JS. (2005). Ultrasound assessment of the splachnic (mesenteric) arteries. In Zwiebel WJ, Pellerito JS (Eds.), In *Introduction to Vascular Ultrasonography 5th ed,* (571-583). Philadelphia: Elsevier Saunders

9. Bowersox JC, Zwolak RM, Walsh DB et al. (1991). Duplex ultrasonography in the diagnosis of celiac and mesenteric artery occlusive disease. *J Vasc Surg* 14:780-788.

10. Rzucidlo EM, Zwolak RM. (2005). Arterial duplex scanning. In *Rutherford Vascular Surgery 6th edition*. (233-253). Philadelphia. Elsevier Saunders.

11. Moneta GL, Lee RW, Yeager RA et al. (1993). Mesenteric duplex scanning: A blinded prospective study. *J Vasc Surg* 17:79-86.

12. Hallett, JW, Brewster DC, Rasmussen TE, (2001) Intestinal ischemia. In *Handbook of Patient Care in Vascular Diseases,* (231-237), Philadelphia: Lippincott Williams & Wilkins .

13. Erden A, Yurdakul M, Cumhur T.(1998).Doppler waveforms of the normal and collateralized inferior mesenteric artery. *Am J Roentgenol* 171:619-627.

Definition

The use of real time B-mode imaging with pulsed and color flow Doppler (duplex scan) to evaluate the portal and hepatic veins for evidence of portal hypertension (PHT). Portal hypertension is the elevation of pressures within the portal circulation.

Etiology

- Portal hypertension and its causes can be divided into pre-hepatic, intrahepatic and post hepatic.
  - Pre-hepatic causes
    - Portal or splenic vein thrombosis
    - Portal or splenic vein invasion or extrinsic compression by tumor
    - Arteriovenous fistula
  - Intrahepatic causes (most common cause of PHT)
    - Pre-sinusoidal (e.g., schistosomiasis)
    - Post-sinusoidal (e.g., cirrhosis, acute hepatitis, congenital hepatic fibrosis)
  - Post-hepatic causes
    - Right sided heart disease
    - Budd Chiari Syndrome
      - Hepatic vein thrombosis (may be associated with hypercoaguable risk factors, including oral contraception)
      - Right atrial tumors
      - IVC webs or obstruction
      - Hepatic veno-occlusive disease

Risk Factors

- Chronic liver disease that precedes fibrosis or cirrhosis
  - Viral hepatitis: chronic hepatitis B or C
  - Alcoholic liver disease
  - Autoimmune disorders: primary biliary cirrhosis, primary sclerosing cholangitis
  - Metabolic & genetic disorders
    - Haemachromatosis
    - Wilson's disease
  - Schistosomiasis
  - Sarcoidosis
  - Non-alcoholic steatohepatitis (NASH)
- Heart disease resulting in increased right sided heart pressures
  - Tricuspid regurgitation
  - Congestive heart failure
  - Constrictive pericarditis

> *Cirrhosis is the most common cause of PHT.*

Indications for Exam

- Suspected or known chronic liver disease
- Acute liver failure
- Unexplained ascites
- Unexplained gastrointestinal bleeding
- Documented gastroesophageal varices or portal hypertensive gastropathy
- Follow-up post trans-jugular intrahepatic portosystemic stent (TIPS)
- Post-liver transplant

Contraindications/Limitations

- Small, contracted liver with abundant ascites
  - Bowel gas and floating bowel in ascites
- Poor patient cooperation (caused by hepatic encephalopathy or otherwise)
- Severe fatty livers (often result in poor image quality)

Anatomy

- The liver can be divided into right and left lobes.
- Nutrient rich blood is delivered from the splenic and mesenteric veins.
- The splenic vein and superior mesenteric veins converge to form the main portal vein.
- The main portal vein divides into the right and left portal vein branches at the liver edge. These further divide into branches that feed each segment of the liver.
- The blood flow from the liver drains through the hepatic veins (right, left, and middle) and into the IVC.
- The caudate lobe drains directly into the IVC via one-four possible veins, and in about 50% of patients there is at least one accessory inferior right hepatic vein.

> *The normal diameter of the main portal vein is 8-12 mm in diameter. The hepatic veins can measure up to 10 mm in diameter.*

Normal Fluid Dynamics

- The liver has a dual blood supply.
  - 80% is delivered via the main portal vein (nutrient rich / oxygen poor).
  - 20% is delivered via the hepatic artery (oxygen rich).
- Portal and hepatic blood mix within the portal sinusoids of the liver.
- The sinusoids drain into terminal hepatic veins and then to the systemic venous system via the main hepatic veins.
- Each hepatic vein drains different portions of the liver.
- If an obstruction to drainage occurs, there is resulting increase in sinusoidal and portal vein pressure, although there is capacity for the hepatic veins to develop collateral pathways of drainage.

Anatomy of the Portal Venous System

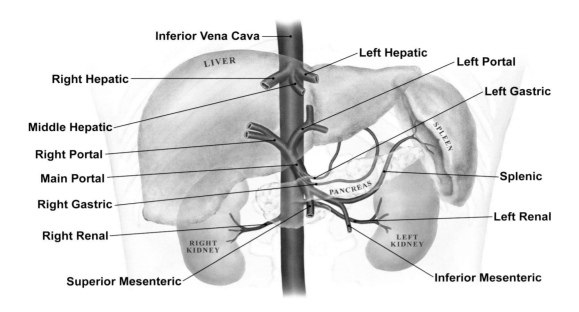

Mechanisms of disease

- Portal hypertension refers to the elevation of portal pressure within the portal circulation caused by an increased resistance to flow, usually within the hepatic parenchyma.
- The portohepatic system naturally attempts to reduce increased pressure by diverting blood away from the liver directly into the systemic system, via portosystemic collaterals (e.g., gastroesophageal varices).
- Rupture of these varices can result in life-threatening hemorrhage.
- Other consequences of portal hypertension are ascites, hepatic encephalopathy, and splenomegaly (in about 50% of patients), which can lead to low platelet counts.

Location of Disease

- Hepatic veins
  - Right hepatic veins
  - Middle hepatic veins
  - Left hepatic veins
- Portal veins
  - Main portal veins
  - Right portal veins
  - Left portal veins

Patient History/Symptoms

- Some patients are asymptomatic
- Abdominal distension from ascites
- Manifestations of liver disease, and conditions associated with its cause (e.g., pancreatitis, if alcohol related)
- Variceal hemorrhage (hematemesis and melena)
- Bacterial peritonitis

Physical Examination

- Jaundice (if liver is sufficiently impaired)
- Splenomegaly
- Dilated abdominal wall veins (including caput medusa around the umbilicus)
- Hepatic encephalopathy (confusion due to poor liver function)

Hepatoportal Duplex Protocol

- Patients should fast 6-12 hours before examination to minimize the presence of air and fluids. A limited volume of clear liquids may be ingested prior to the examination (e.g., to swallow medications).
- Some patients may require the use of a range of transducers; including high-frequency (5-7 MHz) transducer and lower frequency (1-4 MHz) curved linear, phased sector or vector array transducers.
- Multiple patient positions may be used during examination, including:
  - Supine
  - Left lateral decubitus
  - Oblique
- Multiple scanning windows are utilized:
  - Subcostal
  - Substernal
  - Intercostal
- Pulsed-wave (PW) Doppler angle should be at ≤60º with the angle cursor parallel to the vessel walls and the sample volume within the center of the flow stream. Doppler samples are taken at several locations and should include the following observations:
  - Presence and direction of flow
  - Flow velocity and characteristics
  - Vessel diameter measurements

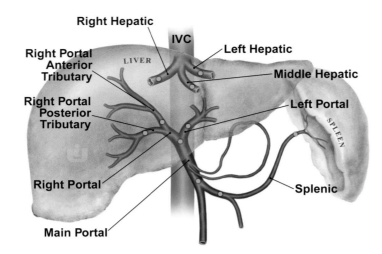

Color and spectral Doppler sample locations

Angle corrected spectral and color Doppler sample locations include:

- **Main portal vein (MPV):** With the patient in a 45º left posterior oblique position, a subcostal approach with the transducer angled superiorly can be used to image the MPV. If the MPV has a flat orientation, a right lateral intercostal approach, angling medially is more favorable for an optimal Doppler angle.
- **Right portal vein (RPV):** A subcostal or intercostal window can be used to image the RPV in the transverse plane.

> *Interrogation of both the right anterior and right posterior branches is necessary, as reverse flow or thrombus may occur in either of these branches.*

- **Left portal vein (LPV):** With the patient supine, a substernal approach is utilized to document the LPV.
- **Splenic vein (SV):** A spectral Doppler trace is obtained from the anterior abdominal wall in midline, with the patient supine. Documentation is also taken at the splenic hilum with the patient in a right lateral decubitus position.
- **Right hepatic vein (RHV):** The RHV is best interrogated with a right lateral intercostal window for an optimal Doppler angle and visualization of the vessel.
- **Middle hepatic vein (MHV):** A substernal or subcostal approach is the best position to document the MHV.

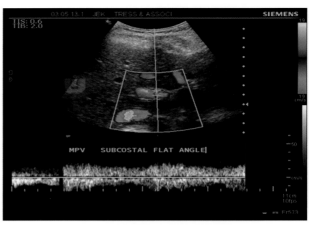

MPV: Using a subcostal approach often results in a 90º Doppler angle

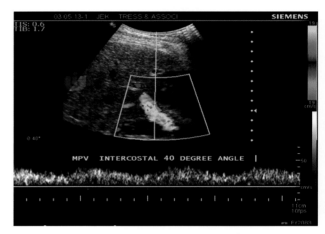

MPV: Intercostal approach is more favorable for an optimal Doppler angle

- **Left hepatic vein (LHV):** With the patient in the supine position, the LHV is examined from a substernal approach, angling superiorly.

> *Hepatic veins should ideally be interrogated during expiration, as deep inspiration can dampen the normal hepatic vein pulsatility.*

- **Inferior vena cava (IVC):** Assessment for thrombus and direction of flow in the IVC can be made in a longitudinal plane.
- **Paraumbilical vein:** This vessel traverses the ligamentum teres within the falciform ligament. It extends anteriorly and inferiorly from the LPV. Assessment for recanalization should be made with color, power and spectral Doppler. (An investigation for a patent paraumbilical vein can be made with a retrograde approach from the umbilicus.)
  - The falciform ligament can be seen on ultrasound as an echogenic band with a hypoechoic channel. It extends superficially and inferiorly from the anterior aspect of the LPV, exits the liver, and travels along the anterior abdominal wall to the umbilical region. If a hypoechoic channel is seen, its diameter is measured.

> *Use a higher frequency transducer for the paraumbilical vein.*

- **Collaterals:** Evidence of other venous collaterals should be documented, e.g., at the splenic hilum, between the spleen and left kidney, midline around the pancreas, gallbladder fossa, anterior abdominal wall towards umbilicus, and along the liver surface.

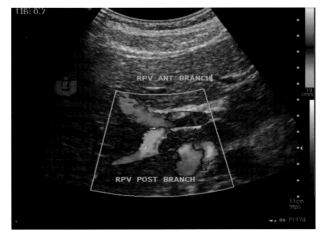

Doppler interrogation of the anterior and posterior branches of the right portal vein (performed to assess for hepatofugal flow or thrombus)

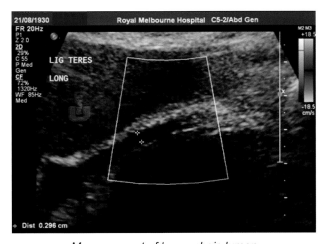

Measurement of hypoechoic lumen within the ligamentum teres

Other Diagnostic Parameters

- **Measure the main portal vein** anterior to the IVC on inspiration
- **Measure splenic length:** A preferred technique is to measure the splenic length in the coronal plane, from the top at the diaphragm to the inferior border of the spleen.
- **Assess for presence of ascites**

> *Use a higher frequency transducer for liver surface assessment.*

- **Liver texture and liver surface:** Examine the liver for coarse echo texture and irregular liver surface seen with cirrhosis. Fibrosis and cirrhosis do not attenuate the ultrasound beam as much as a fatty liver.
- **Hepatic vein surface:** Assess for waviness of the hepatic vein wall, which results from the nodularity of cirrhosis.

> *Carefully examine the entire liver with the focal zone in the near field, and repeat examination with the focal zone in the far field, searching for possible focal liver lesions.*

- **Assess for focal liver lesions:** Cirrhosis is associated with an increased risk of hepatocellular carcinoma (HCC).

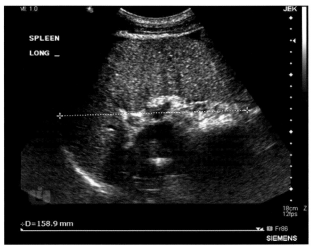

Splenic length measured in the coronal plane

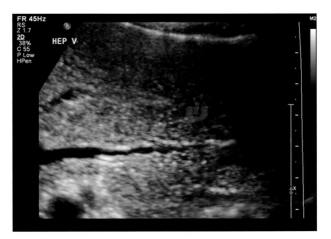

Irregular hepatic vein surface in a cirrhotic liver

- Consider the ultrasound window that you use.
- Do not persist with a gas filled window.
- Attempt all respiratory states, roll the patient, utilize the erect position in a difficult patient.
- Utilize an intercostal approach, especially with small contracted livers.
- Change transducers:
  - Deep attenuating structures or a cirrhotic liver require a lower frequency (e.g., phased array).
  - Surface detail requires a higher frequency transducer.

TABLE 114: Hepatoportal Duplex Protocol Summary

Obtain a PW Doppler peak systolic velocity (PSV) at the following locations:

- Main portal vein (MPV)
- Right portal vein (RPV)
- Left portal vein (LPV)
- Splenic vein (SV)
- Right hepatic vein (RHV)
- Middle hepatic vein (MHV)
- Left hepatic vein (LHV)

IVC

- Assess inferior vena cava (IVC) for thrombus and document flow direction.

Paraumbilical Vein

- Assess for recanalization with color, power and spectral Doppler. Measure the diameter of the hypoechoic channel of the falciform ligament if seen.

Collaterals

- Document any venous collaterals noted (such as between the spleen and left kidney, midline around the pancreas, gallbladder fossa, etc.).

Hepatic Vein

- Assess for waviness of the vein wall.

Liver

- Examine the liver for coarse echo texture and irregular liver surfaces.
- Assess for focal liver lesions.

Measurements

- Main portal vein
- Splenic length

* Include assessment for ascites

Interpretation

TABLE 115: Normal Hepatoportal Doppler Waveform Analysis

Vessel	Wave Characteristics
Main portal vein	Hepatopetal, and continuous
Right portal vein	Hepatopetal and continuous
Left portal vein	Hepatopetal and continuous
Hepatic artery	Hepatopetal and pulsatile (low resistance)
Splenic vein	Continuous
Superior mesenteric vein	Continuous
Right hepatic vein	Multiphasic
Middle hepatic vein	Multiphasic
Left hepatic vein	Multiphasic

- Portal veins demonstrate mild respiratory and cardiac phasicity.

Hepatopetal refers to flow direction towards the liver.

Normal Hepatic Veins Waveforms

- The pulsations from the right heart are reflected in the waveform of the hepatic veins, with a multiphasic flow pattern consisting of two periods of forward flow corresponding to atrial diastole and ventricular systole. The period of transient flow reversal corresponds to the right heart contraction of atrial systole.

Normal hepatic vein waveform

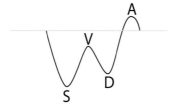

(S) - Filling of RA during ventricular systole
(V) - RA overfilling just before tricuspid valve opens
(D) - Filling of RA during ventricular diastole
(A) - RA contraction reversed flow into liver

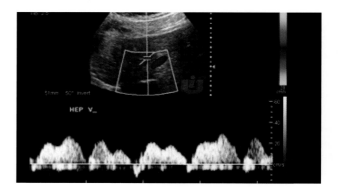

Portal Hypertension

Abnormal Findings

- Hepatofugal flow in the main portal vein or its branches is only seen in advanced PHT cases.

> Both right and left portal veins may show reversed flow, but if there is a large patent paraumbilical vein, the right portal vein may be reversed, while the left and main portal veins are flowing in the normal direction.

- Hepatofugal flow in the splenic vein

- Hepatofugal flow in the SMV (uncommon)

- Enlarged diameter of portal veins (MPV >13 mm) may be found, although is not a sensitive sign of disease (found only in about 40% of patients with PHT).

- Dilated mesenteric or splenic veins >10 mm.

- Acute thrombus identified within the hepatic, portal veins or IVC appears as hypoechoic to echogenic material producing little or no expansion of the lumen of the vessel. No flow is observed with color or spectral Doppler.

> Acute thrombus occurs in up to 5% of patients with PHT due to cirrhosis.

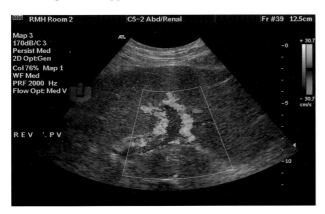

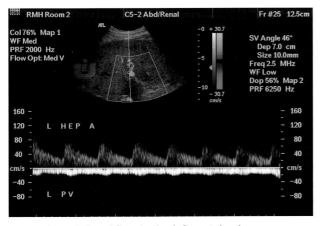

Hepatofugal flow in the left portal vein seen on color and spectral Doppler

- Chronic thrombosis with cavernous transformation appears as a small echogenic lumen with multiple, tortuous collateral channels seen within the porta hepatis. These form a bypass route from the splanchnic veins to the intrahepatic portal veins around the thrombosed portal vein. (This may take up to a year to develop.)

- Echogenic material may be visualized expanding the lumen of the portal vein in cases of malignant thrombus from vascular invasion of hepatocellular carcinoma (HCC). Pulsatile arterial flow may be present within the thrombus. The main portal vein diameter is usually >2 cm in this context, so a large occluded portal vein (or branches) should suggest the presence of HCC.

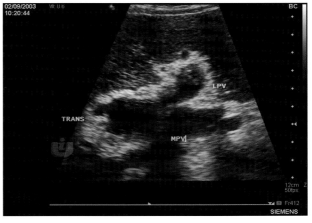

Hepatocellular carcinoma, malignant thrombus extending the portal vein diameters

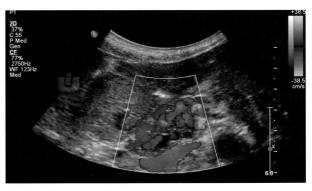

Cavernous transformation in a patient iwth chronic thrombosis of the portal vein

- A spleen diameter >13 cm measured in the coronal plane is a sign of splenomegaly.

- A patent umbilical vein demonstrating hepatofugal venous flow (spectral Doppler is the most reliable measure) is the most sensitive ultrasound sign, seen in up to 85% of patients with PHT. **An umbilical vein diameter** >2.5 mm, also indicates portal hypertension.

> Be aware of transmitted arterial wall thump. This is not umbilical venous flow.

- A mass of tortuous, worm-like vessels, with no accompanying artery and a low-mid velocity, and turbulent Doppler signals suggest gastro-esophageal, splenorenal and/or retroperitoneal collaterals.

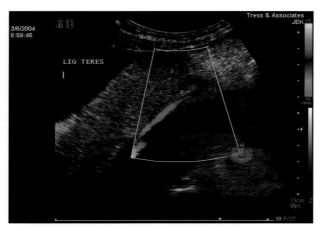

Patent umbilical vein seen on colour Doppler

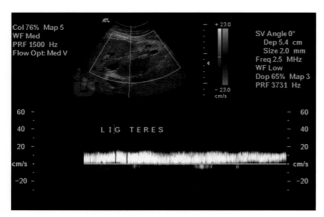

Patent umbilical vein seen on spectral Doppler

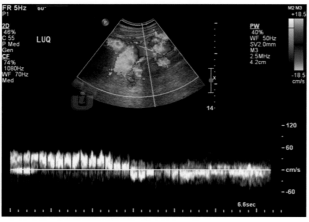

Splenorenal collaterals demonstrated with spectral Doppler.

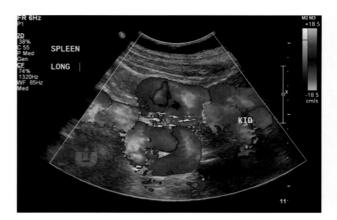

Splenorenal collaterals demonstrated with color Doppler

Budd-Chiari Syndrome

Abnormal Findings

- Decreased, absent, or reversed flow in any of the hepatic veins
- Decreased venous flow, or narrowing of the IVC
- Intrahepatic venovenous collaterals
- Echogenic intralumenal echoes in the hepatic veins or IVC
- Dampened spectral tracing in the hepatic vein if there is an obstructing lesion in the hepatic vein or IVC
- Caudate lobe hypertrophy

TABLE 116: **Normal Hepatoportal Interpretation Summary**
Normal: no detectable hepatoportal disease
• Portal vein
– low velocity hepatopetal flow with respiratory variation
– maximum velocities vary within 15-30 cm/s
• Hepatic artery
– low resistance flow
– PSV range 70-150cm/s
• Hepatic Vein
– multiphasic flow pattern

Source: Robinson, KA, Middleton WD, AL-Sukaiti R, Teefey SA & Dahiya N. (March 2009). Doppler sonography of portal hypertension, *Ultrasound Quarterly.* 25(1), 3-13.

TABLE 117: Normal Hepatoportal Velocity Ranges Reported in the Literature

Results from various studies have shown a great variation in normal maximum portal vein velocity ranges:

Velocity Range	Source
8-18 cm/s (fasting)	Patriquin. et al
26.5 cm/s (± 5.5)	Haag et al
16-31 cm/s	Abu-Yousef et al
11-39 cm/s	Kok et al
20-33 cm/s	Cioni et al

- The large variation in results can be a result of intraobserver variability, diversity in fasting and respiratory states, differing cardiac outputs, and the presence of varied collateral pathways (especially the recanalized paraumbilical vein).
- This variation makes it difficult to rely on velocities as an indicator of portal hypertension. In general, unusually low velocities in the portal vein indicate portal hypertension, although velocities in the normal range do not exclude this diagnosis.

Source: Robinson, KA, Middleton WD, AL-Sukaiti R, Teefey SA & Dahiya N. (March 2009). Doppler sonography of portal hypertension, *Ultrasound Quarterly.* 25(1), 3-13..

TABLE 118: Diagnostic Criteria for Abnormal Hepatoportal Disease

- **Right-sided heart failure/Tricuspid valve regurgitation**
  - Increased hepatic vein pulsatility
  - Pulsatile portal vein
- **Portal Hypertension**
  - Hepatofugal (reverse) flow in the main portal vein or its branches, splenic vein, or SMV
  - Slow portal vein flow
  - Portal flow alternating between retrograde and antegrade flow
  - Main portal vein diameter >13mm
  - Splenic vein diameter >10mm
  - Portal vein thrombosis +/- cavernous transformation
  - Patent paraumbilical vein
  - Paraumbilical vein diameter >2.5mm
  - Presence of other portal systemic collaterals
  - Spleen coronal length >13mm
  - Presence of ascites
- **Budd-Chiari Syndrome**
  - Decreased, absent, or reversed flow in any of the hepatic veins
  - Narrowing of the IVC
  - Intrahepatic hepatic venovenous collaterals
  - Echogenic thrombus in hepatic veins or IVC
  - Damped spectral tracing in hepatic veins
  - Caudate lobe hypertrophy

Source: Robinson, KA, Middleton WD, AL-Sukaiti R, Teefey SA & Dahiya N. (March 2009). Doppler sonography of portal hypertension, *Ultrasound Quarterly.* 25(1), 3-13.

Correlation

- Upper GI series
- CT scan
- MRI
- Endoscopic examination
- Angiography

Medical Treatment

- Managing the cause of portal hypertension (e.g., anticoagulation for hepatic vein thrombosis, treating any identified cause of liver disease).
- Beta-blockers–can reduce portal pressure
- Management of complications:
  - Varices
    - Endoscopic banding
    - Sclerotherapy
  - Ascites
    - Diuretics
    - Salt restriction
    - Paracentesis
    - Treat any supervening bacterial peritonitis

Surgical Management

- Esophageal devascularization
- Liver transplant– considered if liver function is poor
- Portosystemic vascular shunts
  - Distal splenorenal shunt (DSRS)
  - Portocaval shunt (main portal blood flow shunted to the IVC)
  - Mesocaval shunt (blood from the superior mesenteric vein shunted to the IVC)

TIPS (Transjugular Intrahepatic Portosystemic Shunt)

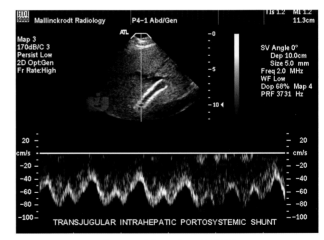

Spectral Doppler of TIPS

> *TIPS is used to treat life threatening varices.*

Under angiographic guidance, a stent is inserted via the right internal jugular vein to connect the hepatic vein with the portal vein (usually RPV to RHV).

- A normal stent on ultrasound appears with echogenic walls and an anechoic lumen.
- Normal flow for a TIPS is 100-190 cm/s.
  - Change in peak velocity of either greater or less than 50 cm/s from the baseline post-procedural ultrasound may indicate stenosis.
  - Greater than 190 cm/s suggests stenosis.
- Normal PV branch flow direction is shunted into the stent (hepatofugal), so a change to hepatopetal flow (away from the stent) is an indirect sign of stent malfunction.

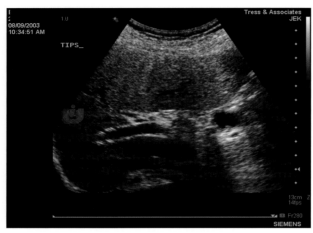

Transjugular intrahepatic portosystemic shunt demonstrated with echogenic corrugated walls on B-mode imaging

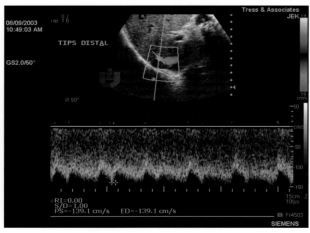

Spectral Doppler of a distal end of a TIPS draining into the right hepatic vein

Points to Remember

- Although numerous vessel velocities and diameters have been reported in various studies, the most reliable and widely used approach for the diagnosis of portal hypertension is the detection of portal systemic collaterals.
- Special consideration needs to be given when evaluating the portal hepatic venous system utilizing Doppler. Patients with PHT often have very slow flow states and Doppler needs to be optimized accordingly to accurately assess direction of flow and to detect portal vein thrombosis. The utilization of color or power Doppler may be a useful tool to evaluate if flow is present.
- The most specific signs of portal hypertension are hepatofugal flow in the portal veins, a patent paraumbilical vein, or other evidence of collateralization.
- Ascites is not a specific sign of PHT as there are multiple causes of ascites.
- Patients with severe fatty livers that result in impaired image quality should have additional imaging with CT or MRI.
- Decreased pulsatility in the hepatic vein may suggest hepatic parenchymal disease or Budd-Chiari syndrome. Pulsatility varies with respiration and it is important to obtain a spectral Doppler tracing on quiet breathing, expiration or shallow inspiration.
- Increased pulsatility in the hepatic vein or portal vein may suggest tricuspid valve insufficiency or right sided heart failure.
- Pulsatile portal vein and nonpulsatile hepatic vein tracings can be seen uncommonly in normal population.
- When the portal pressure is increased, the hepatic artery may carry more blood flow as portal flow decreases.
- Any communication between the systemic and portal veins (portosystemic shunts or fistulas) may lead to a pulsatile portal vein.

References

1. Baxter GM, (2003). Imaging in renal transplantation. Ultrasound quarterly. 19(3) 123-137.
2. Ditchfield MR, Gibson RN, Donlan JD, Gibson PR. (1992). Duplex Doppler ultrasound signs of portal hypertension: relative diagnostic value of examination of paraumbilical vein, portal vein and spleen. Australasian Radiology, 36: 102-105
3. Gibson RN, Gibson PR, Donlan JD, Padmanabhan R. (1993). Modified Doppler flowmetry in the splanchnic circulation. Gastrenterrology; 105:1029-1034.
4. Gibson RN, Gibson PR, Donlan JD, Clunie DA. (1989). Identification of a patent paraumbilical vein using Doppler sonography: importance in the diagnosis of portal hypertension. AJR, 153: 513-516.
5. Irshad A, Ackerman SJ, Campbell AS, A. (2009). An overview of renal transplantation: current practice and use of ultrasound. Seminars in Ultrasound, CT and MRI. 30 (4) 298-314.
6. Robinson, KA, Middleton WD, AL-Sukaiti R, Teefey SA & Dahiya N. (March 2009). Doppler sonography of portal hypertension, Ultrasound Quarterly. 25(1), 3-13.
7. Vessal S, Naidoo S, Hodson J, Stella D, Bibson RN. (2009). Hepatic vein morphology- a new sonographic diagnostic parameter in the investigation of cirrhosis. J Ultrasound Med. 28:1219-1227.
8. Zwiebel, WJ (2005). Ultrasound assessment of the hepatic vasculature. In Zwiebel WJ, Pellerito JS (Eds.), Introduction to Vascular Ultrasonography 5th ed, (586-609). Philadelphia: Elsevier Saunders.

Definition

Combination of real time B-mode imaging with pulse wave and color Doppler to provide monitoring for both early post-operative evaluation and long term follow up of renal transplants

Etiology (of allograft complications)

- Vascular complications
- Parenchymal complications
- Perinephric fluid collections
- Urological complications
- Post biopsy complications

Risk Factors

- Surgical trauma or incorrect surgical technique
- Donor hypotension and prolonged warm ischemic time (acute tubular necrosis (ATN))
- After an episode of acute transient rejection, patients have higher risk for chronic rejection.
- Renal vein thrombosis: hypercoagulable states, acute rejection, and venous compression by fluid collections
- Renal biopsy (increased risk of hemorrhage and arteriovenous fistula (AVF))
- Kinked or tortuous renal arteries
- Atherosclerosis in the donor or recipient's renal or iliac arteries

Indications for Exam

- Routine follow up of post-operative transplant kidney
- Investigation and follow-up of transplant dysfunction or complications
- Suspected renal artery stenosis
  - Hypertension: severe hypertension refractory to medical therapy
  - Renal artery graft bruit
  - Reduction in renal function following ACE inhibitor treatment
- Guide for interventional procedures including biopsy, nephrostomy and drainages

Contraindications/Limitations

- Exam can be time consuming and requires patience.
- Surgical dressings over the suture site immediately post-transplant
- Multiple renal arteries may increase the difficulty of the examination, and the examination time.
- Transplant renal artery may be difficult to assess completely because of its tortuosity.
- To minimize the risk of radiation exposure to the sonographer, avoid examining the patient immediately post-nuclear medicine examination.

Technique of Renal Transplantation

> *Renal transplantation has become the treatment of choice for end-stage renal disease, offering significantly decreased mortality and increased quality of life. Grafts are obtained from cadavers or donated from living donors.*

- The transplanted kidney is commonly placed extraperitoneally into the right or left iliac fossa, anterior to the psoas muscle.
- The donor renal artery and renal vein are anastomosed with an end-to-side configuration to the external iliac artery and vein respectively (less commonly to the internal iliac vessels).

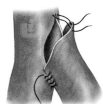

- Renal transplants are typically harvested with an attached portion of the aorta (**Carrel patch**) which is anastomosed end-to-side to the recipient's external iliac artery. When there are multiple renal arteries of the donor kidney, either a long Carrel patch containing both renal artery origins or separate patches are obtained. In the living donor with multiple renal origins, the arteries may be reconstructed to have a common stem.

End to Side Anastomosis

- The anastomosis is formed by attaching the donor ureter to the dome of the bladder. The ureter is tunnelled through the bladder wall to create a pseudo sphincter, and as the bladder fills, the increasing pressure compresses the ureter preventing reflux.

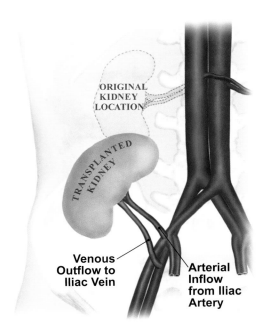

Renal Transplant Anatomy

Mechanisms of disease

Vascular complications

- **Renal artery stenosis (RAS)** is the most common vascular complication of renal transplantation.
  - Early presentation occurs within the first three months. Most stenoses occur at the anastomosis or proximal renal artery and are directly related to surgical technique or kinking of the vessel.
  - Late presentation is generally due to intimal hyperplasia of the artery. Stenosis of the anastomotic site is more common, although mid/distal renal artery stenoses may be due to intimal hyperplasia in response to turbulent flow.
- **Renal artery thrombosis**: occurs within the first week of the post-operative period, and almost invariably leads to graft loss.
  - **Complete occlusion**: usually results from errors in surgical technique, such as kinking or torsion of the artery, or dissection of the arterial wall. Other causes include acute rejection, ATN, and a hypercoagulable state.
  - **Segmental infarction**: results from thrombosis of the intrarenal arterial branches or accessory arteries, or may occur as a result of rejection.
- **Renal vein thrombosis or stenosis** is a rare cause of transplant dysfunction, usually occurring within the first week post-transplant. Causes include surgical technique, renal vein compression by fluid collections, hypercoaguable states and acute rejection.
- **Arteriovenous fistula (AVF)** is usually secondary to vascular trauma during a percutaneous biopsy. AVF forms when a needle penetrates both the artery and vein, creating a communication between them.
  - Small AVFs are usually asymptomatic and resolve spontaneously.
  - Large AVFs may result in renal ischemia due to a "steal" phenomenon or a high output cardiac failure, and this may require urgent treatment.
- **Pseudoaneurysms** may also result from renal biopsy, although only the artery is injured. A communication via a neck is formed between the artery and the pseudoaneurysm. Most are asymptomatic and resolve spontaneously.
- **Extrarenal arteriovenous fistula and pseudoaneurysm** are extremely uncommon, and are usually a consequence of surgical technique rather than percutaneous biopsy. Extrarenal pseudoaneurysms have a high incidence of spontaneous rupture and are potentially catastrophic.

Parenchymal complications

- **Acute rejection** occurs in the first few weeks post-transplant.
- **Chronic rejection** results in a gradual deterioration in graft function beginning at least three months after transplant.
- **Drug nephrotoxicity:** Immunosuppressive agents that are required post-transplant have nephrotoxic potential, which may result in direct damage to the tubules.
- **Acute tubular necrosis (ATN)** is common in the early post-transplant period and usually resolves during the first two weeks. ATN is a result of ischemia of the donor kidney during the process of transplantation (greater risk with cadaveric donors).

- **Post-transplant neoplasm:** the prevalence of cancers is significantly higher in transplant recipients. Risk for primary renal carcinoma may be increased in transplant recipients, with approximately 90% occurring in the native kidneys and approximately 10% in the renal transplant.

Perinephric fluid collections

Peritransplant fluid collections are very common. Many are asymptomatic and are noted during routine sonographic evaluation of the kidney post-operatively.

- **Hematomas** are common immediately post-operative as the result of trauma or biopsy. They are usually small and resolve spontaneously. Large hematomas can displace the allograft and may produce a mass effect.
- **Lymphoceles** are very common. They are a result of intra-operative trauma to lymphatic vessels and they have the potential to produce a mass effect and obstruct the ureter.
- **Urinomas** are relatively rare, occurring within the first 2 months post-transplant. Urinomas are formed by urine leaks, which are secondary to ureteral necrosis from inadequate vascular supply of the distal ureter or from surgical technique.
- **Peritransplant abscesses** are an uncommon complication and may occur secondary to development of pyelonephritis or infection of a perinephric fluid collection.

Urological complications

- **Obstructive hydronephrosis**: early obstruction may be attributable to a blood clot within the ureter or bladder or suboptimal surgical technique. Late obstruction can be due to ureteral stricture of the distal ureter occurring as a result of ischemia, compression by fluid collections, ureteral kinking or renal calculi.
- Transient dilatation of the collecting system as a result of ureteral anastomotic edema frequently occurs immediately after renal transplantation and usually resolves spontaneously.

Patient History

Patient symptoms are often non-specific and may not be helpful in identifying the cause of the dysfunction.

- Fever (may be masked by immunosuppressants)
- Pain over the graft site
- Impaired or delayed renal function
- Oliguria or anuria (decreased or absent urine output)
- Rising creatine levels
- Hematuria
- Proteinuria
- Hypertension: severe hypertension refractory to medical therapy

Physical Examination

- Swelling and tenderness over the graft
- Swelling or "puffiness;" a sign of fluid retention
- Bruit (abnormal sound heard through ausculation caused by turbulent flow)

Renal Transplant Duplex Protocol

- Obtain patient history to include symptoms and risk factors.
- Obtain past surgical reports/records including a general date of surgery.

- Some patients may require the use of a range of transducers; including high-frequency (5-7 MHz) to image anatomical detail and a low frequency curved linear array transducer (2.0-4.0 MHz) depending on body habitus.

Transplant kidney imaging

A post-operative ultrasound examination should be obtained within the first 24-48 hours to establish a baseline for further monitoring. Follow-up examinations are then performed as needed, based on the patient's clinical status.

B-mode imaging

- Grayscale imaging of the transplant, urinary bladder, and perinephric area should be undertaken first with the patient in a supine or oblique position, utilizing an anterolateral approach. In the case of immediate post-operative ultrasound, sterile gel should be used.

- In the longitudinal (sagittal) plane, grayscale images and measurements of the kidney length should be documented. Evaluation should also include:
  - Cortical thickness
  - Renal echogenicity
  - Calyceal dilatation
  - Measurement of any perinephric collections

- Any evidence of distension of the renal pelvis should be documented by measuring the pelvic diameter in the transverse (short axis) plane.

- If the collecting system is dilated, attempt to follow the ureter to the bladder.

- Transverse images of the transplant kidney are also recorded in the upper, mid and lower poles.

- Record grayscale images of the bladder in both longitudinal and transverse planes.

- If there is an indication of ureteric obstruction, color Doppler can be used to look for evidence of a ureteric jet at the transplant vesicoureteric junction.

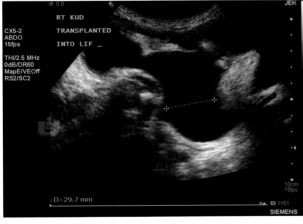

Transplant hydronephrosis. The diameter of the renal pelvis is measured in the longitudinal plane.

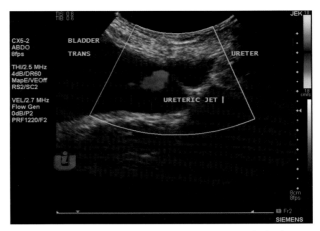

Ureteric jet: Using color Doppler, a ureteric jet is demonstrated at the vesicoureteral junction.

Color and Spectral Doppler

- A baseline Doppler examination is performed to evaluate transplant renal perfusion, as well as vascular flow in the renal and iliac vessels. This will identify any complications that need to be addressed.

- Color, power and spectral Doppler are applied observing for vessel patency, flow direction, waveform characteristics and velocity of blood flow. A Doppler angle of <60° is required for accurate velocity measurement at the following locations:
  - Interlobar arterial branches: upper, mid and lower poles
  - Main renal artery (and accessory arteries): anastomosis, proximal, mid and distal renal artery
  - Main renal vein
  - Ipsilateral external iliac artery: proximal, at, and distal to the anastomosis

- The spectral parameters most commonly assessed include:
  - Peak systolic velocity (PSV)
  - End diastolic velocity (EDV)
  - Acceleration time (AT)
  - Acceleration index (AI)
  - Resistive index (RI)
  - Main transplant artery to iliac artery PSV ratio

> *Resistive Index (RI) measures the resistance to arterial flow within the renal vascular bed. This is a non-specific marker of renal transplant dysfunction.*

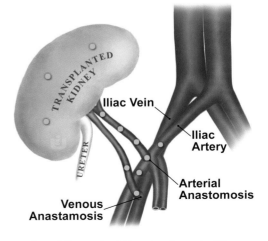

Renal Transplant Doppler Sample Sites

Intrarenal transplant vessels

- Using a longitudinal or transverse plane, interrogate and document the intrarenal vessels using color or power Doppler to assess renal transplant perfusion, in particular cortical perfusion. Using a high frequency linear transducer, a normal transplant should demonstrate flow extending all the way to the renal capsule.

- Spectral Doppler is applied to the distal interlobar or arcuate arteries in the upper, mid and lower portions of the kidney. A resistive index of each of these sections is recorded.

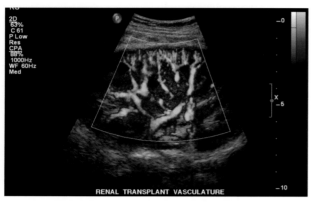

Power Doppler demonstrates renal transplant perfusion, with flow extending to the renal capsule

Image courtesy of Philips Healthcare

Resistive index measurement of an intrarenal artery

Extrarenal transplant vessels

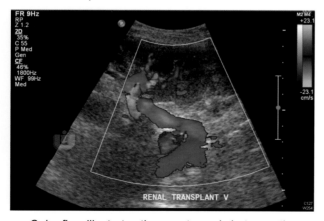

Color flow illustrates the anastomosis between the transplant renal vein and external iliac vein

---

TABLE 119: Renal Transplant Duplex Protocol Summary

B-mode imaging

Transplant kidney
- Sagittal plane: measurements of renal length
- Transverse planes: upper, mid & lower poles

Bladder– sagittal and transverse planes

Perinephric region

Document calyceal or renal pelvis dilatation.

Measure and document evidence of perinephric collections.

Color, power, and spectral Doppler

Assess transplant renal perfusion.

Observe vessel patency, direction, velocity and characteristics of blood flow at the following locations:
- Interlobar arterial branches
- Upper, mid & lower poles
- Main renal artery (and accessory arteries)
- Anastomosis: proximal, mid & distal
- Main renal vein
- Ipsilateral external iliac artery: proximal to anastomosis, at the anastomosis, and distal to anastomosis

- Measure RI (resistive index) at each site.

- In the longitudinal or transverse plane, record a spectral analysis of the main renal vein, assessing it along the entire length to the anastomotic site with the iliac vein. Note the direction of flow and any region of high velocities.

- Assess the main renal artery along the entire length for any indication of stenosis with color Doppler. Measure the PSV and EDV in the distal, mid and proximal portions of the main renal artery, or at regions of high velocities. Careful attention should be given to the anastomosis with the iliac artery. In the presence of renal artery stenosis, document any post-stenotic turbulence.

> *It is often difficult to optimize the angle of insonation relative to the vessel at the arterial anastomosis. The patient may need to be rolled, or alternatively a "heel-toe" technique with the transducer may be necessary.*

Iliac vessels

- Orient the transducer in an oblique plane using the bladder as a window to locate the external and internal iliac vessels. Determine the anastomotic site of the main renal artery and vein.

- Measure the PSV and EDV of the iliac artery (external or internal) proximal to the anastomosis, at the anastomosis, and distal to the anastomosis. Assess the iliac arteries for evidence of stenosis.

Worksheet

- All results may be recorded in a worksheet and included with the examination report.

Interpretation

Normal renal parenchymal appearance

The transplant kidney appears similar to the native kidney, although anatomical detail is better delineated due to the superficial nature of the transplant, and the utilization of a higher frequency transducer.

- The cortex should be homogeneous, with mid to low level echoes and a uniform cortical thickness. The central renal sinus is relatively hyperechoic.

- The renal pyramids are mildly hypoechoic relative to the parenchyma and are regularly spaced with no communication between them (differentiating feature from dilated calyces).

- The renal pelvis may be identified but should not be distended; typically the calyces are collapsed. Over time a mild degree of distension is common presumably because the ureter is denervated and becomes "baggy".

- The kidney size is usually enlarged, with the volume increasing by up to 30% within the first 3 weeks.

- Sometimes the echoes are "real" and indicate pus, blood or debris. Seeing some echoes is preferred to assure that real echoes haven't been removed.

> *Mild hydronephrosis immediately following surgery may reflect ureteral anastomotic edema or denervation of the kidney. This hydronephrosis is transient, resolving over time, and can be reassessed by follow-up examinations.*

Normal Flow Parameters

- Normal transplants can display a wide variation in velocities, and it is important to compare the patient's previous results to indicate a significant change in velocities.

> *Turbulence and increased velocities are often seen at the anastomosis of the renal artery particularly in the immediate post-transplant period.*

- Intrarenal arteries demonstrate cortical perfusion that extends to the renal capsule.

- Normal intra and extra renal arterial flow is represented by a low resistive waveform as they feed a low resistance vascular bed. Normal RI is <0.7.

- The main renal vein is represented by continuous, low-velocity, phasic flow, typically between 40-60 cm/s.

- Iliac arteries display monophasic or biphasic flow proximal to the anastomosis, and triphasic flow distal to the anatomosis.

- Iliac veins display continuous phasic flow.

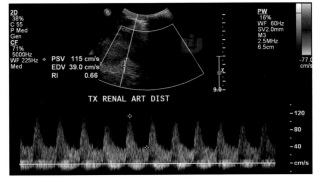

Normal transplant renal artery demonstrating a low resistance waveform

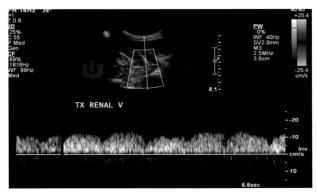

Normal transplant renal vein waveform

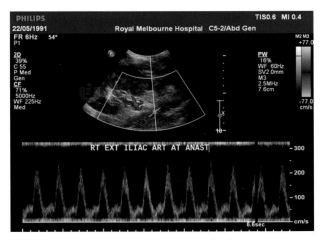

The external iliac artery displays biphasic flow proximal to the anastomosis

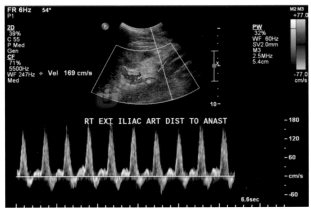

The external iliac artery displays triphasic flow distal to the anastomosis

TABLE 120: **Resistive Index (RI) Severity for Renal Transplant**	
RI	**Severity**
<0.70	Normal
0.70-0.80	Indeterminate
>0.80-0.90	Abnormal

Source: Langer JE, Jones LP. (2007). Sonographic evaluation of the renal transplant. Ultrasound Clinics; 2:73-88.

Renal Transplant Duplex

Abdominal Arterial Testing

Abnormal Vascular Complications

- **Elevated Resistive Index (RI):** An elevated RI may be seen in all forms of graft dysfunction and, although it cannot differentiate the causes, it is a good predictor of immediate graft function.

  - Normal RI <0.7

  - Indeterminate RI 0.7-0.8

  - Abnormal RI >0.8-0.9

  - Serial measurements may determine if there are changes from the patient's baseline values.

- **Renal artery thrombosis**

  - **Complete occlusion**: Absence of arterial flow is seen in the renal arteries and intrarenal vessels on color Doppler examination. Depending on the position of the thrombus, duplex sampling may demonstrate a highly resistive damped waveform, with absent diastolic flow at the proximal renal artery ("thump at the stump" pattern). B-mode imaging may demonstrate an enlarged and hypoechoic kidney.

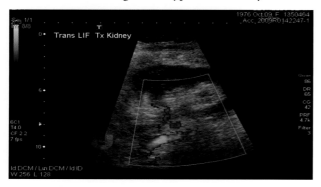

Power Doppler demonstrates occlusion of the intrarenal arteries

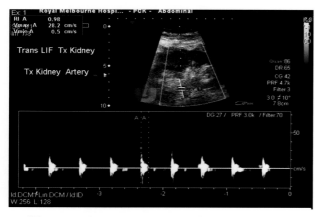

"Thump at the stump" type waveform is seen at the renal hilum, indicating intrarenal artery occlusion

> *It is critical to adjust technical parameters appropriately to avoid a false-positive result. The use of power Doppler may help to demonstrate flow in a technically difficult patient.*

  - **Segmental occlusion**: This may appear as focal hypoechoic wedge-shaped regions in the cortex without any demonstrable flow. Eventually the infarcted segment reduces in volume and forms an echogenic wedge, and finally a linear echogenic focus with a cortical scar.

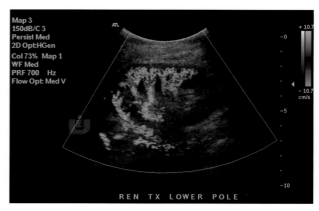

Segmental infarct demonstrated as a loss of flow on color Doppler in the lower pole of the transplant kidney

- **Renal vein thrombosis**

  - A dilated main renal vein, expanded by thrombus may be seen on B-mode. Acute thrombus can appear hypoechoic and is difficult to demonstrate, although this may increase in echogenicity over time.

  - Absent or diminished venous flow is demonstrated on color or spectral Doppler. Non-occlusive thrombus may be seen with partial flow around the thrombus.

  - Elevated resistive index: flow in the renal artery is reduced, with absent or reversed diastolic flow, depending on the extent of the thrombus.

  - B-mode imaging may demonstrate an enlarged and hypoechoic kidney with increased cortical thickness.

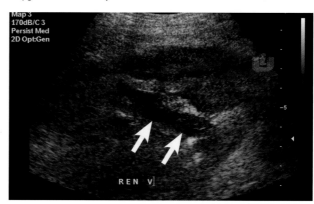

Transplant renal vein thrombosis seen with hypoechoic thrombus distending the main renal vein

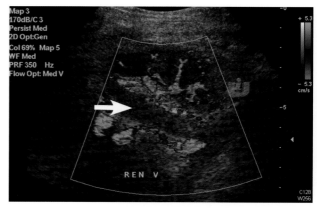

Color Doppler confirming renal vein thrombosis

- **Renal vein stenosis**
  - Visible as an area of narrowing and color aliasing with a three-four fold increase in velocity through the region of stenosis relative to the pre-stenotic region.

Renal Vein Stenosis: figure (a) The renal vein proximal to the anastomosis demonstrates high velocities, which are >4 times in comparison with velocities proximal to the stenosis in figure (b).

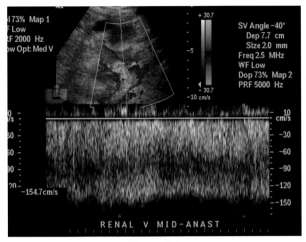

Figure (a)

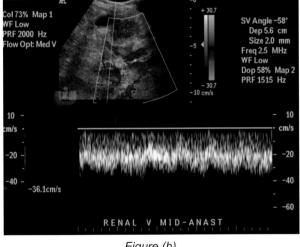

Figure (b)

- **Renal artery stenosis (RAS) (≥50% diameter reduction)**
  - Elevated arterial and venous velocities may be seen immediately post-transplantation and return to normal at one to three months post-transplant. This finding suggests physiologic adaptation rather than true stenosis.

It is important to note that a wide range of parameters for stenosis criteria are used by different laboratories.

- **Direct signs (most sensitive Doppler criteria)**
  - Color aliasing at a focal velocity increase with appropriate Doppler settings.
  - Increased velocities: PSV >200 cm/s with marked spectral broadening, and post-stenotic turbulence
  - Transplant renal artery to iliac artery systolic ratio >2 velocity of stenotic region compared with the pre-stenotic segments in the iliac artery (2 cm upstream from the anastomosis in the iliac artery)

A velocity cut off <250 cm/s improves specificity, but may decrease sensitivity. This cut off reduces the number of patients referred for an unnecessary angiogram.

- **Indirect signs (should be used in conjunction with the direct criteria)**
  - Tardus parvus waveform of the intrarenal arteries or distal to a stenosis (loss of early systolic peak, delayed systolic upstroke).
  - Acceleration Time (AT) >100 msec in the renal or intrarenal arteries and decreased acceleration index <300 cm/s^2

Mimics of renal artery stenosis include tortuosity or transient kinking of the renal artery, which may cause increased velocities and spectral broadening in normal vessels.

Transplant Renal Artery Stenosis

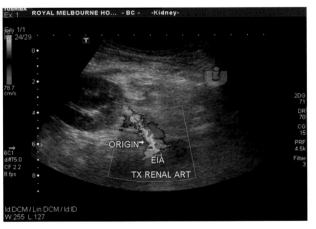

Color aliasing of the transplant renal artery at the anastomosis

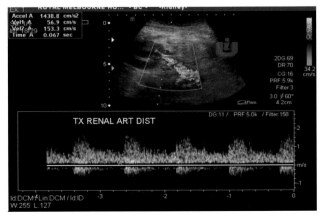

Turbulence is demonstrated in the waveform distal to the stenosis

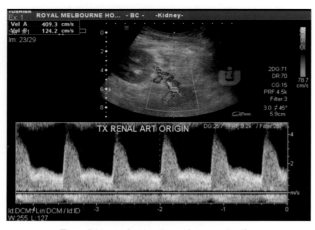

*Renal transplant artery demonstrating
elevated velocities at the anastomosis*

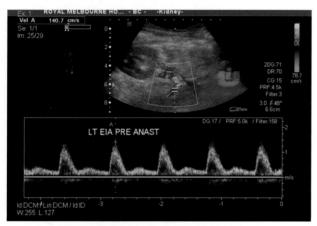

*External iliac arterial velocities are less than
half of the velocities in stenotic region*

- **Arteriovenous Fistula (AVF)**
  - Color Doppler shows aliasing at focal areas of turbulent flow (mosaic appearance).
  - Spectral Doppler demonstrates turbulent flow with high velocities and a low resistance trace at the AVF and in the inflow artery.
  - The draining vein demonstrates pulsatile flow due to arterialization.

Arteriovenous Fistula

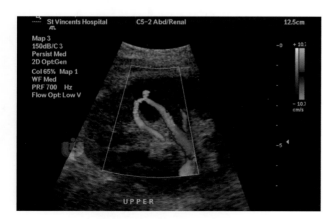

*Color Doppler reveals an AVF is
a feeding artery and draining vein*

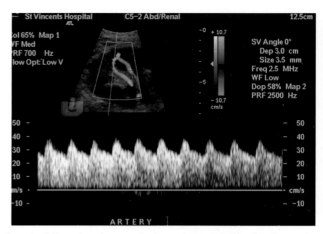

Spectral Doppler demonstrates a low resistive feeding artery

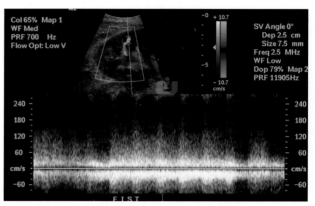

*Spectral Doppler reveals high velocity
and turbulent flow within the AVF*

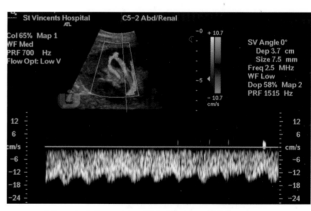

*The draining vein distal to the AVF appears
pulsatile due to arterialization*

- **Pseudoaneurysm**
  - On grayscale imaging it is seen as a simple or complex cystic mass.
  - Color Doppler shows a turbulent and swirling flow pattern.
  - Spectral Doppler reveals a forward and reverse waveform (referred to as the "yin-yang" sign).

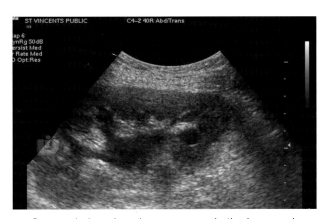

Grayscale imaging shows an area in the lower pole that has the appearances of a simple cyst

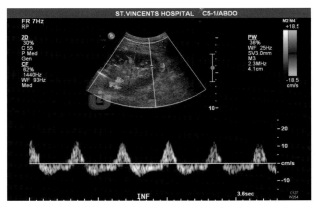

Reverse end-diastolic flow seen in the intrarenal artery of a patient with graft dysfunction

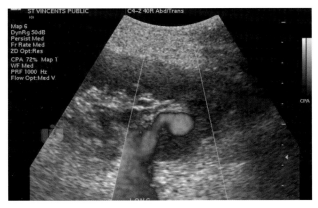

Power Doppler indicates how this region contains flow and is representive of a pseudoaneyrsm

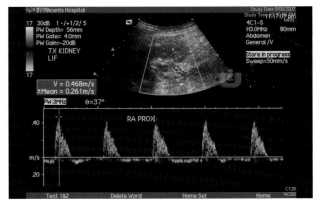

Reverse end-diastolic flow seen in the main renal transplant artery

- **Parenchymal complications**

ATN, rejection and drug nephrotoxicity are difficult to differentiate on imaging and a renal biopsy is required to establish the diagnosis. Several non-specific sonographic findings are demonstrated in patients who have graft dysfunction due to these complications, although these findings may only be apparent in the late stages.

Sonographic findings may include:

- Renal enlargement
- Decreased cortical and renal medullary echogenicity (loss of corticomedullary differentiation)
- Effacement of the renal sinus
- Thickening of uroepithelium
- Absence of diastolic flow or flow reversal (acute rejection)
- Elevated intrarenal RI (ATN, acute rejection)
- Decreased venous flow with severe acute rejection
- Chronic rejection displays a decreased renal size, with a thinned echogenic cortex.

- **Perinephric fluid collections**
    - **Hematomas** are usually hyperechoic and complex in the acute phase, whereas resolving hematomas are typically hypoechoic.
    - **Lymphoceles** are seen as loculated anechoic collections that may have thin septations and internal echoes.
    - **Urinomas** are observed as well defined anechoic fluid collections with occasional septations, usually visualized between the kidney and the bladder. These may rapidly increase in size.
    - **Abscesses** are demonstrated as a complex perirenal cystic mass, which may contain air or a fluid level.

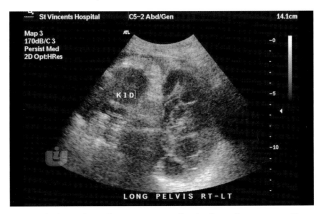

Grayscale imaging shows a complicated cystic mass adjacent to the transplant kidney representative of a urinoma

Renal Transplant Duplex

Abdominal Arterial Testing

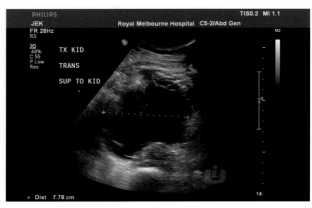

*A lymphocele is seen as an anechoic
collection with internal septations*

- **Urological complications**
  - **Obstructive hydronephrosis** is demonstrated by dilated renal pelvis and calyces. The graft can become distended and edematous, and an increased RI may be apparent.
  - **Pyelonephritis**: the kidney may be enlarged with regions of increased or decreased echogenicity and areas of altered parenchymal flow. Internal echoes within the collecting system may be noted.

Other Pathology

Peritransplant collections

- **Lymphoceles**: most are small and asymptomatic, and intervention is not necessary. Lymphoceles that cause compression of the ureter or vascular pedicle require percutaneous drainage.
- **Urinoma**: large urinomas may rupture, producing urinary ascites, or compress vascular or ureteral structures. These urinomas should be drained percutaneously to relieve extrinsic compression and reduce the risk of infection.
- **Abscess**: prompt surgical or percutaneous drainage, combined with antibiotics is mandatory due to the immunosuppressed state of transplant patients.

Urological complications

- **Urinary leaks**: percutaneous nephrostomy and stent placement can divert urinary flow to allow ureteral healing. Surgical revision is required in some cases.
- **Hydronephrosis** is often managed by percutaneous nephrostomy. Ureteral stenting or balloon dilatation can be utilized if obstruction persists.

Differential Diagnosis

None

Correlation

- Renal transplant biopsy
- Laboratory studies
- Radionuclide imaging (Tc-99 MAG3)
- CTA iodinated contrast avoided due to nephrotoxic effects
- MRA
- Angiography for vascular intervention

Medical Treatment

Acute rejection

- High-dose steroids or antibody therapy
- Plasma exchange for steroid resistant transplant rejection

Chronic rejection(irreversible with no effective treatment)

- Temporary measures include controlling blood pressure and avoiding nephrotoxins.
- Reduce episodes of acute rejection to decrease the risk of chronic rejection.

Surgical Treatment

- Surgical resection and revision of the anastomosis is indicated for recurrent stenoses and those that cannot be treated by or recur after PTA.
- Surgical thrombectomy with arterial/venous repair (in cases of early graft thrombosis)
- Nephrectomy (graft thrombosis that cannot be salvaged)

Endovascular Treatment

- Angioplasty, with or without stenting (for renal artery and venous stenosis
- Intra-arterial directed thrombolysis (early graft thrombosis)
- Coil embolization (post-biopsy bleeds, arteriovenous fistulas, and pseudoaneurysm)

Points to Remember

- A wide range of arterial and venous velocities can be found in the normal renal transplant.
- Doppler of the transplant renal artery can be technically difficult. It may be difficult to obtain a Doppler angle ≤60° at the anastomosis site, or in a tortuous artery. Angles >60° may mimic a renal artery stenosis (elevated velocities and turbulent flow) and produce a false positive result.
- Velocities immediately post-transplant are often elevated with turbulent flow, and revert back to normal at one to three months post-transplant. This suggests a physiological adaptation rather than a true stenosis.
- Turbulence and increased velocities are often seen at the anastomosis of the renal artery, particularly in the immediate post-transplant period.
- The decision to intervene on a renal artery stenosis diagnosed by Doppler is often based on the combination of a high clinical suspicion, the patient's clinical status and biochemical testing.
- Ultrasound appearances of ATN, rejection and drug nephrotoxicity are non-specific as they often have similar sonographic and Doppler features. This can cause a diagnostic dilemma for the interpreting physician, so interpretation of dysfunction should be made based on the time of onset, the patient's clinical status, as well as results of biochemical testing.
- Renal transplant biopsy is generally accepted as the gold standard for clarifying the cause of renal dysfunction.
- Chronic rejection is irreversible and cannot be treated effectively

References

1. Baxter, GM, Imaging in Renal Transplantation, (September 2003). US Quarterly, 19 (3), 123-127.
2. Irshad, A, Ackerman SJ, Campbell AS, & Anis, M (August 2009). An Overview of Renal Transplantation: Current Practice and Use of Ultrasound. US CT and MRI, 30 (4), 298-314.

Defintion

A vascular screening program uses non-invasive ultrasound testing techniques to detect the presence of lower extremity peripheral arterial disease (PAD), carotid arterial disease, abdominal aortic aneurysm (AAA) and cardiovascular disease (CVD).

Rationale

Vascular screening programs are designed to detect the presence or absence of pathology in the vascular system of persons who may be at risk for vascular occlusive or aneurysmal disease. The most common types of vascular screening are ankle/brachial indices (ABIs) for atherosclerotic occlusive disease of the lower extremities, carotid duplex exam for extracranial internal carotid artery stenosis, and aortic duplex for abdominal aortic aneurysm. Vascular screenings may also include other exams, such as carotid intima-media thickness (CIMT), renal artery duplex ultrasound, echocardiography, coronary artery disease and serum cholesterol levels.

Screenings may have a variety of sponsors and be offered in a variety of settings and locations:

Sponsors	Types	Locations
Community groups	Mass screenings	Hospitals
Professional societies	Health fairs	Vascular labs
Hospitals, malls or churches	Individual appointments	
Vascular labs	One-time events	Community centers or hotels
Screening only companies		Vans, or mobile units

Vascular Screening Goals

The four primary goals of any vascular screening program:

- To detect the presence of vascular disease in those who lack signs, symptoms, or indications of disease.
- To increase public awareness of vascular disease.
- To provide educational information about vascular disease to the community.
- To provide information on lifestyle modification for those who are at risk of developing vascular disease.

Screening Versus Diagnostic Exams

- Similar equipment and personnel may be used.
- Screening exams differ from diagnostic exams in many ways, including who gets the exam, what exam they get, how the exams are interpreted and reported, how results are distributed and follow up.
- Selection criteria for screening exams are flexible.

- Testing procedure protocols are very abbreviated and diagnostic criteria are usually broader than for diagnostic exams.
- Results are often shared with the participant immediately after the screening.
- Attendees at screenings are often referred to as "participants", rather than patients, since they are not known to have pathology.
- Most insurance companies do not pay for vascular screening exams and these exams are often paid for by the participant.
- There is no need for a "medically necessary" indication as is required for diagnostic exams reimbursed by insurance claim.

Indications for Screening

- Screening vascular exams, unlike diagnostic vascular exams, do not require specific signs and symptoms of disease.
- The definition of a screening exam is one that is performed in the absence of signs and symptoms of disease.
- It is reasonable to select participants who will benefit most from screening on the basis of age, family history and risk factors.

Contraindications/Limitations

- Participants who have obvious signs and symptoms of vascular disease or who have been previously diagnosed with peripheral vascular or aortic aneurysmal disease are NOT appropriate candidates for vascular screening.
- Those patients who have appropriate indications for more comprehensive diagnostic vascular testing should be encouraged to contact their medical provider.

Participant Selection

Vascular screening programs should have guidelines regarding those who are most appropriate for the screening based on risk factor assessment. Risk factors for screening tests are identical to those for the respective diagnostic exam:

- Age (usually >55 years of age)
- Diabetes
- Hypertension
- Hyperlipidemia
- Obesity
- Smoking
- Family history of PAD
- Family history of AAA

Prior to the Screening

- For large, publicly-advertised screenings, registration of participants is recommended in order to ensure appropriate selection of those "at risk", to redirect inappropriate requests, and to assign appointment times to manage workflow.
- A brief "Risk Factors" checklist may be completed by the participant prior to the test and is often included on the same form where results of the exams(s) are documented.
- When screening events are held in public spaces, privacy for removal of clothing for the ABI and AAA exams may be limited.
- Participants are asked to wear shoes and socks that are easily removed and clothing that can be pulled down at the waist without requiring disrobing.

Personnel

- Technical staff and medical/interpreting staff should be required to be certified and to have adequate training and experience in the performance/interpretation of the respective diagnostic exam.
- Ancillary staff may be necessary to assist with appointment scheduling, registration, completion and maintenance of paperwork, traffic flow, and distribution of educational materials.

Equipment

- Portability of the equipment used for performing these tests is an important consideration if screening is performed outside of the traditional vascular lab.
- Equipment for screening exams must have features and capabilities adequate to provide reliable and accurate data (e.g., Doppler frequencies appropriate for vessel evaluation).
- Spectral and color Doppler are required for carotid duplex exams.
- Spectral and color Doppler are not required for abdominal duplex exams.
- Cuffs of various sizes (adult, large adult, toe cuffs) and some type of detecting device, such as a continuous wave Doppler unit are recommended for ABI exams.
- Computerized-assisted electronic calipers or semiautomatic edge detection software must be used for CIMT measurement.

Education

- Participant education is one of the most important components of a vascular screening program.
- Educational offerings may take many forms (e.g., handouts, brochures, videos, CDs, lectures, individual consultations).
- Printed materials on various vascular topics are available from many national and local community health and professional organizations, or facilities may develop their own educational materials.
  - www.padcoalition.org
  - www.vdf.org
  - www.venousdiseasecoalition.org
  - www.venous-info.com/
  - www.sirweb.org/
  - www.vascularweb.org

Vascular Screening Procedure Protocols

General Considerations

- Written screening procedure protocols promote standardization of technique, consistency in interpretation, and accuracy of results.
- Screening protocols may be created by the sponsoring organization or may be adapted from the protocols used in the respective diagnostic exam in a testing facility.
- Review risk factors and pertinent medical history with participant.
- Removal of appropriate clothing (e.g., shoes and socks).
- Participant is examined in the supine position.

ABI and Analog Pedal Artery Waveforms

- Apply blood pressure cuffs of appropriate width to the upper arm and ankle bilaterally.
- Using a Doppler or other blood flow sensing device, obtain systolic blood pressure recordings in the brachial artery bilaterally and in at least two arteries at the ankle level, usually the dorsalis pedis and posterior tibial arteries bilaterally.
- Calculate the ankle/brachial index (ABI) by dividing the higher of the two brachial pressures into the higher ankle pressure for each ankle. *See Ankle/Brachial Index (ABI) section*
- Doppler waveforms are optional.

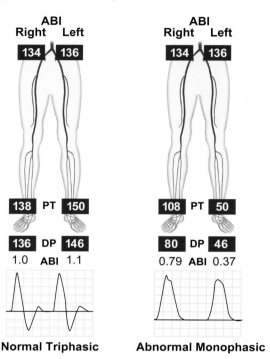

ABI
Right   Left
134   136

138 PT 150

136 DP 146

1.0 **ABI** 1.1

Normal Triphasic

ABI
Right   Left
134   136

108 PT 50

80 DP 46

0.79 **ABI** 0.37

Abnormal Monophasic

Screening Carotid Duplex Ultrasound

- Begin scanning in the common carotid artery in the longitudinal view at the base of the neck, moving up through the bifurcation and into both the ECA and ICA.
- Normal exam - obtain a spectral Doppler velocity waveform in the proximal ICA and measure the peak systolic and end diastolic velocities in cm/s.
- Abnormal exam: obtain a spectral Doppler velocity waveform in the area of maximum velocity and measure the peak systolic and end diastolic velocities in cm/s.
- Repeat the procedure in the contralateral ICA.

Carotid Intima-Medical Thickness (CIMT)

- Begin scanning in the common carotid artery in the longitudinal view at the base of the neck, moving up to the distal CCA.
- All measurements are taken during end diastole.
- Measurements from at least three long imaging planes, one optimal and two complementary imaging planes
  - Anterior
  - Lateral
  - Posterior
- Measurements must be taken from the far wall of the distal 1-2 cm of the CCA.
- Measurements may also be taken from the near wall of the distal CCA.
- Measurements may also be taken from the near and fall wall of the bifurcation and proximal 1 cm of the ICA.
- If plaque is present, characterization and/or dimensions of the plaque should be documented.

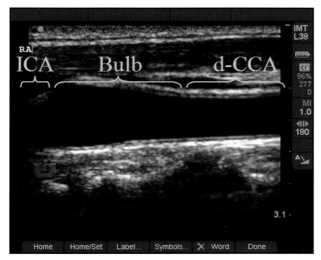

Carotid artery segments

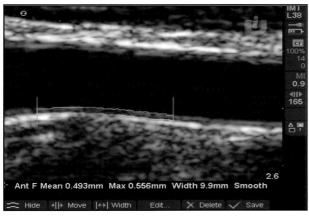

Measurements are performed within the distal CCA, just before the walls start to dilate, beginning in the bulb area on the far wall

Images Courtesy of SonoSite FUJIFILM

Screening AAA Duplex Ultrasound

- Using a duplex imager, begin scanning in the transverse view (short view) from the suprarenal (proximal) abdominal aorta, through the mid aorta to the iliac bifurcation.

> *Maintaining an angle perpendicular to the aorta, measure AP and transverse dimensions from outer wall-to-outer wall.*

- All measurements are taken perpendicular to the long axis of the aorta with measurement documentation from outer wall-to-outer wall.
- In normal exams, measure the maximum diameter of the abdominal aorta in transverse view.
- In abnormal exams, measure the maximum diameter of the dilated abdominal aorta in transverse view and measure the maximum diameter of the non-dilated aorta for comparison.

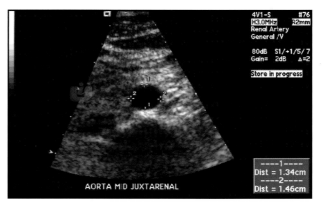

Normal aortic diameters

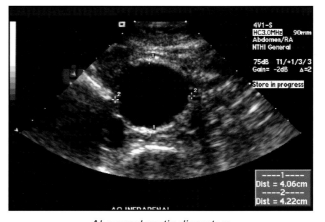

Abnormal aortic diameters

TABLE 121: ABI Screening Protocol Summary

- Take brachial systolic pressures bilaterally
- Take bilateral ankle pressures from the
  - dorsalis pedis artery at ankle level
  - posterior tibial artery at ankle level

TABLE 122: CIMT Screening Protocol Summary

- Take measurements during end diastole
- Measurements from far wall of 1-2 cm of the CCA
  - Anterior
  - Lateral
  - Posterior

TABLE 123: Carotid Duplex Ultrasound Screening Protocol Summary

- Normal: Measure peak systolic and end diastolic velocities in proximal ICA.
- Abnormal: Measure peak systolic and end diastolic velocities in area of disease/pathology.

Perfect carotid imaging technique is important. Keep Doppler angles ≤60°, sample in a straight segment of artery and align cursor to posterior artery wall.

TABLE 124: AAA Duplex Ultrasound Screening Protocol Summary

- Sweep through abdominal aorta in transverse view from proximal portion to iliac bifurcation.
- Normal: Measure maximum diameter of abdominal aorta in transverse view.
- Abnormal: Measure diameter of maximally dilated abdominal aorta in transverse view AND measure maximum diameter of non-dilated aorta for comparison.

Color Doppler is unnecessary for AAA screening ultrasounds.

Interpretation

- There must be written criteria for all screening exams.

To reduce false negative exams, a low threshold for positive exams should be established.

- Diagnostic criteria for interpretation of screening exams are broader, focusing on the presence of gross abnormalities that require further investigation or surveillance.
- Screening diagnostic criteria are often adapted from the typical criteria in use for a diagnostic exam by condensing or consolidating some categories of disease.

TABLE 125: Screening ABI Diagnostic Criteria

Description	ABI Range
Normal or no significant disease	≥0.90
Abnormal or presence of significant disease	<0.90
Non-diagnostic or incompressible	≥1.30

Source: McDermott, et al, (2002). The walking and leg circulation study. *Annals of Internal Medicine.* (873-83). Jun 18;136(12).

TABLE 126: CIMT Diagnostic Criteria

Description	IMT
Normal	<0.8
Abnormal	>0.8

Age, gender and race should be documented for risk assessment.

Source: Stein JH, Fraizer MC, et al. (2004). Vascular age: Integrating carotid intima-media thickness measurements with global coronary risk assessment. *Clin Cardiol.* (388-392) 27.

TABLE 127: Screening Carotid Duplex Diagnostic Criteria

Description	ICA PSV	ICA EDV	Plaque
Normal or no disease	<125	<40	None
<50%, or non-significant disease	<125	<40	Minimal
>50%, or significant disease	>125	>40	Mild-large
Occlusion	no flow detected		

Source: Modified from SRU Consensus Panel; Radiology 229:340-346; 2003.

TABLE 128: Screening AAA Diagnostic Criteria

Description	Range
Normal or no aneurysm	<3.0 cm
Abnormal or aneurysmal	>3.0 cm

Source: U.S. Preventive Services Task Force (USPSTF) recommendations on screening for abdominal aortic aneurysm (AAA)

Reporting Results

Once the screening exam has been performed, results may be distributed in a variety of ways.

- For mass screening events, it is most efficient to route participants to another on-site station to meet with a physician or other medical practitioner to discuss the results and to receive educational information and referral, if indicated.

- For participants with individual appointments, results, education, instructions, and referrals may be transmitted by a second appointment with the interpreter, or by letter, email, or telephone call.

> *Whatever you do to one side of the equation, you MUST do to the other side. Screening results should be discussed with the participant and copies provided for the participant and his/her primary care provider.*

Correlation and Quality Assurance

- You must have a written procedure for regular correlation.

- Separate "Quality Assurance Logs and Matrices" for screening exams should be maintained in a manner similar or identical to the QA logs and matrices for traditional diagnostic testing.

- Although screening exams are abbreviated versions of a traditional diagnostic exam, it is equally important that screening exams be performed accurately.

- Quality screening programs have very few false negative results. This is particularly important since false negatives may cause participants to have an unwarranted sense that all is well, and they may be lost to medical follow up.

- Regular correlation of both positive and negative screening exams with any of the methods below is necessary to ensure consistent accuracy:
  - Duplex ultrasound
  - Angiography
  - CT, CTA
  - MRA
  - Surgical pathology
  - Clinical outcome

> *Randomly selecting participants to undergo a diagnostic exam by a second technical staff member unaware of the screening results may also be used as a correlation method.*

- Follow-up of all positive exams may be achieved by contact through telephone call or letter to the participant.

Record Keeping

- Copies of the screening results, including recommendations for follow-up and disposition, should be maintained according to State medical records law and any other applicable regulations.

- It is not necessary to assign a medical record number or to create a formal chart for participants as long as the records are maintained and can be accessed if necessary.

Points to Remember

- Abbreviated exams can detect the presence or absence of significant vascular disease in at-risk participants who do not have signs, symptoms, or indications for diagnostic testing. If significant disease is found, the participant is referred for appropriate diagnostic testing and all participants receive educational information on risk factor modification.

- Screening cannot replace diagnostic examinations for symptomatic individuals.

- Resist the urge to develop screening protocols that are too lengthy or complicated.

- Yield of positive findings for most screenings is low. Typically only 1-5% of participants will have positive findings, depending on participant selection criteria.

- If screenings are performed in non-medical facilities, consideration must be given to participant safety and provisions must be made for emergency situations.

- Vascular Screening standards are screening guidelines for the appropriate selection of participants, and should be based upon contemporary scientific publications.

This section has been adapted from the 04/2010 ICAVL CAMS* Standards for Accreditation of Medical Screening Examinations.

* Commission for the Accreditation of Medical Screening Services

References

1. Criqui, M.A, et al. (2008). Atherosclerotic peripheral disease symposium II; screening for atherosclerotic vascular diseases: should nationwide programs be instituted? *Circulation*. (2830-2836) 118.

2. Bendick, Phillip, Ph.D. (September 13, 2007). Vascular screening may facilitate early disease detection, management; AuntMinnie.com. (Retrieved from http://www.auntminnie.com/index.asp?sec=ser&sub= def&pag=dis&ItemID=77508). (2-10-11).

3. ICAVL Standards, Screening; Intersocietal Commission for the Accreditation of Vascular Laboratories, April, 2010

4. McDermott, et al. (2002). The walking and leg circulation study. *Annals of Internal Medicine*, (873-83). Jun 18;136(12).

5. Stein JH, Fraizer MC, Aeschlimann SE, Nelson-Worel J, McBride PE, Douglas PS. (2004). Vascular age: Integrating carotid intima-media thickness measurements with global coronary risk assessment. *Clin Cardiol*. 27:388-392.

6. Stein JH, Korcarz CE, et al. (2008). Use of carotid ultrasound to identify subclinical vascular disease and evaluate cardiovascular disease risk: A consensus statement from the American Society of Echocardiography Carotid Intima-Media Thickness Task Force. *Journal of the American Society of Echocardiography*. 21:93-111.

Definition

Alternative testing modalities used to obtain diagnostic information when clinical correlation is suggested after duplex imaging.

Differential Tests Include:

- Computerized Tomography (CT) Scan
- Computerized Tomography Angiography (CTA) Scan
- Magnetic Resonance Imaging (MRI)
- Magnetic Resonance Angiography (MRA)
- Magnetic Resonance Venography (MRV)
- Angiography
- Venography
- D-dimer blood test
- Ventilation/Perfusion Scan (VQ Lung Scan)

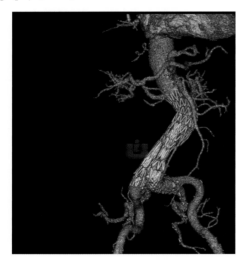

CT angio of an abdominal endograft using 3-D

Computed Tomography (CT) Scan

Tomography is derived from the Greek word "tomo" for slice. A CT scan, also known as a CAT scan, is a non-invasive imaging technique that can obtain diagnostic information of the internal organs, bones, soft tissue, and blood vessels. The patient is placed in the supine position on a movable table into a CT scanner while multiple x-ray beams, combined with a set of electronic x-ray detectors, rotate around the body in a spiral motion. 2 dimensional (2-D) cross sectional images are created and displayed on a computer monitor.

- **Spiral CT/Helical CT**: continuously takes pictures very quickly in a circular motion

> *CT testing is the current gold standard examination to diagnose a PE.*

- **Computerized Tomography Pulmonary Angiogram (CTPA)**: used to diagnose a pulmonary embolism (PE)

- **Computerized Tomography Angiography (CTA) Scan**: a CTA is a procedure used to obtain images of the arteries in the body. A contrast agent is injected to enhance the images.

  - 2-D cross sectional and 3-D images are created and displayed on a computer monitor.

  - Multiplanar reconstruction and 3-D rendering techniques use computer software to provide alternative views of the information gathered from a CT scan.

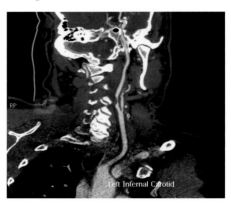

Multiplanar CT angio image of a left ICA stenosis

Indications

- Tumors of the chest, abdomen, and pelvis
- Vascular abnormalities
- Heart conditions
- Diseases of the chest, abdomen, and pelvis

Contraindications/Limitations

- Iodinated contrast allergy
- Kidney failure
- Anaphylactic reaction
- Pregnancy
- Breast feeding
- Arrhythmia

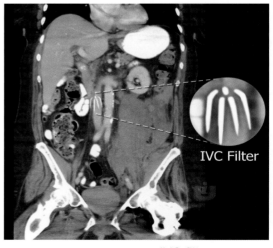

CT imaging of an IVC filter

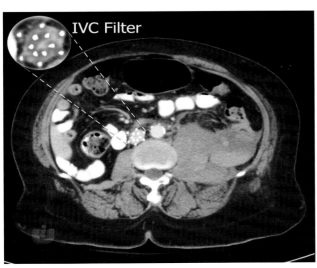

CT imaging of an IVC filter

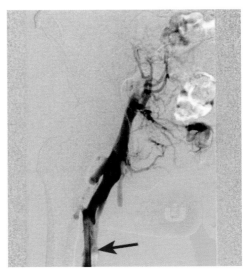

MRV of an iliac vein thrombosis
note: collateral network toward midline

Magnetic Resonance Imaging (MRI)

MRI is a non-invasive imaging technique. The MRI scanner is a large tube surrounded by a giant circular magnet. The patient is placed on a movable bed which is inserted into a magnetic tube. The large, powerful circular magnet and radio frequency pulses of the MRI machine work together to realign the hydrogen protons in the body. The MRI scanner returns radio-waves, storing them as digital images which detail the body's organs, vasculature, muscles and any abnormalities (e.g., tumors etc.) for presentation on a computer monitor.

- **Magnetic Resonance Angiography (MRA)**: a study of the arteries in the brain, kidneys, pelvis, legs, lungs, heart, neck or abdomen. An MRA can be non-invasive or it can be minimally invasive with the use of a contrast agent to enhance images. A 2-D or 3-D image is created for display on a computer monitor.
- **Magnetic Resonance Venography (MRV)**: a study of the veins in the brain, kidneys, pelvis, legs, lungs, heart, neck or abdomen. An MRV uses a contrast agent to enhance images. A 2-D or 3-D image is created on a computer monitor.

Indications

- Vascular abnormalities
- Peripheral arterial insufficiency
- Renal vascular disease
- Aneurysmal disease
- Aortic arch disease
- Abnormal arterial anatomy
- Venous thrombosis
- Venous insufficiency
- Arteriovenous malformation (AVM)
- Tumors of the chest, abdomen, and pelvis
- Diseases of the chest, abdomen, and pelvis
- Heart conditions

Contraindications/Limitations

- Obesity
- Pacemaker
- Metal objects in the body (total replacement joints, pins, clips, valves, etc.)
- Oxygen dependent breathing
- Pregnancy
- Claustrophobia

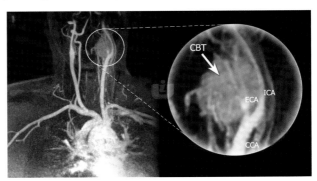

MRI image of a carotid body tumor (CBT)

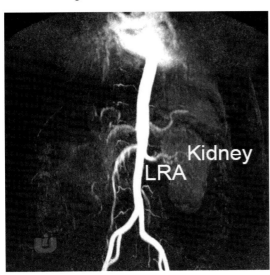

MRA showing a solitary left kidney and patent left renal artery

Angiography

Angiography is derived from the Greek word "angio" for vessel. Angiography is an invasive imaging technique where a radio-opaque contrast material is injected into an artery through a catheter. The contrast makes imaging of the arteries possible with x-ray technology. The images produced provide diagnostic information regarding anatomy and any vascular abnormalities. Images from multiple planes are sometimes necessary for accurate evaluation of any stenotic area.

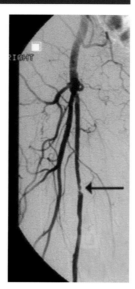

Superficial femoral artery stenosis by angiography

Digital subtraction angiography
(DSA) is an x-ray taken prior to injection of contrast and stored digitally. After injection of a contrast agent, multiple images are taken while the contrast flows through the arteries. The digital information from the original non-contrast image is subtracted from the contrast image, leaving only the contrast image.

Indication

- Peripheral arterial insufficiency
- Renal vascular disease
- Aneurysmal disease
- Aortic arch disease
- Abnormal arterial anatomy
- Arteriovenous malformation (AVM)

Contraindications/Limitations

- Pregnancy
- Allergy to iodinated contrast agent
- Renal failure

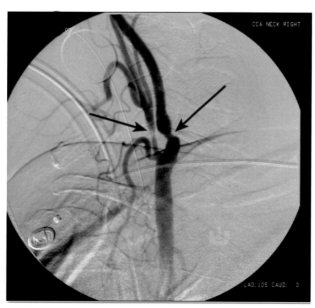

Moderate internal and external carotid artery stenoses by angiography

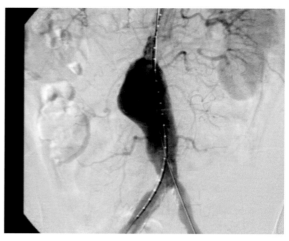

Angiogram of a fusiform aneurysmal abdominal aorta with iliac arteries

Venography

Venography, also known as phlebography, is an invasive imaging technique that injects radio-opaque contrast material into the lumen of a vein (usually in the foot). The contrast makes blood flow visible via x-ray. The x-ray machine emits a burst of radiation that passes through the body and produces an image on photographic film. These films display information regarding venous anatomy and any venous abnormalities.

- There are two types of venography, ascending and descending.
- **Descending venography**: assesses for chronic venous insufficiency
  - The contrast is injected into the common femoral vein (or into a superficial vein in the upper extremity). On the x-ray film, the contrast in the veins either:
    - Returns to the heart (indicating that valves are working normally)
    - Appears to "pool" in the lower extremities (indicating that valves are abnormal)
- **Ascending venography**: assesses for deep vein thrombosis
  - The contrast material is injected into a vein on the top of the foot; the blood clot appears as a deficit in the contrast material on the x-ray image of the veins.
- A method called **digital subtraction venography** may be used to obtain a more intense image of the veins. During this method the surrounding bone and tissue is digitally subtracted, leaving only the veins to be evaluated with greater clarity and detail.

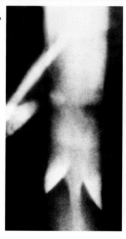

Venous valve on descending venogram
Image courtesy of Terry Needham RVT, FSVU

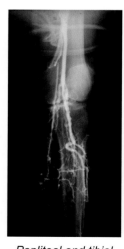

Popliteal and tibial veins on venogram
Image courtesy of Terry Needham RVT, FSVU

Indications

- Deep vein thrombosis (DVT)
- Venous insufficiency
- Vein size (for bypass conduit)
- Arteriovenous malformation (AVM)

Contraindications/Limitations

- Active cellulitis
- Iodinated contrast allergy
- Renal insufficiency

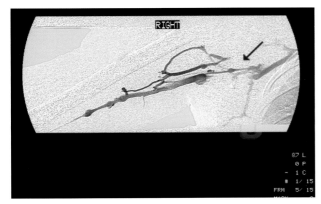

Abnormal venogram SCV occlusion with collaterals

D-dimer Blood Test[5]

A blood sample is obtained intravenously from a patient's arm in order to measure fibrinolytic activity in the blood.

- Fibrinolytic activity reflects the breakdown of fibrin, a protein involved in blood clot formation.
- Fragments called "D-dimer" are a degradation product of fibrin. The D-dimer test is a predictive value for active blood clot (thrombus) formation. An elevated D-dimer level suggests blood clot formation. A low D-dimer value indicates there is likely no activity of blood clot formation in the body.
- A normal D-dimer result, indicating lack of fibrinolytic activity and clotting, is more useful than a positive D-dimer value. See the "Contraindications/Limitation" section.
- A D-dimer value is reported in units of parts per million (ng/ml or ug/ml).
- D-dimer can be helpful in predicting the likelihood of a recurrent thrombosis after 6 months of treatment of an unprovoked venous thrombosis.
- D-dimer is measured on anticoagulant therapy, if normal, the anticoagulants can be stopped and the test repeated in 30 days. If the test remains normal, the risk of recurrent thrombosis is low (about 3% per year). If the test is positive, the risk is > 10% per year. Anticoagulation should be repeated in 3 months.

Indications

- Suspicion of deep vein thrombosis (DVT)
- Suspicion of pulmonary embolism (PE)

Contraindications/Limitations

- Patients may have increased coagulation factors due to conditions other than DVT (e.g., cancer, liver disease, high rheumatoid factor, trauma, pregnancy, advancing age). A false positive test will be the result.

Component Results

Component	Value	Flag	Reference Range	Status
D Dimer Assay	5.98	H	<0.40 ug/ml	Final

Comment:

Note: The literature cut-off for exclusion of DVT/PE for this assay is 0.5

RESULT DOUBLE CHECKED

Abnormal D-dimer Laboratory Report

TABLE 129: **D-dimer Criteria**

Fibrinolytic Blood Values	
Normal range	<500 ng/ml
Elevated range	>500 ng/ml
ng/ml= nanograms per milliliter	

Source: Dunn KL, Wolf JP, Dorfman DM, Fitzpatrick P, Baker JL, Goldhaber SZ. (2002). Normal D-dimer levels in emergency department patients suspected of acute pulmonary embolism. J Am Coll Cardiology, 40, 1475-1478.

Ventilation/Perfusion (VQ) Scan

A VQ scan is a test comprised of two nuclear scans. The first portion of the exam is known as the *ventilation scan*. The second portion of the exam is known as the *perfusion scan*.

Ventilation scan: uses a radioactive gas, such as radionuclide xenon or diethylene triamine pentaacetic acid (DTPA), which is inhaled into the lungs through a mask. A nuclear scan, known as a scintigraphy scan, is performed to identify the areas of the lungs that are not receiving enough air.

Perfusion scan: a radioactive contrast is injected into a vein in the arm which travels to the lungs to identify the areas that are not receiving enough blood flow. Multiple images of the patient's chest are taken at different angles to detect if a blood clot is blocking blood flow through the lungs.

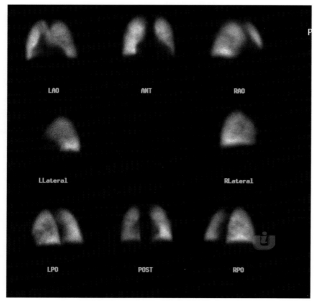

Normal VQ scan

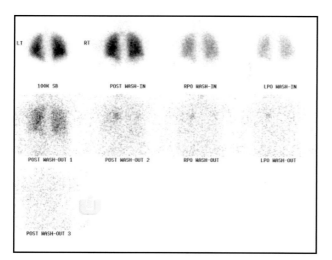

Abnormal VQ scan

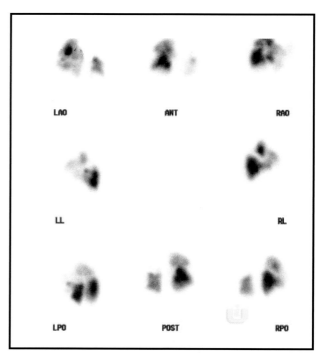

Abnormal perfusion scan

The ventilation images show a uniform distribution of activity on single-breath and wash-in images. There is abnormal Xe-133 retention during the wash-out phase focally in the right upper lung zone.

The perfusion images show multiple medium and large sized segmental defects which in sum make this a high probability examination for pulmonary embolism. These include the right upper posterior segment, and the left upper anterior and apical posterior segments as well as the left lower anterior medial basal segment and lateral basal segment.

IMPRESSION: High probability examination for pulmonary embolism.

Official report for abnormal VQ and perfusion image above

Indications

- Pulmonary embolism (PE)
- Lung function
- Evaluates blood flow (perfusion) through the lungs
- Evaluates air circulation (ventilation) through the lungs

Contraindications/Limitations

- Pregnancy
- Breast feeding
- Treatment using barium contrast within 4 days of the VQ scan

Scoring for Risk of DVT

TABLE 130: Clinical Prediction Criteria for Deep Venous Thrombosis (Wells Criteria)

Condition	# Points Assigned
Cancer treatment or palliative care in past 6 mos.	+1
Paralysis, paresis or recent LE immobilization	+1
Bedridden for >3 days or major surgery within past 4 wks	+1
LE tenderness along deep venous tract	+1
LE swelling of entire limb	+1
Unilateral calf swelling >3 cm	+1
Pitting edema of symptomatic leg	+1
Superficial collaterals	+1
Alternative diagnosis as likely or more likely than DVT	-2

Use total number of points to assess risk

Note: When both legs are symptomatic, use more symptomatic limb

Interpretation of risk according to point total:

High >3 pts
Moderate 1-2 pts
Low <1 pts

Source: Wells PS, Anderson DR, Bormanis J, Guy F, Mitchell M, Gray L, Clement C, Robinson KS, Lewandowski B. (1999). Application of a diagnostic clinical model for the management of hospitalized patients with suspected deep-vein thrombosis. Thromb Haemost, Volume 81:493-7

See also **TABLE 80:** Risk Factors for Acute Deep Venous Thrombosis (Caprini DVT Risk Score) on page 217

TABLE 131: Clinical Prediction Criteria for Pulmonary Embolism

Condition	# Points Assigned
Clinical DVT symptoms	+ 3
Alternative diagnosis as likely or more than DVT	+ 3
Heart rate >100 beats/min	+ 1.5
Major surgery/trauma within past 4 weeks	+ 1.5
History of DVT/PE	+ 1.5
Hemoptysis	+ 1
Malignancy	+ 1

Interpretation of risk according to point total:

High	≥6 pts
Moderate	2-6 pts
Low	≤2 pts

Source: Line JA, Wells PS. (2003). Methodology for a rapid protocol to rule out pulmonary embolism in the emergency department. Annal Emerg Med; 42:266-275.

TABLE 132: Pioped Criteria (Prospective Investigation of Pulmonary Embolism Diagnosis)

The **p**rospective **i**nvestigation **o**f **p**ulmonary **e**mbolism **d**iagnosis (PIOPED) criteria states ranges for diagnosing the likelihood of a pulmonary embolism (PE) by VQ scan:

Probability	Likelihood of PE
High	80-100%
Intermediate	20-80%
Low	0-20%

Source: Medoff, B. (9-13-2008). Pulmonary ventilation/perfusion scan-overview. Retrieved from http://www.umm.edu/ency/article/003828.htm

References:

1. Medoff, B. (9-13-2008). Pulmonary ventilation/perfusion scan-overview. Retrieved from http://www.umm.edu/ency/article/003828.htm.

2. Dunn KL, Wolf JP, Dorfman DM, Fitzpatrick P, Baker JL, Goldhaber SZ. (2002). Normal D-dimer levels in emergency department patients suspected of acute pulmonary embolism. J Am Coll Cardiology, 40, 1475-1478.

3. American Association for Clinical Chemistry. (June 18, 2010) D-dimer. Retrieved from http://www.labtestsonline.org/understanding/analytes/d_dimer/test.html

4. Wells PS, Anderson DR, Rodger M, et al. (2003). Evaluation of D-dimer in the diagnosis of suspected deep-vein thrombosis". N. Engl. J. Med. 349 (13): 1227–35.

5. Kutinsky H, Blakely S, Roche V. (1999). Normal D-dimer levels in patients with pulmonary embolism. Arch Intern Med. 159, 1569-1572.

6. RadiologyInfo.org (March 15, 2010). Retrieved from http://www.radiologyinfo.org

Purpose

Optimizing your image is a way of putting your stamp of approval on a study. Many factors come together in image optimization. General optimization techniques include:

- Ensure the comfort of your patient in terms of environment and positioning. Results of certain vascular studies, such as preoperative vein mapping, can be directly related to environment and patient comfort.
- Choose the transducer which is most appropriate for the study.
  - Abdominal studies should be performed using a lower frequency transducer, such as a curved probe.
  - Evaluate the patient's body habitus as well identifying any swelling or edema in the extremities, as this could lead to the use of lower frequency transducers.

Optimization of Settings

- **Depth**: The depth of the image is shown by the markers on the side of the screen.
  - The vessel or structure of interest should be adjusted to the center of the screen eliminating any excess space above or below the image.
  - The depth is directly related to the pulse repetition period (PRP).

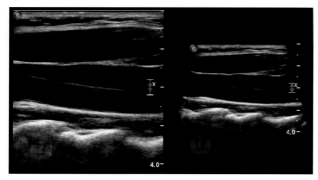

Decreased depth   Increased depth

*Note: decreasing the depth improves
the resolution of the vessel*

- **Gain**: The gain adjusts the overall "brightness" of the image.

  - The gains need to be adjusted appropriately to demonstrate the area of interest without obscuring the image with too many echoes.

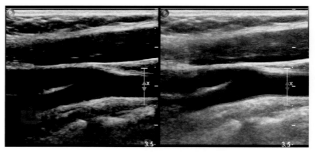

(Figure 1) Appropriately adjusted gain on the left and high gain on the right (sometimes referred to as over gaining) which can obscure the image.

- **Time Gain Compensation (TGC)**: The TGC allows for adjustment of different reflecting echoes at different depths and in return produces an image that is consistent in appearance.
  - Careful attention should be taken not to eliminate low-level echoes, resulting in elimination of soft/ homogeneous appearing plaque.
  - The TGC controls aid in creating a uniform brightness from top to bottom in the image.

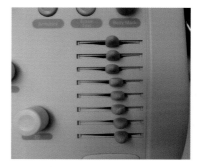

(Figure 2) Typical TGC controls on a duplex machine

- **Focus (focal zones)**: The focal zone(s) should be placed beside the vessel or structure of interest.
  - This is the point at which the ultrasound beam becomes the most intense.
  - This feature is adjustable so it can "focus" on a particular point in the image and provide the highest quality detail possible. (Figure 3)

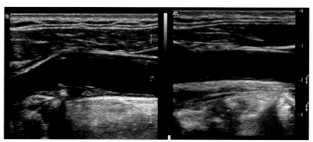

(Figure 3) The focal zone(s) are usually placed just below or next to the structure of interest

Active Gains

Active gains include color/power Doppler and spectral Doppler.

- **Color Doppler:** Color should fill the lumen of the vessel or structure without "bleeding" outside of the vessel. (Figure 4).

  - Adjusting the wall filter can eliminate any low frequency Doppler shifts outside the vessel wall.

  - It is important to be able to visualize any intralumenal wall irregularities that may be present.

  - It may be necessary to decrease the scale to fill in low flow state vessels or increase the scale in areas of higher velocities.

  - While it is important to eliminate excess color outside the vessel wall, it is equally important to ensure the lumen of the vessel fills with color. (Figure 5)

  - If the lumen is not filling with color, it could be suggestive of obstruction. It is important to apply power Doppler (color angio) to evaluate for low flow states or occlusions.

  > *Spectral Doppler should also be used to determine an obstruction.*

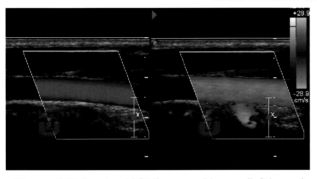

(Figure 4) Color should fill the vessel lumen (left image) without spilling out the vessel wall (right image)

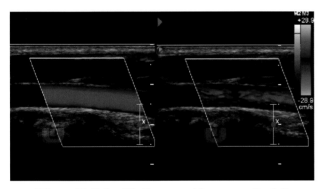

(Figure 5) Color fills the vessel lumen on the left. Having the color gain set too low causes poor color filling within the vessel lumen (right)

- **Spectral Doppler**: It is important to demonstrate the silhouette of the Doppler waveform. Over gained waveforms can overestimate the velocity as under gained waveforms can underestimate the velocity. (Figure 6 & 7)

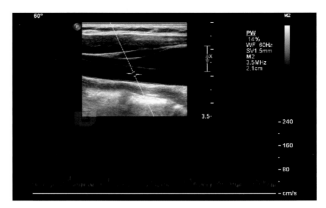

(Figure 6) Under-gained Doppler waveforms are difficult to measure.

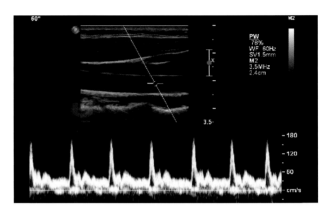

(Figure 7) Over-gained Doppler waveform creates spectral broadening and can over estimate velocities.

- Aliasing occurs when the sampled velocity is too high in comparison to the setting of the scale.

  - The Doppler waveform appears at the bottom of Doppler scale, in turn making the measurement inaccurate. (Figure 8)

  - The scale needs to be increased to allow for the higher velocities in order to eliminate aliasing.

  - Adjusting the baseline is also another option.

> HINT: In many cases where aliasing occurs, a combination of increasing the scale and adjusting the baseline is necessary to optimize the spectral waveform.

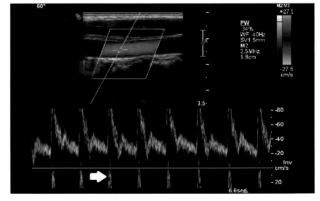

(Figure 8) Doppler aliasing

- **Frame rate**: A desirable image has a higher frame rate which increases the temporal resolution. Frame rate is affected by multiple factors:
  - Focal zones
  - Sector width of the image
  - Color box
  - Depth

> *Note: Multiple frame rates, larger color boxes, increased depth and width of the image will slow down the frame rate. Try to reduce as many of these as possible.*

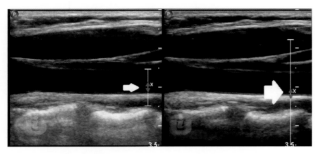

One, smaller focal zone | Multiple, larger focal zones

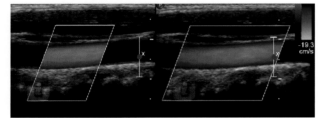

Narrow color box/ sector width | Wider color box/sector width

- **Compression**: Compression alters the appearance of the grey scale image allowing it to be in range of the human eye.
  - Compression is adjustable by the sonographer.
  - An image with higher compression demonstrates more shades of grey. (Figure 9)
  - An image with lower compression demonstrates less shades of grey. (Figure 9).

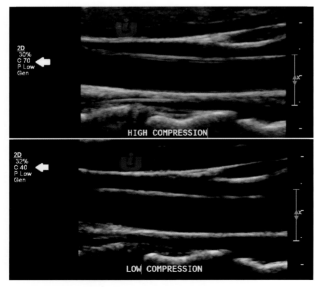

(Figure 9) Examples of high and low compression

- **Doppler Angle**: The Doppler cursor should be placed in the middle of the vessel and be parallel to the flow within the vessel.
- **Angle of the color Doppler box**: Due to the cosine of the angle, correct steering of the color box will ensure maximum color fill. (Figure 10)
  - The cosine of the angle is in reference to the beam of the ultrasound and the blood flow.
  - Incorrect steering of the color box prevents complete color fill of the vessel lumen. (Figures 11-12)

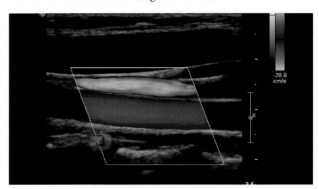

(Figure 10) Correct steering of the color box optimizes color filling

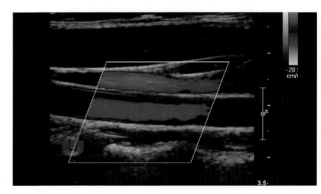

(Figure 11) Suboptimal color flow noted when the color box angle is poorly optimized

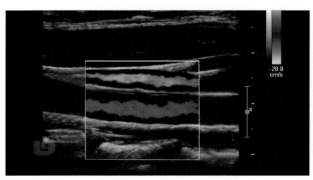

(Figure 12) Minimal or no color flow is detected when the color box is perpendicular to flow

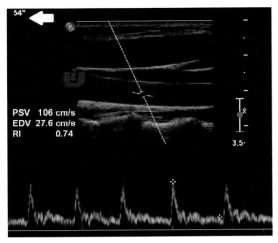

Doppler angle <60°: Velocity underestimated

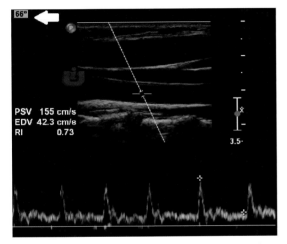

Doppler angle >60°: Velocity overestimated

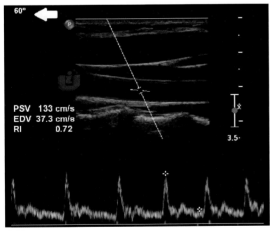

Doppler angle at 60°: Optimal velocity

Points to Remember

- Be familiar with your ultrasound machine and its capabilities, this is essential to optimize the image. The ultrasound machine is only as useful as you make it.

- A brief, initial evaluation of your patient and decisions about what type of probe and examination presets will be used are the first few steps in ensuring an optimal study.

- Prior to capturing each image, perform a quick run through, evaluating each of the settings. This will help optimize your images.

- Capturing an accurate velocity is one of the most important components in vascular ultrasound.

- Remain perpendicular to your vessel when scanning in B-mode.

- Try to keep the sample volume gate at 1.5 mm and the sample gate centered in the lumen whenever possible.

- If there are reverberations throughout the vessel, change the B-mode gain.

- Adequate color flow in the vertebral arteries may be difficult. Try the following adjustments:
  - Increase the color gain
  - Decrease the color scale
  - Increase the color gate
  - Increase the color filter

- A quality image of the distal SFA can be difficult to obtain. Try "harmonics" to make the vessel stand out. Enlarge the image and create a smaller color box. Apply pressure to omit any venous flow interference.

- The subclavian artery can also be difficult to image:
  - Recall your anatomy. The mid subclavian vessels run underneath the clavicle bone. Start with the transducer at the clavicular area (supraclavicular is suggested).
  - Begin with the transducer in sagittal and with the notch towards the head. The opposite end of the transducer should touch the clavicle.
  - Using enough gel, a longitudinal view of both the proximal and distal subclavian vessels can often be visualized in a single image.

- If you are not getting adequate color flow through a vessel, try the following adjustments:
  - Turn up the gain. Increase all the way up till you see color "speckles" and decrease from there.
  - Decrease the scale (especially for calf veins)
  - Decrease the frequency
  - Increase the color filter
  - Increase the size of the color gate
  - Change transducers (use an abdominal probe for difficult/ obese patients)
  - Place the patient in reverse Trendelenberg while imaging lower extremity veins

References

1. Non Invasive Vascular Diagnostics, *A Practical Guide to Therapy , 2nd Edition*, Ali F. AbuRahma MD, FACS, FRCS, RVT, RPVI, John J Bergan MD, FACS, Hon FRCS; Springer-Verlag London Limited 2007; ISBN-13: 978-1-84628-446-5; Pg 262 graft surveys

2. Vascular Technology, *An Illustrated Review, 3Rd Edition*, Claudia Rumwell RN, RVT, FSVU, Michalene McPharlin RN, RVT, FSVU, Davies Publishing, Inc 2006, ISBN-0-941022-69-2

3. Understanding Ultrasound Physics, 3rd Edition, Sidney Edelman, Ph.D., Copyright 2007, ISBN 0-9626444-4-7

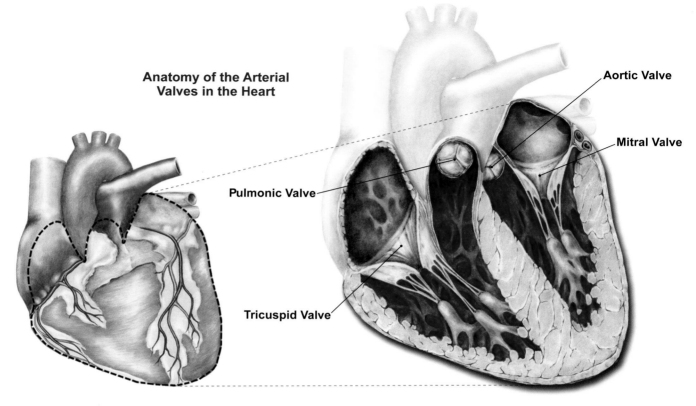

Anatomy of the Arterial Valves in the Heart

Aortic Valve

Mitral Valve

Pulmonic Valve

Tricuspid Valve

Image courtesy of Echo-web.com

Introduction

According to the American Heart Association, cardiovascular disease is still the leading cause of death for U.S. men and women and risk factors are on the rise. When performing a vascular exam in the aging population, heart disease must be considered and a general knowledge of how heart disease affects the Doppler waveform in the vascular examination should be understood. Abnormal Doppler spectral waveforms may not always be associated with vascular disease. Certain conditions can either over estimate or under estimate the stenosis. Using a combination of velocities and velocity ratios, along with an algorithm, weighting the findings of each should be used.

TABLE 133: **Summary of Cardiac Effect on Spectral Doppler Vascular Waveforms**	
Over Estimate Stenosis: High Cardiac Output	**Under Estimate Stenosis: Low Cardiac Output**
Chronic anemia	Congestive heart failure
Chronic hypercapnia	Cardiac valvular problems
Sepsis	Coronary artery disease
Beriberi heart disease	Cardiac diastolic dysfunction
Sickle cell anemia	Pericarditis
Pregnancy	Congenital heart disease
Obesity	Cardiomyopathy
Hepatic disease	Systemic hypertension
Carcinoid syndrome	Anemia
Paget's disease	Cardiac arrhythmias
Multiple myeloma	Atrial fibrillation
Cardiac arrhythmias	Cardiac tamponade

High Cardiac Output

An increase in cardiac output (normal range: 4 to 6 liters per minute (Lpm)) may result in an increase in peak systolic velocities. The ICA/CCA ratio may be useful to calculate when the B-mode information does not match the increased systolic velocities. The following disease states are associated with increased cardiac output:

- Chronic anemia
- Chronic hypercapnia
- Sepsis
- Beriberi heart disease
- Pregnancy
- Obesity
- Hepatic disease
- Carcinoid syndrome
- Paget's disease
- Multiple myeloma
- Cardiac volume overload diseases
- Cardiac arrhythmias (compensatory beats)

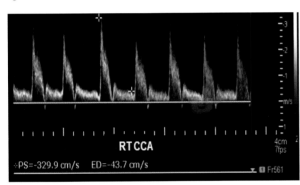

Spectral Doppler waveform of the CCA in a patient with high cardiac output. This waveform will be noted in the CCA bilaterally.

Low Cardiac Output

A reduction in cardiac output may result in a decrease in peak systolic velocities. The ICA/CCA ratio may be useful to calculate when the B-mode information does not match the decreased peak systolic velocity. Low cardiac output is defined as a cardiac output below 4 lpm. The following disease states are associated with low cardiac output:

- Congestive heart failure
- Low ejection fraction (EF%)
- Coronary artery disease
- Cardiac diastolic dysfunction
- Pericarditis
- Congenital heart disease
- Cardiomyopathy
- Systemic hypertension
- Anemia

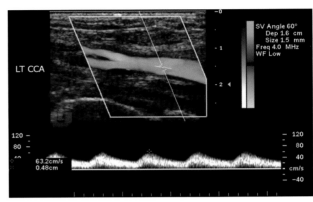

Spectral Doppler waveform of low cardiac output from a patient with severe congestive heart failure. This waveform will be noted in the CCA bilaterally and should not be confused with a waveform that is found with a proximal high grade stenosis.

> Hint: The low cardiac output will be seen in all the vessels examined and should not be confused with proximal high grade stenosis.

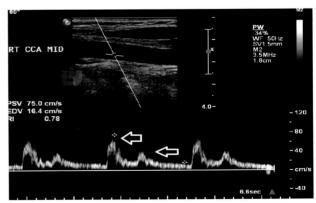

Pulsus Alternans is usually caused by idiopathic dilated cardiomyopathy and cardiac tamponade. The peak systolic velocity of the vessel alternates between two levels on sequential beats; notice the rhythm is regular within the cardiac cycle. This rhythm can also be associated with hypocalcemia, or IVC compression.[1]

> Hint: When performing vascular exams on patients with significant cardiac disease, the velocity ratio is usually more useful than the peak systolic velocity (PSV) in the exam interpretation when the abnormality is found throughout the cardiac cycle.

Aortic Regurgitation (AR)

Aortic regurgitation is defined as the back flow of blood through the aortic valve during ventricular diastole into the ventricle. Some labs may refer to aortic regurgitation as aortic insufficiency.

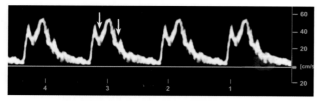

Pulsus Bisferiens is seen in approximately 50% of patients with aortic valvular disease and can also be associated with hypertrophic cardiomyopathy.

- Aortic regurgitation may be acute or chronic.
- An echocardiogram will be required to ascertain the presence, etiology and quantification of aortic regurgitation.
- Severe aortic regurgitation results in a volume overload of the left ventricle.
- Increased pressures may inhibit pulmonary return.
- AR can result in dilation of the left ventricle.
- Doppler waveforms of the aorta and the great vessels may show holo-diastolic flow reversal characteristics.
- When aortic regurgitation or stenosis is present, a "double peaked" vascular waveform may be seen.

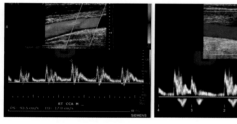

Bisferiens waveform from two separate patients with aortic valvular disease.

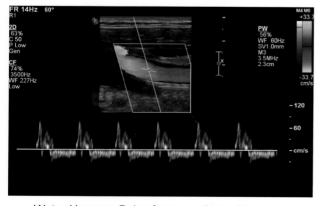

Water-Hammer Pulse from a patient with severe aortic regurgitation. The end diastolic flow is actually reversed due to the severe regurgitation.

Aortic Stenosis (AS)

Aortic stenosis is the narrowing and restriction of antegrade blood flow through the aortic valve.

- The most common etiologies of aortic stenosis are as follows:
  - Congenital (e.g., bicuspid aortic valve)
  - Degenerative and rheumatic. Severe aortic stenosis is defined as the narrowing of the aortic valve area <1.0 cm^2.
  - Doppler interrogation of the ascending aorta will usually show increased velocities.
  - In cases of severe aortic stenosis, Doppler interrogation of the common carotid artery may only show a low amplitude, turbulent PW waveform with a prolonged acceleration time. This finding may be most apparent in the proximal common carotid artery spectral tracing.
  - Severe AS is associated with a BSA <.06 cm^2

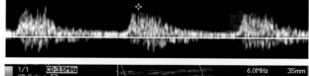

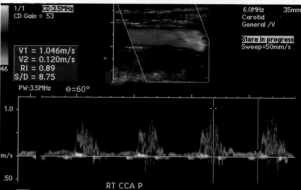

Low amplitude and turbulent spectral Doppler waveforms of the CCA. These waveforms should be noted in the CCA bilaterally and should not be confused with a stenosis.

> *Hint: In a patient with aortic stenosis the PSV will be underestimated; use the ratio for interpretation of disease.*

- The ICA/CCA ratio may be useful to calculate when the B-mode information does not match the decreased peak systolic velocity.
- Overall systemic circulation will be reduced and low amplitude signals will be present.
- Low brachial blood pressures may be seen bilaterally. (If unilateral, you should suspect subclavian stenosis.)

Mitral Stenosis (MS)

Mitral Stenosis is the narrowing and restriction of antegrade blood flow through the mitral valve.

- Severe MS will cause a pressure overload in the left atrium and reduced filling of the left ventricle.
- Doppler waveforms of the aorta and carotid arteries may show low amplitude signals as a secondary result of MS.

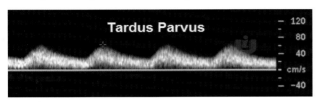

A low amplitude Doppler waveform can result in the CCA secondary to severe mitral stenosis characterized by a rounded, prolonged peak with diminished amplitude. Parvus tardus waveforms are often identified distal to a severe stenosis.

Mitral Regurgitation (MR)

Mitral regurgitation is the abnormal back flow of blood through the mitral valve.

- Severe mitral regurgitation results in a volume overload of the left atrium (LA) which in turn will result in increased pressures in the left atrium and pulmonary capillary wedge.
- Increased pressures will inhibit pulmonary venous return.
- MR can result in dilation of pulmonic veins. (There are 4 pulmonary veins that return blood into the LA.)
- Doppler waveforms of the pulmonary veins show marked reversal characteristics during systole, particularly in the systolic pulmonary vein waveform.
- MR does not usually affect the spectral Doppler in vascular exams.

Tricuspid Regurgitation (TR)

Tricuspid regurgitation is the abnormal back flow of blood through the tricuspid valve.

- Severe tricuspid regurgitation results in a volume overload of the right atrium.
- Increased pressures in the right atrium (RA) will restrict/inhibit venous return.
- TR can result in dilation of the RA, IVC and hepatic veins.
- Doppler waveforms of the hepatic veins and IVC may show marked reversal characteristics during systole.
- Jugular vein distention may be also be present.
- Systolic murmur maybe present

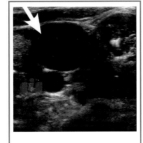

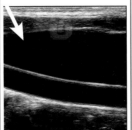

Dilated internal jugular vein caused from elevated pressures within the right side of the heart.

- Increased or elevated pressures within the right side of the heart may result in pulsatility of hepatic, portal, internal jugular vein and peripheral veins.

Pulmonary Regurgitation (PR)

Pulmonary regurgitation is the abnormal back flow of blood through the pulmonic valve. Some labs refer to pulmonary regurgitation as pulmonic insufficiency.

Severe pulmonary regurgitation results in a volume overload of the right ventricle.

- Increased pressures can inhibit venous return.
- PR can result in dilation of the right ventricle.
- Doppler waveforms of the pulmonary arteries may show marked flow reversal components during diastole.
- Increased or elevated pressures within the right side of the heart may result in pulsatility of peripheral veins.

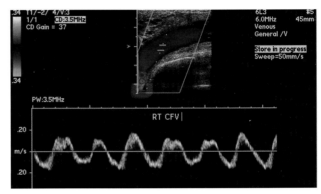

Increased pulsatility noted in a common femoral vein caused from elevated pressure within the right side of the heart.

Pulmonic Stenosis (PS)

Pulmonic stenosis is the narrowing and restriction of antegrade blood flow through the pulmonic valve.

- Severe pulmonic stenosis will cause a pressure overload in the right ventricle and reduced flow to the pulmonary arteries.
- Doppler waveforms of the pulmonary arteries may show increased amplitude and turbulent waveform patterns.
- Increased or elevated pressures within the right side of the heart may result in pulsatility of peripheral veins.

Tricuspid Stenosis (TS)

Tricuspid stenosis is the narrowing and restriction of antegrade blood flow through the tricuspid valve.

- Severe tricuspid stenosis will cause a pressure overload in the right atrium and reduced filling of the right ventricle.
- Doppler waveforms of the main pulmonary artery may exhibit a turbulent waveform pattern.
- IVC and hepatic veins may become dilated.

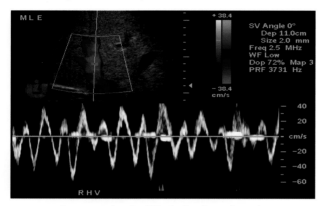

Increased pulsatility in the hepatic vein

Cardiac Tamponade

Cardiac tamponade is an emergent cardiac finding. There is a reduction in diastolic filling of the heart due to increase intrapericardial pressures from the accumulation of fluid or blood around the heart (pericardial effusion).

- Patients with cardiac tamponade are considered to have emergent findings and should be addressed immediately.
- The classic clinical finding for cardiac tamponade is *pulsus paradoxus*, defined as a drop in systolic blood pressure by greater than 10mmHg upon inspiration. This drop in blood pressure is due to a reduction of left ventricular filling during inspiration.
- Consequently the carotid PW Doppler spectral tracing will demonstrate a decrease in peak systolic carotid Doppler signal.
- Conversely, there is an increase in left ventricular filling with expiration resulting in an augmented peak systolic carotid Doppler signal velocity during expiration. This is referred to as *respiratory variation*.

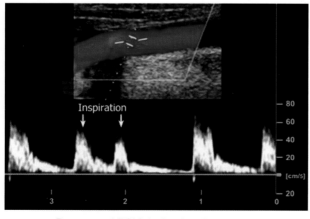

Decreased PSV during inspiration and increased PSV during expiration

Constrictive Pericarditis

Constrictive pericarditis is the thickening of the pericardium due to inflammation which interferes with the diastolic filling of the heart.

IVC dilation without inspiratory collapse is a very helpful sign of constrictive pericarditis.

- Commonly seen in post-cardiac surgery
- Distension of the internal jugular vein, IVC and peripheral edema is usually present.
- The resultant carotid PW Doppler spectral tracing will demonstrate a decrease in peak systolic velocity upon inspiration.

Cardiac Arrhythmias

Cardiac arrhythmias exhibit irregular spectral Doppler waveforms that correspond with the heart rhythm and rate.

- Vascular labs have adopted several different methods of measuring velocities when arrhythmias are present.
- A common technique used when an irregular rhythm is present is to take the measurement of the most consistent beats. This may be a string of three or more.
- In cases where the rhythm present is "irregularly irregular" (no pattern that can be followed), it becomes more difficult. An average of the 3-5 most consistent beats may be taken. This is more subjective and care should be taken when reporting results using this method. Diameter and area reduction tools may prove extremely useful in cases of irregularly irregular arrhythmias.
- In cases where an intraortic balloon pump is being used, it may be difficult to determine underlying rhythm.

> *Some physicians will allow the balloon pump to be turned off for brief periods so underlying rhythms can be seen and measurements taken.*
> **This should NOT be done by the sonographer!**

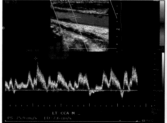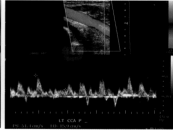

Spectral waveform from a patient on a intra-aortic balloon pump (IABP)

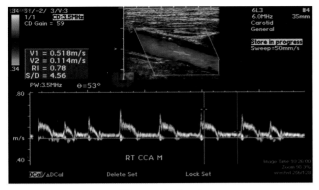

Sinus arrhythmia

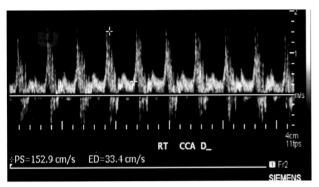

Sinus tachycardia

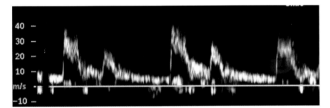

Bigeminy rhythm

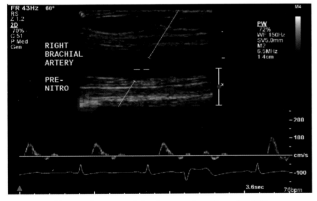

Premature ventricular contraction (PVC)

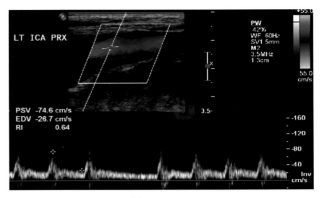

Sinus pause

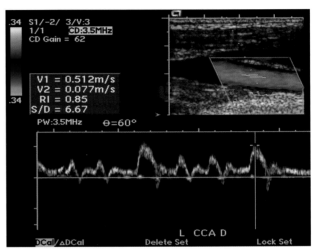

Trigeminy

Atrial Fibrillation

Atrial fibrillation is a common cardiac arrhythmia which may result in a mixture of short and long R-R cardiac cycles. It is the fibrillation of the two upper chambers of the heart (atria). The carotid PW Doppler spectral waveform may appear to have a variety of peak systolic velocities due to the varying R-R intervals. It is recommended to measure 3 to 5 beats and average.

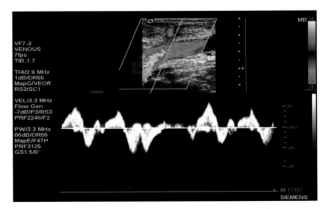

Atrial fibrillation noted in the venous waveform

Cardiac Rhythm Diagnosis

Normal Pulse
smooth upstroke

"Water-hammer Pulse"
associated with aortic insufficiency
Note: rapid upstroke and rapid fall in diastole

Anacrotic Pulse
associated with aortic stenosis
Note: delayed upstroke

Dicrotic Pulse
associated with decreased arterial tone
Note: accentuated secondary pulse wave
(may feel like heart rate is twice as fast as normal)
use direct method with stethoscope

Pulsus Bisferiens
associated with combined aortic stenosis and insufficiency
Note: double peaks

Pulsus Alternans
usually associated with heart failure
Note: large pulse wave followed by small secondary wave

Pulsus Paradoxus
usually associated with cardiac
tamponade or constrictive pericarditis
Note: diminished pulses during inspiration

Image courtesy of Echo-web.com

TABLE 134: Effects of Cardiac Diseases on the Spectral Waveform

Disease	Effect on Spectral Waveform
High cardiac output	Increased systolic velocity
Low cardiac output	Decreased systolic velocity
Aortic Regurgitation	Double peaked waveform and/or reversal during diastole; diminished or absent dicrotic notch
Aortic Stenosis	Low amplitude and/or turbulent waveform; parvus-tardus
Mitral Stenosis	Low amplitude
Mitral Regurgitation	No effect usually in the vascular exam
Tricuspid Regurgitation	Increased pulsatility in the venous waveform
Pulmonic Regurgitation	Increased pulsatility in the venous waveform
Pulmonary Stenosis	Increased pulsatility in the venous waveform
Tricuspid Stenosis	Increased pulsatility in the venous waveform
Cardiac Tamponade	Decreased peak systolic velocity during inspiration and increased peak systolic velocity during expiration
Constrictive Pericarditis	Decreased peak systolic velocity during inspiration and increased peak systolic during expiration
Cardiac Arrhythmia	Varying peak systolic velocity

TABLE 135: Cardiac Diseases and Symptoms

Condition	Mitral Stenosis	Mitral Regurgitation	Aortic Stenosis	Aortic Regurgitation	Mitral Valve Prolapse
General Complaints	Fatigue; DOE; palpations; hemoptysis; hoarseness; orthopnea; PND	Dyspnea; fatigue; exercise intolerance; orthopnea; palpitations	Fatigue; dyspnea; orthopnea; angina pectoris; dizziness; syncope	Dyspnea on exertion; palpitation; orthopnea; exertional chest pain	Dyspnea; syncope; palpitations; sharp chest pain unrelated to exercise; fatigue
Physical Examination	Resting tachycardia; irregular pulse; jugular venous distention in the presence of RV failure; pulmonary hypertension except in atrial fibrillation	Irregular pulse; sharp upstroke of arterial pulse; jugular venous distention in presence of RV failure; prominent "A" wave in presence of increased RV pressure	Early: normal blood pressure; late-systolic blood pressure decreased; narrow pulse pressure; carotid pulse is slow with small pulse volume	Arterial pulsation; bounding pulse with rapid rise and fall (waterhammer pulse); widened pulse pressure; head bobbing (Musset's sign); skin warm, damp and flushed	May not be any particular signs of cardiac disease unless regurgitation becomes detectable. Most patients are young women.
Palpation	Diastolic thrill at apex	Apical impulse forceful and downwardly displaced to left	Systolic thrill palpable at base of heart; apical pulse strong and sustained throughout systole	Diastolic thrill along left sternal border; laterally displaced apically; systolic thrill in jugular notch and along carotid arteries	May not be any particular signs of cardiac disease unless regurgitation becomes detectable
Auscultation	Loud S1; opening snap; low snap; low pitched, rumbling diastolic murmur	Diminished or absent S1; wide splitting of S2; presence of S3; presence of S4 heard in severe regurgitation; holosystolic murmur heard best at apex	Diminished or absent A2; harsh crescendo-decrescendo systolic murmur heart best at base (second intercostal space to right of sternum); aortic ejection sound	Decrescendo diastolic murmur (blowing); high pitched and heard best at base	Systolic click and apical systolic murmur usually high pitched and quite musical
EKG	LA enlargement; notched P wave (P Mitral); RV hypertrophy	LA enlargement; LV hypertrophy; atrial fibrillation	LV hypertrophy; conduction defects; first degree AV block; LBBB	LV hypertrophy	Normal; may show ST segments and T wave abnormalities, especially in inferior leads or prominent U waves; dysrhythmias; supraventricular tachyarrhymias; premature atrial or ventricular beats
Chest X-Ray	LA and RV enlargement; pulmonary venous congestion; pulmonary edema	LA and LV enlargement; pulmonary vascular congestion	Post-stenotic; dilatation of aorta; aorta valve calcification	Aortic valve calcification; LV enlargement; dilation of ascending aorta	Identifies or confirms presence of skeletal abnormalities
Echocardiogram	Decreased excursion of mitral leaflets; diminished E-F slope; enlarged LA	LA enlargement; hyperdynamic LV	Nonrestricted movement of aortic valve; thickening of LV wall	LV dilated; diastolic flutter of anterior leaflet of mitral; vibration of septal wall	Mild to moderate: anterior and/or posterior mitral leaflets separation at the coaptation point of the cusps; enlarged LA size; chordal rupture
Cardiac Cath	Pressure gradient across mitral valve; LA and PAW pressure increased; low cardiac output (fixed)	LVEDP increased; LA pressure increased; angiography with contrast media performed to quantify regurgitation	LVEDP increased; pressure gradient across the aortic valve	Pulse pressure increased; LVEDP increased; LA pressure increased; angiography with contrast media performed to quantify regurgitation	Normal unless mitral regurgitation present; LV angiogram shows the prolapsed mitral valve

Courtesy of Echo-web.com

Points to Remember

- Left ventricular and aortic valve abnormalities mainly affect arterial hemodynamics (pulse contour and pressure).
- Right ventricular and tricuspid valve abnormalities mainly affect venous hemodynamics.
- If the spectral waveform abnormality stems from cardiac issues, the waveform abnormality is usually seen throughout the vascular exam, it is important to compare waveforms bilaterally.
- Increased cardiac pressures can result in increased recorded velocities (e.g., hyperdynamic left ventricle).
- Decreased cardiac pressures can result in decreased recorded velocities (e.g., low ejection fraction, aortic stenosis).
- Increased or elevated right sided cardiac pressures may result in pulsatility in peripheral veins (e.g., CHF).
- If pulsatile venous flow is noted in the lower extremities, clinical correlation should be considered for pulmonary embolism (PE).
- When a cardiac arrhythmia is encountered, consider waiting for a short period of time to begin or continue exam, as these can be intermittent in some patients.
- Pulsatility of hepatic and subclavian veins is normal due to the proximity to the heart. Peripheral veins will normally exhibit phasic respiratory flow.
- Carotid intimal thickening is considered an indicator of coronary artery disease (CAD) when greater than 1 mm. These patients may not have CAD but will be considered high risk for CAD.
- High resistant arterial waveforms that have a diminished or absent dicrotic notch indicate aortic valve disease may be present (e.g. AR).
- Paradoxical embolism occurs when an emboli crosses from the right side of the heart to the left through a defect in the septum resulting in a stroke. Septum defects fall into two categories. Atrial septal defect (ASD) is when there is a "hole" in the septum dividing the two atria. Ventricular septal defect (VSD) is when there is a "hole" in the septum dividing the two ventricles. PFO (Patent Foramen Ovale) can also be a source of embolism.
- Cardiomyopathies are diseases that affect the myocardial (muscular) layer of the heart. There are several types. This disease can affect the heart globally and segmentally. Cardiomyopathies may affect ejection fraction, cardiac output and pressures within the heart.
- Any cardiac disease present may have effect on the vascular system. These effects can be seen in the arterial and venous waveforms. Careful examination of patient history will prove useful.
- Cardiac valvular problems can be congenital, genetic, inflammatory, stress or structural based.

References

1. Rohren, Eric, Kliewer, Mark et al. (2003). A Spectrum of Doppler Waveforms in the Carotid and Vertebral Arteries. AJR, 181:1695-1704.
2. Bendick, Phillip, Cardiac Effects on Peripheral Vascular Doppler Waveforms, Journal for Vascular Ultrasound, 35(4):237-243, 2011.
3. Reynolds, Terry. (2008). The Echocardiographers' Pocket Reference, 3rd edition. Phoenix, School of Cardiac Ultrasound.
4. Reynolds, Terry. (1997). Cardiovascular Principles: A registry Exam Preparation Guide. Phoenix, School of Cardiac Ultrasound.
5. Kaddoura, Sam. (2002). In Echo Made Easy Philadelphia: Elsevier Saunders.
6. http://www.cdc.gov/heartdisease/facts.htm. 2012
7. http://www.echo-web.com

Aneurysm

- The main treatment is corrective surgery.
- Antihypertensives are sometimes used to control blood pressure and thus enlargement of the aneurysm.

Aortic Coarctation

- Antihypertensives are often used before and after surgery to control blood pressure.
- Infants may receive alprostadil to help keep the ductus arteriosus open to serve as a bypass until the coarctation is repaired.

Arterial Dissection

- Although main treatment is surgery, IV esmolol is often used to decrease the rate of rise of left ventricular pressure (dP/dt), then nitropresside to reduce afterload if blood pressure is still too high.
- Heparin and/or warfarin are often used to prevent clot formation in dissected area.

Arteritis *see vasculitis*

Atherosclerosis

There is no direct treatment, just management of risk factors.

For patients with hyperlipidemia

- Statin
- Niacin
- Cholesterol absorption inhibitors
- Fibrates
- Bile acid resins

For diabetic patients:

- Sulfonulureas
- Meglitinides
- Biguanides
- Thiazolidinediones
- Alpha-glucosidase inhibitors
- Insulin
- DPP-4 inhibitors
- Bile acid sequestrants
- Incretin mimetics
- Amylin analogues

For hypertensive patients:

- Diuretics
- Beta blockers
- ACE inhibitors
- ARBs
- CCBs
- Alpha blockers
- Central alpha agonists
- Direct renin inhibitors

Other agents include:

- Antiplatelets
- Anticoagulants
- Thrombolytics
- Steroids

Carotid Body Tumor

Treatment is surgical.

Cerebrovascular Events (TIA/Stroke)

- If blood pressure is too high, IV labetolol is first line.
- Alteplase is the only FDA-approved thrombolytic for stroke.
- No antiplatelets or anticoagulants should be given for 24 hours.
- May use heparin or low molecular weight heparin (LMWH) for VTE prophylaxis after 48 hours.
- For non-cardioembolic stroke, antiplatelets are recommended for secondary prevention.
- For cardioembolic stroke, ASA is recommended for low risk patients, and warfarin for high-risk patients for secondary prevention.
- For ischemic stroke, Factor VIIa is sometimes used, but there is a lack of evidence of efficacy.
- Supportive care is often the only treatment, including:
  - Blood pressure control
  - VTE prophylaxis
  - Seizure prophylaxis
  - Reduction of ICP

Fibromuscular Dysplasia

- Daily aspirin is generally considered first-line treatment.
- Plavix or Aggrenox can be substituted/added as necessary.

Lymphedema

- Diuretics have been used somewhat successfully, but the oncotic pressure of lymph quickly causes recurrence of edema.
- Benzopyrones have also been used, but are no longer recommended.
- Refractory pain can be managed with analgesics, concomitant TCA, corticosteroids, anticonvulsants, and local anesthetics.

May-Thurner Syndrome

Prescribed medications include those to treat venous thrombosis.

TABLE 136: Anticoagulants and Thrombolytics

Class	Agents
Anticoagulants (clot prevention)	Warfarin
Thrombolytics (clot treatment)	Streptokinase, Urokinase, Anistreplse, Alteplase, Reteplase, Tenecteplase

Mesenteric Ischemia

- The vasodilator papverine is often given if the condition is discovered during angiography, or during and after surgery to repair this condition.
- Heparin, warfarin, and thrombolytics are often used to treat and prevent clot formation.

Neointimal Hyperplasia

- The current treatment regimen involves the placement of drug-eluding stents.

Phlegmasia Alba or Cerulea Dolens
see venous thromboembolism

Popliteal Artery Entrapment Syndrome

- No drug therapy indicated unless thrombus is present. If present, options include:
- Streptokinase
- Reteplase
- Anistreplase
- Tenecteplase
- Alteplase

Popliteal Cystic Disease

- Pharmaceutical treatment is strictly supportive, likely corticosteroids.

Portal Hypertension

- Primary prophylaxis is with non-selective beta adrenergic blockers. Agents include:
  - Propranolol
  - Nadolol
- For acute variceal bleeding:
  - Somatostatin
  - Octreotide
  - Vasopressin

Postphlebitic Syndrome/ Venous Insufficiency

- There is no indication for pharmacologic treatment of postphlebitic syndrome.
- Proper anticoagulation after VTE may prevent the onset of the condition.

Pseudoaneurysm

- Preliminary evidence suggests that sonographically-directed percutanous injection of thrombin is safe and effective.
  - Overall success rate of 96%
  - Usual dose of 1-5 mL of thrombin

Raynaud's Phenomenon

- Medications may be prescribed to dilate blood vessels.

TABLE 137: Pharmacology

Class	Agents
Dihydropyridine calcium channel blockers	Nifedipine, amlodipine, felodipine, isradipine
Angiotensin receptor antagonist	Losartan
Selective serotonin reuptake inhibitor	Fluoxetine
Alpha adrenergic antagonists	Prazosin
Prostaglandins	Epoprostenol, alprostadil

Alternatives include: nitroglycerin ointment and pentoxyfylline

Renovascular Hypertension

- This condition is often treated surgically.
- Renal function may deteriorate even with controlled blood pressure. Agents often used include:
  - ACEIs (first line)
  - CCBs (slightly less effective but safer)

Subclavian Steal Syndrome

- No pharmacological treatment is known to be of value in the treatment of this syndrome.

Superior Vena Cava Syndrome

- Diuretics are often used to reduce the pressure on the vena cava. Furosemide is most common.
- Steroids are sometimes used to decrease the swelling of any tumors exerting pressure.
- Anticoagulants and thrombolytics are used to treat and prevent clot formation.

Thoracic Outlet Compression Syndrome

- Anti-inflammatory, pain medication and muscle relaxants are commonly prescribed.

TABLE 138: Anti-inflammatory

Class	Agents
NSAIDS	ASA, naproxen, IBU, diclofenac
Anticoagulant	Warfarin
Muscle relaxants	Baclofen, carisoprodol, cyclobenzaprine

Alternatives include:
Nerve block and thrombolytics for acute blockage

Varicose Veins

- Sclerotherapy is the standard treatment.
- Additional agents include:
  – Sotradecol
  – Scleromate
  – Polidocanol (not FDA approved for use in the U.S.)

Vasculitis

- Standard treatment is corticosteroids, including prednisone and methylprednisone.
- Controversial agents include non-steroidal anti-inflammatory drugs (NSAIDs), azathioprine, cyclophosphamide, dapsone, methotrexate.

Venous Thromboembolism / Pulmonary Embolism

- Empiric treatment should be started in all patients with suspected DVT or PE.
- "Unfractionated heparin" (UFH, class = antithrombotic) and subqutaneous low-molecular weight heparin (LMWH) are common drugs used in treatment.
- Initially give IV UFH or SQ LMWH; overlap with warfarin therapy.
- LMWH (e.g., Enoxaparin, Dalteparin, Tinzaparin, Lovenox) should be stopped once patient is on therapy for at least 5 days and INR >2 for 24 hours.
- Warfarin (class = anticoagulant) should be continued for a minimum of 3 months.
- Fondaparinux is an agent of the drug class, factor X inhibitor.

TABLE 139: Recommendations for Treatment of DVT and PE

Caprini Score	Risk	VTE Incidence	Recommended Prophylaxis	Duration
0 - 2	Very low to low	< 1.5%[1]	Early ambulation, IPC	During hospitalization
3 - 4	Moderate	3%[1]	LMWH; UFH; or IPC. If high bleeding risk, IPC until bleeding risk diminishes.	At least 5 - 7 days
5 - 8	High	6%[1]	LMWH + IPC; or UFH + IPC. If high bleeding risk, IPC until bleeding risk diminishes.	At least 5 - 7 days*
> 8	Very high	6.5 to 18.3%[2,3,4]	LMWH + IPC; or UFH + IPC. If high bleeding risk, IPC until bleeding risk diminishes.	Consider extended prophylaxis (e.g., 14-30 days)

* Abdominal or pelvic surgery for cancer should receive extended VTE prophylaxis with LMWH x 30 days.[1]

IPC = intermittent pneumatic compression, LMWH = low molecular weight heparin
UFH = unfractionated heparin

1. Gould MK, Garcia DA, Wren SM, et.al. Prevention of VTE in nonorthopedic surgical patients: antithrombotic therapy and prevention of thrombosis, 9th ed: Americal College of Chest Physicians Evidence-Based Clinical Practice Guidelines. Chest. 2012; 141(2)(Suppl): e227S-e277S.
2. Bahl V, Hu HM, Henke PK, et.al. A validation study of a retrospective venous thromboembolism risk scoring method. Ann Surg. 2010; 251(2): 344-350.
3. Pannucci CJ, Bailey SH, Dreszer G, et.al. Validation of the Caprini risk assessment model in plastic and reconstructive surgery patients. J Am Coll Surg. 2011 January; 212 (1): 101-112.
4. Shuman AG, Hu HM, Pannucci CJ, et al. Stratifying the risk of venous thromboembolism in otolaryngology. Otolaryngology - Head and Neck Surgery 2012;146:719-724

Reprinted with permission from J. A. Caprini, MD.

References:

1. Third Report of the Expert Panel on Detection, Evaluation, and Treatment of High Blood Cholesterol in Adults. Sept 2002. JAMA. www.nhibi.nih.gov. Accessed 13 Nov 2009.
2. The Seventh Report of the Joint National Committee on Prevention, Detection, Evaluation, and Treatment of High Blood Pressure. 21 May 2003. JAMA. www.nhibi.nig.gov. Accessed 13 Nov 2009.
3. Aneurysm. www.mayoclinic.org. Accessed 10 Oct 2009.
4. Pazzullo JA, Dupuy DE, Cronan JJ. Percutaneous injection of thrombin for the treatment of pseudoaneurysm after catheterization. AJR 200; 175:1035-1040.
5. Vega, Jose MD. Arterial dissection and stroke.
6. Moon, Marc MD. Approach to the treatment of aortic dissection. Surgical Clinics of North America. 2009 Aug 89(4): 869-93.
7. Schmidt, WA. Current diagnosis and treatment of temporal arteritis. Current Treatment Options in Cardiovascular Medicine. 2006 April; 8(2): 125-51.
8. Drug therapy of temporal arteritis and polymyalgia rheumatica. DRUGDEX Consults.
9. Wigley, Frederick M. Reynaud's Phenomenon. NEJM. 2002 Sept; Vol 347: 1001-8.
10. Coarctation of the aorta. www.mayoclinic.org. Accessed 1 Nov 2009.
11. Wright LB, Matchett JW, Cruz CP, et al. Popliteal artery disease: diagnosis and treatment. RadioGraphics. 2004 March; 24(2):467-79.
12. Drug Facts and Comparisons
13. Popliteal Cystic Disease. www.mayclinic.org. Accessed 29 Sept 2009.
14. Adams, HP, del Zoppo G, Alberts MJ et al. Guidelines for the early management of adults with ischemic stroke. Stroke 2007;38:1655-1711.
15. Adams RJ, Albers H, Alberts MH et al. Update to the AHA/ASA recommendations for the prevention of stroke in patients with stroke and transient ischemic attack. Stroke 2008;39:1647-52.
16. Sahid MS, Hamilton G, Baker DM. A Multicenter review of carotid body tumor management. European Journal of Vascular and Endovascular Surgery. 2007 Aug 34(2): 127-30.
17. Wilson, James. Fibromuscular dysplasia: treatment & medication. The Fibromuscular Dysplasia Society of America. www.fmdsa.org. Accessed 3 Nov 2009.
18. McIntrye, Keneth. Subclavian Steal Syndrome. Medscape. www.medscape.com. Accessed 3 Nov 2009.
19. Schachner T, Steger C, Heiss S et al. Paclitaxel treatment reduces neointimal hyperplasia in cultured human saphenous veins. European Journal of Cardio-Thoracic Surgery. 2007 Dec; 32(6):906-11.
20. Chronic venous insufficiency and postphlebitic syndrome. The Merck Manual. www.merck.com. Accessed 3, Nov 2009.
21. Shebel ND, Whalen CC. Diagnosis and management of iliac vein compression syndrome. J Vasc. Nurs. 2005 Mar; 23(1):10-17.
22. Antithrombotic and thrombolytic therapy, 8th Ed: ACCP Guidelines. Accessed 01 Oct 2009 Drug Facts and Comparisons
23. Bhalla A, D'Cruz S, Lehl SS, Singh R. Renovascular hypertension - its evaluation and management. JIACM 2003; 4(2): 139-46.
24. Acute Mesenteric Ischemia. The Merck Manual Online. www.merck.com. Accessed 12 Nov 2009. Depiro seventh edition.
25. Tajani S, Sanoski C. Davis's Pocket Clinical Drug Reference. 2009 F.A. Davis Company.
26. Harris SR, Hugi MR, Olivotto IA, et al. Clinical practice guidelines for the care and treatment of breast cancer: 11. Lymphedema. CMAJ 2001 Jan 23; 154(2):191-9.

Math Symbols

Symbols	Meaning	Example
+	Add to	5 + 5 = 10
-	Subtract from	9 – 5 = 4
x	Multiply	4 x 2 = 8
*	Multiply	4 * 2 = 8
( )	Multiply	4 (2) = 8
·	Multiply	4 · 2 = 8
÷	Divide by	8 ÷ 2 = 4
/	Divide by	8 / 2 = 4
=	Equal to	5 = 5
≠	Not equal to	5 – 4 ≠ 8 - 2
±	Plus or minus (answer may deviate in a certain range)	The results of the study showed 36% ± 2% of those examined…
∞	Infinity	Never ending string of numbers
≈	Approximately/almost equal to	5.24 + 5.66 ≈ 11
~	Approximately/almost equal to	5.24 + 5.66 ~ 11
>	Greater than	8 >2
<	Less than	4 <9
≤	Less than or equal to	In 6 ≤6 the number to the left may be less than (<) or equal to (=) to the number on the right
≥	Greater than or equal to	In 6 ≥6 the number to the left may be greater than (>) or equal to (=) the number on the right
μ	Micro (millionth)	The speed of sound through soft tissue is 1.54 mm/μs.
π	Pi	3.14
λ	Lambda	Wavelength (λ) = c/f
:	Colon	The ratio of females to males in the class is 4:1
Δ	Change	ΔP = change in pressure
∝	Proportional to	Power is proportional to amplitude[2]

Order of Operations

A specific order of operations must be followed when multiple techniques are used to solve a problem:

> The acronym PEMDAS (**P**lease **E**xcuse **M**y **D**ear **A**unt **S**ally) is often used to remember the order of operations.

- **P**arenthesis (solve all portions of the equation in parenthesis first).
- **E**xponents (solve all portions of the equation containing exponents next).
- **M**ultiplication and **D**ivision (working left to right, solve all portions of the equation that use multiplication and division next).
- **A**ddition and **S**ubtraction (working left to right, solve all portions of an equation using addition and subtraction next).

   Example: $4^2 + (2 \times 6) + 9 - 6 =$

   $4^2 + 12 + 9 - 6 =$

   $16 + 12 + 9 - 6 =$

   $37 - 6 =$

   $37 - 6 = 31$

   Additional example: The equation $4v^2$ refers to a simplified calculation to determine pressure:

   $4v^2$ if v=2, then the calculation is as follows:

   $4 * 2^2 = 4 * 4 = 16$ (correct answer)

If the order of operations was not followed and multiplication was performed first instead of calculating exponents, the result would be dramatically different.

   $4 * 2^2 \neq 8^2 = 64$ (incorrect answer)

> *If the order of operations are not followed, the calculation will produce an incorrect answer.*

Variables

- Symbols (usually letters) are used to represent a value.
- When variables are placed next to a number, it implies multiplication should be performed.
   Example: $4a = 4 \times a$

Distributive Property

- When expressions use more than one math function, it can be viewed or solved in more than one way.
   Example: $a (b + c) = ab + ac$

   If we assign each variable a value:

   $a = 2$

   $b = 3$

   $c = 7$

   $2 (3 + 7) = (2) (3) + (2) (7)$

   $2 (10) = 6 + 14$

   $20 = 20$

Integers

Adding Integers

- When adding positive and negative integers, there are a certain set of rules to follow.
   - When adding similar signs, add the absolute values and give the result using the same sign.
      Examples: $(+4) + (+4) = 8$
      $(-4) + (-4) = -8$
      $(-4) + (-2) = -6$
   - When adding opposite signs, subtract the smaller value and use the sign from the larger integer.
      Examples: $(+5) + (-2) = 3$
      $(+4) + (-4) = 0$

   Additional Example:
      If a brachial pressure is measured at 120 mmHg and hydrostatic pressure is estimated at -30 mmHg, what is the measured pressure? Using the equation:

   circulatory pressure + hydrostatic pressure = measured pressure

   $(+120 \text{ mmHg}) + (-30 \text{ mmHg}) = 90 \text{ mmHg}$

Subtracting Integers

- When subtracting integers, add "its opposite":
   Examples:
   $(-7) - (+2) = -9$ (add "negative" 2 to the negative 7)

Remember that two negatives combined make a positive:
   $(-6) - (-6) = 0$ (add "positive" 6 to the negative 6)

   $(+4) - (-6) = 10$ (add "positive" 6 to the positive 4)

Multiplication and Division of Integers

- When multiplying or dividing positive and negative integers, rules include:
   - **A positive (+) and positive (+) will result in a positive (+) number.**

      - ***Example:***
         (+ 4) divided by (+ 2) is equal to (+ 2).

   - **A positive (+) and negative (-) will result in a negative (-) number.**

      - ***Example:***
         (+ 4) multiplied by (- 4) is equal to (-16).

   - **A negative (-) and negative (-) will result in a positive (+) number.**

      - ***Example:***
         (- 4) multiplied by (- 4) is equal to (+ 16).

> *When multiplying the same sign, the answer is positive. When the signs are different, the result will be negative.*

Fractions

- Any whole number can be treated as a fraction.
- May be written several different ways:

  number ÷ number   or   number/number

- Any number divided by 1 will equal the original number.

  Example: 25/1 = 25   16/1 = 16

- Zero divided by any number is zero.

  Example: 0/25 = 0

  0/16 = 0

- Any number divided by itself equals 1.

  Example: 25/25 = 1   16/16 = 1

- Fractions may be reduced by dividing the numerator and denominator by the same number (any common denominator that can divide into both numbers).

  Example: *both the numerator and denominator can be divided by 5*

  5/10 = 1/2

  because 5 divided by 5 equals 1 and 10 divided by 5 equals 2

- Multiplying fractions- when multiplying fractions, both numerator and denominator are multiplied.

  Example:

  $$\frac{5}{8} * \frac{2}{5} = \frac{10}{40} = \frac{1}{4}$$

- "Cancelling out" is a shortcut that can also be used to reduce fractions, when the numerator and denominator are the same, you can cancel out both variables.

  Example:

  $$\frac{\cancel{5}}{8} * \frac{2}{\cancel{5}} = \frac{2}{8} = \frac{1}{4}$$

  Although cancelling out is a shortcut, it does not change the answer that would have been given if the expanded work was completed as referenced below:

  Expanded work shown:

  $$\frac{5}{8} * \frac{2}{5} = \frac{5*2}{8*5}$$

  $$\frac{5*2}{8*5} = \frac{2*5}{8*5}$$

  $$\frac{2*\cancel{5}}{8*\cancel{5}} = \frac{2*1}{8*1}$$

  $$\frac{2}{8} * \frac{1}{1} = \frac{2}{8}$$

  $$\frac{2}{8} = \frac{1}{4}$$

> *Remember any number or variable divided by itself = 1.*

Conversions

Fraction and Decimal Conversions

- To convert a fraction to a decimal, divide the numerator by the denominator.

  Example: ½ =1 ÷ 2 = 0.5

- To convert a decimal to fraction, use the place value to create a fraction, then reduce if necessary.

  Examples:

  0.5 = 5/10   5/10 = ½

  0.75 = 75/100   75/100 = ¾
  (reduced by the common denominator of 25)

- When converting to a fraction, the denominator can usually be reduced since it is based on a system of tens.

> *If the conversion is done correctly, the resulting decimal will equal less than 1 when the numerator is less than the denominator. If the numerator is greater than the denominator, the resulting conversion will be >1.*

TABLE 140: **Fraction to Decimal Conversion/Equivalent**			
1/10	.1	3/5	.6
1/8	.125	5/8	.625
1/6	.16666…	2/3	.666…
1/5	.2	7/10	.7
1/4	.25	3/4	.75
3/10	.3	4/5	.8
1/3	.3333…	5/6	.8333…
3/8	.375	7/8	.875
2/5	.4	9/10	.9
1/2	.5	1/1	1

Practice example:

$$\text{ABI (ankle brachial index)} = \frac{\text{Highest ankle pressure}}{\text{Highest brachial pressure}}$$

If the ankle pressure is measured at 105 mmHg and the brachial pressure is measured at 120 mmHg, the ABI equation will produce a fraction of 105/120. ABIs are reported in the form of a decimal, so a conversion is necessary. 105 divided by 120 yields a decimal conversion of .875 (Rounded to .88).

Metric Conversions

- This system is used to represent weight (grams), distance (meters), area (square meters), and volume (liters).

  - These units can be further represented by larger or smaller numbers simply by adding a prefix (e.g., centi-, kilo-). The prefixes used in the metric system change the place value of the decimal.

  - The movement of the decimal placement changes the value of a number by factors of ten.

  ### Example:

  1 kilometer = 1000 meters

  Kilo stands for 1000. In this case, it gives the instruction to move the decimal 3 placements. Three decimal placements to the right increases any number by a thousand (because you add three 0s).

TABLE 141: Prefix Definitions			
Mega- (M)	million	(1,000,000)	10^6
Kilo- (k)	thousand	(1,000)	10^4
Hecto- (h)	hundred	(100)	10^2
Deka- (da)	ten	(10)	10^1
Deci- (d)	one-tenth	(.1) = 1/10	10^{-1}
Centi- (c)	one-hundredth	(.01) = 1/100	10^{-2}
Milli- (m)	one-thousandth	(.001) = 1/1000	10^{-3}
Micro- (μ)	one-millionth	(.000001) = 1/1000000	10^{-6}

- It is sometimes necessary to convert from one unit to another. Converting from one form to another is done by examining the prefix and moving the decimal the correct number of places.

- When converting, you need to understand what number/unit you are starting with and to what form you are converting.

  ### Question:

  How many "kilo" are in a "mega"?

  ### Solution:

  "Kilo" means 1000 and "mega" means million. Thus, the question becomes how many 1000s make up a million? The answer is 1000 kilos are in 1 mega.

  How do you convert? The difference from kilo to mega is 3 decimal places. Since this conversion is from larger (mega) to smaller (kilo), the resulting number will be larger. This means 3 decimal places are added to the right (add three 0s).

  ### Example:

  1000 kilo = 1,000,000 (1 mega)
  (kilo means a thousand, so
  1000 kilo is equal to
  1000 x 1000 or 1,000 x 1,000 = 1,000,000
  (multiplying by 1000 = adding 3 zeros to the right)

Practice examples:

Question:

Let's say we measure the kidney at 100 mm on its longest axis. The physician wants you to write on the tech sheet in centimeters. How do we convert centi to milli?

Solution:

We know that centi means 100th and that milli means a thousandth. There is one decimal place difference between the two. The next question is which way to move the decimal; left or right? Since we are converting from a smaller to larger number, the resulting number will be smaller. The answer to this question is 100 mm = 10 cm.

Question:

How do you calculate the wavelength of a 1 MHz transducer in soft tissue? $λ = c/f$

Solution:

We know that the average speed of sound (c) in soft tissue is 1540 m/s and the frequency, 1 MHz equals 1×10^6 cm/s. We must convert both figures to a similar unit:

$$λ = 1540 \times 10^0 \text{ m/s} \div 1 \times 10^6 \text{ cm/s}$$

$$= 1540 \times 10^{-6} \text{ m} = 1.54 \times 10^{-3} \text{ m} = 1.54 \text{ mm}$$

Examining differences in prefixes

> When converting from a smaller to larger prefix, the resulting number will be smaller.

- centi = 0.01
- milli = 0.001
- mm < cm
- 1/1000 is smaller than 1/100.
- 100 mm = 100 X .001 (milli = .001) = 0.1 meters
- 10 cm = 10 X .01 (centi = .01) = 0.1 meters
- (If the conversion was done properly, they should be equal)

Temperature Conversion

- From Fahrenheit to Celsius: $C = (F - 32) \times 5/9$
- From Celsius to Fahrenheit: $F = 9/5\, C + 32$

TABLE 142: American-Metric Conversion	
American unit	**Metric equivalent unit**
2.2 lbs (pounds)	1 kilogram
1 lb (pound)	0.454 kilogram
1 inch	2.54 centimeters
0.394 inches	1 centimeter
1 mile	1.61 kilometers
0.62 mile	1 kilometer

Exponents

- Exponential notation is used to express numbers that are multiplied by themselves. It is a kind of shorthand that is used in mathematics to represent large numbers.

  Example:

  $10^2 = 10 \times 10$

  $10^4 = 10 \times 10 \times 10 \times 10$

- **Multiplication of exponents**: When exponents have the same base number, the exponents are simply added together. This technique can also be used when the two exponents have the same variable.

  Example:

  $10^4 \times 10^2 = 10^6$

  Example:

  $a^4 \times a^2 = a^6$

- **Dividing exponents**: When exponents have the same base number, the exponents are simply subtracted. This technique can also be used when the two exponents have the same variable.

  Example:

  $10^5 / 10^2 = 10^3$

  Example:

  $a^5 / a^2 = a^3$

- A negative exponent is equivalent to the inverse of the number with a positive exponent.

  Examples:

  $a^{-3} = 1 / a^3$

  $10^{-3} = 1 / 10^3$

  $10^{-6} = 1 / 10^6$

- Any number with an exponent to the power of 0 will equal 1.
  Example: $5^0 = 1$

Formulas

> Area reduction versus diameter reduction calculations will yield different percentages of change.
> *For example:* 50% diameter reduction = 75% area reduction.

Proportionality

- Direct-In a direct relationship, when one factor or variable is manipulated, another is affected in the same way.

  Example:

  $A = \dfrac{B}{C}$ Therefore, B is proportional to A.

> If the numerator (B) is increased, the sum (A) will also be increased. If the numerator (B) is increased, the sum (A) will also be increased.

- Inverse-In an inverse or opposite relationship, when one factor or variable is manipulated, another is affected in the opposite way.

  Example:

  $A = \dfrac{B}{C}$

  Therefore, C is inversely proportional to A.

> When approaching equations, the denominator and the sum are inversely proportional. The numerator and sum are directly proportional.

> If the denominator (C) is increased, the sum (A) will be decreased.

Additional Examples:

$$\uparrow A = \frac{B\uparrow}{C} \qquad \downarrow A = \frac{B\downarrow}{C} \qquad \downarrow A = \frac{B}{C\uparrow} \qquad \uparrow A = \frac{B}{C\downarrow}$$

$5 = \dfrac{10}{2}$ If 10 is increased to 20, the resulting effect to 5 will be to increase to 10 $10 = \dfrac{20}{2}$

(directly proportional)

Linear Versus Non-Linear Proportionality

- Linear
  - If two variables have linear proportionality, each variable is affected the same way.

    Power is proportional to intensity.

  Example:

  If power is increased, intensity is also increased. If power is decreased, intensity is also decreased.

  If power is increased by a factor of 2, intensity is increased by a factor of 2. If power is decreased by a factor of 2, intensity is decreased by a factor of 2.

- Non-linear
  - If two variables have non-linear proportionality, each variable is not affected the same way.

  Example:

  Power is proportional to amplitude squared. If amplitude is increased by a factor of 2, power is increased by a factor 2^2 or a factor of 4. Both variables are affected, but not equally (non-linear).

Decibels

- Decibels are used commonly in word problems when describing a change in power or intensity.

Question: Initial power is 2 watts. If the power is increased by a factor of 16, what is the change in decibels?

> *Reminder: When a word problem states: "increase by a factor", it is asking you to use multiplication. When a word problem states: "decrease by a factor", it is asking for the use of division.*

Answer: +12 dB

Question: What is the final power for the question above?

Answer: The final power is 32 watts

2 watts multiplied by 16 (12 dB change) = 32 watts

Question: Initial power is 5 watts. If there is a +12 dB change, what is the final power?

Answer: 80 watts

5 watts multiplied by 16 (12 dB change) = 80 watts

Question: Initial intensity is 8 w/cm^2. If there is a decrease in intensity by a factor of 6 dB, what is the final intensity?

Answer: 2 w/cm^2

8 w/cm^2 divided by 4 (6 dB change)= 2 w/cm^2

Cosine

Mathematically, cosine angles are used when calculating frequency shifts.

TABLE 144: **Commonly Used Cosines**	
Cos (0°)	1
Cos (30°)	0.87
Cos (45°)	0.71
Cos (60°)	0.50
Cos (90°)	0

Example:

Doppler Shift =

$$\frac{2 \text{ (speed of blood) (operating frequency) cos } (\theta)}{\text{propagation speed}}$$

TABLE 143: **Decibel Chart**	
Decibel change	**Meaning or instruction**
3 dB	Multiply by 2 (increase by a factor) or divide by 2 (decrease by a factor)
6 dB	Multiply by 4 (increase by a factor) or divide by 4 (decrease by a factor)
9 dB	Multiply by 8 (increase by a factor)or divide by 8 (decrease by a factor)
10 dB	Multiply by 10 (increase by a factor) or divide by 10 (decrease by a factor)
12 dB	Multiply by 16 (increase by a factor) or divide by 16 (decrease by a factor)
15 dB	Multiply by 32 (increase by a factor) or divide by 32 (decrease by a factor)
20 dB	Multiply by 100 (increase by a factor) or divide by 100 (decrease by a factor)
30 dB	Multiply by 1,000 (increase by a factor) or divide by 1,000 (decrease by a factor)
40 dB	Multiply by 10,000 (increase by a factor) or divide by 10,000 (decrease by a factor)
50 dB	Multiply by 100,000 (increase by a factor) or divide by 100,000 (decrease by a factor)

Reynolds Number	$Re = \dfrac{V\rho 2r}{\eta}$ *Reminder: The Reynolds number is considered "dimensionless"(no unit of measure). A Reynolds number greater than 2000 is an indication of flow disturbance (turbulence).*	Re= Reynolds number V= velocity ρ= density of fluid r=radius of vessel η =viscosity of fluid within the vessel
Resistance equation *Reminder: Changes in radius will have the greatest effect on resistance.*	$R = \dfrac{8\,L\,\eta}{\pi\,r^4}$	R = resistance L = length of the vessel r = radius of vessel π = 3.14 η = viscosity of fluid
Attenuation coefficient for soft tissue	$\approx$ .5 dB/cm/MHz	
Nyquist limit	$\dfrac{\text{pulse repetition frequency (PRF)}}{2}$	
Doppler equation	$f_{Dop} = \dfrac{2\,f_o\,v\,\cos(\theta)}{c}$	
The Doppler equation may also be seen as	$\dfrac{2\,(\text{speed of blood})\,(\text{operating frequency})\,\cos(\theta)}{\text{propagation speed}}$	
Change in pressure (simplified equation)	volume flow x resistance	
Ohm's law	voltage = current x resistance	
Measured pressure	circulatory pressure + hydrostatic pressure	*Note:* (hydrostatic pressure is 0 mmHg @ heart level)
Poiseuille's law	$Q = \dfrac{\Delta P\,\pi\,r^4}{8\,L\,\eta}$	Q= volume flow ΔP= change in pressure ($P_1 - P_2$) r=radius L=length of vessel η =viscosity of fluid π=3.14
Simplified Bernoulli equation	Pressure (mmHg)= $4v^2$	When calculating a change in pressure, Δ Pressure(mmHg)= $4(v_2{}^2 - v_1{}^2)$
Ankle Brachial Index (ABI)	$\dfrac{\text{highest ankle pressure}}{\text{highest brachial pressure}}$	

Reminder: ABIs are typically performed bilaterally. Two pressures are taken from each ankle artery (PTA and DPA). The highest ankle pressure from the right leg is used for the right ABI. The highest ankle pressure from the left leg is used for the left ABI. Bilateral brachial arm pressures are taken. However, only the higher of the two brachial pressures is used for the ABI calculation.

Area	πr^2
Area reduction*	$(\%) = (1 - \pi r_2^2 / \pi r_1^2) \times 100$
	r_1 represents true lumenal radius of the native vessel
	r_2 represents residual lumenal radius of the narrowed lumen
Circumference	$2\pi r$
Diameter	$2r$
Diameter reduction*	$(\%) = (1 - D_2 / D_1) \times 100$
	D_1 represents the true lumenal diameter of native vessel
	D_2 represents the residual lumenal diameter of narrowed lumen
Volume	$4/3 \, \pi r^3$

Manipulating Equations

- To separate a variable, utilize division or multiplication to isolate the variable to one side of the equation.

> *There is one very important rule that must be followed when manipulating an equation. Whatever you do to one side of the equation, you MUST do to the other side.*

Example:

Given the equation:

$$A = \frac{B}{C}$$

To isolate B, multiply each side by C

$$C * A = \frac{B * C}{C}$$

Since "C" cancels out, you are left with the equation:

$$C * A = B \text{ or } B = C*A$$

To isolate C:

$$B = C * A$$

Divide each side by A

$$\frac{B}{A} = \frac{C*A}{A}$$

Since "A" cancels out, you are left with the equation:

$$\frac{B}{A} = C \text{ or } C = \frac{B}{A}$$

Example:

Manipulate an equation utilizing addition and subtraction:

$$8A - 2 = 30$$

To isolate variable A, add 2 to each side to isolate 8A by itself:

$$8A - 2 = 30$$
$$2 + 8A - 2 = 30 \, (+ 2)$$

The +2 and -2 on the left side of the equation cancel out and you are left with:

$$8A = 32$$

To isolate A by itself, divide each side by 8, you are then left with:

$$\frac{8A}{8} = \frac{32}{8} \qquad (8/8 \text{ cancels out})$$

$$A = \frac{32}{8} \text{ or } A = 4$$

References

1. Bello I. (2006). Introductory Algebra, A Real-World Approach 2nd edition. McGraw Hill.
2. Hutchison, Bergman B, Baratto. (2005). Basic Mathematical Skills with Geometry 6th edition. McGraw Hill.
3. Slater, TJ. (2002). Basic College Mathematics 4th edition. Pearson/Prentice Hall.
4. Shulte AP, Peterson RE, (1986). Preparing to use Algebra 4th edition. Laidlaw Brothers.
5. Kime LA, Clark J, Michael BK. (2005). Explorations in College Algebra 3rd Edition. John Wiley & Sons, Inc.
6. Smith KJ. (2006). Mathematics: Its Power and Utility. Thomson Brooks/Cole..
7. Edelman, SK. (2005). Understanding Ultrasound Physics. ESP Ultrasound.
8. Miele FR. (2006). Ultrasound Physics and Instrumentation Vol.1 & 2. Pegasus Lectures Inc.

Math Review

Rationale

One of the main objectives for any non-invasive vascular laboratory is to provide accurate test results. Physicians expect that a positive exam truly means that their patient has disease and a negative exam truly means the patient has no significant disease. Exams should also have a high degree of reliability and repeatability.

Regular, ongoing correlations by the non-invasive lab with gold standard procedures ensure the highest quality of service to patients and their referring physicians.

Definitions

- **Gold standard**: A well accepted standard used during the comparison of diagnostic information derived from the non-invasive vascular lab exam. Examples of gold standard exams include, but are not limited to:

  - **Peripheral arterial:** Angiograms, CT scans, operative findings, MRA, surgical pathology reports

  - **Extracranial/intracranial:** CT scans, angiography

  - **Peripheral venous:** Venograms, repeat non-invasive exams, MRV

  - **Visceral:** CT scans, angiography

Terms Used in Accuracy Measurements

Positive and negative levels of disease must be defined to determine true and false/positive and negative comparisons.

For instance, if a positive carotid is any exam with a stenosis >50% (including occlusions) and a CTA shows a 40% stenosis, the duplex would correlate as a false positive non-invasive exam. Though both exams demonstrate disease, the degree by CTA is considered "not significant", since the stenosis is < 50%. Separate correlations must be done for differing levels of disease, e.g., >50%, >70%, or 80-99%, etc.

- **True Positive (TP)**: Significant disease is present by both the gold standard and the non-invasive exam.

- **True Negative (TN)**: No no significant disease present by either the gold standard or the non-invasive exam.

- **False Positive (FP)**: Although significant disease is suggested by the non-invasive exam, the gold standard detected no significant disease.

- **False Negative (FN)**: No disease was suggested by the non-invasive exam, though the gold standard indicated significant disease was present.

- **Sensitivity**: The ability of the non-invasive exam to detect disease.

- **Specificity**: The ability of the non-invasive exam to detect the lack of disease.

- **Positive Predictive Value (PPV)**: How often any positive non-invasive exam truly indicates the presence of significant disease.

- **Negative Predictive Value (NPV)**: How often a negative non-invasive exam is found to be truly negative by the gold standard

- **Overestimation**: The non-invasive exam suggested disease or a disease category that was greater than diagnosed by the gold standard.

- **Underestimation**: The non-invasive exam graded the disease in a lower category than the gold standard.

- **Sample size (n)**: The number of examinations used in analysis.

Formulas

- **Sensitivity** = $\dfrac{\text{True Positive non-invasive exams}}{\text{All positive gold standard exams}}$

- **Specificity** = $\dfrac{\text{True Negative non-invasive exams}}{\text{All negative gold standard exams}}$

- **PPV** = $\dfrac{\text{True Positive non-invasive exams}}{\text{All positive non-invasive exams}}$

- **NPV** = $\dfrac{\text{True Negative non-invasive exams}}{\text{All negative non-invasive exams}}$

- **Overall Accuracy (OA)** = $\dfrac{\text{TP + TN}}{\text{TP+TN+FN+FP}}$

Protocol for Gathering Statistical Correlation

- Gather data throughout the year to be used for quality assurance (QA) analysis.

  - Keep logs of all results. Keeping a list of abnormal results only will skew the data. Normals are important to identify and are comparable too. They may improve statistics.

  - Determine if any patients tested by a non-invasive exam were also referred for a correlating exam.

  - Specifically for venous correlations, designated "repeat exam" days are scheduled throughout the month. On these days, two technologists will scan the patient during the visit.

    - Ask the patient if they would mind taking part in a quality assurance study. Explain that a second examiner will perform a quick repeat exam and the results will be compared to ensure the quality of work in the office.

    - The first technologist/sonographer performs the exam and writes a preliminary report.

    - The second technologist/sonographer repeats the examination without knowing the results of the first examiner's work. The second examiner should write their own preliminary results.

    - Designate a third person to compare both results and log agreement/disagreement.

Date	Name	1st TECH Venous Right Leg	1st TECH Venous Left Leg	2nd TECH Venous Right Leg	2nd TECH Venous Left Leg	Agree? Yes/No **RIGHT**	Agree? Yes/No **LEFT**	Comments
	DVT/SVT							
	CVI							
	DVT/SVT							
	CVI							
	DVT/SVT							
	CVI							

Sample log for the repeat venous examination method of correlation

Statistical Correlation

- 2 x 2 table or chi-square tables are helpful when organizing data and calculating accuracies. Typically, the gold standard can be plotted along the x-axis and the non-invasive exam can be plotted along the y-axis:

Gold Standard Test Results

		+	−
Non-invasive Test Results	+	True Positive (TP)	False Positive (FP)
	−	False Negative (FN)	True Negative (TN)

Practical examples of statistical calculations:

Question:

How accurately did our lab identify carotid stenosis in the 50-79% range?

> The acceptable time frame between the non-invasive test and the gold standard is typically no more than 3-6 months, depending on the type of disease.

Solution:

The question is best answered with the percent agreement plotted on a matrix.

150 carotid arteries scanned during the year were found to have a corresponding CT scan on record at our hospital.

– The results of the non-invasive and CT scans for each carotid were plotted onto a matrix. *The various ranges of carotid disease (0-49%) (50-79%) (80-99%) and (100%) used in this particular institution were considered.*

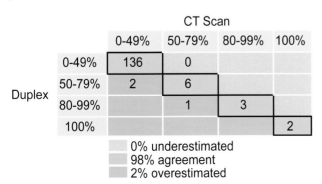

Expanded version of a 2 x 2 table used to tabulate TN, TP, FP and FN

The total number of TP, TN, FP and FN were calculated:

Gold Standard Test Results

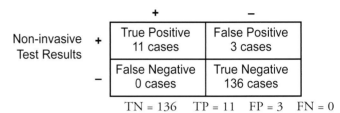

		+	−
Non-invasive Test Results	+	True Positive 11 cases	False Positive 3 cases
	−	False Negative 0 cases	True Negative 136 cases

TN = 136   TP = 11   FP = 3   FN = 0

Using these values in the statistical formulas for sensitivity, specificity, PPV, NPV and OA, the following percentages were calculated:

$$\textbf{Sensitivity} = \frac{TP}{\text{All positive CT scans}} = \frac{11}{11 + 0} \times 100 = 100\%$$

$$\textbf{Specificity} = \frac{TN}{\text{All negative CT scans}} = \frac{136}{136 + 3} \times 100 = 98\%$$

$$\textbf{PPV} = \frac{TP}{\text{All positive duplex scans}} = \frac{11}{11 + 3} \times 100 = 79\%$$

$$\textbf{NPV} = \frac{TN}{\text{All negative duplex scans}} = \frac{136}{136 + 0} \times 100 = 100\%$$

$$\textbf{OA} = \frac{TN + TP}{TP + TN + FN + FP} = \frac{136 + 11}{136 + 11 + 3 + 0} \times 100 = 98\% \text{ OA}$$

Question:

Of all the stenoses in the 80-99% range, what is the most predictable peak systolic velocity (PSV) to indicate the presence of disease ≥80%?

Solution:

There are commercial software programs available for biomedical researchers which use ROC (receiver operating characteristic) curve analysis that can help determine the most accurate velocity to use for diagnosing disease in a certain patient population, establishing a new threshold for your lab.

- Accurate diagnosis by "level of disease" (aortoiliac, versus, femoropopliteal versus infrapopliteal versus multilevel disease) can be a useful analysis.
- After correlations are completed, it is important to find ways to improve any areas of concern.

Patient Name	Medical Record #	Side	Date of Vascular Lab Studies	B-Mode Diameter Reduction	PSV	EDV	% Stenosis in conclusion	Date of CTA	CTA Results	Correlation	Notes
Smith, McKenzie	12345798	R	12/30/2008		61	25	0-49%	1/2/2009	No stenosis	TN	
Smith, McKenzie	12345798	L	12/30/2008		98	34	0-49%	1/2/2009	No stenosis	TN	
Thomas, Tom	9876541	R	1/23/2009		80	42	0-49%	1/25/2009	No stenosis	TN	
Thomas, Tom	9876541	L	1/23/2009	82%	422	223	80-99%	1/25/2009	80-90% stenosis	TP	
Manning, Ted	7095312	R	7/7/2009	64%	202	51	50-79%	7/16/2009	50% stenosis	TP	
Manning, Ted	7095312	L	7/7/2009		40	4	0-49%	7/16/2009	40% stenosis	TN	
Kromer, Blair	7772213	R	4/16/2009		273	76	50-79%	4/16/2009	Heavily calcified	FP	When CT remeasured a 73% stenosis was found in the RICA and this correlates with duplex findings
Kromer, Blair	7772213	L	4/16/2009		261	65	50-79%	4/16/2009	Heavily calcified	FP	When CT remeasured a 54% stenosis was found in the LICA and this correlates with duplex findings

Excerpt from a QA log for the year

Question:

Why is the OA lower for predicting disease at the aortoiliac level compared to the femoropopliteal segment?

Considerations: The femoropopliteal segment is imaged directly using duplex scanning. Common femoral artery waveforms alone are all that is considered when predicting aortoiliac disease.

Possible Solution:

Add additional testing, such as volume pulse recording, to gather supporting evidence of aortoiliac obstruction. Add direct imaging of the aortoiliac segment to look for stenosis/occlusion and re-study to see if accuracies improve. You may consider better ways to interpret the duplex common femoral artery waveform to identify aorto-iliac obstruction.

Points to Remember

- The non-invasive examination should have been performed before the gold standard test for the most honest comparison.

- Be sure that no therapeutic procedures were done between the non-invasive and gold standard exams.

- Use all results regardless of agreement with the non-invasive exam to eliminate bias. Test results should not be altered after review of the correlating examination. Instead, concentrate on how to improve testing methods for the future. In addition, keep a list of uninterpretable non-invasive exams.

- Each laboratory should have a written policy outlining the procedure used to collect data, frequency of analysis, personnel responsible and how results are disseminated to staff.

- Different radiologists within the same institution may use different methods for measuring stenosis (on an angiogram for example). Different percent stenosis may be calculated on an imaging study depending on whether the observer used the distal ICA or residual lumen at the point of stenosis. Ensure that the same method was used for the patient population being considered for QA study whenever possible.[1]

- Statistical analysis can also be calculated for each modality used in a particular area of testing. For example, QA data can be generated for segmental pressures, volume pulse recording and arterial duplex separately. This may provide insight into which modality is the most reliable in your laboratory.

- Each aspect of the diagnostic criteria used can also be analyzed. For example, carotid QA may include accuracy calculations for:
  - B-mode image
  - ICA peak systolic velocity
  - ICA end-diastolic velocity
  - ICA/CCA peak velocity ratio
  - ICA/CCA end diastolic velocity ratio

- CPT charge reports can be a useful tool to identify which patients have had a study that can be used for correlation.

- The time frame between the non-invasive exam and the gold standard may need to be less than 3 - 4 months when rapidly progressing disease is involved (e.g., transcranial imaging for vasospasms).[2]

- There may be difficulty accessing gold standard test results for use in comparisons, especially in non-hospital based laboratories. Telephone surveys or follow-up letters to the referring physicians may help to gather this information.

Dr. Tyler
4321 N. Gravel Road
Chicago, IL 60637

Dear Dr. Tyler:

A venous duplex exam was performed on your patient, Dave
Bowl on May 1, 2011 at ABC Hospital.

Since our laboratory is interested in maintaining the highest quality of service
for you and your patients, we are asking for your assistance by providing
information on clinical outcomes.

Did your patient demonstrate any of the following?

	YES	NO
Documented resolution of thrombus?		
Development of insufficiency		
Progression of DVT following treatment?		

Please have your office forward a copy of this questionnaire via fax or mail
using the enclosed, self-addressed stamped envelope.

Thank you,
Non-invasive Vascular Laboratory
Department of Vascular Surgery
1234 Stone Road
Chicago, IL 60637
(800) 123-4567
(800) 777-9999 Fax

Dr. Tyler
4321 N. Gravel Road
Chicago, IL 60637

Dear Dr. Tyler:

A mesenteric duplex exam was performed on your patient, Betty Who on
March 1, 2011 at ABC Hospital.

Since our laboratory is interested in maintaining the highest quality of service
for you and your patients, we are asking for your assistance by providing the
following information:

1. Was an invasive procedure performed for this patient within the past
    6 months?

2. If so, please specify the type of procedure and have your office forward a
    copy of the exam report via fax or mail using the enclosed, self-addressed
    stamped envelope.

We thank you for your cooperation.

Thank you,
Non-invasive Vascular Laboratory
Department of Vascular Surgery
1234 Stone Road
Chicago, IL 60637
(800) 123-4567
(800) 777-9999 Fax

- Consider combining QA data for upper and lower extremity venous exams in order to reach the minimum ICAVL requirement of 30 limbs necessary for correlation.

- It is important to try and account for any false negative or false positive results in the vascular lab in order to improve the quality of testing.

- Consider engaging all technologists in the ongoing quality assurance initiative in your lab. Rotate who maintains the logs, collects the correlating studies and calculates the statistics each year. This enables the team to have a greater appreciation for the QA process and accuracy of their work. Participation also provides a better understanding of what specific areas of testing may need attention in order to improve.

- ICAVL standards state that a minimum of two vascular QA meetings must be held yearly in accredited laboratories. Calculating accuracy statistics is fairly useless without subsequent analysis, discussion, and action plans to improve accuracy. Meeting minutes and attendance should be kept and agenda items should include, but are not limited to: [2]

  - Discussion of QA results

  - Discussion of any discrepancies (e.g. FP or FN exams)

  - Review of challenging cases

  - Discussion of QA issues identified within the laboratory

- A goal for percent agreement should be at least 70% for any given exam.[2]

- Finding exams to use for venous correlation can be challenging. Besides venography and surgical pathology, ICAVL standards suggest the following as acceptable methods for correlation:[2]

  - Case Peer Review by a second interpreting physician; documenting technical adequacy, Interpretation accuracy and final report completeness

  - Comparison of repeat venous exams performed on the same patient within 3 days of initial exam

  - Gathering information about a patient's clinical outcome

- Since surgical specimens can shrink, care should be taken to arrange for any specimens to remain under fixed pressure.[1]

- When using several gold standards to assess accuracy for a given exam (e.g., CT scan and carotid angiography), calculate sensitivity, specificity, PPV, NPV and OA for each group separately. Do not combine gold standards.

Example:

- **Accuracy for hemodynamically significant arterial obstruction using angiograms**:

  TN = 33

  TP = 64

  FN = 0

  FP = 6

  $$\text{Sensitivity} = \frac{TP}{TP+FN} = \frac{64}{64+0} \times 100 = 100\%$$

  $$\text{Specificity} = \frac{TN}{FP+TN} = \frac{33}{6+33} \times 100 = 85\%$$

  $$\text{Positive Predictive Value} = \frac{TP}{TP+FP} = \frac{64}{64+6} \times 100 = 91\%$$

  $$\text{Negative Predictive Value} = \frac{TN}{TN+FN} = \frac{33}{33+0} \times 100 = 100\%$$

  $$\text{OA} = \frac{TP+TN}{TP+TN+FP+FN} = \frac{64+33}{64+33+6+0} \times 100 = 94\%$$

- **Accuracy using Infused CTs**:

  TN=40

  TP=0

  FN=0

  FP=5

  $$\text{Sensitivity} = \frac{TP}{TP+FN} = \text{Not applicable. No data.}$$

  $$\text{Specificity} = \frac{TN}{FP+TN} = \frac{40}{5+40} \times 100 = 89\%$$

  $$\text{Positive Predictive Value} = \frac{TP}{FN+FP} = \text{Not applicable}$$

  $$\text{Negative Predictive Value} = \frac{TN}{TN+FN} = \frac{40}{40+0} \times 100 = 100\%$$

  $$\text{OA} = \frac{TP+TN}{TP+TN+FP+FN} = \frac{0+40}{0+40+5+0} \times 100 = 89\%$$

References

1. Gerlock AJ. (1988). Accuracy of measurement determinations. In Application of Non-invasive Vascular Techniques. (526-530). W.B. Saunders Company.
2. Intersocietal Commission for the Accreditation of Vascular Laboratories. ICAVL standards for accreditation in non-invasive testing. Retrieved from http://icavl.org/icavl/standards/2010_ICAVL_Standards.pdf (accessed 1/8/12)

Additional References

Hayes AC. "Calculation and implication of accuracy measurements". Bruit. 9:178-182, July 1985.
Lambeth A. "Statistics in the vascular laboratory" Bruit. 6:47-48, June 1982.

Arterial (Lower Extremity)

Ankle Brachial Index (ABI): When narrowing of the arterial lumen reaches a critical level, distal arterial flow and pressure decrease significantly. Ankle brachial indices (ABIs) define the resulting decrease in blood flow to the extremity at the ankle level.

Ankle Brachial Index (ABI)

Calculate by dividing the higher of the ankle pressures by the higher of the two brachial pressures:

$$\frac{\text{Higher ankle pressure}}{\text{Higher brachial pressure}}$$

Toe Brachial Index (TBI)

Calculate by dividing the digital pressure by the higher brachial pressure to determine the digital brachial index:

$$\frac{\text{Toe pressure}}{\text{Higher brachial pressure}}$$

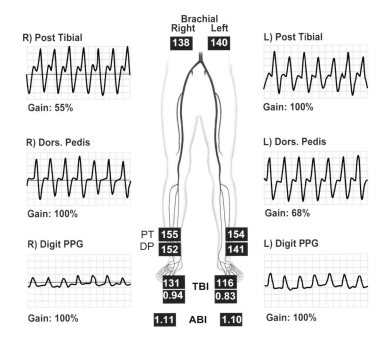

Normal ABI and TBI Physiologic Report

TABLE 147: Disease Categorization for ABI/TBI

ABI		TBI
≥1.0	Normal	>0.70
0.90-<1.0	Mild	0.60-0.69
0.50-0.90	Moderate	0.59-0.40
0.30-0.50	Severe	<0.39
<0.30	Critical	-

ABI Data Source: Modified from AbuRahma AF. (2000). Segmental Doppler pressures and Doppler waveform analysis in peripheral vascular disease of the lower extremities. In AbuRahma AF, Bergan JJ (Eds). Non-invasive Vascular Diagnosis. (213-229). London: Springer.

TBI Data Source: Source: Internally validated at the University of Chicago Medicine Vascular Laboratory

Calculation Examples:

Calculate the right ankle brachial index (ABI):

155 ÷ 140 = 1.1 categorizing the right ABI as normal

Calculate the right toe brachial index (TBI):

131 ÷ 140 = 0.94 categorizing the right TBI as normal

Calculate the left ankle brachial index (ABI):

154 ÷ 140 = 1.1 categorizing the left ABI as normal

Calculate the left toe brachial index (TBI):

116 ÷ 140 = 0.83 categorizing the left TBI as normal

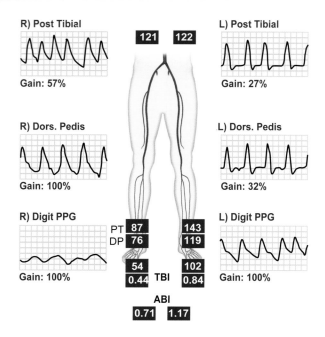

Abnormal ABI and TBI Physiologic Report

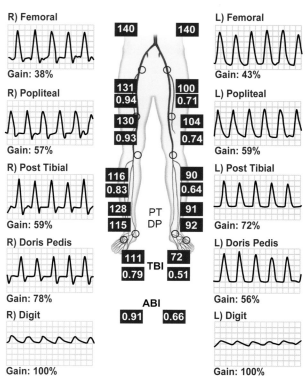

Segmental Pressures Physiologic Report

Calculation Examples:

Calculate the right ankle brachial index (ABI):
87 ÷ 122 = 0.71 categorizing the right ABI as moderate

Calculate the right toe brachial index (TBI):
54 ÷ 122 = 0.44 categorizing the right TBI as moderate

Calculate the left ankle brachial index (ABI):
143 ÷ 122 = 1.17 categorizing the left ABI as normal

Calculate the left toe brachial index (TBI):
102 ÷ 122 = 0.84 categorizing the left TBI as normal

Lower Extremity Segmental Pressures

Segmental pressures define the level of disease by comparing the limb and brachial pressures from one level to the next. A pressure gradient (pressure difference) of 20-30 mmHg indicates a significant stenosis or occlusion between cuff levels. Higher gradients most likely represent an occlusion, rather than a stenosis. Doppler waveforms from the lower extremity arteries normally demonstrate a high resistance waveform pattern, whereas waveforms distal to a significant obstruction typically reflect a low resistance configuration.

Values calculated by dividing the segmental pressure by the higher of the two brachial pressures:

$$\frac{\text{Segmental pressure}}{\text{Higher brachial pressure}}$$

Calculation Examples:

Calculate the right ankle brachial index (ABI):
128 ÷ 140 = 0.91 categorizing the right ABI as mild

Calculate the right high thigh index:
131 ÷ 140 = 0.94

Calculate the right low thigh index:
130 ÷ 140 = 0.93

Calculate the right calf index:
116 ÷ 140 = 0.83

Calculate the right toe brachial index (TBI):
111 ÷ 140 = 0.79 categorizing the right TBI as normal

Calculate the left ankle brachial index (ABI):
92 ÷ 140 = 0.66 categorizing the left ABI as moderate

Calculate the left high thigh index:
100 ÷ 140 = 0.71

Calculate the left low thigh index:
104 ÷ 140 = 0.74

Calculate the left calf index:
90 ÷ 140 = 0.64

Calculate the left toe brachial index (TBI):
72 ÷ 140 = 0.51 categorizing the left TBI as moderate

Exercise and Stress Ankle/Brachial Indices (ABIs)

Upon exercise, an individual's distal vascular bed vasodilates, decreasing resistance and increasing blood flow in response to the demand. If a patient cannot exercise, the reactive hyperemia technique is an alternative means of increasing blood flow in order to elicit a pressure gradient that is not present at rest. The ankle pressure will decrease in the presence of increased flow and a significant arterial obstruction.

TABLE 148: Treadmill Testing Protocol Summary

- Apply pneumatic cuffs on the arm and ankle.
- Measure pre-exercise ankle-brachial indices (ABI).
- Have the patient walk on the treadmill at a 10% grade and speed of 2 mph for 5 minutes or until claudication or other restrictions occur.
- Quickly re-measure ABI within the first minute post-exercise.
- Retake the ABI every 2 minutes until ankle pressures return to within 10 mmHg of the baseline pressure or for 5-10 minutes (whichever comes first).
- Determine classification of disease according to laboratory diagnostic criteria.

> Determine classification of disease according to laboratory diagnostic criteria.

TABLE 149: ABI Response to Exercise

Normal Response

- There should be little to no drop in ankle pressure after 5 minutes of exercise.
- The ABI may increase.
- Brachial pressures should increase post-exercise.
- Drop in post-exercise systolic ankle pressure should be <20% of the resting pressure and should return to baseline within 3 minutes after exercise.

Abnormal Response

- A recovery time between 2-6 minutes suggests single level disease.
- Multilevel disease typically requires 6-12 minutes before pressures return to baseline levels.
- The drop in post-exercise systolic ankle pressure should be >20% of the resting pressure and take >3 minutes to return to baseline after exercise.

Exercise Pressure Measurement							
	Rest	Imm	1	2	3	4	5
R Ankle:	130	134	135	132	130	131	132
L Ankle:	128	60	62	64	63	64	62
Brachial:	126	129	130	128	127	127	128
R ABI	1.03	1.04	1.04	1.03	1.02	1.03	1.03
L ABI	1.02	0.47	0.48	0.50	0.50	0.50	0.48

Exercise Pressure Measurement Report

Percent Pressure Drop Calculation

Calculate the ABI response to exercise:

Calculated by 1 - (post exercise pressure) x 100

Calculation Examples:

Calculate the percent drop using the 3 minute post exercise mark

Calculate the right post exercise exam:

Resting pressure – 130 mmHg

3 minute post exercise pressure -130 mmHg

130/130 =1

1 – 1 = 0

0 x 100 = 0% drop

Categorizing the right exercise stress test as normal

Calculate the left post exercise exam:

Resting pressure: 128 mmHg

3 minute post exercise pressure: 63 mmHg

63 ÷ 128 = 0.49

1 – 0.49 = 0.51

0.51 x 100 = 51

A sustained drop of 51% at three minutes categorizing the left exercise stress test as abnormal.

TABLE 150: Diagnostic Criteria for Post-Treadmill Exercise Ankle-Brachial Indices and Recovery Times

Recovery Time	Classification
<3 minutes *	Normal
2-6 minutes **	Single-level disease
6-12 minutes **	Multi-level disease
>15 minutes **	Severe occlusive disease

* The post-exercise systolic ankle pressure drops <20% compared to the resting systolic pressure.

** The post-exercise systolic ankle pressure drops >20% compared to the resting systolic pressure.

Source: Modified from Strandess DE, Zierler RE. (1993). Exercise ankle pressure measurements in arterial disease. In Bernstein EF (Ed.), Vascular Diagnosis (54 553). St. Louis: Mosby.

Arterial (Upper Extremity)

Wrist Brachial Index (WBI): Non-invasive physiological tests which compare the systolic pressure at the level of the brachial artery to the systolic pressure at the level of the digits in the hand (DBI) and detect arterial pulsations in the terminal portions of the digits (PPG). A pressure gradient (pressure difference) of 20-30 mmHg indicates a significant stenosis or occlusion between cuff levels. Calculated by dividing the higher wrist pressure by the higher brachial pressure:

$$\frac{\text{Higher wrist pressure}}{\text{Higher brachial pressure}}$$

> There should be no >20 mmHg difference between the right and left brachial pressures.

Digital Brachial Index (DBI)

Calculated by dividing the digit pressure by the higher brachial pressure:

$$\frac{\text{Digit pressure}}{\text{Higher brachial pressure}}$$

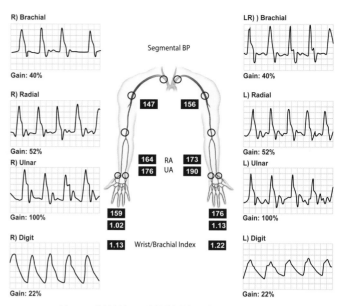

Normal WBI and DBI Physiologic Report

Calculation Example

Calculate the right wrist brachial index (WBI):

176 ÷ 156 = 1.13 categorizing the right WBI as normal

Calculate the right digital brachial index (DBI):

159 ÷ 156 = 1.02 categorizing the right DBI as normal

Calculate the left wrist brachial index (WBI):

190 ÷ 156 = 1.22 categorizing the left WBI as normal

Calculate the left digital brachial index (DBI):

176 ÷ 156 = 1.13 categorizing the left DBI as normal

TABLE 151: Diagnostic Criteria for WBI/DBI

WBI		DBI
≥1.0	**Normal**	>0.70
0.9 to <1.0	**Mild**	0.60-0.69
0.5 - 0.9	**Moderate**	0.59-0.40
0.30 - 0.5	**Severe**	<0.39
<0.30	**Critical**	

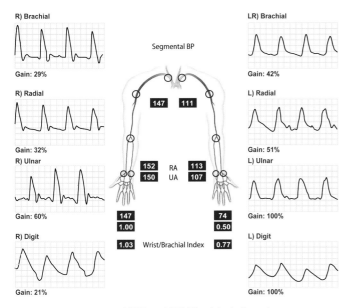

R) Brachial — Gain: 29%
R) Radial — Gain: 32%
R) Ulnar — Gain: 60%
R) Digit — Gain: 21%

LR) Brachial — Gain: 42%
L) Radial — Gain: 51%
L) Ulnar — Gain: 100%
L) Digit — Gain: 100%

Segmental BP

147 111

152 RA 113
150 UA 107

147   74
1.00   0.50

1.03 Wrist/Brachial Index 0.77

Abnormal WBI and DBI Physiologic Report

Left brachial pressure gradient

Calculation Example:

Calculate the right wrist brachial index (WBI):

152 ÷ 147 = 1.03 categorizing the right WBI as normal

Calculate the right digital brachial index (DBI):

147 ÷ 147 = 1.00 categorizing the right DBI as normal

Calculate the left wrist brachial index (WBI):

113 ÷ 147 = 0.77 categorizing the left WBI as moderate

Calculate the left digital brachial index (DBI):

74 ÷ 147 = 0.57 categorizing the left DBI as moderate

Penile

Penile Brachial Index (PBI): Non-invasive physiological testing which compares systolic blood pressures to evaluate the penile arterial system.

Calculated by dividing the penile pressure by the highest brachial pressure:

$$\frac{\text{Penile Pressure}}{\text{Higher Brachial Pressure}}$$

TABLE 152: **Diagnostic Criteria for Penile Bracial Index (PBI)**	
Disease Category	**PBI**
Normal	>0.75
Marginal	0.6 - 0.74
Abnormal	<0.60

Source: Modified from Zierler RE, Sumner DS. (2005). Physiologic assessment of peripheral arterial occlusive disease. In Rutherford Vascular Surgery 6th edition. (197-222). Philadelphia. Elsevier Saunders

Calculation Example:

Right brachial pressure of 128 mmHg

Left brachial pressure of 132 mmHg,

Cavernosal pressure #1- 91 mmHg

Cavernosal pressure #2- 95 mmHg

95 ÷ 132 = 0.72
categorizing the PBI as marginally reduced

Example

Right brachial pressure of 126 mmHg

Left brachial pressure of 122 mmHg,

Cavernosal pressure #1- 98 mmHg,

Cavernosal pressure #2- 96 mmHg

98 ÷ 126 = 0.78 categorizing the PBI as normal

Velocity Ratio

- Calculated by dividing the maximum PSV of the stenosis into the normal proximal segment of the vessel:

$$\frac{\text{Maximum PSV}}{\text{Pre-stenotic PSV}}$$

- For increased accuracy when assessing disease, measure in B-mode whenever possible and consider reductions together with Doppler velocity ratios.

TABLE 153: Velocity Ratio Vs Diameter Reduction

Velocity Ratio	Diameter Reduction
<2.1	<50%
2.1-4.1	50-74%
>4.1	>75%

Source: Cossman DV, Ellison JE, et al (1989). Comparison of contrast arteriography to arterial mapping with color flow duplex imaging in the lower extremity The Journal of Vascular Surgery, Nov; 10(5):522-8; discussion 528-9.

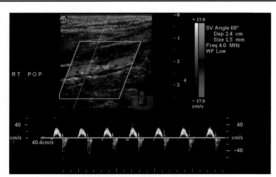

Pre stenosis spectral tracing

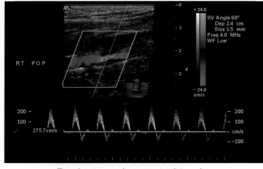

Peak stenosis spectral tracing

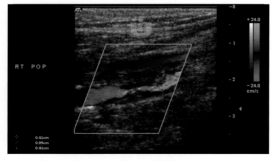

Diameter reduction (DR) at stenosis

Calculation of velocity ratio:
276 ÷ 40 = 6.9
categorizing the velocity ratio as >4.1 (>75% DR)

Diameter Reduction

Diameter reduction is a percent stenosis calculation. Diameter reduction measurements should only be used in conjunction with peak systolic velocity measurements. Diameter and area reduction tools may prove extremely useful in cases of irregularly irregular arrhythmias.

TABLE 154: Calculating Stenosis by Diameter Vs Area

Diameter Reduction	Cross Sectional (Area Reduction)
$1 - (d/D) \times 100$	$1 - (d^2/D^2) \times 100$

Calculation Example:

Diameter reduction:

$$D=0.41$$
$$d=0.09$$
$$1-(0.09 \div 0.41) \times 100$$

- Step One: $0.09 \div 0.41 = 0.22$
- Step Two: $1 - 0.22 = 0.78$
- Step Three: $0.78 \times 100 = 78$
- 78 % diameter reduction

Cross Sectional Area (Area Reduction):

$$D=0.41$$
$$d=0.09$$
$$1-(0.09^2 \div 0.41^2) \times 100$$

- Step One: $(0.0081 \div 0.1681) = 0.048$
- Step Two: $1-0.048 = 0.95$
- Step Three: $0.95 \times 100 = 95$
- 95% area reduction

Pulsatility Index

Pulsatility Index (PI): Provides information regarding the resistance in distal vascular beds. It is expected that the ratio increases from the central to peripheral arteries.

Calculate by:

$$\frac{\text{PSV} - \text{EDV}}{\text{MV}}$$

TABLE 155: Pulsatility Index and Resistance Relationship

Higher Pulsatility Index	Increased Vascular Resistance
Lower Pulsatility Index	Decreased Vascular Resistance

Peripheral Venous

Venous Insufficiency: Reflux means to "flow backward". Venous reflux is venous flow moving in the wrong direction, either away from the heart or from the deep to the superficial system through the perforating veins.

- Duplex ultrasound can identify the presence, exact location, extent, and severity of venous reflux.
- Evaluated by measuring the time in seconds for the purpose of assessing reflux for significance

TABLE 156: Diagnostic Criteria for Venous Reflux by Duplex

System	Normal	Abnormal
Superficial	<0.5 Sec	>0.5 Sec
Deep	<1 Sec	≥1 Sec
Perforators	<0.35 Sec	≥0.35 Sec

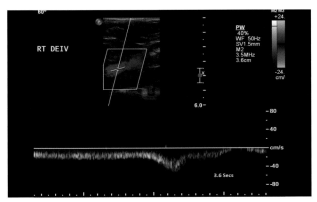

Normal: No venous insufficiency

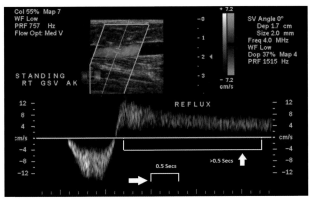

Significant venous insufficiency

Venous Refill Time (VRT): Measurement reflecting volume changes (venous emptying and filling) as a result of the calf muscle pump in the leg.

- ≥20 seconds (sec) is considered normal; legs completely empty and the veins refill by the arterial system within normal limits.
- <20 sec are associated with chronic venous insufficiency (CVI). The calf veins do not empty properly due to venous obstruction and incompetent venous valves allow for retrograde flow (back flow).

TABLE 157: Venous Refill Time (VRT)

Normal	Abnormal
≥20 seconds	<20 seconds

Renal

Renal Aortic Ratio (RAR): The renal to aortic ratio may provide additional information and can be useful when the B-mode information does not match the increased systolic velocities.

Calculated by dividing the:

$$\frac{\text{Highest renal artery PSV}}{\text{Highest PSV in the suprarenal abdominal aortic segment}}$$

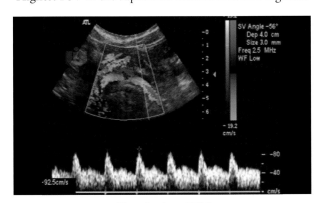

Renal artery PSV

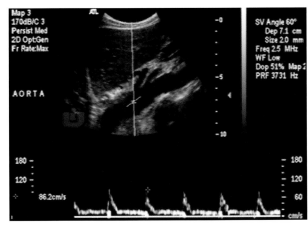

Suprarenal Aortic PSV

Example:

93 ÷ 86 = 1.1 categorizing the RAR as normal

TABLE 158: **Diagnostic Criteria for Disease According Renal-to-Aortic-Ratio (RAR)**		
Renal-to-Aortic Ratio (RAR)		
<3.5	Normal	<60% Diameter Reduction
>3.5	Abnormal	>60% Diameter Reduction

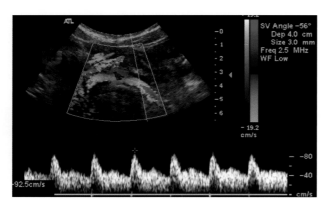

Normal renal artery PSV

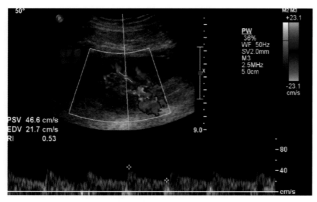

Intrarenal arterial spectral tracing

Resistive Index (RI): Measures the resistance to arterial flow within the renal vascular bed. The (RI) provides information regarding the presence of intrinsic kidney disease.

Calculated by:

$$\frac{PSV - EDV}{PSV}$$

Example:

$$\frac{47 - 22}{47} = 0.53$$

Categorizing the renovascular resistance as normal (low)

TABLE 159: **Resistive Index (RI)**	
<0.70	Normal
0.70 – 0.80	Indeterminate
>0.80	Abnormal

End-diastolic-ratio (EDR): Provides additional information regarding the arterial resistance within the kidney.

Calculated by dividing the end diastolic velocity by the peak systolic velocity

$$\frac{End\ Diastolic\ Velocity}{Peak\ Systolic\ Velocity}$$

TABLE 160: **Interpretation of End-Diastolic Ratio (EDR)**	
>0.2	Normal
<0.2	Abnormal: Indicates an increase in resistance within the kidney

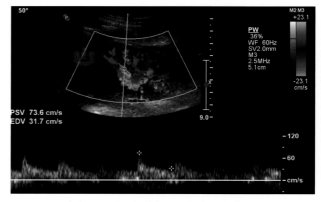

Intrarenal arterial spectral waveform

Example:

32 ÷ 74 = 0.43 categorizing the EDR ratio as normal

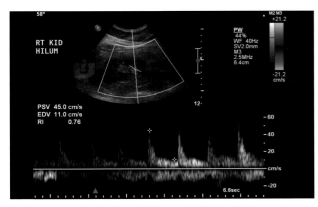

Intrarenal arterial spectral waveform

Example:

$$11 \div 45 = 0.24 \text{ categorizing the EDR ratio as}$$
borderline abnormal

Extracranial Cerebrovascular

ICA/CCA Ratio: The ICA/CCA ratio may provide additional information and can be useful when the B-mode information does not match the increased systolic velocities.

Calculate by dividing the:

$$\frac{\text{Maximum PSV from the proximal ICA}}{\text{PSV from the distal CCA}}$$

• The ICA/CCA ratio may be unreliable if significant CCA disease is present.

TABLE 161: Ratio Correlation to Diameter Reduction

ICA/CCA Ratio	Diameter Reduction
<2	<50%
2-4	50-69%
>4	70-99%

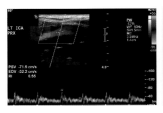 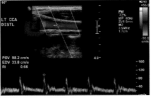

Example: 72 ÷ 98 = 0.73
categorizing the ICA/CCA ratio as <2 (<50% DR)

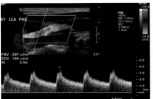 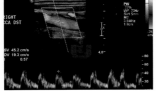

Example: 397 ÷ 45 = 8.8
categorizing the ICA/CCA ratio of >4 (70-99% DR)

Hemodialysis AVF/Prosthetic Graft

Hemodialysis requires high flow in a vessel that is easily accessible and can withstand multiple punctures with the dialysis catheters.

To accomplish this, an arteriovenous fistula is often created surgically by connecting an artery and a vein together, so that a high flow situation is created as blood flows directly from a large high pressure artery to the vein.

When an AVF is not an option, an AV graft may be surgically inserted, which also connects an artery to a vein for hemodialysis access using a prosthetic graft or transposing a vein as conduit.

• Calculate velocity ratios through the AVF/AVG by

$$\frac{\text{PSV (V}_2\text{) distal}}{\text{PSV (V}_1\text{) proximal ratio}}$$

TABLE 162: Diagnostic Criteria for Hemodialysis AVF

Hemodynamically significant stenosis (arterial inflow or venous outflow)	>2
Hemodynamically significant stenosis at the anastomosis	>3
Occlusion	Absent signal

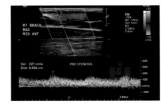 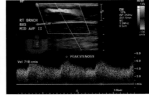

Hemodialysis AVF

Example:

$$718 \div 227 = 3.2 \text{ categorizing the ratio as a}$$
hemodynamically significant stenosis

Calculated by

$$\frac{\text{PSV (V}_2\text{) distal}}{\text{PSV (V}_1\text{) proximal ratio}}$$

TABLE 163: Diagnostic Criteria for Prosthetic Hemodialysis Graft (AVG)

Location/Disease	Ratio/Velocity
Within Normal Limits (0-49% Stenosis)	<2
Hemodynamically Significant (50-74%)	<2
Hemodynamically Significant (>75%)	>3
Venous Anastomosis	>400 cm/s
Occlusion	——

Prosthetic Hemodialysis Graft

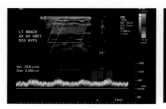 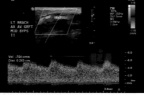

Example: 704 ÷ 79 = 8.9 categorizing the ratio as
a hemodynamically significant stenosis

Volume Flow

- Calculate the volume flow using a straight, non-tapering segment of the access.
- Activate the "time average maximum" calculation or its equivalent on the duplex scanner.
- Measure the diameter of the segment, placing the calipers perpendicular to the vessel wall.
- At the same location, open the Doppler gate to include the entire width of the vessel.
- Measure at least one cycle (PSV to PSV or EDV to EDV) on the spectral tracing to obtain volume flow (mL/min). Use complete cycles if measuring more than one.
  - Optimal volume flow in a hemodialysis AVF should be >500 mL/min
  - Optimal volume flow in a prosthetic hemodialysis graft should be >800 mL/min

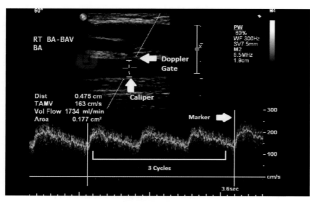

Volume flow

Identifying and Analyzing Atypical Spectral Doppler Waveforms

Various Cardiac Arrhythmias

An average of the most consistent beats may be taken. Avoid measuring the Doppler waveform directly after the irregular beat (Avoiding any erroneous focal spike in velocity)

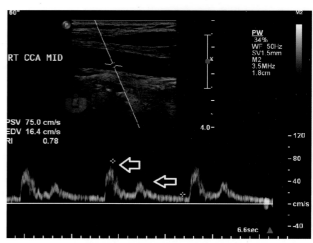

Pulsus Alternans: *Demonstrates alternating peak systolic velocities. This type of spectral Doppler waveform is often associated with cardiac abnormalities.*

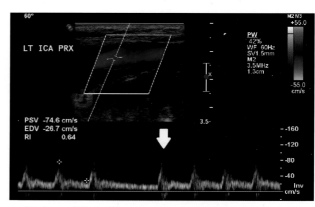

Pulsus Bisferiens: *Demonstrates two prominent systolic peaks. This type of spectral Doppler waveform is often associated with cardiac abnormalities.*

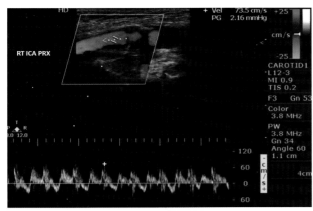

Intra-Aortic Balloon Pump (IABP): *This alters the arterial waveform demonstrating a cyclical flow pattern from the inflation and deflation of the balloon pump. This complicates accurately identifying the PSV and EDV and identifying any possible underlying carotid disease. An attempt should be made to measure the most consistent PSV and EDV.*

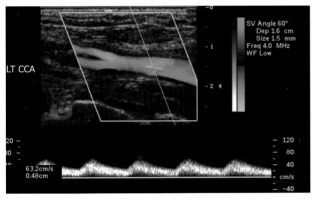

Tardus Parvus: *Characterized by a rounded, prolonged peak with diminished amplitude. Tardus parvus waveforms are often identified distal to a severe stenosis.*

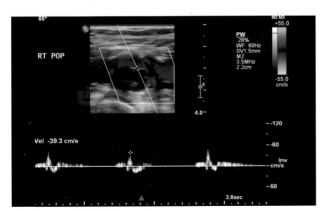

Helical Flow: *A flow pattern that describes a "spiral flow" often identified in aneurysmal segments or within an active pseudoaneurysm. There is often no EDV to measure.*

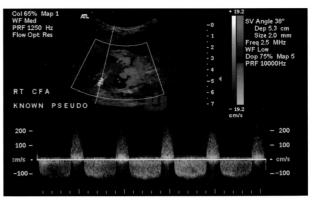

To-and-Fro-Flow from the neck of a pseudoaneurysm: *To-fro Doppler flow patterns will be apparent within the "neck" of the pseudoaneurysm. If possible, obtain a measurement of the PSV, although aliasing often occurs due to the high velocities within the pseudoaneurysm neck.*

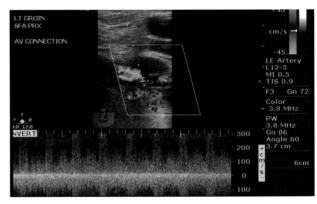

Arteriovenous Connection: *An AV fistula is an abnormal connection between an artery and a vein causing a turbulent spectral Doppler waveform with both arterial and venous characteristics. It is often difficult to decipher the arterial component from the venous component of the spectral Doppler, making it complicated to accurately measure PSV and EDV.*

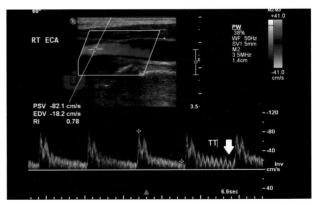

Temporal Taps: *Avoid measuring the PSV and EDV of the spectral Doppler waveform where the interruption is from the "temporal tap" maneuver.*

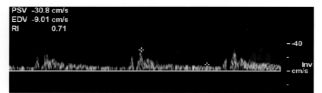

"Presteal Flow (Bunny waveform)": *The stage where the spectral Doppler takes on the appearance of the "bunny" type waveform. This is the stage prior to the flow becoming retrograde. Attempt should be made to measure the most consistent PSV and EDV portion of the waveform.*

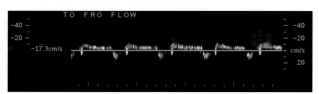

Bidirectional "To-Fro-Flow": *In terms of the vertebral artery, bidirectional flow may occur in the vertebral artery if there is a hemodynamically significant stenosis in the ipsilateral subclavian artery at its ostia. Measure the PSV of the antegrade portion of the spectral Doppler waveform.*

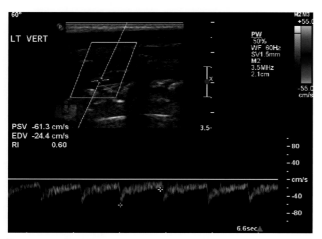

Retrograde Flow: *Vertebral artery flow reverses (flow is a retrograde direction) in an attempt to provide circulation to the upper extremity when the subclavian or right innominate artery is severely stenosed or occluded. PSV and EVD should still be obtained to document the retrograde velocity.*

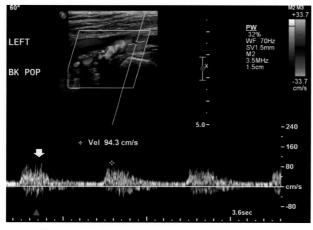

Post-stenotic turbulence: *Obtain a PSV and EDV (If present) measurement of the most consistent portion of the Doppler waveform, avoiding any erroneous peaks within the waveform.*

References

1. Non Invasive Vascular Diagnostics A Practical Guide to Therapy , 2nd Edition
2. Ali F. AbuRahma MD, FACS, FRCS, RVT, RPVI John J Bergan MD, FACS, Hon FRCS
3. Springer-Verlag London Limited 2007 Pg 262 graft surveys (mean velocity for failing graft)
4. Rumwell C., McPharlin, M. Vascular Technology An illustrated review 3rd Edition, Davies Publishing, Inc 2006
5. Edelman, S, Understanding Ultrasound Physics, 3rd Edition . Vortex Communications 2007

References

Glossary of Terms

(Printed with permission from the Society of Vascular Ultrasound)

Terminology for the Vascular Ultrasound Technologist/ Sonographer

The VOICE for the Vascular Ultrasound Profession

Copyright © 2005 Society for Vascular Ultrasound

Acknowledgements

The *Glossary of Terms* for the Vascular Technologists as first compiled in 1983 by the Education Committee of the then Society of Non-Invasive Vascular Technology, Mary Jane Pomajzl, Chair. The Glossary has since been updated three times. The second edition was published in 1989 under the direction of Paula A. Heggerick, RDMS RVT FSVU, Chair, SVT Publication Committee. The third edition was published in 1995; Joanne E. Drago, LPN RVT, Chair. The fourth edition was revised and updated in 2001 due to the efforts of Jean White, RVT, Chair, and Allene Woodley, RN RVT; Joanne Spindell, RVT RDCS; Paula Gehr, RVT; Cathy Brown, BSCVN RN RVT RDCVS; and Michael Sampson, RVT. This fifth edition has been revised and updated in 2005 due to the efforts of Products Committee Chair Michel Comeaux, RN RVT RDMS FSVU; Tom Baer, MBA RVT RDMS RDCS; Debbie Pirt, AS RVT; William Harkrider, MD RVT; and Bill Zang, BS RVT RDMS.

© Copyright 2005 Society for Vascular Ultrasound
4601 Presidents Drive, Suite 260 Lanham, MD 20706-4831
Tel. 301-459-7550
Fax: 301-459-5651
Web: www.svunet.org

A

A-C coupling (Alternating Current): Type of output signal to graphic display connection which responds to changes faster than 0.5Hz. This reduces baseline shifts and results in a stable graphic tracing.

A-mode: A mode of operation in which the display plots time along a horizontal axis and echo amplitude along a vertical axis. In ultrasound, this is referred to as the amplitude mode.

Abdominal aorta: The abdominal aorta is a portion of the descending aorta and is located at the level of the diaphragm and extends to its bifurcation (the common iliac arteries).

Abdominal Aortic Aneurysm (AAA): A focal dilation of the aorta. Most common location is infrarenal.

Abduction: Drawing away from the midline, opposite of adduction.

Abscess: A localized collection of pus surrounded by inflamed tissue.

Absorption: A process of conversion of acoustic energy to heat, resulting in a loss of energy. Absorption is a factor in attenuation.

Acceleration Index (AI): This is the systolic acceleration of the Doppler spectral waveform determined by the change in distance between the onset of systolic flow and the peak systolic velocity (cm/s), divided by the acceleration time (AT). The acceleration index (AI) is reported in frequency units as KHz/sec/MHz or velocity units as cm/s^2 Acceleration Time (AT): This is the time interval from the onset of flow to the initial peak—not peak systole Achrocyanosis: Coldness and blueness of an extremity; a vasospastic condition. Symptoms include a symmetrical, mottled cyanosis of the hands and feet, cold seat on the digits. Cold accentuates, warmth relieves the symptoms.

Acoustic: Having to do with sound.

Acoustic field: The distribution pattern of sound energy in space and time.

Acoustic impedance: Property of a medium equal to the product of density and propagation speed. The intensity of reflection (echo production) is related to the ratio of difference in acoustic impedance at an interface. The greater the difference in impedance the greater the intensity of reflection.

Acoustic shadow: Loss of acoustic properties of targets lying behind an attenuating structure. In the arteries, the most common cause of acoustic shadowing is calcified plaque (see calcification).

Acoustic variables: Pressure, density, temperature, and particle motion. Sound is identified as the rhythmical cycling of acoustic variables.

Acute: Short, severe symptoms of sudden onset or short duration; i.e., not chronic.

Adduction: Drawing toward the midline.

Adventitia: The outermost layer of an artery.

Aliasing: A phenomenon associated with pulsed Doppler; a misrepresentation of the Doppler shift in a negative direction occurs when the Doppler shift exceeds half the pulse repetition frequency.

Allen test: A test performed to check the continuity of the palmar arch normally supplied by both the radial and ulnar arteries. The test may be performed using a Doppler, a PPG, or Strain Gauge Plethysmograph.

Amaurosis fugax: Temporary blindness (partial or total) resulting from transient ischemia of the retinal arteries secondary to cerebral arterial disease. The most likely etiology is embolic.

Ampere: A unit of electromotive force; one volt acting against the resistance of one ohm (see Ohm's law).

Amplifier: An electronic device for increasing the amplitude of a signal.

Amplitude: The maximum variation in an acoustic variable. It is the difference between the average value and the maximum value of an acoustic variable. Units used with amplitude coincide with the acoustic variable used.

Amputation: The cutting off (traumatic or surgical) of all or part of an appendage.

AK amputation: Above the knee, BK amputation: below the knee, Syme's amputation: foot amputation with heel pad intact, Transmetatarsal amputation: toe amputation (across the metatarsals).

Amputee: One who has had an amputation.

Analgesia: Loss of painful sensation.

Analogue signal: A signal which is measured along a scale rather than by numerical values. The Doppler waveform derived from a chart recorder is a type of analogue signal (see digital signal).

Anastomosis: The natural or surgically-created communication between blood vessels or prosthetic graft and blood vessel as in a bypass graft. Anastomosis can then be referred to as proximal or distal.

Anechoic: Describes the property of being echo-free or without echoes (i.e., fluid-filled cyst).

Anesthesia: Loss of sensation.

Aneurysm: Dilation of a blood vessel, as a result of degeneration and weakening of the vessel wall. The most common cause of aneurysm formation is atherosclerosis.

Aneurysm, dissecting: Rupture of the intima allows blood between layers of the vessel wall, expanding the vessel while separating the layers. Extensive extravasation can occlude the lumen.

Aneurysm, pseudo: An encapsulated hematoma occurring at the site of an anastamosis, or a ruptured artery, or following an iatrogenic procedure. The pulsing mass resembles an aneurysm, i.e., it is a "false" aneurysm.

Angiectasis: Abnormal dilation of blood vessels.

Angiogram: A series of x-rays taken of a blood vessel following the injection of a radiopaque substance into the vessel (arteriogram).

Angioplasty: Dilation of an artery by a balloon tipped catheter. Often referred to as percutaneous transluminal angioplasty (PTA).

Angle of incidence: The angle at which an ultrasound beam strikes an interface (with respect to the normal or perpendicular angle). In reference to Doppler, it is the angle of the beam with respect to the flow axis.

Ankle-arm pressure index: The ratio of ankle systolic pressure to highest arm systolic pressure. The numerical index serves as an indicator of arterial insufficiency. Normal value is 1.0 or greater; the ratio decreases as arterial insufficiency increases. Usually referred to as ABI.

Annular array: Array made up of ring-shaped elements arranged concentrically.

Anomaly: A marked deviation from the normal standard.

Anoxia: Absence of oxygen to the tissues.

Antecubital fossa: A triangular area located at the bend of the elbow that contains the cephalic, median cubital and basilic veins.

Antegrade: Proceeding toward.

Antegrade flow: Proceeding towards or forward. Opposite of retrograde or reversed.

Anterior: Situated in the frontal plane, in the front of.

Anterior tibial artery (ATA): A terminal branch of the popliteal artery located along the lateral surface of the tibia and continues onto the dorsum of the foot as the dorsalis pedis artery.

Anticoagulant: Substances which prohibit or delay the normal blood clotting mechanism, e.g., Coumadin and heparin.

Aorta: The main trunk of the arterial system with its origin off the surface of the left ventricle. It is usually described in several portions, the ascending aorta, the aortic arch, and the descending aorta (thoracic and abdominal).

Aphasia: Impairment of speech due to cerebral dysfunction.
  Sensory aphasia: inability to recognize written or spoken words.
  Motor aphasia: Loss of ability to articulate language.

Arcus senilis: An opaque ring around the cornea, seen in the elderly.

Array: Transducer array.

Arrhythmia: Abnormal heart rhythm.

Arterial compliance: The expansile and contractile properties of an artery.

Arterial inflow: Pertaining to blood flow into the lower extremities proximal to the level of the common femoral arteries.

Arterial insufficiency: Reduction in blood flow within the arterial system. Inadequate blood flow results in hypoxia; the symptoms produced by arterial insufficiency vary with the end organ site.

Arterial occlusion: Complete blockage of an artery.

Arterial outflow: Normally pertaining to the medium size blood vessels, common femoral through the popli. Outflow could also pertain to the vessels carrying blood away from a bypass graft.

Arterial runoff: The infra-popliteal vessels (tibial and distal vessels).

Arterial ulceration: A local defect or excavation which is produced by sloughing of inflammatory necrotic tissue.

Arteriography: A radiologic procedure in which an opaque substance is injected into an artery and subsequent x-ray films are taken in order to visualize the arterial system. Arteriography is an invasive procedure with a small but definite associated morbidity and mortality.

Arteriole: A minute artery whose distal end leads to a capillary.

Arteriosclerosis: Degenerative changes in the artery associated with aging.

Arteriotomy: Incision into an artery.

Arteriovenous malformation: congenital anomalies resulting from faulty development of arterial, capillary, venous or lymphatic structures or any combination thereof. These lesions are though to be present from birth and do not represent neoplasms.

Arteritis: A disease characterized by inflammation of the walls of the blood vessels (vasculitis). The vessels affected are the arteries (hence the name "arteritis") This usually affects patients over 50 years of age. Cranial arteritis is also known as temporal arteritis or giant cell arteritis. It can lead to blindness and/or stroke.

Artery: Any of the blood vessels which carry blood from the heart to the other parts of the body. With the exception of the pulmonary and umbilical arteries, arteries transport oxygenated blood.

Arteries are composed of three layers: the intima, media, and adventitia.

Artifact: In ultrasound usage, refers to an echo which does not correspond to a real target. In general, refers to any artificial finding which may resemble the expected findings. artifacts may be intrinsic, e.g., reverberation or extrinsic, e.g., probe or limb movement during an examination. Cuff artifact refers to abnormally high pressures associated with the use of cuffs which are proportionately too narrow for the limb they are encircling.

Ascites: Accumulation of serous fluid in spaces between tissues and organs in the abdominal cavity.

Atheroma: Fatty degeneration or thickening of the arterial intima.

Atherosclerosis: Disease of the arterial intima, characterized by intimal proliferation (hyperplasia), deposition of fatty substances and luminal reduction.

Atrophy: Diminution in size or function, wasting.

Attenuation: Reduction in amplitude and intensity as a sound wave passes through a medium. Factors contributing to attenuation include: absorption, reflection, refraction, and scattering.

Augmentation: To cause to augment or increase. When used in conjunction with Doppler examinations of the venous or cerebral systems, refer to the increased flow velocity which is noted after one or more compression/ release maneuvers.

Auscultation: Listening to body sounds with a stethoscope.

Autologous vein graft: Self generation vein specimen (your own vein), used for bypass conduit, same as autogenous.

Axilla: Pertains to the armpit.

Axillary artery: A continuation of the subclavian artery that begins at the outer border of the first rib and terminates at the lower border of the teres major muscle and becomes the brachial artery.

Axial resolution: Separation required to distinguish two reflectors along the same longitudinal plane, i.e., parallel to the beam axis. Axial resolution is equal to one-half the spatial pulse length.

B

B-Mode: A method of operation in which the intensity of the returning echo is displayed as a spot, brightening for each pulse; brightness mode.

Bandwidth: The range of frequency components within a signal. When referring to a device or system, bandwidth is the range of the frequencies that the system is capable of processing.

Basilic vein: Large vein on the inner side of the arm (medial), near the brachial veins, a superficial vein.

Beam: The acoustic field produced by a transducer.

Bernouilli effect: The reduction in pressure which accompanies an increase in velocity of fluid flow.

Bernouilli equation: The equation which states that the total fluid energy along a streamline of fluid flow is constant. This is a form of the more general law of conservation of energy.

Bi-Directional Doppler: A Doppler instrument capable of determining whether the frequency of the Doppler shift is above or below the transmission frequency, permitting determination of blood flow towards or away from the probe.

Bifurcation: That location where a vessel branches; a frequent site of atherosclerosis.

Bilateral: On both sides.

Biphasic: Having two phases or variations having a forward and reverse component.

Blood pressure (BP): Pressure within the arterial system, quantified in millimeters of mercury (mm Hg); includes systolic pressure (during heart contraction), diastolic pressure (during cardiac relaxation) or mean blood pressure. Blood pressure is usually expressed as systolic over diastolic pressure.

Blood urea nitrogen (BUN): Waste product that accumulates in the blood stream when the kidneys are not working properly. Levels above 25 are abnormal.

Boundary layer: A thin layer of stationary fluid that is in contact with the vessel walls.

Brachial artery: Main artery of the arm, continuation of the axillary artery, on the inside of the arm, used to take the blood pressure.

Brachial veins: A paired set of veins which accompany the brachial artery. They are formed at the elbow by the union of the radial and ulnar veins. They drain the same area that the brachial artery supplies.

Brachiocephalic (Innominate): Right artery arising from the arch of the aorta, dividing into the right subclavian and right common carotid arteries.

Bradycardia: Abnormally low heart rate, generally less than 60 beats per minute.

Bruit: Auscultory sound produced by turbulent or disturbed blood flow.

Budd-Chiari syndrome: Venous outflow obstruction or occlusion, located at any level from the hepatic venules to the inferior vena cava (IVC), associated with ascites and liver failure.

Buerger's disease: Inflammatory disease of the arteries and veins, also called thromboangiitis obliterans Symptoms produced are those of arterial insufficiency which can ultimately progress to gangrene Young males are the most commonly affected Smoking is a very definite factor in the development of this disease.

Bypass: An alternate route, a surgically created pathway within the arterial or venous system used to avoid an obstruction.

C

Calcification: Deposition of calcium salts within an organic substance causing hardening; a normal process in bone but pathological in the arteries. Medial calcification is known as Monckeberg's sclerosis Arterial calcification hampers Doppler ultrasonic evaluation of blood flow because of the high reflectivity of calcium. In ultrasound, acoustic shadowing occurs distal to a calcified plaque because most of the ultrasound is reflected back to the transducer. Calcified structures have a higher acoustic impedance than the surrounding tissues.

Calf: The fleshy mass formed by the gastrocnemius muscle at the back of the leg below the knee.

Callosity or Callus: A thickening of the skin, due to friction, pressure or other irritation.

Capillary: A minute vessel that connects the arterioles and venules forming a network, in all parts of the body.

Cardiac: Pertaining to the heart.

Cardiovascular: Pertaining to the heart and blood vessels.

Carotid body: An oval mass of cells within the carotid sinus. This area acts as a chemoreceptor site and responds to changes in oxygen and carbon dioxide concentrations within the blood.

Carotid phonoangiography: A process of recording bruits and analyzing their frequency components. device consists of a sensitive microphone and a storage oscilloscope commonly called CPA.

Carotid sinus: A slight dilation of the carotid bifurcation area which contains pressure receptors (baroreceptors) that respond to changes in blood pressure by altering the heart rate.

Catheterization: Passage of a small catheter into the artery or vein to obtain blood samples, used with interventional and diagnostic procedures on the arteries in the heart or the body.

Catheter: A tube passed through the body for evacuating fluid or injecting them into the body cavities. Typically made of elastic, elastic web, rubber, glass, metal, or plastic.

Cathode Ray Tube (CRT): A television, or a large vacuum tube. The inner surface of the CRT screen is coated with phosphors that glow when struck with electrodes.

Caval: Pertaining to the vena cava.

Cavity: A hollow space.

Caudad: In a direction toward the feet (or tail), the opposite of cephalad.

Caudate lobe: The lobe of the liver that lies anterior to the inferior vena cava and posterior to the left lobe.

Causalgia: Severe neuralgic pain; also called reflex sympathetic dystrophy.

Celiac artery: First branch of the abdominal aorta. The branches of the celiac artery (left gastric, hepatic, and splenic arteries) supply blood to the stomach, liver, spleen, duodenum, and pancreas.

Cellulitis: Inflammation of cellular or connective tissue. An infection in or close to the skin is usually localized by the body defense mechanisms.

Centimeter: One hundredth of a meter.

Cephalad: Toward the head.

Cephalic: Cranial; superior in position.

Cephalic vein: A superficial vein that ascends from the dorsal aspect of the radial border of the forearm, to the anterior surface and subcutaneously up the arm and ends in the axillary vein near the clavicle. Frequently used for arteriovenous fistula formation for dialysis access.

Cerebral: Pertaining to the brain.

Cerebrovascular: Pertaining to the blood supply and blood vessels to the brain.

Cerebrovascular accident (CVA): Catastrophic event in which cerebral ischemia results in a neurologic deficit (lasting longer than 48 hours). The type of symptoms depends upon the cerebral hemisphere and territory involved. The etiology of CVA can be thrombotic, hemorrhagic, or embolic.

Cervical rib: An extra rib in the cervical region; may cause symptoms by compression of the brachial plexus (see thoracic outlet syndrome).

Cholesterol: Ammohydric alcohol; a sterol widely distributed in animal tissues and occurring in egg yolks, various oils, fats, the nerve tissue of the brain and spinal cord, the liver, kidneys and adrenal glands.

Chronic: Of long duration, or occurring with repeated frequency; opposite of acute. Occurring over a long period of time, old versus new.

Circle of Willis: Arterial circle of the cerebrum composed of left and right internal, anterior, posterior, and middle cerebral arteries as well as anterior and posterior communicating arteries. This important anastomosis connects the bilateral carotid circulation with the vertebral circulation and may be a source of collateralization in internal carotid occlusive disease.

Circulation: The continuous passage of blood throughout the arterial and venous systems.

Cirrhosis: A chronic disease of the liver; dense connective tissue forms, liver cells cease to function.

Claudication: Literally, "to limp" symptoms associated with arterial insufficiency of the extremity; intermittent leg pain (ache, cramp, etc.) brought on by exercise and relieved by rest.

Coagulate: To become clotted or congealed.

Coagulation: To change from a fluid to a semi solid mass.

Coapt: To meet or join. When performing a venous duplex exam, with light probe pressure, the walls of normal veins collapse and come together (compression).

Coarctation: A stricture or narrowing of a vessel, usually of a congenital nature.

Collagen disease: Any of various clinical syndromes characterized by widespread alterations of connective tissue including inflammation and degeneration. Included are polyarteritis, systemic lupus erythematosus, Marfan's syndrome.

Collateral circulation: An alternate, natural circulatory pathway. When there is interference in the arterial supply because of obstruction, communicating channels develop to accommodate blood flow. The peripheral resistance of the collateral vessels is higher because of the smaller diameter of the vessels.

Colon: The large intestine from the terminal ileum to the rectum; divided into ascending, transverse, descending, and sigmoid colon.

Common bile duct (CBD): Passes very obliquely through the muscular wall of the duodenum and joins with the pancreatic duct to form the ampulla of vater; carries bile to the duodenum and after receiving it from the cystic duct of the gall bladder and the hepatic ducts from the liver.

Common Carotid Artery: The common carotid artery (CCA) is the main artery that supplies the head and neck. It arises from the innominate (brachiocephalic) artery on the right and from the aorta on the left CCA. Each CCA branches into the internal and external carotid arteries.

Compartment syndrome: This syndrome occurs when increased pressure in the noncompliant fascia compromises circulation and neuromuscular function in that anatomic space.

Competence: In the normal vein no retrograde flow is detected, either with Valsalva maneuver, with proximal compression, or with the release of distal compression. Absence of retrograde flow confirms adequate venous valve closure.

Composite bypass: An arterial bypass graft constructed by using composites of autogenous vein and dacron or synthetic graft material interchangeably.

Compression: The act of pressing or squeezing; the condition of being pressed together.

Conduction: The transmission of waves (light or sound) through a medium.

Congenital: Present at birth.

Congested: Containing an abnormal amount of blood in the tissue.

Congestive heart failure (CHF): A chronic cardiac condition in which the heart is unable to maintain adequate output of blood resulting in congestion of blood in the veins and other organs of the body.

Constriction: The narrowing of a vessel opening.

Continuous flow: In abnormal veins the respiratory phasicity is lost, resulting in a steady flow signal. When coupled with very low velocity, continuous flow indicates proximal (except in the Portal system) obstruction that is preventing the normal fluctuations in flow that occurs during respiration. It is not always possible to distinguish between extrinsic vein compression and intrinsic obstruction (DVT), most especially in the iliac segments.

Continuous wave: A wave in which cycles repeat indefinitely.

Continuous wave Doppler (CW): A Doppler which uses separate transmitting and receiving piezoelectric crystals, each operating without interruption. The reflected sound waves are processed continuously.

Contralateral: On the opposite side.

Contrast medium: The use of a foreign substance to provide a difference in density (contrast) so that the tissue or organ can be better visualized.

Cord: A string like structure. A firm elongated structure consistent with a thrombosed vein.

Coronary artery bypass surgery: Surgical establishment of a shunt that permits blood to travel from the aorta to a branch of the coronary artery at a point past an obstruction.

Coronary Artery Disease (CAD): Narrowing of the arteries sufficient to prevent adequate blood supply to the myocardium.

Cortex: The outer layer of an organ as distinguished from the inner medulla, as in the kidney, ovary, lymph nodes, etc.

Costoclavicular: Pertains to the ribs and the clavicle.

Costotomy: Incision or division of a rib or part of one.

Coumadin anticoagulant: One of a group of natural and synthetic compounds that antagonize the biosynthesis of vitamin K dependent on coagulation factors in the liver.

Coupling medium: Normally an aqueous based gel. Used due to its high impedance match with tissue which allows for rapid passage of the sound beam into the tissue, with very little refraction.

Cramp: Spasmodic muscle contraction; term often used by patients to describe claudication pain.

Creatine: The decompression product of the metabolism of phosphocreatine, a source of energy for muscle contraction. Increased quantities of it are found in advanced stages of renal disease.

Credentialing: Recognition by licensure and/ or certification that an individual has met a certain criteria.

Crescendo TIAs: TIAs that are increasing in frequency over a given period of time.

Critical stenosis: A stenosis of sufficient diameter reduction that flow rate and pressure are significantly affected. Sometimes called "hemodynamically significant" stenosis.

Crosstalk: Occurs when a strong Doppler signal in one direction channel passes into the other channel. This can produce the Doppler mirror-image artifact.

Cuff artifact: Consistently high segmental blood pressure in the lower extremity resulting from the use of narrow segmental cuffs which may not completely transmit cuff pressure to the vessels in the central part of the limb (i.e., femoral artery). This effect is most pronounced in the upper thigh. Cuff artifact must be considered to avoid false negative examinations.

Cyanosis: A slight bluish, grayish, slate like or dark purple discoloration of the skin caused by reduced amounts of hemoglobin in the blood. Etiology: a deficiency of oxygen.

Cycle: A complete variation of an acoustic variable.

Cyst: A closed sac or pouch, with a definite wall, contains fluid, semi fluid, or solid material. A simple cyst is usually spherical, with echo enhancement posterior to cyst. Complex cysts can have internal debris and septations.

D

D-C coupled (Direct Current): Type of output signal to graphic display connection which responds to steady state conditions; results in baseline shifts.

Damping: A technique used to reduce the amplitude of an ultrasound pulse at its point of origin in the transducer or upon its return to the transducer.

Damping factor: The ratio of proximal and distal pulsitility indices (Gosling). DF = Proximal PI Distal PI Damping material (backing material): A material that is bonded to the backside of the active element and acts to limit the "ringing" of the crystal.

D-Dimer: D-Dimer is formed as fibrin is broken down. Lab testing can reveal its presence in the blood. Positive levels are suggestive of a thrombotic event such as deep vein thrombosis or pulmonary embolism. Negative levels can virtually rule out the presence of DVT or PE, sparing the patient further expensive, uncomfortable and/or invasive testing Dead zone: The region close to the transducer that cannot be imaged accurately.

Deceleration: A decrease in velocity.

Decibel (dB): The unit for expressing logarithmically the pressure or power (intensity or loudness) of sound.

Decubitus, lateral: Refers to a patient lying on their side.

Deep vein thrombosis (DVT): Obstruction of the deep veins by blood clot. At one time referred to as phlebothrombosis; DVT is a non-inflammatory process. The possibility of the loosely attached thrombus dislodging is always present. DVT can lead to valvular destruction, post-phlebitic syndrome, and pulmonary embolism.

Demarcation: A distinct dividing line that is visually noted, separating living and necrotic tissue.

Dependent rubor: Abnormal redness noted of the toes (filling of the small vessels) and forefoot when the leg is in the dependent position. This is usually noted in patients with severe occlusive disease.

Depth of penetration: That depth wherein echoes are no longer detectable; a function of the operating frequency of the transducer.

Dermatitis: Inflammation of skin evidenced by itching, redness, and various skin lesions.

Diabetes mellitus: A chronic disease characterized by hyperglycemia secondary to inadequate production or reduced effectiveness of insulin. Juvenile onset diabetes develops before the age of 40 and is associated with lack of insulin. Adult-onset diabetes occurs later in life, primarily in the obese; these patients have inadequate insulin supply but can usually be managed by dietary treatment or oral hypoglycemic agents. Diabetes accelerates the atherosclerotic process and in its later stages results in a variety of vascular complications. Medial-wall calcification is commonly found in diabetic patients.

Diagnosis: The art of identifying a disease.

Diaphragm: A musculomembranous wall separating the abdomen from the thoracic cavity. It contracts and expands with respiration.

Diastole: Relaxation period of the cardiac cycle.

Diastolic bruit: A bruit which extends into diastole. This is indicative of a very severe stenosis.

Diastolic pressure: The period of least pressure in the arterial vascular system.

Dicrotic notch: A brief, abrupt upswing in pressure during the deceleration phase of systole, forming a "notch" in the pressure and velocity waveforms. This marks the closure of the semiliunar valves, sometimes used as a marker for the end of systole.

Digit: A toe or finger.

Digital signal: A signal which occurs in discrete steps over time and in sequence; signals converted into numerical values or multiples of the numerical. Digital data information is then translated (e.g., through a digital scan converter) for display purposes.

Digital subtraction angiography (DSA): An invasive computerized radiologic procedure performed to visualize major vessels, the bone and soft tissue is subtracted electronically to enhance the images. This procedure can be intra-arterial or intravenous.

Dilatation: A vessel is stretched beyond normal dimensions.

Dissecting aneurysm: Splitting or dissection of an arterial wall by blood entering through an intimal tear or interwall hemorrhage. Usually in aortic arch and thoracic aorta.

Dissection: Separation of tissues; usually surgically (see aneurysm, dissecting).

Disseminated intravascular coagulation (DIC): A pathological form of coagulation that is diffuse rather than localized, as would be the case of normal coagulation. The process damages rather than protects the area involved, and several clotting factors are consumed to such extent that generalized bleeding may occur.

Distal: Farthest from the center from medial line, or from the trunk; opposite of proximal.

Distance: The space between two objects.

Distortion: Variation in amplitude or frequency of a signal that may be caused by overdriving the amplifier in the circuit.

Divergence: The spreading out of a beam that results from a source of small physical dimensions or diffraction's or scattering. Divergence degrades the ultrasound image by creating loss of beam intensity.

Doppler: A diagnostic instrument which emits an ultrasonic beam into the body. This ultrasound is reflected back from moving structures within the body at a frequency higher or lower than this transmitted frequency (Doppler shift). This shift is amplified and presented as a sound or graphic (chart) display.

Doppler angle: The angle between the direction of propagation of the ultrasound and the direction of flow. As an approximation, the angle between the axis of the ultrasound beam and the axis of the vessel lumen is generally used.

Doppler effect: Observed frequency change of reflected sound due to reflector movement to the source or the observer.

Doppler scanning: A scanning technique based on the Doppler effect to indicate the presence or absence of motion.

Doppler shift: The frequency shift created between the transmitted frequency and received frequency by an interface moving with velocity at an angle to the sound source.

Doppler shift formula:

$F = 2\,ft\,V\,(\cos\theta)\,C$

F = Frequency shift
ft = transmitting frequency
V = velocity of target
θ = angle of incidence
C = velocity of sound in tissue.

Doppler shifted frequency: The change in frequency equal to reflected frequency minus incident frequency.

Doppler waveform: The time display of the spectrum of the Doppler signal.

Dorsal: Indicating a position toward the rear part, pertaining to the back: opposed to ventral.

Dorsalis pedis artery: The extension of the anterior tibial artery, distal to the ankle joint, along the dorsum of the foot.

Drop attacks: A symptom of vertebrobasilar insufficiency manifested by loss of postural control resulting in sudden periodic falling, not associated with vertigo or unconsciousness.

Duct: A narrow or tubular vessel or channel, especially one that conveys secretions from a gland.

Duodenum: The first part of the small intestine, connecting with the pylorus of the stomach and extending to the jejunum.

Duplex scan: An ultrasound technology which combines two-dimensional B-Mode imaging with time-velocity spectral analysis.

Duplex scanner: Instrument that combines static Bmode or real-time imaging with Doppler flow detection.

Duty factor: Amount of time that the ultrasound system is on.

Dynamic range: The ratio of the largest and smallest signals that a system can handle simultaneously; expressed in decibels.

Dysarthria: A speech disorder in which the pronunciation is unclear although the linguistic content and meaning are normal.

Dysesthesia: Abnormal sensations on the skin, such as feelings of numbness, tingling, prickling, or a burning or cutting pain.

Dysfunction: Abnormal, inadequate, or impaired action of an organ or part.

Dyskinesia: A defect in the ability to perform voluntary movement.

Dysphagia: A condition in which the action of swallowing is either difficult to perform, painful, or in which swallowed material seems to be held up in passage to the stomach.

Dysphasia: Lack of coordination of speech, and failure to arrange words in an understandable way; related to cortical damage.

E

Ecchymosis: A skin discoloration consisting of large irregularity formed hemorrhagic areas.

Echo: Reflection of acoustic energy.

Echogenic: The acoustic property of a medium which renders it capable of producing echoes.

Echoic: The area of an ultrasound image that depicts strong echoes created by strong interfaces.

Ectatic: Distended or stretched.

Ectopic: In an abnormal position. Originating in an area of the heart other than the sinoatrial node causing an ectopic heart beat.

Edema: A local or generalized condition in which the body tissues contain an excessive amount of tissue fluid.

Elasticity: Willingness of a medium to distort from its original size and shape and restore to its original form after the external influence is removed.

Elevation pallor: Pallor induced by elevation of the limb.

Embolectomy: Removal of an embolus from a vessel.

Embolism: An obstruction in a vessel from a foreign substance or blood clot.

Embolus: A mass of undissolved matter present in a blood or lymphatic vessel and carried there by the blood or lymph current.

Endarterectomy: Surgical removal of atherosclerotic material and intimal lining from within an artery.

Endarteritis: Inflammation of the innermost layer (intima) of an artery.

Endograft: A graft placed within a vessel.

Endoleak: Endoleak is a term that describes the presence of persistent flow of blood into the aneurysm sac after device placement. There are 4 types of endoleaks dependent on their etiology Endoleak, attachment (Type I): A type I endoleak, is due to an incompetent seal at either the proximal or distal attachment site.

Endoleak, branch (Type II): Type II endoleaks are the most prevalent type and describe flow into and out of the aneurysm sac from patent branch vessels. They are most often identified on the post procedural CT, appearing as collections of contrast outside of the endograft, but within the aneurysm sac. The most frequent sources of type II endoleaks are collateral back flow through patent lumbar arteries and a patent inferior mesenteric artery. Because the sac fills through a collateral network, the endoleak may not be visualized on the arterial phase of CT scanning; thus, delayed imaging is required.

Endoleak (Type III): These endoleaks are less common and represent flow into the aneurysm sac from separation between components of a modular system, or tears in the endograft fabric.

Endoleak (Type IV): These endoleaks are due to egress of blood through the pores in the fabric.

Endotension: An enlarging of the aneurismal sac without a visible endoleak.

Endothelium: A form of squamous epithelium consisting of flat cells that line the blood and lymphatic vessels.

Endovascular: A catheter-based, imaging-guided procedure that allows one to work within a vessel Enhancement: An image artifact created behind a low attenuating medium.

Erythema: Reddening of the skin.

Erythrocyte: A mature red blood cell (RBC) or corpuscle.

Esophageal varices: Varicosities of the branches of the azygos vein that anastomose with the tributaries of the portal vein in the lower esophagus; occurs in patients with portal hypertension.

Ethics: A code of moral principles, individually or collectively defined; derived from a set of values or beliefs.

Etiology: Study of the causation of disease.

Eversion: To turn inside out.

Exogenous: Originating outside an organ or part.

External carotid artery (ECA): The vessel which arise from the common carotid artery at the carotid bulb and course anteromedially, supplying the exterior of the head, the face, and the greater part of the neck (normally has eight branches).

External iliac artery: The branch of the iliac bifurcation that arises from the common iliac artery that supplies the pelvic and genital organs. This artery is also known as the hypogastric artery.

Extracranial: Outside of the skull, usually used in reference to vessels or structures outside of the cranium.

Extravasation: Discharge or escape, as of blood or other substance from within a vessel into the tissue.

Extrinsic: Originating from without, opposite of intrinsic.

F

Faint: A state of temporary unconsciousness.

Falciform ligament: A wide, sickle-shaped extension of the peritoneum that serves as the principal attachment of the liver to the diaphragm and separates the right from the left lobes of the liver.

False aneurysm: See aneurysm, pseudo.

False negative rate: Rate at which a diagnostic test produces negative results when disease is actually present. False Neg. Rate = FN × 100 = % TP + FN FN = false negative, TP = true positive False positive rate: Rate at which a diagnostic test produces positive results when disease is not present.

False Pos. Rate: FP × 100 = % TN + FP TN = true negative, FP = false positive Far zone (far field, Fraunhofer): Distance from a focused transducer to the center of the focal region; in an unfocused transducer, that area where the beam begins to diverge.

Fasciotomy: A surgical procedure which involves the incision and division of the fascia in order to relieve pressure within the muscle compartments (compartment syndrome).

Fast Fourier transformation: A mathematical formula used to analyze amplitude frequency profile.

Fibromuscular dysplasia: An abnormal development of tissue composed of fibrous and muscular tissue (usually found, distal internal carotid and mid to distal renal arteries).

Field: That region propagated by an ultrasonic wave.

Field of view: That plane seen by specific ultrasound transducer.

Filter: An electronic circuit designed to allow signals of certain frequencies to pass and to stop signals of other frequencies.

Fistula, arteriovenous: Communication between an artery and a vein. It may be congenital, traumatic, or surgically created for dialysis access.

Focal length: The distance from the focused transducer to the center of the focal region.

Focal region: That region where beam diameter and area are minimum.

Frame rate: Number of television frames displayed by a system per second. Standard television format is 30 frames per seconds. The field rate is 60 frames per second (2 fields make up 1 frame).

Frame: The display produced by one scan of an ultrasound beam.

Frequency: Number of cycles per unit of time (usually seconds); expressed in Hertz (Hz): l Hz = 1 cycle per second, Kilohertz (KHz): l KHz = 1,000 Hz, or Megahertz (MHz): l MHz = 1,000,000 Hz or 1,000,000 cycles per second.

Friable: Easily crumpled; term is occasionally used to describe atherosclerotic plaque.

Fusiform: uniform circumferential dilatation; spindle shaped.

G

Gain: The ratio of output to input in an amplifying system.

Gaiter area zone: The region of the medial lower leg just above the ankle. It is this area where signs of venous stasis are most evident.

Gallbladder: A pear shaped sac on the underside of the right lobe of the liver; it stores bile from the liver, concentrates the bile by removing water from it, and discharges the bile through the cystic duct.

Gangrene: Tissue death, usually as a result of inadequate blood supply; occasionally due to infection. Lack of blood supply may be due to atherosclerosis, embolism, spasm, frostbite, tourniquets, etc.

Gastric: Pertaining to the stomach.

Gastric artery: Arises from the celiac axis; usually the first branch; divides into right and left; supplies blood to the stomach.

Gastro-duodenal artery: Arises from the common hepatic trunk and supplies the stomach and duodenum.

Gastrointestinal (GI): Pertaining to the stomach and intestine.

Gastrocnemius: That large muscle of the posterior portion of the lower leg that propels venous blood up the leg as it contracts. Commonly referred to as the calf muscle pump, this superficial muscle extends the foot and helps to flex the knee.

Gate: Electronically controlled device which controls transmission or reception of a signal.

Glaucoma: An ocular disease characterized by increased intraocular pressure. Presence of this disease should be noted prior to performing OPG or OPG-G testing.

Glomerulonephritis: A variety of nephritis characterized by inflammation of the capillary loops in the glomeruli of the kidney. It occurs in acute, subacute, and chronic forms and is usually secondary to an infection, especially with the hemolytic streptococcus.

Graft: The material used, either organic or inorganic, that is surgically inserted to replace a defect in the body.

Gravitational: Pertaining to the force of gravity.

Gray scale: A display format in which the intensity information is recorded as changes in brightness. Also known as B-mode.

Greater saphenous vein (GSV): One of the two major superficial veins of the lower limb. It originates on the dorsum of the foot, ascends medially along the calf and thigh, and drains into the common femoral vein. It is the longest vein in the body and is the vessel of choice for lower extremity bypass procedures and is also used for coronary artery bypass.

H

Hard copy: A method of preserving or recording observed data, e.g., Polaroid pictures of images, analog tracings of Doppler shifted signals and digital images.

Heat: Energy resulting from thermal molecular motion.

Hemangioma: A tumor, growth, or abnormal mass composed of blood vessels.

Hematoma: A blood-filled swelling.

Hemianopia: Blindness in one-half of the visual field; may affect one or both eyes.

Hemiparesis: Muscular weakness affecting one side of the body.

Hemiparalysis: Paralysis of one side of the body; may be permanent (stroke) or temporary (TIA).

Hemiplegia: Paralysis of one side of the body.

Hemispheric: Pertaining to one side of the brain. Stroke is referred to as being right or left hemispheric; this is in relation to the side of the brain that is affected, not the side of the body that is afflicted.

Hemodynamics: Pertaining to the physical principles governing blood flow (i.e., blood pressure, blood flow, vascular volumes, heart rate, ventricular function).

Hemoglobin: The iron containing pigment of the red blood cells. Its function is to carry oxygen from the lungs to the tissues. The amount of hemoglobin in the blood averages 14-16 grams per 100ml.

Hemorrhage: Escape of blood from a vessel (arterial or venous). Abnormal bleeding.

Heparin: Substance used to inhibit coagulation of blood; frequently used in the treatment of deep venous thrombosis.

Hepatic artery (common): Arises from the celiac trunk and supplies the stomach, pancreas, duodenum, liver, gallbladder, and greater omentum. Divides into proper hepatic and gastroduodenal arteries.

Hepatic artery (proper): Arises from the common hepatic artery and supplies the liver and gallbladder.

Hepatic veins: Drain blood flow from the liver into the inferior vena cava. There are three main veins, the left, middle and the right.

Hepatofugal flow: Directed or flowing away from the liver.

Hepatopetal flow: Directed or flowing toward the liver.

Hertz (Hz): The basic unit of frequency, equal to one cycle per second.

Heterogeneous: Of different kind or species; used in ultrasound to describe sonographic characteristics of atherosclerotic plaque; opposite of homogeneous.

Hilum: A depression or pit at that portion of an organ where vessels, ducts, and nerves enter. The indented part of the kidney.

Histogram: A graphic representation of a frequency distribution.

Holosystolic: Throughout systole, used interchangeably with pansystolic.

Holosystolic bruit: A bruit which extends throughout the period of systole from the first to the second heart sound; consistent with a severe stenosis.

Homan's sign: Pain in the calf muscle resulting from passive dorsiflexion of the foot. Is sometimes indicative of deep venous thrombosis; of limited accuracy.

Homogeneous: Uniform in structure, of the same composition.

Homologous vein graft: A graft which is similar in structure and origin to the native vessel and is donated from another human being or specimen (Bovine).

Homonymous: Of corresponding halves; see hemianopia.

Homonymous hemianopia: Blindness in the same visual fields in both eyes (see hemianopia).

Horseshoe kidney: A congenital abnormality in which both kidneys are joined at their lower poles.

Hunter's canal: A triangular space lying in the distal thigh beneath the sartorius muscle and between the adductor longus and the vastus medialis muscle. It is at this location that the femoral vessels and the saphenous nerve are transmitted. This change in the course of the superficial femoral vein may cause difficulty in evaluating the compressibility of that vessel during a venous imaging procedure.

Hydronephrosis: Obstruction of the outflow from the kidney somewhere in the ureter, bladder, or urethra, causing dilation of the kidney's collecting system.

Hydrostatic pressure: A pressure created in a fluid system, such as the circulatory system.

Hypercholesterolemia: Excessive cholesterol in the blood.

Hyperchromic: Excessive pigmentation or coloration; term may be used to describe venous stasis changes.

Hyperechoic: Producing echoes of higher amplitude than normal for the surrounding medium.

Hyperemia: Increased blood in an area. May be active, i.e., caused by increased flow or passive, i.e., increased flow that occurs in response to a previous restriction of flow (see reactive hyperemia).

Hyperlipemia: Excessive fat in the blood.

Hyperplasia: Excessive cell formation.

Hypertension: Abnormally elevated blood pressure: may be essential (etiology unknown) or secondary to another condition (e.g., renal disease, pregnancy). Although there is no universal agreement, 140 systolic and 90 diastolic are considered the upper limits of normal. Hypertension is a major risk factor in the development of atherosclerosis. Control of hypertension is an important consideration; some sequelae of hypertension include stroke, small vessel damage, and congestive heart failure.

Hypertrophy: Abnormal tissue or structural size.

Hypervolemia: Excessive blood volume.

Hypoechoic: Producing echoes of lower amplitude than normal for the surrounding medium.

Hypoesthesia: Diminished sensation.

Hypogastric artery: Another name for the internal iliac artery, which supplies the pelvic viscera and musculature.

Hypoplastic: Incomplete development or underdeveloped (artery or organ).

Hypotension: Abnormally low blood pressure; may be primary, secondary, or postural.

Hypovolemia: Decreased blood volume.

Hypoxia: Diminished oxygen content in the tissues.

I

Iatrogenic: Refers to any condition which arises from the treatment of another condition by a physician or surgeon, e.g., damage to the artery during an arteriographic procedure.

Iliac artery: Originates at the terminal bifurcation of the abdominal aorta forming the right and left iliac arteries.

The common iliac branches into the external and internal iliac arteries.

Iliac vein: Formed by the union of the internal iliac vein which drains the pelvis and the external iliac vein which is a continuation of the common femoral vein. The right and left common iliac veins unite to form the inferior vena cava.

Image update: The ability of a duplex scanner to alternate between the two functions of imaging and Doppler.

Impedance: Electrical resistance; changes in impedance (or resistance) are measured by impedance plethysmography (IPG) and strain gauge plethysmography (SPG) (see acoustic impedance for ultrasound usage).

Impedance plethysmography: A noninvasive diagnostic technique used in the diagnosis of deep venous thrombosis. Four electrodes are placed around the calf and a small electrical current is sent through the underlying tissues. A recording is made of changes in venous capacitance occurring during a period of obstruction to venous outflow (via an occluding thigh cuff). Since the current is held constant any changes in resistance (or impedance) detected by the skin electrodes are associated with volume changes in the calf. By plotting venous filling (capacitance) and venous emptying (outflow) on a graph, conclusions can be drawn about the patency of the venous system (see Ohm's law).

Impotence: In the male, inability to achieve penile erection. The etiology can be neurogenic, metabolic, vasculogenic, or psychogenic. Identification of the primary etiology is complex and involves serum hormonal studies, nocturnal tumescence study, and noninvasive vascular examination (see penile-brachial index).

In situ: In position. Used to describe a vascular surgery procedure where the greater saphenous vein remains in its anatomical position as the vessel is transformed into an arterial conduit. The valves are surgically removed and the branches are ligated before the proximal and distal anastomoses are made.

Incidence angle: Angle between propagated sound beam direction and line perpendicular to media boundary.

Incompetent: Unable to perform natural function. Used to refer to venous valves which no longer close completely, permitting blood to flow in a backward direction.

Incompressible vessel: Inability to eliminate the arterial flow signal with maximal cuff pressures most likely due to medial calcification of the arterial wall and resulting in falsely high pressures.

Inertia: Resistance to acceleration.

Infarct: A localized area of ischemic tissue necrosis due to inadequate arterial blood supply.

Infarction: An event occurring when there is an arterial occlusion or stenosis to the point of insufficient blood flow to an organ.

Inflow obstruction: Arterial blood flow is severely restricted due to a proximal obstructing lesion.

Inferior: Lower than, beneath.

Inferior mesenteric artery (IMA): Originates from the distal aorta and supplies the left portion of the transverse colon, the descending colon, the sigmoid colon, and part of the rectum.

Inferior mesenteric vein (IMV): Is usually small in size and runs to the left of the superior mesenteric vein to join the splenic vein.

Inferior vena cava (IVC): Originates from the union of the right and left iliac veins terminating in the right atrium of the heart.

Infrapopliteal: Located below the popliteal artery or popliteal space.

Infrarenal: Located below the renal artery.

Inguinal ligament: A fibrous band extending from the anterior superficial iliac spine to the pubis tubercle in the groin.

Innominate artery: Arising from the arch of the aorta, dividing into the right subclavian and right common carotid arteries.

Innominate vein: Formed by the union of the internal jugular with the subclavian vein.

Insonate: To expose to ultrasound waves, to examine utilizing sound waves.

Insulin: Pancreatic hormone required for carbohydrate metabolism (see diabetes).

Intensity: Total energy in an acoustic wave as it travels through a space per unit time; equal to the power in the wave divided by the area over which the power is spread.

Intensity = power (watts) area (CM2) Interface: Surface forming the boundary between two media having different properties/densities (i.e., acoustic impedance).

Intermittent: Occurring at intervals, not constant. Used when describing claudication.

Internal: Inside, opposite of external.

Internal carotid artery (ICA): The internal carotid artery arises from the common carotid artery at the carotid bulb, and courses posterolaterally to the base of the skull where it gives rise to vessels which feed the brain, nose, orbit, internal ear, and forehead. It is divided into four parts: cervical, petrous, cavernous, and cerebral.

Interosseous artery: A branch of the ulnar artery, which in some individuals continues to the wrist.

Intima: Innermost layer of an artery; comprised of an endothelial lining, a thin layer of connective tissue, and an internal elastic membrane.

Intima media thickness (IMT): A statistical measurement/ parameter used to define the extent of atherogenesis in its early phase (discrimination threshold in the resolution area of ultrasound equipment: >100um).

Intimal flap: A loosened portion of the innermost wall of the artery.

Intracranial: Within the skull; used to refer to those structures and blood vessels within the cranium. Opposite of extracranial.

Intraluminal thrombus: Soft clot (usually poorly echogenic), which is contained within the walls of a blood vessel.

Intravascular sonography: The introduction of suitable transducers into the blood vessel.

Intrinsic: From within, inside. Opposite of extrinsic.

Invasive: Penetrating into the body tissues; e.g., an invasive procedure is one in which a substance or an instrument enters the body.

Iodine-125 fibrinogen uptake: Radio labeled fibrinogen is injected into the blood stream and is "taken up" or incorporated into any active clot formation.

Ipsilateral: On the same side, opposite of contralateral.

Ischemia: Deficient local blood supply to body tissues; due to obstruction of arterial inflow. Symptoms of ischemia include coldness, pallor, pain, impairment of function and ultimately tissue necrosis (gangrene).

J

Jugular vein: Major neck vein subdivided into anterior, external, and internal jugular veins bilaterally.

Jugular vein anterior: Originates from the veins draining the lower jaw, descends anteriorly, and terminates in the external jugular vein.

Jugular vein external: Drains the exterior of the cranium and deep parts of the face, runs perpendicularly in the neck to empty into the subclavian, internal jugular, or brachiocephalic vein.

Jugular vein internal: Continues from the transverse sinus at the base of the skull, runs vertically in the neck to unite with the subclavian vein to form the brachiocephalic vein.

Juxtarenal: Adjacent to, side by side, or in close proximity to the renal structures.

K

Kilohertz (KHz): 1,000 Hertz or cycles per second (see Hertz, frequency).

Kinetic: Pertaining to motion; e.g., kinetic energy is that energy associated with movement.

L

Lacunar infarct/Lacunes: Important, but poorly understood, irregularly/jagged cavities in the brain (0.5 to 15 mm in size) believed to be small, deep cerebral infarcts.

Lamina: A thin layer.

Laminar flow: Blood flowing in thin layers in a streamline direction parallel to the vessel wall. The highest velocities are at center stream; slowest along the wall. In laminar flow, red blood cells tend to migrate toward center stream, leaving the less viscous plasma along the wall.

Lateral: Away from the mid-line, to the side.

Lateral resolution: That separation required to distinguish two reflectors along a path perpendicular to the sound beam path; a function of beam width.

Left gastric artery: Originates from the celiac artery and supplies the stomach.

Lens, acoustic: A transparent material placed in front of a transducer used to focus an ultrasound beam.

Lesion: Any pathological change in a body tissue, e.g., a venous ulcer is a lesion, atherosclerotic plaque may be referred to as a lesion.

Lesser saphenous vein (LSV): One of two major superficial veins of the lower limb. Originating on the lateral side of the foot, it extends along the posterior aspect of the calf. The termination of the LSV varies; terminations include the popliteal 2-4 cms near knee crease, distal SFV, or GSV (either directly or via a perforating vein).

Ligamentum teres: Echogenic structure in the left lobe of the liver (a remnant of the ductus venosum) in which the umbilical vein runs.

Ligate: To tie off, e.g., to tie off a blood vessel at surgery.

Light reflection rheography (LRR): An instrument, similar to the photoplethysmograph, which measures, by means of three infrared lights and a receiving diode, changes in skin blood perfusion. This instrument is used to assess venous disease (i.e., venous reflux, obstruction).

Linear: Relating to, consisting of, or resembling a line. Linear transducer; multiple elements arranged in a line.

Linear array: An electronically steered real time transducer composed of multiple transducer elements, each element can be fired independently or in combination.

Linear phased array: Is operated by applying voltage pulses to all elements with small time variants. This allows the beam to be shaped and steered.

Linear switched array: Operated by applying voltage pulses to groups of elements in succession.

Lipid: Generic term used to describe any of the water soluble fats.

Lobe: A well-defined portion of any organ, usually a lobe is demarcated in some way.

Longitudinal: Along the path of a sound beam; or along a lengthwise course, as in a longitudinal scan.

Longitudinal resolution: Same as axial resolution.

Lumen: The space inside a tube, blood vessel, or duct.

Lymph: Transparent fluid, comprised of white blood cells (lymphocytes), conveyed in the lymphatic vessels.

Lymphangitis: Inflammation of a lymph vessel.

Lymphedema: Fluid retention in the tissues as a result of obstruction in the lymphatic system. Can present symptoms similar to deep venous thrombosis.

Lymphoceles: Fluid collections, which result from lymphatic leakage from, disrupted channels along the iliac vessels.

M

M-Mode: Method of display in which a brightening spot for each pulse produces a one-dimensional time display of reflector position; motion mode.

Manometer: An instrument for measuring pressure.

Matching layer: The material placed in front of the front face of the transducer element to reduce the reflection at the transducer element face.

Maximum venous outflow: Describes the maximum rate of venous emptying which occurs in a limb following rapid cuff deflation post venous occlusion.

Mean: Midway between two points or measurements; the arithmetic average.

Mechanical scanners: A single transducer or several transducers are oscillated within the scan head steering the sound beam over the region of interest.

Media: Middle layer of an artery.

Medial: Toward the midline, opposite of lateral.

Median: The middle number in a distribution, half of the numbers will be above and half of the numbers will be below it.

Median cubital vein: Located in the antecubital fossa and crosses from the medial to the lateral side of the fossa and connects the basilic and cephalic veins.

Medium: Substance through which a sound wave travels.

Medulla: The inner part of the kidney containing the renal pyramids which appear hyperechoic on ultrasound.

Megahertz (MHz): 1,000,000 Hertz or cycles per second (see Hertz, frequency). Most clinical Doppler instruments operate between 2-20 MHz.

Membrane: A thin lining or covering.

Memory: A collection of integrated circuits in which data is stored. Binary data is stored as electrical signals.

Menu: A list of all the programs that can be used with the system or a listing of all the functions within a program. The menu lists the options available to the operator; options are selected by pressing a key. Mesenteric artery, superior (SMA): The SMA arises from the abdominal aorta, approximately 1 cm below the celiac trunk. The SMA and its branches (inferior pancreatic, duodenal, colic, ileocolic and intestinal arteries) supply blood to the small intestines and to the proximal half of the colon.

Mesenteric artery, inferior (IMA): The IMA arises from the abdominal aorta approximately at the level of the 3rd and 4th vertebra. The IMA and its branches (left colic, sigmoid and superior rectus arteries) supply blood to the descending colon, sigmoid colon and rectum.

Microprocessor: An integrated circuit that performs basic data processing operations; i.e., the processing of electronic signals.

Migraine: Periodic, throbbing headache, often unilateral.

Mirror image artifact: Identical representation of an object on the other side of a strong reflector (sonography). Identical representation of the spectrum on the other side of the baseline (Doppler).

Mode frequency: Indicates the frequency with the highest amplitude and is the value that can be measured most reliably.

Monckeberg's sclerosis: Degenerative arteriosclerotic change in which calcium is deposited in the media of small and middle-sized arteries. Medial calcification results in a rigid artery which does not compress under ordinary pressure. In such cases, abnormally higher pressure must be exerted with a blood pressure cuff in order to obliterate the arterial signal. Pressures measured in this way are artifactually elevated.

Monocular: Pertaining to one eye; e.g., amaurosis fugax may produce monocular symptoms.

Monophasic: A monophasic pattern as a readily distinguishable systolic pulse but a lack of oscillatory activity during diastole. Such patterns demonstrate diminished arterial compliance. They may indicate a stenosis proximal to the examination site and low resistance in distal vessels.

Morbidity: The ratio of unhealthy individuals to the total population of a given group; a state of being sick/ diseased.

Mortality: The ratio or total number of deaths to the total number of a given group.

Motor: Pertaining to motion, action.

Mottling: A condition that is marked by discolored areas.

Mural: Refers to the wall of a cavity, organ, or vessel.

Murmur: Abnormal sound heard on auscultation of the heart, associated with turbulent blood flow. Synonymous with bruit, but is limited to the heart.

Muscle pump: A mechanism to direct blood from the lower extremities towards the heart. The contracting muscles of the leg, especially the calf, act as a power source to propel the venous drainage collected in the soleal sinusoids. Competent valves prevent the reflux of blood. When the muscles relax, the space created in the now-emptied deep veins draws blood from the superficial veins into the deep system via the perforators.

Myocardial infarction (MI): Damage or death to an area of heart muscle resulting from reduction of blood supply; a heart attack.

N

Near zone (near field, Fresnel zone): The region of a sound beam in which the beam diameter decreases as the distance from the transducer increases.

Necrosis: Localized tissue death; when due to arterial insufficiency is called ischemic necrosis; often used interchangeably with the term gangrene.

Negative predicted value: The likelihood that a negative test result actually implies the absence of disease.

Negative predictive value: The ability of a test to anticipate (predict) normal findings. Neg. Pred. Value = TN × 100 = % TN + FN TN = true negative, FN = false negative Neointimal hyperplasia: The narrowing of an endarterectomized artery by smooth muscle and fibrous overgrowth of the tissue layer that replaces the intima after surgery.

Nephrology: Science of the structure and function of the kidney.

Neurogenic: Originating within the nervous system, may be used to describe claudication or impotence when the etiology is nervous rather than vascular.

Neuropathy: A functional disturbance or pathological change in the nervous system. Can be related to peripheral vascular disease in the diabetic patient, sensory, motor, autonomic, and mixed varieties.

Nocturnal: Occurring during the night. May be used to describe rest pain which causes awakening from sleep.

Noise: Any signal that conveys unwanted information; may refer to unwanted echoes that are due to reverberation. Electronic noise may originate in the transducer and the electrical components of a system.

Nondirectional: A Doppler instrument which assesses flow, via frequency shift, without regard for direction of blood flow.

Noninvasive: Refers to any procedure or examination in which the body is not penetrated by a substance or instrument. Plethysmographic and ultrasonic examinations are examples of noninvasive examinations. Venography or arteriography are examples of invasive examinations.

Nonocclusive: Not totally obstructed.

Normotensive: Of normal pressure.

North America Symptomatic Carotid Endarterectomy Trial (NASCET): A technique for measuring a carotid stenosis using the smallest residual internal carotid artery diameter in the stenosis (a) divided by the normal ICA diameter beyond the stenosis (b). Percent stenosis = a/b × 100.

Nyquist limit: The highest frequency in a sampled signal that can be represented unambiguously; equal to one-half the pulse repetition frequency.

Nystagmus: Involuntary, repetitive, jerky movements of the eye.

O

Objective: Pertains to things or events that are external to one's self. Objective tests are those in which the results can be observed by individuals other than the examiner. Objective signs are those which can be noted by an observer, as opposed to those signs (such as pain) which are described by a patient. Opposite of subjective.

Obstructive Raynaud's syndrome: Episodic attacks of vasospasm resulting in the closure of small arteries and arterioles of the distal extremities in response to cold or stress with obstruction of the palmar and digital arteries.

Occlusion: The complete closure of an opening, duct or vessel.

Ocular: Pertaining to the eye.

Oculoplethysmography: A noninvasive diagnostic procedure designed to detect flow reducing lesions of the internal carotid artery. Changes in ocular volume are related to changes in arterial blood flow. These changes in volume are detected (via small corneal eye cups attached to a transducer) and recorded (ocular pulse recordings). A delay in ocular pulse arrival time is associated with a hemodynamic stenosis. This is an indirect measurement of internal carotid artery status.

Oculopneumoplethysmography: A noninvasive diagnostic procedure designed to detect flow reducing lesions of the internal carotid artery. Intraocular pressure is measured by placing small cups (which are attached to a transducer) on the sclera. A negative vacuum is applied to obliterate arterial inflow. The degree of vacuum corresponds to a specific intraocular pressure. As the vacuum is released, ocular pulsations return and the intraocular pressure is recorded. Differences in intraocular pressure between the eyes is associated with a hemodynamic stenosis. Like the OPG, this is an indirect measurement of internal carotid artery status.

Ohm: Unit of electrical resistance; one ohm is the resistance which permits one ampere of current to flow under an electromotive force of one volt.

Ohm's law: States that voltage equals current multiplied by resistance (impedance). Voltage = Current × Resistance This is the basis for strain gauge and impedance plethysmographic testing. When voltage and current are held constant, the changes in resistance can only be due to changes in limb volume.

Ophthalmic: Pertaining to the eye.

Ophthalmic artery: Arises from the internal carotid artery, just as that vessel is emerging from the cavernous sinus, on the inner side of the anterior clinoid process, and enters the orbit through the optic foramen, below and on the outer side of the optic nerve.

Ophthalmoscope: An illuminating instrument used to examine the interior of the eye.

Origin: The source or starting point; i.e., the point where an artery begins.

Orthostatic hypotension: A fall in blood pressure that is associated with standing upright.

Orthotic: Any device (including prostheses) applied to the body in the management of disability or impairment. For example, the special implements used to facilitate eating in the stroke patient are orthotic devices.

Oscillation: Vibration.

Overall accuracy: Sum of true positive tests and true negative tests divided by the total number of tests performed.

P

Pallor: Abnormal paleness or lack of color in the skin.

Palmar: Pertaining to the palm of the hand, as in palmar arch. The palmar arch is formed by the anastomoses of ulnar and radial arteries, both superficial and deep.

Palpation: The act of examining by touch, manually. To assess skin temperature or pulses by touch is to palpate.

Pancreas: A large elongated gland, located behind the stomach, it stretches transversely between the spleen and duodenum. Produces digestive enzymes and insulin.

Pansystolic: Extending throughout systole, as in pansystolic bruit. Used interchangeably with holosystolic.

Papaverine: A vasodilating agent used in patients with suspected vasculogenic impotence. The intracavernosal injection bypasses the psychoerotic and neurologic pathways that normally induce an erection.

Papilledema: Edema of the optic disc (choked disc); indicates increased intracranial pressure.

Paralysis: Complete or incomplete loss of nervous function to the body or body part, may be motor or sensory or both. Stroke is only one of the many causes of paralysis.

Paraplegia: Paralysis of the lower extremities, may include bowel and bladder paralysis also.

Parasympathetic: A division of the autonomic nervous system involved primarily with restorative functions. The parasympathetic nerves are derived from intracranial and sacral nerves and travel via the vagus nerves. The vagi participate in visceral reflexes including pressures and chemical receptors located in the aortic arch. Parasympathetic activity is mediated by acetylcholine.

Parenchyma: The essential elements of an organ; used in anatomical nomenclature as a general term to designate the functional elements of an organ as distinguished from its framework.

Paresis: Partial or incomplete paralysis.

Paresthesia: Abnormal sensation without objective cause, such as numbness, prickling and tingling ---a heightened sensitivity. Experienced in central and peripheral nerve lesions and in locomotor ataxia.

Patency: The state of being open. A venous characteristic assessed in the venous Doppler examination.

Patent: Open, not occluded.

Pathogenesis: The origin and development of a disease.

Pathology: The study of the essential nature of disease, especially of the structural and functional changes in tissues and organs of the body which cause or are caused by disease, the structural and functional manifestations of disease.

Pedal: Pertaining to the foot as in pedal pulses, the pulses of the foot.

Penile brachial index (PBI): An index derived by dividing the penile blood pressure by the brachial blood pressure. An abnormal pressure ratio suggests a decreased blood flow which may explain urologic symptoms.

Penile implant: A semi rigid rod or inflatable device implanted in the penis to provide an erection in men with organic impotence.

Percent window: A measure of spectral broadening, integrated over systole. The measure is normalized so that 100% indicates no spectral broadening or a "clear" window.

Percutaneous: Effected through the skin, as in injection, or to inject through the skin.

Perforating veins (communicating veins): Veins that link the superficial veins of the leg to the deep venous system.

Perfusion: The passage of blood through the vessels of a specific organ.

Periarteritis: Inflammation of the outer lining of an artery and the surrounding tissues.

Perigraft fluid: An accumulation of fluid adjacent to an allograft in the post-operative period. Possibilities include serous fluid (seroma), blood (hematoma), pus (abscess), urine (urinoma) and lymph (lymphocele.)

Periorbital: Surrounding the eye (orbit).

Periorbital Doppler examination: The terminal branches of the ophthalmic artery (derived from the internal carotid artery) are assessed via a directional Doppler probe. Normal flow is antegrade out of the orbit of the eye and can be obliterated with ipsilateral common carotid artery compression. In the presence of a flow reducing lesion, flow may be retrograde into the orbit of the eye (the source of flow derived from the external carotid artery), or normal in direction but not obliterated with ipsilateral common carotid artery compression.

Peripheral vascular resistance: That resistance (or impedance) to blood flow in the systemic arterial system. Resistance to blood flow is determined primarily by the caliber of small arterioles, i.e., the smaller the vessel the greater the resistance. Other factors affecting resistance include the length of the vessel and viscosity. It is vascular resistance which contributes to the brief period of flow reversal in the peripheral vessels.

Peripheral: Pertaining to the outer boundaries, away from the center. Peripheral vascular refers to those vessels away from the center, i.e., excluding the heart.

Perivascular: Surrounding a blood vessel.

Peroneal artery: Arising about 2.5 cm below the bifurcation of the popliteal artery, it is the largest branch of the posterior tibial artery. It follows the medial edge of the fibula and remains in close relation with the posterior aspect of the bone and with the interosseous membrane throughout the rest of its course.

Perm Cath catheter: Used for acute dialysis access. These catheters may be used immediately. Their softer material is better tolerated by patients and allows the catheter to remain in place for prolonged periods. Petechia: A very small hemorrhagic spot.

Pevronie's disease: A condition when scarring thickens and may even calcify the tunica albuginea that surrounds the corpora cavernosa. Symptoms include painless curvature with erection or sometimes enough pain with erection that detumescence results.

Phantom: Materials used with similar characteristics of normal tissue (e.g., scattering or attenuation).

Phased array: A type of electronically steered transducer in which there are multiple transducer elements. The ultrasound energy from a phased array is steered by pulsing all of the elements as a group but with a small time (or phase) difference between the elements. A phased array produces a sector B-scan.

Phasicity: Normal venous flow increases and decreases in response to respiration. In a normal lower extremity, flow will diminish or cease with respiration. Phasicity is reversed in the upper extremity veins.

Phlebitis: Inflammation of a vein.

Phlebography: Radiologic procedure in which an opaque substance is injected into a vein; subsequent x-ray pictures are taken in order to visualize the venous system. Synonymous with venography.

Phleborheography (PRG): A noninvasive diagnostic technique used to identify the presence of deep venous thrombosis. This is a plethysmographic technique in which air-filled cuffs are placed on the extremity and the volume changes associated with the respiratory variability of venous blood flow are recorded. In the absence of venous obstruction, respiratory waves are present in the limb. Compression of the limb distal to the recording cuffs should produce no change in the baseline recordings.

Phlebothrombosis: Term used to describe occlusion of vein by clot in the absence of an inflammatory process (see deep venous thrombosis).

Phlegmasia Cerulea Dolens: When DVT involves the major veins proximal to the inguinal ligament. Commonly referred to as iliofemoral thrombosis.

Phonoangiography: See carotid phonoangiography (CPA).

Photoplethysmograph (PPG): A device (transducer) which assesses minute changes in skin blood perfusion. Infrared light is emitted from a transmitting diode and reflected back to a receiving diode; changes in red blood cell density associated with arterial pulsation are detected by the transducer. Thus, PPG detects changes in red blood cell volume; the signal output is in the form of a pulse wave form. PPG is used in a number of noninvasive diagnostic examinations; venous reflux plethysmography, supraorbital plethysmography, digital pressures, Allen's test, and thoracic outlet maneuvers to name a few. Piezoelectric (from the Greek piezo, meaning pressure): The property of certain crystals cause them to emit electricity when deformed or squeezed. When electricity is applied to the crystal, the crystal changes its shape and the crystal vibrates; this is the source of the ultrasound wave.

Piezoelectric effect: Changing of mechanical to electrical energy and vice versa.

Pignoli's double line measurement: Characteristic double lines on images that represent the combined thickness of the intima and media of the arterial wall.

Pixel: The individual picture cell on a television screen. A screen is divided into many horizontal scan lines, which are in turn divided into pixels. The result is a grid made of many, many pixels.

Plantar: Pertaining to the sole of the foot.

Plaque: Generic term used to describe an atherosclerotic lesion. It can consist of platelets, fibrin, lipids, and calcium.

Plasma: Fluid portion of the blood.

Platelet: A round or oval disk, 1/3 to 1/2 the size of an erythrocyte found in the blood. Platelets number from 150,000 to 450,000 per cc. Function: Platelets play an important role in blood coagulation, hemostasis and blood thrombus formation. When a vessel is injured, platelets adhere to each other and the edges of the injury and form a plug which covers the area. The plug or blood clot formed soon retract and stops the loss of blood. Plethysmograph (from the Greek plethys, meaning volume): Any device, instrument, or transducer which measures volume changes in size or amount. Air plethysmographs include: phleborheography, volume pulse recordings, and ocular pulse recordings. Water plethysmography is typified by the OPG. Impedance plethysmography and strain gauge are similar in concept and detect changes in calf size associated with venous filling of a limb. Photoplethysmography detects the volume of red blood cells in the skin.

Poiseuille's law: Formula describing the relationship between flow, pressure, and resistance in a laminar flow system. The following formula is an abbreviated version the pressure/volume flow relationship. Q = P R Q = Flow, P = Pressure, R = Resistance Polycystic disease: Multiple cysts of varying sizes found in the kidneys and the liver.

Polytetrafloroethylene (PTFE): A synthetic or prosthetic graft or material used for bypass or patching arteries.

Popliteal artery: Originates as a continuation of the femoral artery in the popliteal space, bifurcating at the lower border of the popliteus muscle into the anterior and posterior tibials. Its branches also include the lateral and medial superior geniculars, middle genicular, the lateral and medial inferior genicular, and gastrocnemius arteries.

Portacaval shunt: The surgical creation of an anastomosis between the portal vein and vena cava.

Porta hepatis: The transverse fissure on the visceral surface of the liver where the common bile duct exits the liver and the hepatic artery and portal vein enter the liver.

Portal hypertension: Increased portal venous pressure, usually due to liver disease. Can cause the dilatation or thrombosis of the portal vein, superior mesenteric vein, splenic vein, and the formation of varices.

Portal system: Consists of the portal vein, splenic vein, and inferior and superior mesenteric veins.

Portal vein (PV): Collects blood from the digestive tract and empties into the liver to be detoxified. Formed by the junction of the splenic vein and the superior mesenteric vein.

Portosystemic Shunt: An expandable metallic stent between the right hepatic vein and right portal vein for the treatment of portal hypertension, variceal bleeding, and refractory ascites.

Positive predictive value: The ability of a test to anticipate (predict) abnormal findings.

Pos. Pred. Value = P × 100 = % TP + FP TP = true positive, FP = False positive Posterior: Refers to the back; or dorsal side of the body; opposite of anterior.

Posterior tibial artery (PTA): The larger and more directly continuous of the two terminal branches of the popliteal artery. Its branches are the peroneal, nutrient of the fibula, lateral and medial posterior malleolar, nutrient of the tibia, and the lateral and medial plantar.

Postphlebitic syndrome: Chronic venous insufficiency secondary to previous deep venous thrombosis. Venous thrombosis damages the valves and renders them incompetent. The physical signs include edema, stasis pigmentation changes, pain, and ulceration.

Potential energy: Capable of doing or being although not yet doing or being; possible but not actual. Latent energy, energy of position, the energy existing in a body by virtue of its state of existence, which is not exerted at the time.

Pourcelot index (resistance index): An index of pulsatility of blood flow. The difference between the maximum and minimum Doppler frequency shifts, divided by the maximum Doppler frequency shift, represents the Pourcelot index.

Power: Rate of flow of energy in the direction of propagation; expressed in watt units. Power is proportional to the square of amplitude.

Precursor: Forerunner.

Profunda femoris artery (deep femoral artery): Deep artery of the thigh which originates from the common femoral artery. Its branches include the lateral circumflex femoral and the median circumflex femoral. It terminates in three or four perforating branches in the mid-thigh (major source of collateral flow in the presence of an occluded superficial femoral artery).

Profundaplasty: Reconstruction of the occluded or stenosed deep femoral artery.

Proliferate: To increase by cell division, e.g., the early lesions of atherosclerosis are marked by intimal proliferation.

Prone: Lying on the abdomen with the face downward, opposite of supine.

Propagation speed: Velocity of an acoustic wave; equal to the product of frequency and wavelength.

Prophylaxis: Pertaining to any measures designed to prevent disease development.

Prosthesis: An artificial part or device used as a substitute for one that is missing; e.g., after a limb amputation, a prosthesis is fitted to the stump.

Proximal: Nearest to a point of reference. Opposite of distal.

Pseudoaneurysm: See aneurysm, pseudo.

Pseudoclaudication: Term used to describe a syndrome of symptoms resembling claudication but not of a vascular origin. The most common etiology is neurogenic. Pseudoclaudication can be differentiated from true claudication by the nature of the presenting symptoms. The exercise-pain-rest-relief cycle is not present in pseudoclaudication.

Psychogenic: Arising from the psyche or the mind; i.e., not organic in nature.

Pulmonary embolus: Embolus (blood clot, air, fat) which is carried through the venous system ultimately lodging in the pulmonary vasculature. PE is a serious and occasionally fatal complication of deep venous thrombosis.

Pulsatility index (PI): A parameter used to convey the pulsatility of a time varying waveform such as the maximum Doppler shift frequency of the signal from an artery. Indices of pulsatility are usually ratios of Doppler shift frequencies and are hence independent of Doppler angle. The most common definition of pulsatility index (PI) of a waveform such as that defined by the maxi mum Doppler shift frequency, is the difference between the maximum and minimum value, divided by the mean value of the waveform over the cardiac cycle. PI = Peak to Peak Velocity Mean Pulse: The regular, palpable wave of distention or volume change transmitted to the arteries. This is due to blood ejected from the heart during ventricular contraction.

Pulse pressure: The difference between the peak systolic and minimum diastolic pressure in the cardiac cycle.

Pulse reappearance time: An index of arterial insufficiency defined by Fronek; the time period required for the return of toe pulse waves (via strain gauge or PPG) after four minutes of arterial occlusion by cuff.

Pulse repetition frequency (pulse repetition rate): The rate of repetition of pulses per unit time; in a pulsed system, the number of pulses generated every second. Not to be confused with frequency, PRF is the rate of pulse repetition.

Pulse volume recorder (PVR): Plethysmographic technique in which air filled cuffs are placed segmentally on an extremity; changes in limb volume associated with arterial pulsation are translated in pulse waveforms. Alterations in the shape of the waveform at each level are associated with obstruction proximal to the cuff.

Pulse wave Doppler (PW): Timed bursts of ultrasound (pulses); a single transducer alternately transmits and receives impulses. Permits more discrete sampling from a select depth and volume. Sample volume is selected through the process of range gating, i.e., receiving reflections after a defined time period has elapsed (see gate, sample volume).

Pulsed wave: Refers to an intermittent wave of sound (frequency) produced by applying short bursts of electrical impulses to an ultrasound transducer.

Pulseless Disease: Takayasu's disease; progressive obliterative arteritis.

Pulsus tardus/pulsus parvus: Terms used to describe dampened, post obstructive waveforms. Tardus refers to delayed arrival of the systolic peak, and parvus refers to overall low velocity.

Pyelonephritis (chronic): Repeated infections of the kidneys that cause scaring in some areas of the parenchyma.

Pyramids: Conical structures within the medulla of the kidney where blood is filtered and absorbed, leaving urine behind.

Q

Q's law: Quality before quantity.

Quadriplegia: Paralysis of all four limbs.

Qualitative: A non-objective measurement relating to quality; descriptive assessment of attributes, traits, or characteristics. Measurements in which an exact numerical value cannot be assigned; scales or grades can be used.

Quantitative: An observable quantity which can be described in objective, measurable terms, i.e., numbers.

R

Radial artery: It begins at the division of the brachial artery below the bend of the elbow, and passes along the radial side of the forearm to the wrist where the pulse is readily palpated.

Radiography: Generic terms referring to any type of xray procedure; venography, arteriography are two types of radiographic techniques.

Range: The distance between the reflector (target) and the transducer; equal to one half of the total ultrasound path length.

Range ambiguity: Occurs when the pulse repetition frequency is too high, causing misrepresentation of echoes ranges.

Range gating: With range gating the transducer will only accept echoes from a selected depth based on echo arrival times.

Raster: On a cathode ray tube, the pattern of horizontal lines beginning at the top of the screen and progressing from left to right. Each line is made of many pixels.

Raynaud's disease: Vasospastic disease characterized by intermittent pallor, cyanosis and rubor of the digits; rarely results in tissue necrosis. Symptoms are induced by exposure to cold or emotional upset. Raynaud's disease is a primary condition and exists in the absence of arterial obstruction and has no clear-cut association with any other systemic disease. Syndromes with similar symptoms, but with secondary etiology, are referred to as Raynaud's phenomenon.

Raynaud's phenomenon: Describes any number of conditions which present symptoms suggestive of digital arterial vasospasm (see Raynaud's disease). The phenomenon follows the color sequence of pallor, cyanosis, rubor. Pain may be present and occasionally there may be gangrene of the digital tips. The underlying etiology may include; collagen vascular disease, nerve compressions, occupational trauma, and arterial obstruction.

Reactive hyperemia: Response to ischemia characterized by rapid increase in blood flow following cessation of a period of induced ischemia. A technique to assess the degree of functional arterial impairment. Resting ankle pressures are recorded prior to the application of an occlusive cuff to the thigh. Following a period of ischemia, the cuff is deflated and ankle pressures are measured. The degree of drop in ankle pressure immediately following release is indicative of the degree of impairment. This technique is sometimes used in lieu of exercise/treadmill testing.

Real-Time display: Display system in which an image is continuously up-dated and reviewed as the target changes or moves.

Recanalization: The formation of a new canal or channel of blood flow through an obstruction, such as blood clot or thrombus (deep vein thrombosis).

Reconstitution: When a main artery is again patent distal to a segment of occlusion (SFA/POP) due to collateral flow.

Reflection: The acoustic energy returned (reflected) back to the transducer from a structure (target). The intensity of the reflection is dependent upon the acoustic impedance ratio at the tissue interface. The greater the impedance ratio the greater the reflection.

Reflex sympathetic dystrophy (RSD): A condition characterized by diffuse pain, swelling, and limitation of movement that follows an injury such as a fracture in an arm or leg. The symptoms are way out of proportion to the injury and may linger long after the injury has healed.

Reflux: Backward flow. A characteristic noted on the venous Doppler examination during proximal limb compression; indicative of valvular dysfunction.

Refraction: The change in direction of an acoustic wave at an interface; the bending of an acoustic wave; refraction occurs when the angle of incidence is not normal (perpendicular) or as the wave passes through media of different densities (acoustic impedances).

Regeneration: The natural renewal of a structure, tissue, organ, or part.

Rehabilitation: A planned program of therapy designed to restore a patient who is disabled to maximum physical and psychological functioning.

Rejection: The body's immune response against foreign bodies, or grafted tissue, that results in the failure of the grafted tissue or organ to survive.

Renal arteries: Originates off the aorta just below the level of the superior mesenteric artery. They supply the kidneys, adrenals, and the ureters.

Renal veins: Drain the kidney and empty into the inferior vena cava. The left renal vein is longer than the right renal vein.

Renovascular hypertension: High blood pressure pertaining to or affecting blood vessels of the kidney, or hypertension produced by renal artery flow reducing stenosis or occlusion.

Resistance: The opposition to blood flow occurring in the vascular system (see peripheral vascular resistance). The opposition to flow of current in an electrical circuit (see impedance, Ohm's law).

Resistance index (RI): (see Pourcelot index).

Rest pain: A sign of severe arterial obstruction resulting in pronounced ischemia of an extremity. Arterial compromise is such that pain occurs at rest; often causing night-time wakefulness (due to recumbency and the reduced cardiac output of sleep). The pain is confined to the digit and dorsum of the foot and symptoms are relieved, in part, by dependency of the limb. Generally two or more segments of the arterial tree are involved and ABI values are below 0.5. If left untreated, rest pain will progress to gangrene.

Retrograde: Proceeding away from or backward; opposite of antegrade or forward.

Retrograde flow: Blood flowing moving backwards or against the usual direction of flow.

Reverberation: Multiple reflections within a confined space or from the same target; a source of false echo information in real time imaging (see artifact).

Reynolds number: Predicts the onset of turbulence based on flow speed and viscosity.

RIND: Refers to Reversible (or resolving) Ischemic Neurologic Deficit.

Rubor: Redness; term used to describe inflammation.

Dependent rubor: Describes the classic redness which occurs in an ischemic limb on dependency following a period of elevation.

Rupture: Tearing apart; bursting.

S

Saccular: Having the shape of or resembling a sac, an out pouching.

Sagittal: In the anterior-posterior plane of the body.

Sample volume: With a pulsed Doppler system, describes the site of flow detection; size of the sample volume is determined by beam diameter and length of the ultrasound pulse (see pulsed Doppler, gate).

Saphenous vein: There are two veins that serve as the principal superficial venous outflow, the greater saphenous and lesser saphenous. The greater (long) saphenous vein runs from the foot to the groin where it confluences with the common femoral vein. The lesser saphenous vein (short) runs from the posterior lateral malleolus (lateral to the Achilles' tendon, near ankle) along the posterior leg and usually joins the popliteal vein in the space behind the knee.

Scattering: Diffuse reflection and refraction of an acoustic wave in many directions; caused by irregular interfaces, heterogeneous media, or particle suspensions (blood).

Scleroderma: A disease of the connective tissue in which the skin forms scar tissue (fibrous tissue). This may also occur in other organs of the body.

Sclerosis: Generic term used to describe an abnormal hardening or fibrosis of an artery (see atherosclerosis, Monckeberg's sclerosis, calcification, diabetes).

Segmental blood pressures: Obtaining blood pressure measurements at different levels of the upper or lower extremities, the comparison of pressure change across each segment of the limb in order to determine the level of occlusive disease.

Sensitivity: The ability of a diagnostic technique to identify the presence of disease when disease is actually present. Sens. = TP × 100 = % TP + FN TP = true positive, FN = false negative Sequential bypass: Arterial bypasses in series; a continuation and/or additional bypass performed to maintain patency of previous surgery.

Serum creatinine: When the kidneys do not work properly this waste product accumulates in the blood. Levels above 1.0 are considered to be elevated and abnormal in a female. Levels above 1.3 are considered elevated and abnormal in a male.

Shadowing: Reduction in reflection amplitude from reflectors that lie behind a strongly reflecting or attenuating structure.

Shunt: Term used to describe a pathway other than the usual to divert blood from one point to another; may be a natural channel, i.e., an arteriovenous fistula or a surgically created channel, i.e., a bypass graft. In carotid endarterectomy a shunt is often used to divert blood from the common carotid artery to the internal system during the procedure. Shunt is synonymous with bypass.

Side effect: Any physiological change (other than the expected one) which occurs as a result of a prescribed treatment or procedure.

Sinus: The renal sinus contains the collecting system, renal arteries and veins, lymphatics, fat and fibrous tissue. The renal sinus has an ultrasound appearance that is highly echodense.

Snell's law (simplified): In ultrasound, states that the angle of reflection is equal to the angle of incidence.

Spatial pulse length: Distance traveled by an ultrasound pulse; equal to the product of wavelength and the number of cycles in a pulse.

Specificity: The ability of a diagnostic technique to identify the absence of disease (normalcy) when no disease is actually present. Spec. = TN × 100 = % TN + FP TN = true negative, FP = false positive Spectral analysis: A method of analyzing and/or displaying the Doppler signal output. The Doppler shifted signal is made up of a range of frequencies. Spectral analysis, using a microprocessor, is capable of analyzing and displaying the complete range of frequencies in each waveform. This technique may be used with pulsed or continuous wave Doppler systems. Time is displayed on the horizontal axis, frequency on the vertical axis and amplitude of the signal by the intensity of the gray scale. Spectral analysis provides the most complete assessment of the Doppler waveform and is a useful technique for quantifying degree of arterial stenosis.

Spectral broadening: The width of the Doppler spectrum on a sonogram display corresponds to the range of Doppler shift frequencies present at a given time. Spectral broadening will be seen when this range is increased; an example is the Doppler signal obtained when laminar flow with a blunt flow profile becomes disturbed.

Spindle: Hour glass shaped.

Spleen: A large, glandlike and ductless organ; situated in the upper abdomen; disintegrates red blood cells and sets free hemoglobin which the liver transforms to bilirubin; creates red blood cells in the fetus and in the newborn; produces lymphocytes and plasma, etc.

Splenic artery: Originates from the celiac artery and supplies the pancreas, spleen, stomach, and greater omentum.

Splenic vein: Collects blood from the spleen and part of the stomach and joins with the superior mesenteric vein to form the portal vein.

Spontaneity: In normal veins flow occurs passively. It should be detectable in all major veins.

Stasis: Refers to the stagnation of blood; cessation of normal blood flow. In the venous system of the lower extremity, stagnant blood flow as the result of immobility contributes to venous thrombosis. Stagnation of venous blood in the extremity because of valvular dysfunction (or post-phlebitic syndrome) results in pigmentation changes and ulceration.

Stenosis: The narrowing or constriction of a tube, specifically the lumen of an arterial blood vessel.

Plural, stenoses: A stenosis of sufficient caliber to reduce blood flow is termed a hemodynamically significant stenosis. This is equal to a 75% area reduction or a 50% diameter reduction.

Stent: A tube made of metal or plastic that is inserted into a vessel or passage to keep it open and prevent closure due to a stricture or external compression.

Stent Graft: A stent-graft is an intraluminal device that consists of a supporting framework (currently made of metal such as stainless steel or nitinol) and a synthetic graft material. Stent-grafts can be either self-expanding or balloon-expandable, depending on the type of metal in the stent. The stent may be located inside, outside, or within the graft material, and it may be along the entire length of the graft or restricted to the ends. To deliver the stent-graft through a small vascular access, the device is compacted onto a catheter or compressed into a sheath. With the use of imaging guidance, the device is advanced into an appropriate location in the aorta from a remote access site and deployed.

Stethoscope: An instrument used to listen to body sounds; an auscultatory device. Most stethoscopes have dual components, a diaphragm and a bell. Bruits are best assessed with the bell of the stethoscope.

Stokes-Adams syndrome: Syncope of cardiac origin occurring most often in patients with a pulse rate of less than 40 beats/minute and complete atrioventricular heart block.

Strain gauge plethysmography (SPG): A noninvasive diagnostic technique used primarily for the detection of deep venous thrombosis. The strain gauge consists of an electroconductive material enclosed in a thin elastic tubing. The strain gauge is placed around an extremity and limb volume changes are detected by measuring changes in impedance. Strain gauge is most often used to record maximum venous capacitance/outflow ratios as in impedance plethysmography but may also be used for venous reflux plethysmography and digital arterial waveforms (see Ohm's law, impedance plethysmography).

Streptokinase: A protein produced B-hemolytic streptococci. It is used as a thrombolytic agent; used topically on surface lesions or by instillation in closed body cavities to remove clotted blood.

Stricture: A narrowing of a tube, usually due to scar tissue formation.

Stroke: Popular term for cerebrovascular accident.

Subclavian artery: Originates on the right from the brachiocephalic (innominate) artery and on the left from the aortic arch. As it continues under the scapula, it continues as the axillary artery at the lateral border of the first rib. The major branches are the vertebral, thyrocervical, internal thoracic and costocervical arteries.

Subclavian vein: The direct continuation of the axillary vein at the lateral border of the first rib, it passes medially to join the internal jugular vein and form the brachiocephalic veins bilaterally.

Subjective: Pertains to things or events which are internal, not observable by others. Subjective tests are those in which the results can only be observed by the examiner, e.g., the venous Doppler exam. Opposite of objective. Symptoms are subjective, physical signs are objective.

Superior mesenteric artery (SMA): Originates off the aorta just below the level of the celiac artery. This artery supplies the small bowel, cecum, ascending colon, and part of the transverse colon.

Superior mesenteric vein (SMV): Drains the cecum, transverse and sigmoid colon, and small bowel.

Superficial femoral artery (SFA): It originates from the common femoral artery at its bifurcation with the deep femoral artery (1-2" below the inguinal ligament), and continues through the thigh and Hunter's canal (adductor canal) to then become the popliteal artery.

Superior vena cava (SVC): Returns blood from the head and neck, upper limbs and thorax, and is formed by the union of the two brachiocephalic veins (innominate veins).

Supine: Lying on the back with face upwards, opposite of prone.

Supraorbital: Above the orbit of the eye; term is not synonymous with periorbital.

Supraorbital plethysmography: A noninvasive diagnostic technique used in the assessment of carotid occlusive disease. PPG transducers are placed on the supraorbital region, waveforms are recorded, and the response to compression of the external branch arteries and common carotid arteries are noted. The physiological basis for this technique is similar to the cerebrovascular Doppler exam.

Suprarenal: Located above the level of the renal artery.

Suprasystolic: Above systolic pressure.

Symes amputation: Amputation of the foot at the ankle joint with removal of both malleoli, and creating a flap with the soft parts of the heel.

Sympathectomy: Surgical interruption (excision) or chemical block of part of the sympathetic nervous system. Sympathectomy is used in the treatment of severe arterial occlusive disease (where vasoconstriction is a factor) to produce vasodilation and thereby enhance blood flow to an extremity.

Sympathetic: A division of the autonomic nervous system involved primarily with emergency responses and muscular activity. It is the sympathetic system which mediates homeostasis and vascular smooth muscle response, i.e., vasodilation and vasoconstriction.

Symptom: A subjective manifestation of disease, e.g., pain.

Syncope: A brief loss of consciousness; caused by reduction in cerebral blood flow; etiology may be due to extreme vasodilation brought on by emotions or secondary to hypotension, heart block, or arrhythmia.

Syndrome: A group of signs and/or symptoms, which when occurring together characterize a disease.

Systole: The contraction phase of the cardiac cycle.

T

Tachycardia: Excessively rapid heart rate, usually over 100 beats per minute.

Takayasu's arteritis: Progressive obliteration of the brachiocephalic trunk and the subclavian and common carotid arteries above their origins in the aortic arch; leading to loss of pulse in both arms and carotids and to one or more symptoms associated with ischemia of the brain, eyes, and kidneys.

Temporal arteritis: Also called giant cell arteritis or cranial arteritis. (See arteritis)

Test object: Device used to measure some characteristics of an imaging system without having tissue-like properties.

Testicular torsion: A condition in which the testicle is twisted on its mesentery, impairing blood supply and causing pain.

Thermal biofeedback: A technique used in the treatment of Raynaud's phenomenon; used when symptoms are related to stress or anxiety; patients are taught to increase skin temperature through biofeedback techniques.

Thermocouple: A device that converts temperature to a voltage.

Thermography: Diagnostic technique in which body temperature differences are recorded on photographic paper; temperature differences associated with reduced blood flow can be documented in this manner.

Thoracic outlet syndrome (TOS): A symptom complex associated with compression of the arteries, veins, or nerves of the upper extremity at the outlet from the thoracic cavity. Symptoms include numbness or pain of the arm associated with activity, elevation, or hyperabduction. The cause is usually related to brachial nerve plexus compression rather than arterial compression. To identify or rule out arterial compression, Doppler, or PPG may be used to document obliteration of flow during specific arm movements.

Thrombectomy: Surgical removal of a blood clot from a vessel.

Thromboangiitis: Clot formation within an inflamed vessel; Buerger's disease was referred to as thromboangiitis obliterans.

Thromboendarterectomy: Surgical removal of a blood clot from within an artery.

Thrombogenic: Capable of causing blood clotting.

Thrombolysis: The breaking up of thrombus.

Thrombolytic: Capable of disintegrating a blood clot. TPA, Streptokinase and Urokinase are used to dissolve clots. This agent acts by stimulating the conversion of plasminogen to plasmin (an enzyme which breaks down fibrin). Thrombolytic therapy is used successfully in the treatment of deep venous thrombosis, for acute arterial thrombosis, and graft occlusion.

Thrombophlebitis: Inflammation of a vein with secondary thrombosis in the involved segment.

Thrombosis: The formation of an intravascular blood clot formation.

Thrombus: An intravascular blood clot; plural, thrombi.

Time gain compensation: Selective gain amplification over time used in real-time imaging to compensate for loss in echo intensity due to attenuation; permits echoes from greater depths to have the same intensity as those from shallow sites. Increases the gain in the far field without saturating the echoes in the near field.

Tortuous: Twisting or turning of the vessel. Sometimes making it difficult to interrogate throughout its length with Doppler.

Tourniquet: An apparatus which encircles a limb for the purpose of compressing blood vessels to occlude flow. May be a simple rubber strip or a pneumatic cuff.

Tissue plasminogen activator (TPA): A generic term for a group of substances that have the ability to cleave to plasminogen and convert it to plasmin in its active form; it is used for therapeutic thrombolysis.

Transcranial Doppler (TCD): Doppler evaluation of the major intracerebral arteries via a cranial "window" (transorbital, transtemporal, suboccipital). The method utilizes a pulsed Doppler combined with spectral analysis to obtain velocities of the major vessels.

Transcutaneous: Transdermal, entering through skin as in the administration of a drug applied to the skin in ointment or patch form.

Transducer: Any device which converts one form of energy to another, e.g., pressure to electrical, acoustic to electrical, electrical to acoustic.

Transient ischemic attack (TIA): Fleeting neurological dysfunction without residual symptoms lasts less than 24 hours, more typically 15-30 minutes. Depending on the cerebral territory involved, symptoms may include: sensory/motor dysfunction of an arm/leg, speech impairment (aphasia), and visual disturbances (amaurosis fugax); etiology is usually embolic. TIA is often the precursor of a cerebrovascular accident.

Transluminal angioplasty: Dilatation of a blood vessel by means of a balloon catheter inserted through the skin and through the lumen of the vessel to the site of narrowing, where the balloon is inflated to compress plaque against the arterial wall.

Transmetatarsal amputation: Removal of one or all of the toes across the end of the metatarsal heads.

Transplant: To transfer tissue or organs from one part of the body to another or from one body to another.

Transposition: the state of being transposed, or being on the wrong side of the body.

Transverse: Cross-sectional.

Trifurcation: The site of separation into three branches.

Triphasic: Having three phases or variations; forward flow in systole, brief reverse flow, and a third forward flow component (multiphasic).

Trophic: Pertaining to nutrition; trophic changes on an extremity (e.g., nail thickening, atrophied skin) are the results of ischemia or lack of nutrition to the skin.

Tumor: A growth of tissue in which the multiplication of cells is uncontrolled and progressive; can be neoplasm.

Tunica: A coat; lining membrane, as in tunica intima, tunica media, tunica adventitia.

Turbulence: The disruption of the normal laminar flow within a tube or vessel; disturbed blood flow in which whirls and eddies occur; usually due to obstruction to blood flow; a source of bruits.

U

Ulcer: An open sore or lesion on a body surface. The etiology of lower extremity ulceration may be arterial (ischemic or necrotic ulcer), venous (varicose ulcer or secondary to post-phlebitic syndrome), or neurogenic (as in diabetes). An ulcer in an atherosclerotic plaque may range from a slight irregular and roughened surface to a pronounced lesion within the atheroma. Ulcerative plaques have the potential to produce embolic material.

Ulnar artery: Artery that originates at the division of the brachial artery below the bend of the elbow and travels along the ulnar aspect of the forearm to the wrist.

Ultrasonography: Production of images or audio display for diagnostic purposes through the use of ultrasound.

Ultrasound: Sound above the range of human hearing, greater than 20 KHz. Clinical ultrasound ranges from 2-20MHz.

Umbilical vein: Not usually visualized but may dilate in portal hypertension.

Uniform insonation method: An ultrasonic method for the estimation of volume flow rate in single vessels. The average value of the product of the spatial mean velocity and the cross-sectional area is calculated over several cardiac cycles.

Unilateral: Pertaining to one side.

Ureter: The tube that conducts urine from the kidney to the bladder. It begins in the pelvis of the kidney as a widened area that looks like a funnel; it empties into the bladder and is approximately 16-18 inches long.

V

Valsalva maneuver: Forced expiration against the closed glottis impeding blood flow through the pulmonary capillary bed and increasing intrathoracic pressure. This maneuver impedes venous return and is used in the venous Doppler examination to assess venous flow and valvular competency.

Valve: A membrane within a tube or vessel allowing flow to move in one direction only. The venous valves are bicuspid and open towards the heart to prevent reflux. Damaged or incompetent valves allow retrograde venous flow.

Varices: Enlarged tortuous vessel; the vessels can be veins or lymphatic vessels.

Varicocele: Varicosity of the veins of the spermatic cord. A common cause of infertility in the male. Diagnosis can be made by palpation or (in subclinical presentation) by Doppler ultrasound. Venous reflux during Valsalva maneuver is found in the presence of varicocele.

Varicose veins: Veins that are distended, lengthened, and tortuous. The superficial veins (saphenous veins) of the legs are most commonly affected. There is an inherited tendency to varicose veins (primary) but obstruction to blood flow or incompetent valves, which permit backflow of venous blood (secondary), also may be responsible. Treatment may include elastic support stockings, elevation, sclerotherpy, or vein stripping.

Vascular: Pertaining to the blood vessels.

Vascular steal: Diversion of blood via alternate routes or reversed flow from the vascularized tissue to one deprived by proximal arterial obstruction.

Vasculogenic: Of a vascular origin.

Vasoconstriction: Narrowing of the vessel lumen caused by contraction of the muscular vessel wall.

Vasodilation: Enlarging of the vessel wall caused by relaxation of the muscular vessel wall.

Vasospasm: Spasmodic constricting of a vessel wall.

Vein: A blood vessel which conveys blood from the capillaries back to the heart. Veins are composed of three layers, intima, media, and adventitia. The media of the vein is less muscular than an artery. Veins are more compliant than arteries and are equipped with one-way valves to prevent reflux of blood.

Velocity: Speed of an acoustic wave per unit time in a specific direction.

Velocity: The rate at which an object moves in a specified direction.

Velocity detector: An ultrasound Doppler instrument which detects the velocity of blood flow transcutaneously.

Vena cava filter: A device placed in the IVC to catch emboli and prevent them from getting to the lungs.

Venography: A radiographic procedure in which an opaque substance is injected into the veins. Subsequent x-ray pictures are taken for the purpose of visualizing the venous system (see phlebography).

Venous: Pertaining to the veins.

Venous air embolism: An air bubble which may enter the venous system during any surgical procedure in which the surgical site is above the level of the right atrium. Doppler ultrasound is the most sensitive method of detection of air emboli in the right atrium.

Venous insufficiency: Condition in which faulty or damaged venous valves permit retrograde or backward flow of blood. Stagnant venous blood in the lower extremity may result in pigmentation changes, edema, pain, and ulceration (see post phlebitic syndrome).

Venule: A small vein.

Vertebral artery: First branch arising from the subclavian artery, coursing through the posterior neck and terminating in the basilar artery. Along with the internal carotid arteries, the vertebral arteries are the source of blood supply to the brain.

Vertigo: Dizziness or giddiness; feeling of spinning.

Vessel: A tube, duct, or canal which holds or conveys a fluid.

Virchow's triad: The three mechanisms of thrombosis-- injury to the vessel wall, decrease in blood flow (stasis), and blood hypercoagulability.

Viscosity: Resistance of a fluid to flow when a pressure is applied.

Volt: A unit of electrical force.

Vortices: Areas of circular flow which are present in turbulence.

W

Wallfilter: An electrical filter that removes strong low frequency Doppler shifts (e.g., pulsating heart or vessel walls) while allowing frequencies above a certain level to pass.

Waveform: A curve or undulation traced by a recording device and reflecting alterations in electrical activity; the shape of a wave on a graph (see triphasic).

Wavelength: Distance required for a complete cycle.

Wrap around: An incorrect shift of Doppler information to the other side of base line (caused by aliasing).

XYZ

Xanthaloma: Cholesterol deposition under the skin producing a yellowish lesion.

Xiphoid process: The pointed part of cartilage located at the lower end of the sternum.

Zero-Crossing device: A method of processing a Doppler signal whereby the incoming signal passes through a zero point and produces an output proportional to the average frequency at which the crossing occurs. The output information is both antegrade and retrograde (above or below the zero point); however, the output is an average of the frequencies at any given point in time and therefore not as accurate as spectral analysis.

Prefixes and Suffixes

Prefixes

Prefix	Meaning	Example
sub-	below	subacute
supra-	above	supraorbital
tachy-	rapid	tachycardia
thermo-	temperature	thermography
thrombo-	blood clot	thrombophlebitis
trans-	across	transverse
ultra-	from, beyond, to above	ultrasound
uni-	one	unidirectional
vaso-	vessel	vasospasm

Suffixes

Suffix	Meaning	Example
-algia	pain	causalgia
-ectomy	removal of	thrombectomy
-emia	blood	anemia
-esthesia	sensation	parasthesia
-genesis	origin	thrombogenesis
-genic	causation	vasculogenic
-graphy	writing	plethysmography
-itis	inflammation	arteritis
-logy	study of	physiology
-meter	measure	manometer
-otomy	opening	arteriotomy
-ous	like	atheromatous
-pathy	disease	cardiopathy
-penia	lack of	thrombocytopenia
-phagia	swallowing	dysphasia
-phasia	speech	aphasia
-plegia	paralysis	paraplegia
-rhage	burst forth	hemorrhage
-sonic	sound	ultrasonic
-stasis	stagnation	hemostasis

Acronyms

A

AAA: Abdominal Aortic Aneurysm

ABI: Ankle-Brachial Index

ACAS: Asymptomatic Carotid Atherosclerosis Study

ACC: American College of Cardiology

ACR: American College of Radiology

AEUS: American Emergency Ultrasonographic Society

AHA: American Hospital Association

AI: Acceleration Index

AIUM: American Institute of Ultrasound in Medicine

AMA: American Medical Association

ARDMS: American Registry of Diagnostic Medical Sonography

ARRT: American Registry of Radiologic Technologists

ASE: American Society of Echocardiography

ASN: American Society of Neuroimaging

ASRT: American Society of Radiologic Technologists

AT: Acceleration Time

ATA: Anterior Tibial Artery

ATV: Anterior Tibial Vein

AVA: American Vascular Association

AVIR: Association of Vascular and Interventional Radiographers

B

BUN: Blood Urea Nitrogen

BP: Blood Pressure

C

CAAHEP: Commission on Accreditation of Allied Health Education Programs

CABG: Coronary Artery Bypass Graft

CAC: Carrier Advisory Committee

CAD: Coronary Artery Disease

CBD: Common Bile Duct

CCA: Common Carotid Artery

CCI: Cardiovascular Credentialing International

CFA: Common Femoral Artery

CFV: Common Femoral Vein

CHF: Congestive Heart Failure

CIA: Common Iliac Artery

CMD: Carrier Medical Director

CME: Continuing Medical Education units

CMS: Centers for Medicare and Medicaid Services

CQU: Coalition for Quality in Ultrasound

CVA: Cerebrovascular Accident

D

DHHS: Dept. of Health and Human Services

DBI: Digit-Brachial Index

DIC: Disseminated Intravascular Coagulation

DOL: Dept. of Labor

DVT: Deep Vein Thrombosis

E

ECA: External Carotid Artery

EIA: External Iliac Artery

G

GSV: Greater Saphenous Vein

GI: Gastrointestinal

References

Glossary of Terms

H

HBP: High Blood Pressure

HCT: Hematocrit

HGB: Hemoglobin

HIPAA: Health Insurance Portability and Accountability Act of 1996

I

ICA: Internal Carotid Artery

ICAEL: Intersocietal Commission for the Accreditation of Echocardiography Laboratories

ICAVL: Intersocietal Commission for the Accreditation of Vascular Laboratories

IDTF: Independent Diagnostic Testing Facility

IMA: Inferior Mesenteric Artery

IMT: Intimal Medial Thickness

IVC: Inferior Vena Cava

IVUS: Intravascular Ultrasound

J

JDMS: Journal of Diagnostic Medical Sonography

JRC-CVT: Joint Review Committee on Education in Cardiovascular Technology

JRC-DMS: Joint Review Committee on Education in Diagnostic Medical Sonography

JVU: Journal for Vascular Ultrasound

K

KHz: Kilohertz

L

LCD: Local Coverage Determination

LMRP: Local Medical Review Policy

LSV: Lesser Saphenous Vein

M

MedPAC: Medicare Payment Advisory Commission

MHz: Megahertz

MI: Myocardial Infarction

N

NAA: National Aneurysm Alliance

NASCET: North American Symptomatic Carotid Endarterectomy Trial

O

OSHA: Occupational Safety & Health Administration

P

PAD: Peripheral Arterial Disease

PBI: Penile Brachial Index

PE: Pulmonary Embolus

PI: Pulsitility Index

POP: Popliteal

PPG: Photoplethysmography

PRG: Phleborheography

PTA: Posterior Tibial Artery

PTFE: Polytetrafloroethylene

PTV: Posterior Tibial Vein

PV: Portal Vein

PVD: Peripheral Vascular Disease

PVR: Pulse Volume Recording

R

RA: Renal Artery

RAR: Renal Aortic Ratio

RDCS: Registered Diagnostic Cardiac Sonographer

RDMS: Registered Diagnostic Medical Sonographer

RI: Resistive Index

RIND: Reversible Ischemic Neurological Deficit

RSD: Reflex Sympathetic Dystrophy

RV: Renal Vein

RVS: Registered Vascular Specialist

RVT: Registered Vascular Technologist

ROUB: Registered Ophthalmic Ultrasound Biometrics

S

SDMS: Society of Diagnostic Medical Sonography

SFV: Superficial Femoral Vein

SIR: Society of Interventional Radiology

SMA: Superior Mesenteric Artery

SMV: Superior Mesenteric Vein

SVMB: Society for Vascular Medicine and Biology

SVN: Society for Vascular Nursing

SVS: Society for Vascular Surgery

SVU: Society for Vascular Ultrasound

T

TBI: Toe-Brachial Index

TCD: Transcranial Doppler

TCPO2: Transcutaneous Pulse Oximetry

TIA: Transient Ischemic Attack

TOS: Thoracic Outlet Syndrome

TPA: Tissue Plasminogen Activator

U

USPSTF: United States Preventative Services Task Force

V

VDF: Vascular Disease Foundation

VPR: Volume Pulse Recording

References

Index